B9186
1/23/06

D1474385

Neural Development and Stem Cells

Contemporary Neuroscience

Neural Development and Stem Cells

Second Edition

Edited by

Mahendra S. Rao, MBBS, PhD

National Institute on Aging, Baltimore, MD

HUMANA PRESS ✳ TOTOWA, NEW JERSEY

© 2006 Humana Press Inc.
999 Riverview Drive, Suite 208
Totowa, New Jersey 07512

www.humanapress.com

All rights reserved.

No part of this book may be reproduced, stored in a retrieval system, or transmitted in any form or by any means, electronic, mechanical, photocopying, microfilming, recording, or otherwise without written permission from the Publisher.

All papers, comments, opinions, conclusions, or recommendations are those of the author(s), and do not necessarily reflect the views of the publisher.

For additional copies, pricing for bulk purchases, and/or information about other Humana titles, contact Humana at the above address or at any of the following numbers: Tel.: 973-256-1699; Fax: 973-256-8341; E-mail: orders@humanapr.com, or visit our Website: www.humanapress.com

This publication is printed on acid-free paper. ∞
ANSI Z39.48-1984 (American Standards Institute) Permanence of Paper for Printed Library Materials.

Cover illustration: Figure 4 from Chapter 13, "Embryonic Stem Cells and Neurogenesis" by Robin L. Wesselschmidt and John W. McDonald

Cover design by Patricia F. Cleary.

Photocopy Authorization Policy:
Authorization to photocopy items for internal or personal use, or the internal or personal use of specific clients, is granted by Humana Press Inc., provided that the base fee of US $30 is paid directly to the Copyright Clearance Center at 222 Rosewood Drive, Danvers, MA 01923. For those organizations that have been granted a photocopy license from the CCC, a separate system of payment has been arranged and is acceptable to Humana Press Inc. The fee code for users of the Transactional Reporting Service is: [1-58829-481-1/06 $30].

Printed in China. 10 9 8 7 6 5 4 3 2 1

Library of Congress Cataloging-in-Publication Data

Neural development and stem cells / edited by Mahendra S. Rao.— 2nd ed.
    p. cm. — (Contemporary neuroscience)
    Includes bibliographical references and index.
    ISBN 1-58829-481-1 (alk. paper) EISBN 1-59259-914-1
    1. Developmental neurobiology. 2. Stem cells. I. Rao, Mahendra S. II. Series.
    QP363.5.S75 2005
    612.8—dc22   2004024052

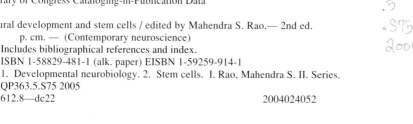

Preface

Developing the second edition of *Neural Development and Stem Cells* was necessitated by the rapid increase in our knowledge of the development of the nervous system. It has become increasingly clear that stem cells are a heterogeneous population that changes extensively during development. Perhaps the most important advance in our understanding of stem cell behavior has been the realization that regionalization of stem cells occurs early in development and this bias toward differentiation in phenotypes of neurons or cells characteristic of a particular part of the brain appears to persist even after prolonged culture. We have therefore included additional chapters on olfactory epithelial stem cells and retinal stem cells, both of which differ in their properties from ventricular zone and subventricular zone–derived neural stem cells. It is also now clear from an analysis of mutants and transgenics where the death or self-renewal pathway is altered that cell death regulates stem cell number. As a consequence, this second edition includes a separate chapter on cell death that summarizes the important changes in the death pathway that occur as stem cells mature. The existing chapters in the book have also been extensively revised and updated by experts who have generously contributed their time and expertise.

The chapters have been organized along the lines of our understanding of how the nervous system develops (Fig.1, on p. vi). Stem cells are present early in development, well before the onset of neurogenesis and gliogenesis. Stem cells proliferate and respond to extrinsic cues to mature as adult stem cells, undergo cell death, enter a state of quiescence, or differentiate. Stem cells appear to become regionally specified and their differentiation potential depends on the region that they have been isolated from.

I thank the authors for their efforts in ensuring that their manuscripts are as up to date as possible, and we all hope that this second edition of *Neural Development and Stem Cells* will serve as a handy guide for a course on stem cell biology in the nervous system for the novice and expert alike.

Mahendra S. Rao, MBBS, PhD

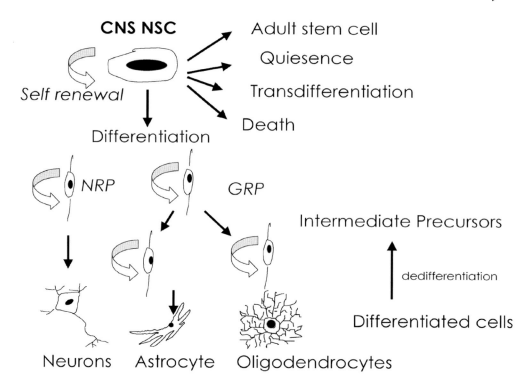

Fig. 1. Multipotent stem cells (NSC) can undergo self-renewal, enter a quiescent state, mature into adult stem cells, die, or respond to signals to differentiate. Differentiation appears to occur via a progressive set of fate choices that include the generation of dividing precursors with a restricted set of fate choices. These precursor cells present during development and, in the adult, mature to generate fully differentiated neurons, astrocytes, and oligodendrocytes. A limited set of data suggest that mature cells or intermediate precursors can dedifferentiate to reenter the cell cycle and acquire the characteristics of NSC.

Contents

Contributors

IQBAL AHMAD • *Department of Ophthalmology and Visual Sciences, University of Nebraska Medical Center, Omaha, NE*

RIZWAN S. AKHTAR • *Departments of Pathology and Neurobiology, Division of Neuropathology, University of Alabama at Birmingham, Birmingham, AL*

ARTURO ALVAREZ-BUYLLA • *Program in Developmental and Stem Cell Biology, Department of Neurological Surgery, University of California, San Francisco, CA*

MICHAEL BONAGUIDI • *Department of Neurology, Northwestern University Feinberg School of Medicine, Chicago, IL*

MARIANNE BRONNER-FRASER • *Division of Biology, California Institute of Technology, Pasadena, CA*

ANI V. DAS • *Department of Ophthalmology and Visual Sciences, University of Nebraska Medical Center, Omaha, NE*

SREEKUMARAN EDAKKOT • *Department of Ophthalmology and Visual Sciences, University of Nebraska Medical Center, Omaha, NE*

DOUGLAS L. FALLS • *Department of Cell Biology, Emory University School of Medicine, Atlanta, GA*

FRED H. GAGE • *Laboratory of Genetics, The Salk Institute for Biological Studies, La Jolla, CA*

STEVEN A. GOLDMAN • *Department of Neurology, Division of Cell and Gene Therapy, University of Rochester Medical Center, Rochester, NY*

CAITILIN HAMILL • *Department of Neurology, Northwestern University Feinberg School of Medicine, Chicago, IL*

HOUMAN D. HEMMATI • *Division of Biology, California Institute of Technology, Pasadena, CA*

JAIME IMITOLA • *Center for Neurologic Diseases, Brigham and Women's Hospital, Harvard Medical School, Boston, MA*

ALI JALALI • *Department of Neurology, Northwestern University Feinberg School of Medicine, Chicago, IL*

JACKSON JAMES • *Department of Ophthalmology and Visual Sciences, University of Nebraska Medical Center, Omaha, NE*

WOOCHAN JANG • *Department of Anatomy and Cellular Biology, Tufts University School of Medicine, Boston, MA*

JOHN A. KESSLER • *Department of Neurology, Northwestern University Feinberg School of Medicine, Chicago, IL*

DANIEL A. LIM • *Program in Developmental and Stem Cell Biology, Department of Neurological Surgery, University of California, San Francisco, CA*

YING LIU • *Laboratory of Neurosciences, National Institute on Aging, Baltimore, MD*

MARLA B. LUSKIN • *Department of Cell Biology, Emory University School of Medicine, Atlanta, GA*

MARGOT MAYER-PRÖSCHEL • *Center for Cancer Biology, University of Rochester Medical Center, Rochester, NY*

JOHN W. MCDONALD • *International Center for Spinal Cord Injury, Kennedy-Krieger Institute, Baltimore, MD*

TANYA A. MORENO • *Division of Biology, California Institute of Technology, Pasadena, CA*

MARK NOBLE • *Center for Cancer Biology, University of Rochester Medical Center, Rochester, NY*

VACLAV OUREDNIK • *Department of Biomedical Sciences, VetMed, Iowa State University, Ames, IA*

THEO D. PALMER • *Department of Neurosurgery, Stanford University, Palo Alto, CA*

KOOK IN PARK • *Department of Pediatrics, Pharmacology, and Brain, Korea 21 Project for Medical Sciences, Yonsei University College of Medicine, Seoul, Korea*

LARYSA HALYNA PEVNY • *Neuroscience Center, Department of Genetics, University of North Carolina, Chapel Hill, NC*

MAHENDRA S. RAO • *Laboratory of Neurosciences, National Institute on Aging, Baltimore, MD*

KEVIN A. ROTH • *Departments of Pathology and Neurobiology, Division of Neuropathology, University of Alabama at Birmingham, Birmingham, AL*

JAMES E. SCHWOB • *Department of Anatomy and Cellular Biology, Tufts University School of Medicine, Boston, MA*

RICHARD L. SIDMAN • *Bullard Professor of Neuropathology (Neuroscience), Emeritus, Harvard Medical School and Department of Neurology, Beth Israel Deaconess Medical Center, Boston, MA*

EVAN Y. SNYDER • *Program in Developmental and Regenerative Cell Biology, The Burnham Institute, La Jolla, CA*

SALLY TEMPLE • *Center for Neuroscience and Neuropharmacology, Albany Medical Center, Albany, NY*

YANG D. TENG • *Department of Neurosurgery, Brigham and Women's Hospital and Children's Hospital, Boston, and Harvard Medical School, Boston, MA*

ROBIN L. WESSELSCHMIDT • *Primogenix Inc., St. Louis MO*

1

Defining Neural Stem Cells and Their Role in Normal Development of the Nervous System

Sally Temple

INTRODUCTION

Stem cells are key players in the development and maintenance of specific mammalian tissues, and their presence has been long established in blood, skin, and intestine. The discovery of stem cells in the central and peripheral nervous systems (CNS and PNS) is a relatively recent event. First, continued neurogenesis (neuron generation) in the adult pointed to a long-lived progenitor cell *(1)*. Isolation of stem-like cells from the embryonic CNS, including basal forebrain *(2,3)*, cerebral cortex *(4)*, hippocampus *(5)*, spinal cord *(6)*, and the PNS *(7)* as well as evidence for multipotent, stem-like progenitors in vivo *(8–10)* indicated that they are important components of the developing nervous system (Fig. 1). Much excitement surrounded the isolation of adult stem cells from known neurogenic (neuron-generating) zones (the subventricular zone and hippocampal dentate gyrus) in rat, primate, and human (reviewed in ref. *11*). More recent evidence for continued presence of stem cells in areas not previously considered to be neurogenic, such as the spinal cord *(12,13)* and neocortex *(14,15)*, suggests that stem cells may be a more widespread feature of the adult nervous system than previously imagined (Fig. 1).

Current research is focused on identifying the characteristics and functions of neural stem cells, in both developing and adult systems, to reveal their place in CNS biology and to facilitate the harnessing of these remarkable cells for repairing damaged nervous systems. To help us understand more about neural stem cells, we can explore a wealth of knowledge concerning stem cells in other systems and organisms, looking for common themes that might explain the essential stem cell state, as well as differences that might reveal the uniqueness of neural stem cells.

The term *stem cell* has a number of different meanings—depending on the system being analyzed and the perspective of the researcher using the term. A general definition is "a cell that is capable of both self-renewal and differentiation." Most researchers in the stem cell field would agree with this baseline definition. In this chapter, *progenitor* is used as a blanket term to describe any dividing cell that can generate differentiated progeny, whether or not it can self-renew, and the term *precursor* is used to describe a cell that is committed to a specific fate.

From: *Neural Development and Stem Cells, Second Edition*
Edited by: M. S. Rao © Humana Press Inc., Totowa, NJ

1

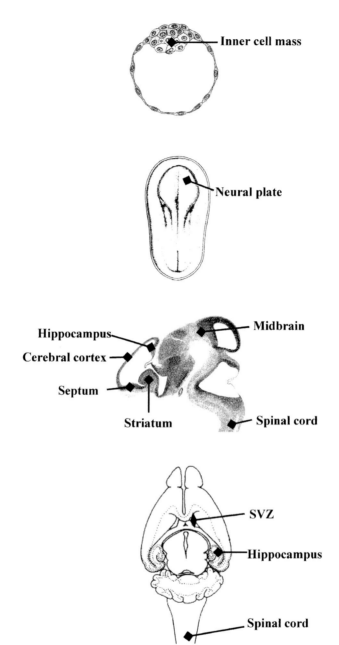

Fig. 1. Multipotent stem cells generating neurons and glia have been isolated at all stages from the early embryo through to adult.

Besides the two fundamental features, self-renewal and differentiation, other specific characteristics have been attributed to stem cells, some of which apply only to stem cells in particular systems, rather than being a general feature of all stem cells, as illustrated in a review *(16)*. This chapter discusses some of the general terminology used to describe and define stem cells, focusing on the terms that apply to neural stem cells, especially during normal neural development.

DOES THE NERVOUS SYSTEM ARISE FROM A SINGLE STEM CELL TYPE?

The *potency* of a progenitor cell represents the range of cell types it can generate. In a general model, stem cells are the basic cell type from which all others emanate through restriction of potency. The most primitive cells are considered *totipotent*—able to generate an entire organism or an entire tissue; for example, cells of the eight-cell-stage mammalian embryo are totipotent. Subsequent restriction of potency can occur within a stem lineage, so that stem cells may be *pluripotent* or *multipotent* (making many different cell types, but not all), *oligopotent* (having a few choices), or *unipotent* (making one type of progeny). The epidermal stem cell in the adult skin is thought of as unipotent, as it appears to generate solely keratinocytes. Stem cells may also release multipotent or oligopotent or unipotent restricted progenitor cells, which serve as transit populations to expand the stem cell progeny prior to terminal differentiation. Formation of blood is believed to follow this general model, in which a primitive hemopoietic stem cell proceeds via restriction of potency within its stem and progenitor progeny toward final hemopoietic cell fates *(17)*.

It is not clear at this point whether there is a stem cell type that is totipotent and can give rise to the entire nervous system with its wealth of neuronal and glial cell types. Embryonic stem cells (ES), which are considered pluripotent, can generate neural stem-like cells *(18)*. In tissue culture, or on transplantation into the embryo, the neural derivatives of ES cells can generate a wide variety of cell types *(19–22)* and these early neural stem cells may emerge as the most plastic. A stem cell that can generate both PNS and CNS derivatives exists in the early embryo, suggesting it has a broad range of potency *(23)*, but its full range has not yet been studied. Multipotent stem cells have been isolated from various regions of the developing and adult CNS (reviewed in ref. *24* and *25–30*) and from the neural crest, which gives rise to the PNS *(31–33)*. Dissociated embryonic neural progenitor populations that include some stem cells can be transplanted from one region of the developing CNS into other regions and show remarkable properties of integration *(34)*, producing cells that resemble those endogenous to the transplant site.

The use of mixed populations of stem and progenitor cells in these transplant studies precludes an accurate description of the contribution of donor stem cells vs donor progenitor cells to the differentiated cells in the host site, and more definitive descriptions of stem cell potency will depend on the ability to isolate pure populations of neural stem cells, as described later. Despite this limitation, these data suggest that neural stem cells may be somewhat plastic, being able to integrate heterotypically, respond to the new regional environmental information and differentiate accordingly; however, the results of some studies indicate that stem cell potency may be limited. After transplantation, differentiating cells may acquire the morphology typical of their new location but do not always express its characteristic molecular markers, suggesting a lack of complete integration. For example, telencephalic cells grafted into the embryonic diencephalon or mesencephalon continue to express telencephalic markers, even into adulthood *(35)*. Similarly, hippocampus-derived stem cells, on transplantation into the adult retina, expressed appropriate neuronal and glial morphologies but not end-stage markers of retinal differentiation *(36)*. Furthermore, cells from one CNS region may incorporate more successfully into some regions than others. In one study, mouse progenitor cells from the lateral ganglionic eminence (LGE) or from the ventral mesen-cephalon (VM) were dissociated and injected into the lateral ventricles of embryonic rats at a similar stage of development. The LGE cells preferentially incorporated into the striatum, whereas the VM cells preferentially incorporated into the hypothalamus and midbrain. None of these cells, derived from basal CNS regions, incorporated effi-ciently into dorsal structures such as the cerebral cortex and hippocampus *(37)*.

Similarly, there is evidence for temporal restriction in potency. Progenitor cells from embryonic ferret cerebral cortex transplanted into an older cortex can produce age-appropriate cells, but cells from an older cortex, on transplantation into a younger cor-tex, are unable to make younger cell types *(38)*. Similarly, mid-hindbrain progenitors show a wider degree of regional incorporation at embryonic day (E)10.5 than at E13.5 *(39)*. Temporal limitations to potency have particular significance when we consider the potential of adult neural stem cells. They can generate neurons, astrocytes, and oligodendrocytes, but the types of neurons and glia generated may be limited. In vivo, adult neural stem cells are primed to generate interneurons, and this appears to be their behavior after transplantation to adult neurogenic zones *(40,41)*. Furthermore, adult neural stem cells cultured for long periods may become increasingly biased toward production of glial cells, in some cases eventually losing neurogenic potential *(42)*. However, when placed in developing nervous system areas, adult stem cells can gener-ate more cell types than they can after transplantation into the adult, as in studies of the retina *(36)*. It is important to establish whether adult stem cells are capable of generat-ing the major projection neurons in the CNS, most of which arise early in embryonic development.

Besides generating a wide variety of neural cells, stem cells derived from the ner-vous system may also be capable of producing cells of other tissues. In one remarkable study, it was shown that a stem cell derived from the adult CNS could generate blood cells after transplantation into the bone marrow of an irradiated host *(43)*. In another study, incorporation of neural stem cells into early embryo blastulas resulted in a chi-meras and apparent differentiation into a variety of somatic cells *(44)*, but interestingly no neural cells. Although we marvel at the plasticity of the stem cell involved, these experiments do not speak to its potency in generating *neural* cell types. Also, it was not clear what the characteristics of the starting cell were. Was it a neural stem cell that acquired the features of other somatic cells through transdifferentiation or dedifferen-tiation? Or could there be a small population of totipotent stem cells in the brain, per-haps even derivatives of migratory germ cells that did not reach the germinal ridges *(45)*, that was responsible for blood cell production in this experiment? If the cell was indeed a neural stem cell, is its remarkable plasticity a reflection of its normal biology, or could it be the result of growing for long periods in tissue culture prior to transplan-tation? Undoubtedly answers to these questions will be found soon and will help us understand the types of stem cells present in the adult brain, their normal potency, and how long-term cell culture might alter them. Finally, transplantation studies in general have to be viewed cautiously, considering the surprising discovery that implanted stem cells can fuse with extant neural cells, and thus appear to generate new neuronal or glial progeny, when in fact they have created a chimera *(46)*.

The idea that normal development might proceed through gradual restriction of potency, as occurs in the blood system, is supported by studies of developing nervous system stem cells. In the CNS and PNS, multipotent progenitors generate restricted progenitors for neurons and glial cells *(29)*. Forebrain stem cells change during development becoming less neurogenic and more gliogenic *(47–50)*. The heterochronic cortical transplantation studies mentioned previously also support this model. How might restriction of potency occur within the stem cell? It has been suggested for stem cells in a number of systems that the more primitive stem cells express a wide variety of transcripts at a low level, perhaps maintaining genes in an "open" chromatin configuration that is poised for transcription. Restriction of potency would proceed by turning off some genes and enhancing expression of others *(51,52)*. For the nervous system, this might explain why fetal glutamatergic and γ-aminobutyric acid (GABA)ergic cortical neurons both express glutamic acid decarboxylase (GAD) transcripts *(53)*, or why neural progenitor cells in the spinal cord express genes characteristic of both interneurons and motorneurons before selecting one or the other phenotype *(54,55)*. Restriction of potency might involve a hierarchy of transcription factors that drive the cell toward a particular fate. In *Drosophila*, proneural genes, for example, *achaete/scute*, and *atonal*, confer competence for neural differentiation, via a chain of transcription factor activation *(56)*.

Homologs of these genes may operate similarly in vertebrates. For example, *Mash1*, a mouse homolog of *Drosophila achaete/scute*, stimulates expression of the transcription factor Phox2a, which in turn stimulates expression of panneuronal properties and of the receptor c-RET, specifying subtypes of autonomic lineage cells *(32,57,58)*. *Mash1* initiates a cascade with different components in the olfactory system *(59)*. It also appears important for generating neurons in the ventral embryonic forebrain, perhaps via influence on Notch signaling *(60,61)*. Given the prevalence of *achaete/ scute* and *atonal* homologs as well as other members of the basic helix–loop–helix (bHLH) transcription factor family, in the developing vertebrate nervous system, there is undoubtedly much to be learned about how these factors might interact within stem cell lineages to generate diverse neural cell fates.

Environmental factors play an important role in influencing potency via these transcription factors. The normal switch from neuronal to glial generation that occurs in CNS stem cells is stimulated by fibroblast growth factor-2 (FGF-2) and inhibited by bone morphogenic protein (BMP) at early stages of development *(47,62)*. Gliogenesis is also stimulated by leukemia inhibitory factor (LIF) and ciliary neurotrophic factor (CNTF), primarily via the Jak/Stat signaling pathway *(63,64)*. Surprisingly, given its early neurogenic role, BMP stimulates late stage progenitors to acquire an astrocyte fate *(65)* via Smad activation *(66)*. In late stage cells, the BMP and LIF/CNTF pathways converge to promote gliogenesis by interacting with the transcriptional coactivators CBP (signal transducer and activator of transcription/CRE binding protein) and p300. The STAT/CBPp300/Smad complex acts at the STAT binding element in the GFAP promoter to stimulate astrogenesis *(67)*. Moreover, the fate choice-point is regulated by the bHLH factor Neurogenin1, which can draw the CBP/Smad complex away from the astrocyte pathway, promoting the transcription of the bHLH gene *NeuroD* and thus stimulating neuron formation and inhibiting glial formation *(68)*. Therefore, at early stages, Neurogenin and BMP activation promote neuron generation. Factors that diminish Neurogenin activity at later stages of development will stimulate the transition from neuronal to glial cell production, and turn BMP into a gliogenic factor.

FGF-2 augments the action of CNTF in astrocyte generation by facilitating access of the STAT/CBPp300 complex STAT binding site of the glial fibrillary acidic protein (GFAP) promoter by chromatin remodeling: inducing Lys4 methylation and suppressing Lys9 methylation of histone H3 *(69)*.

We may conclude, then, that there are different populations of stem cells in the developing nervous system that vary in their developmental potential. It is important to understand the role these various stem cell types have in regional and temporally aspects of CNS development.

STEM CELL POTENCY AND REGIONAL IDENTITY WITHIN THE EMERGING NERVOUS SYSTEM

It is important to note that potency is empirically determined—a cell is challenged with specific environmental signals, and we examine what types of cells it can generate. Hence, a cell present in the cerebellum may be found to be capable of making motor neurons if transplanted into the spinal cord. Importantly, it cannot be concluded from such a result that early neural stem cells are undifferentiated and do not possess regional information, only that the information that they might have can be changed. In fact, it is likely that stem cells normally acquire regional information very early. If progenitor cells are removed from different regions of the early embryonic nervous system and placed in tissue culture, they develop into cell types characteristic of the region from which they were derived. Thus embryonic retina progenitors give retinal cells, embryonic cerebellar progenitors produce cerebellar cells, and embryonic neural crest progenitors generate typical PNS derivatives.

We know that in normal neural development positional information that presages regionalization of the nervous system is imparted very early, probably concomitantly with the neural induction process in the gastrula *(70)*. Given their behavior after isolation in tissue culture, one can hypothesize that positional information is embodied in neural stem cells. Thus, an important role of stem cells in normal development might be to interpret positional information and to read it out by generating cells appropriate to their location. The plasticity that we see exhibited in transplantation experiments may be important in normal development, for example, in the initial interpretation of positional signals, in designating the fate of progenitor cells at the borders between neural regions, or in regulative events that coordinate development throughout the embryo. It may also help the embryo compensate for disease or damage that in the natural environment are normal developmental events. In fact, the evolution of developmental mechanisms may be closely linked with the evolution of repair processes, as suggested by the similarity of some signaling pathways operating in disease and development in *Drosophila (71)*.

We can ask further whether, within each region of the developing nervous system, there is one fundamental type of progenitor cell (e.g., a regional stem cell) that is specified at the beginning of development—one type of cerebellar progenitor cell, one type of cortical progenitor, and so forth—or a number of types with different specificities. In the early cerebral cortex, for example, the cells cycle with apparently uniform dynamics, and there are no overt features that suggest diversity within the population. However, even at early stages, clonal analysis reveals that only about 10% of the cells behave like stem cells in culture *(72,73)*; the remaining behave like restricted progenitor cells. Perhaps this is a shortcoming of the clonal culture system, which might not allow the stem cell phenotype to be fully expressed. Alternatively, this could indicate that stem cells are in fact a subpopulation, even in the primitive neuroepithelium. Similar to the early cerebral cortex, the neural crest contains a mixture of different types of progenitor cells *(33)*. Are these crest progenitors related by a more primitive common precursor, or did they arise from the dorsal neuroepithelium as distinct entities? If the latter, the vertebrate neuroepithelium might be more like that of *Drosophila*. In the fly, each neuroblast has a discrete identity—based on which segment it is in, and where in the segment it arises—and generates appropriate types and numbers of progeny accordingly *(74)*. One can speculate that the vertebrate neuroepithelium also contains from the earliest stage (perhaps designated by positional information), distinct types of neural stem cells. There may also be, from the earliest stage, restricted progenitor cell types that produce certain classes of neural cells that eventually interweave with stem cell products. Rather than being a sheet of equivalent, uncommitted cells, perhaps the early neuroepithelium is a mosaic of progenitor types with defined roles influenced by positional information and with limited developmental plasticity that is necessary to generate a complete functioning organism.

SELF-RENEWAL AND TEMPORAL CHANGES
IN STEM CELLS DURING NEURAL DEVELOPMENT

The central defining feature ascribed to stem cells is the ability to self-renew, sometimes called self-maintenance *(16,75,76)*. This is the essence of the stem cell state—maintaining the ability to generate more stem cells for future generations of progeny. Self-renewal may be a feature of each individual stem cell. Alternatively, it might be an emergent property of a population of stem cells in which, for example, there is a certain probability of dividing or differentiating, so that the maintenance of the stem cell state may be stochastically determined by the dynamics of the population. Demonstration of self-renewal is the litmus test—the functional definition—of stem cells. In the nervous system, self-renewal has been demonstrated in vitro by allowing a stem cell to develop, and then subcloning its progeny to show that it made at least some progeny that behave as stem cells. This has been done in adhesion-based culture systems, by showing that the subcloned cells make secondary clones, and in non–adhesion-based culture systems by showing that the subcloned cells make secondary neurospheres—the large floating spheres of cells that are believed to represent stem cell products *(77)*.

Two ideas are implied by the term *self-renewal*: first, that the stem cell maintains its developmental potency (i.e., the range of types of progeny it is capable of generating) and second, that it maintains its proliferative capacity. These features, which are interrelated, perhaps describe an ideal stem cell, but they are not represented by normal stem cells. Regarding potency, as discussed earlier, production of diverse blood cell types appears to involve successive restriction of stem cell potency from a totipotent cell; this also appears true of the developing neural stem cell.

Formation of the nervous system is an exquisitely orchestrated process in which precise timing of production of different cell types is key. For any individual of a given species, it is possible to predict, within a few hours, the birthdate of a particular neuronal cell type. How the progenitor populations in the developing CNS achieve this remarkable scheduling is an important topic of research. As described earlier, it is clear from transplantation studies that stem cells in the developing nervous system vary over time. Stem cells isolated from early ages have a greater neuronal potency and those isolated from later ages have a greater glial potency. It seems highly likely that temporal changes in stem cells are critical for normal CNS development to ensure that the right types of progeny arise at the right times, and in fact that these changes drive the developmental process—providing a temporal blueprint, just as stem cells are also involved in providing the regional blueprint.

Thus, rather than the exact maintenance of potency, changes in this property may actually be central to stem cell function during tissue formation. In the adult, the situation may be different because the main role of adult cells is to maintain homeostasis rather than to generate different types of progeny in a set sequence, which is a function of stem cells in development. Consequently, adult stem cells may have to maintain their potency more rigidly to ensure that the same range of cell phenotypes is available throughout life.

The proliferative capacity of stem cells is also not perfectly maintained during the lifetime of stem cells. Blood stem cells can be transplanted into, and repopulate, a new host, but this repopulation can be accomplished only a certain number of times, indicating that the stem cell's impressive proliferative capacity is finite *(16)*. In fact, different types of blood stem cells defined by surface markers have specific characteristic proliferative capacities, implying that it is both a finite and an intrinsically determined characteristic *(16)*. Blood stem cells present in the embryo have a larger division potential than those of the adult *(78)*. Both embryonic and adult neural stem cells can be maintained for long periods in tissue culture, but the limits of this maintenance, and comparison of the two stages, have not been fully explored. A recent study indicates that most fetal spinal cord-derived stem cells divide for just three to six passages, and the few cells that divide for longer periods become biased toward generating nonneuronal progeny *(42)*. Changes in potency and/or proliferative capacity in stem cell systems appear to be the norm in many tissues. Besides the examples given, there are age-related changes in stem cells, observed, for example, in the adult intestinal crypt *(79)* and in neurogenic cells in the adult hippocampus *(80)*, that further dispute the concept of perfect self-renewal.

Employment of a strict definition of self-renewal has challenged the inclusion of certain types of cells in the stem cell class. It has been suggested by some researchers that *Drosophila* neuroblasts are not really stem cells because they change over time and because they undergo a limited number of asymmetric divisions *(81)*. Others call them stem cells because they are multipotent, undergo asymmetric division, and are the primary source of CNS tissue. Instead of using the austere definition, one might think of self-renewal as the finite capacity of a stem cell to maintain the stem cell state, rather than the stem cell *per se*. This allows for changes in potency that might be critical for normal development and repair, as well as age-related changes that might be inevitable. We can think of self-renewal as a modifiable property of stem cells that is tailored to the job that the stem cell has to accomplish—to make appropriate progeny according to the demands of the developing or the adult system.

The extent of self-renewal might be linked to telomerase activity. In most dividing somatic cells successive divisions involve progressive shortening of the telomeres at the ends of chromosomes, and telomere erosion correlates with cessation of cell division. In contrast, telomere shortening progresses much more slowly in certain types of stem cells, such as those in the germline, owing to the activity of a specific telomerase enzyme. The telomerase holoenzyme consists of an RNA template and protein components, including a cellular reverse transcriptase *(82)*. Its activity is high in certain proliferative cells and in the vast majority of neoplasms, including neural tumors, again providing a correlation with extended proliferative capacity *(83–85)*. Transfection of telomerase has in some cases conferred immortalization and allowed the establishment of cell lines, for example, from skin *(86)* and more recently from the nervous system *(87)*. Expression of telomerase has been reported in the developing nervous system, although expression significantly downregulates after birth, and activity may be undetectable in the adult *(85,88)*. However, it is possible that rare stem cells in the adult nervous system may retain a low level of expression, as do blood stem cells *(89)*. There are indications that telomerase activity is required for maintenance of normal nervous system development. Mice that lack telomerase RNA show progressively worse symptoms with generations, largely associated with defects in highly proliferative tissues *(90)*. After around six generations, the embryos die very early and show defects in neural tube closure *(41)*.

THE SIGNIFICANCE OF QUIESCENCE AND PROLIFERATION RATE TO THE STEM CELL STATE

It has been suggested that embryonic neural stem cells are not truly stem cells because they divide too rapidly, whereas stem cells are slowly dividing or quiescent, but this concept is erroneous. In fact, proliferation rates among stem cells vary widely. Intestinal crypt stem cells divide about once a day; other stem cells, such as hemopoietic and epidermal cells, divide much more slowly; others, such as the muscle satellite cell, may be genuinely quiescent *(16,91)*. Furthermore, the idea that when actively dividing stem cells are lost they are replaced by a quiescent population of dormant reserve stem cells might be an overgeneralization. Although in blood, plant meristem, and muscle this may be the case *(92–94)*, reserve stem cells in the intestinal crypt are actually rapidly dividing progeny of stem cells that can dedifferentiate and revert to the stem cell state. In the adult subventricular zone (SVZ), type B astrocyte-like stem cells generate rapidly dividing type C transit amplifying neuroblasts that in turn give rise to typeA neuroblasts *(95–97)*. After infusion of epidermal growth factor (EGF) in vivo, type C cells can revert to a type B state, indicating that a similar transition from rapidly dividing progenitor back to stem cell can occur in the nervous system *(98)*.

Given the large proliferative capacity of stem cells, it is clear that the rate of stem cell division must normally be highly regulated. In the intestinal crypt, there are a small number of stem cells, perhaps between five and seven. This is tightly controlled: one cell too many or one cell too few is detected and fixed by apoptosis or cell division *(99)*. Exactly how the changes in stem cell number are detected is unclear, but environmental factors must be key. This is true in the blood system, where quiescent blood stem cells can be rapidly stimulated to divide by cytokines *(100)*.

During normal development of the nervous system, the rates of proliferation of cells in germinal zones change with region and with time. Division rates within the neural germinal zones may be as rapid as every 7–10 hours *(101)* but may be as infrequent as 18 hours by late gestation *(102)*. Adult stem cells may have a cycle time that is on the order of many days *(96,103,104)*. It seems likely then that the proliferation rate of neural stem cells changes during normal neural development, in different regions of the embryo and into adulthood. How these regulative events are accomplished is not clear. They most likely involve regional and age-related changes in environmental factors, such as stem cell mitogens. FGF2 and EGF or the related factor transforming growth factor-α (TGF-α) are present in the CNS throughout life and profoundly stimulate neural stem cell proliferation in vitro and in vivo *(105)*. There are likely to be a large number of as yet undiscovered regulatory molecules that stimulate or inhibit neural stem cell division and hold the promise for expanding stem cells in vivo or in vitro; perhaps they also inhibit division of neural tumors.

THE ROLE OF ASYMMETRIC AND SYMMETRIC CELL DIVISIONS DURING NORMAL NEURAL DEVELOPMENT

Mitotic cell divisions produce two daughter cells that acquire identical genetic material but not necessarily identical epigenetic components. These components may include *cytoplasmic determinants*—molecules that can direct cell fate. Hence, by altering the way these molecules are distributed during the cell division process, it is possible to generate diverse cell fates. When a progenitor cell divides to generate two daughters with essentially the same fate, the process is called *symmetric cell division*; when it divides to generate two daughters with different fates, it is called *asymmetric cell division*. Sometimes a cell division generating two equivalent daughters that subsequently differentiate differently because of environmental influences has been called asymmetric. However, this may be an overextension of the definition, the crux of which is to show that the division process itself is actively involved in producing two distinct daughter cells.

The ability to divide asymmetrically is often described as a fundamental feature of a stem cell. If stem cells are to undergo both self-renewal and the generation of differentiated progeny, one way to do this is to divide asymmetrically. However, there are other ways to achieve this end. For example, self-renewal may be a stochastically determined, intrinsic property of a population of stem cells in which each cell has a given probability to make more stem cells or generate differentiated daughters. In this case, the two functions result from a population, rather than a single stem cell lineage, so it is not necessary to invoke asymmetric divisions to achieve them. Another way is for the stem cell to generate equivalent daughters that move into different environments, some promoting self-renewal and others promoting differentiation.

Nevertheless, asymmetric cell division may be utilized by stem cells, and there is direct evidence for asymmetric cell division within a few stem cell populations. In some species the lineages of progenitor cells have been reconstructed, providing direct evidence for asymmetric cell divisions. For example, in the *Drosophila* CNS, asymmetric cell divisions of the stem-like neuroblast result in the production of a smaller daughter called the ganglion mother cell (GMC) that goes on to generate two neurons or glial cells and another neuroblast. Repeated divisions of the neuroblast result in a chain of GMCs, each forming a pair of differentiated daughter cells *(74)*.

Well-characterized asymmetric cell lineages in *Drosophila* and *Caenorhabditis elegans* nervous systems render them ideal models for understanding how asymmetric divisions are achieved. Studies of mutations in both systems have revealed genes that are involved in this process (Fig. 2). In *Drosophila* neural development, Prospero and

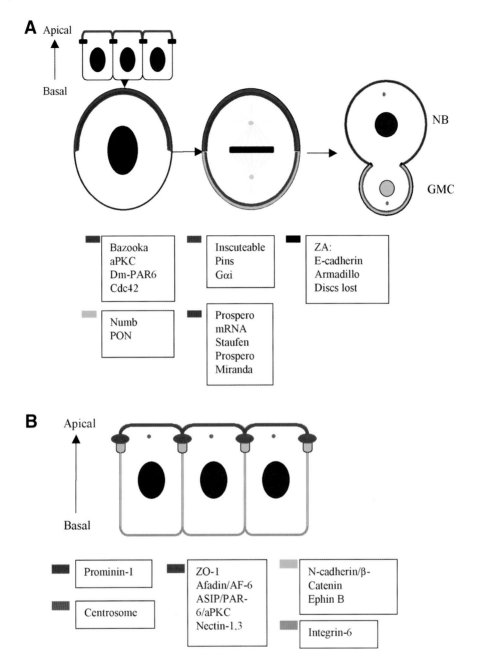

	Bazooka		Inscuteable		ZA:
	aPKC		Pins		E-cadherin
	Dm-PAR6		Gαi		Armadillo
	Cdc42				Discs lost

	Numb		Prospero
	PON		mRNA
			Staufen
			Prospero
			Miranda

	Prominin-1		ZO-1		N-cadherin/β-
			Afadin/AF-6		Catenin
			ASIP/PAR-		Ephin B
	Centrosome		6/aPKC		
			Nectin-1,3		Integrin-6

Fig. 2. **(A)** Asymmetric division of neuroblasts (NBs) in *Drosophila*: the subcellular localization of several polarity molecules in the neuroepithelium and a single dividing NB is indicated in
different colors (see legend). The early neuroepithelium has apical-basal polarity, and Bazooka,
PAR/aPKC complex are concentrated in the apical region. After delaminating, the NB enters into
mitosis. PAR/aPKC complex recruits Inscuteable and its partner, Pins. Miranda, Prospero, Staufen
and Prospero mRNA transiently localize to the apical pole, then quickly move to the basal pole,
forming a basal polarity complex with Numb and PON at metaphase. Later in anaphase and
telophase, these polarity molecules are segregated into the NB and the GMC respectively.
(B) The apical-basal polarity of the mammalian neuroepithelium (NE): each protein or complex
is indicated with different colors (see legend). The NE membrane is subdivided into apical and
basolateral regions. Prominin-1 is localized in the apical region. Components of the adhesion
junction and ASIP/PAR/aPKC complex are concentrated at the apical side of the lateral membrane.

Numb proteins are cell fate determinants that directly influence neural fate decisions at asymmetric cell divisions. Prospero is a transcription factor with a homeodomain, and Numb is an adapter protein with a phosphotyrosine binding (PTB) domain. Both proteins become asymmetrically localized in the basal cortex of the stem cell neuroblast at metaphase and then preferentially segregate into the GMC *(106,107)*. In addition, *prospero* mRNA is localized in a basal crescent at mitosis and segregated into the GMC. Once in the GMC, Prospero is released from the cortex and translocates into the nucleus, where it controls transcription of certain neuroblast- and GMC-specific genes *(108)*. Prospero also prevents cell division and stimulates differentiation so that the GMC only divides once, generating two neurons or glia *(109)*. Numb's function in the GMC is not clear; however, at the following division, Numb segregates asymmetrically into the two daughter cells, where it can create two different neuronal fates by inhibiting Notch function in one cell, but not in the other *(110–113)*.

Complexes of cytoplasmic components bring about the asymmetric localization of Prospero and Numb. Bazooka and Inscuteable are required for correct mitotic spindle orientation in the neuroblast and maintain apical-basal polarity from epithelial cells to neuroblasts *(114–116)*. They are themselves localized asymmetrically at the apical side of the neuroblast before mitosis, forming a complex with DmPAR6, atypical protein kinase C (aPKC), partner of Inscuteable (Pins) and G protein subunit Gαi *(114,115, 117–119)*, and thus providing the positional information necessary for other components (Miranda, Staufen, Prospero, Partner of Numb [PON], and Numb) to be localized basally at mitosis and to be further preferentially segregated into the GMC (Fig. 2) *(120)*.

The asymmetric distribution of the Prospero complex is cell cycle dependent. At interphase, Inscuteable forms a prominent crescent along the apical cell cortex. Miranda, a membrane-associated, multidomain adapter protein, interacts with Inscuteable and Prospero and tethers Staufen, which in turn binds *prospero* mRNA *(121)*. When the neuroblast enters metaphase, Miranda, Staufen, Prospero, and *prospero* mRNA move as a group to the basal side of the dividing neuroblast. After mitosis, this complex of protein and mRNA is segregated into the GMC *(122–124)*. It is not clear how the movement of this complex occurs. Similarly, apical localization of Inscuteable provides a positional guide for the Numb complex, which concentrates at the basal side of the neuroblast during mitosis. Although Miranda can interact with Numb protein in vitro, it is not necessary for asymmetric numb localization. PON colocalizes with Numb at the basal cortex of the mitotic neuroblast and loss of *pon* function causes defects in asymmetric Numb localization *(125)*.

Although a number of the apical components that are retained in the neuroblast rather than moving into the GMC have been isolated, none of them have been shown to be cytoplasmic determinants of the neuroblast fate. It would be very interesting to find such molecules, if they exist, because they might tell us which gene functions are essential to maintain the stem cell state. It is hoped that these molecules will be uncovered in the near future, as we build on knowledge of the basal neuroblast complexes.

As in *Drosophila*, mammalian neuroepithelial (NE) cells (including radial glial cells) also show an apical–basal polarity (reviewed in ref. *126*). In contrast to *Drosophila* NBs, mammalian NE cells do not delaminate when CNS neurons are being generated. The apical plasma membrane selectively contains transmembrane proteins, such as prominin-1 *(127)* and the localization of centrosomes beneath the apical cell membrane *(128)*. Junctional complexes are found at the apical end of the lateral plasma membrane, and these recruit cytoplasmic proteins such as ZO-1, afadin/AF-6, ASIP/ PAR-3/Bazooka, PAR-6, and aPKC *(129–131)*. Even within the lateral plasma membrane, gradients of transmembrane proteins in the apical-basal direction can be detected, such as those of N-cadherin *(129)* or ephrin B1 *(132)*. Interestingly, prior to the onset of neurogenesis (E10), NE cells lose tight junctions *(129)* but with an up-regulation of ZO-1. So, indeed the adhesion junction plays a major role in maintaining neuroepithelium (NE) cell polarity, as evidenced by the mislocation of prominin-1 to the basolateral membrane in afadin/AF-6 knock out mice *(130)* and the binding of PAR-3 to Nectin-1,3 *(133)*. However, Numb exhibits species difference, apical in mouse *(134)* and basal in avian *(135)* neuroepithelium. Whether these polarity molecules have functions similar to those in *Drosophila* need to be further explored.

Studies of the dynamics of cell proliferation within vertebrate CNS proliferative zones suggest that early cell divisions are largely symmetric, perhaps allowing expansion of the stem cell population; as neurogenesis gets under way, cell divisions appear to become largely asymmetric. An interesting correlation has been noted between this purported change in the type of cell division and the direction of the plane of division of mitotic cells at the ventricular surface *(136,137)*. Early divisions usually have the division plane oriented perpendicular to the ventricular surface, whereas later divisions have the plane oriented preferentially in the horizontal direction. Perhaps the perpendicular divisions are symmetric and the horizontal divisions asymmetric? In slices of ferret cortex it has been shown that at least at early stages the products of perpendicular divisions appear to behave similarly, migrating at similar rates within the ventricular zone, whereas the products of horizontal divisions do not *(136)*. It will be important to follow these cells for longer periods to establish whether the change in division plane correlates with final symmetric or asymmetric cell fates. There are situations in which it does not; for example, in plant meristem the division plane alters when progenitor cells generate different types of products, yet the cell divisions involved are asymmetric *(93)*.

In the vertebrate, especially in mammalian systems that develop *in utero*, it is currently impossible to follow the lineage trees of progenitor cells in vivo. We can identify the components of a clone that developed in vivo, for example, by labeling individual cells within the ventricular zone of the CNS using retroviral markers, waiting for a period, and then revealing the clonal contents by a histochemical technique. In labeling experiments conducted in the developing cerebral cortex, clone distribution is sometimes spread between cortical layers, suggesting a stem-like lineage tree with repeated asymmetric divisions, and sometimes confined to a single layer, suggesting a symmetric, proliferative type of lineage tree *(138–141)*. Recently, long-term time-lapse imaging of clonal cells in murine cortical slices has shed some light on the division pattern of radial glial progenitor cells, now understood to be principle neuronal and glial progenitor cells in the developing CNS. Such recordings indicate that radial glia undergo repeated asymmetric cell divisions *(142–144)*. However, we cannot yet determine with these methods exactly how symmetric and asymmetric divisions contribute to clonal development, or how these clone members are generated over time in the animal.

In tissue culture, it has been possible to follow the development of individual isolated embryonic mouse ventricular zone cells for long periods. Continuous recording of the divisions of these cells, combined with immunostaining of the progeny, provides

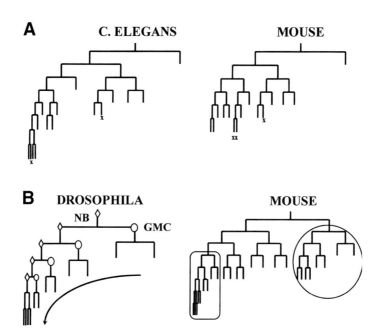

Fig. 3. (**A,B**) Mouse embryonic cortical progenitor cells undergo asymmetric division patterns, resulting in lineage trees that resemble those of invertebrate neural lineages.

lineage trees for mammalian cells developing in vitro. These data show directly that mouse cortical progenitor cells undergo largely asymmetric cell divisions when generating neurons *(145)*. The major neuroblast divides to give a minor neuroblast that produces a small "packet" of about 10 neurons and another stem-like progenitor that divides asymmetrically again, producing another "packet" of neurons, and so on (Fig. 3). Occasionally the minor neuroblast clones appear to have a symmetric lineage, generating their progeny at the same time. (Perhaps these are equivalent to the retrovirally labeled clones that reside within a cortical layer.) Symmetric lineages are associated with the expansion of glioblast clones. However, in the vast majority of cases the neuroblast clones are generated by asymmetric cell divisions. Interestingly, the lineage trees of these cortical neuroblasts are similar to those described for neural progenitors in *C. elegans* and *Drosophila*, suggesting an evolutionary conservation of the mechanisms underlying neural cell generation *(73)*.

It will be important to find out whether the division patterns actually play a role in defining neural cell types in mammals, as they do in invertebrates. It will also be important to establish the mechanisms for generating asymmetric cell divisions in vertebrates. Homologs of Numb have been described and appear to segregate unevenly within dividing cells in the cortical ventricular zone *(134,146,147)* and in sibling daughter cells from isolated cortical progenitor cells *(146)*. Moreover, as in *Drosophila*, asymmetric segregation of mouse Numb has been correlated with binary cell fate choice during cortical neurogenesis *(146–148)*. Interestingly, the fact that the asymmetric mouse cortical lineage trees are seen in a culture setting devoid of normal environmental cues suggests that the presence of other cells may not be necessary for the asymmetry in CNS progenitor cell divisions to occur. The same has been shown for *Drosophila*:

cultured neuroblasts retain an asymmetric lineage pattern in vitro *(149,150)*. However, this is not to say that incorporation into the normal epithelium could not modulate the division process: in *Drosophila* disruption of adherens junctions can convert symmetric epithelial divisions into asymmetric divisions *(151)*.

It is surprising that in a highly regulative embryo such as the mouse, in which cell–cell signaling allows for plasticity in the molding of the final organism, invertebrate-type lineage trees, which are thought of as invariant and characteristic of mosaic development, are employed in making the CNS. One has to remember, however, that although cell division-based mechanisms might operate to generate neural cell types, these processes may still be environmentally responsive and capable of change.

STEM CELL NICHE

From extensive studies of blood stem cells and other stem cell types, it has become clear that the immediate environment of a stem cell—its niche—is critical for determining its behavior. It is in this primary environment that the stem cell acquires information about whether or not to divide and what types of progeny to generate. Blood stem cells need to be kept in a bone marrow stromal niche to maintain their self-renewal. The bone marrow niche is a complex environment of extracellular matrix components, for example, tenascin, and growth factors including stem cell factor, granulocyte/macrophage colony stimulating factor, and FGFs. Specific cytokines release blood stem cells from their adhesion in the niche, mobilizing them for circulation and proliferation *(100)*. In other systems, stem cells also reside in complex niches that regulate their behavior *(152)*.

During normal development of the nervous system, neural stem cells reside in the germinal zones—notably the ventricular zone and the subventricular zone. In the adult, neurogenesis is limited primarily to a few specific areas of the CNS, around the lateral ventricles and in the dentate gyrus (Fig. 1) *(153)*. As reviewed elsewhere *(27,154–157)*, many extracellular matrix molecules (including tenascin) and growth factors (such as EGF and FGFs) have been described in these areas. Clearly, there are also region-specific niche molecules—as shown by the ability of cells in a particular region to dictate new differentiation programs in transplanted cells. Removal of surface components from embryonic progenitor cells prior to transplantation can alter their ability to recognize regional signals *(158)*.

In the adult nervous system, although there are defined areas of neurogenesis, stem cells can be isolated from nonneurogenic areas, such as the spinal cord, and grown in culture to generate both neurons and glial progeny. However, when put back into the spinal cord, these stem cells make only glia. When placed in a neurogenic area such as the SVZ, these spinal cord stem cells can make neurons as well as glia *(159)*. This implies that key environmental molecules within different adult CNS niches regulate the ability of stem cells to generate neuronal or glial products. The search for factors that define the niche (and allow the specification of stem cells, their self-renewal and regulation) is a key area for study: the niche may ultimately define the stem cell. BMP may be a critical niche component in adults that affects the neuron-glial choice, as it does in embryonic progenitor cells. Noggin, expressed by ependymal cells, binds BMP in the adult SVZ, thus inhibiting gliogenesis and promoting neurogenesis *(160,161)*.

In the murine SVZ and hippocampus, and the songbird higher vocal center, neural stem cells have been seen to lie close to blood vessels, raising the possibility that vascular cells provide an important niche *(162–164)*. Indeed, endothelial cell coculture with embryonic and adult SVZ stem cells promotes their self-renewal, maintains their developmental potential, and increases their ability to make neurons *(165)*. Future studies will reveal the niche factors responsible for this effect.

IS THERE A MOLECULAR DEFINITION OF THE NEURAL STEM CELL?

Molecular characterization of stem cells allows the identification of cell components that are critical for stem cell regulation and that help us understand stem cell biology. In addition, employment of these markers for cell selection allows researchers to study a purer population of stem cells and to provide a uniform population for therapeutic use. Hence, considerable efforts have been made to find markers for stem cells, especially surface markers that allow live cell isolation. Hemopoietic stem cells are probably the best characterized at this point, and they can be isolated (based on the expression of particular surface antigens) for study and transplantation *(17)*. Epidermal stem cells have high levels of β1-integrin, which also allows their selection *(166)*.

Characterization of stem cells from a number of systems reveals some common features that help define the general class. For example, the Notch signaling system, initially identified in *Drosophila*, appears to play a role in regulating a variety of stem cells. Notch is expressed on blood stem cells, and Jagged is expressed in the bone marrow; activation of the receptor might keep the blood stem cell in a quiescent state *(166–170)*. Notch is expressed in muscle cell precursors and also regulates their differentiation *(171)*. In the nervous system of *Drosophila*, Notch is involved in switching epidermal progenitor cells between two alternative fates, nonneural vs the neuroblast fate, or between two types of neuron *(172,173)*. By feedback regulation (called lateral inhibition) between Notch and its ligand Delta, the number and placement of neuroblasts in the neuroepithelial sheet are determined. In the vertebrate nervous system, Notch1 and its ligands Delta and Jagged are widely expressed in germinal zones during development. Constitutive expression in the embryonic mouse forebrain ventricular zone results in maintenance of the radial glial state, now known as a principle CNS progenitor that can have stem cell features and give rise to type B astrocyte stem cells in the SVZ *(174)*. In the adult CNS, Notch is present in neurogenic zones *(175,176)*. Notch is also expressed on long-lived adult oligodendrocyte O-2A progenitors that have stem cell-like properties, and Jagged is expressed by mature oligodendrocytes and neurons. Activation of Notch on the adult O-2A may maintain them in an immature state *(177)*.

There are other examples of common features shared by stem cells from a variety of sources. For example, FGF-1 and -2, closely related members of the FGF family, EGF, or its relative TGF-α appear mitogenic for a wide variety of stem cells, including epidermal, bone, blood, gut, and neural stem cells as well as primordial germ cells. Similarly, members of the BMP family influence cell division in these stem cell systems, often negatively *(178–186)*. Components of these signaling pathways may thus help identify a number of classes of stem cells.

Other markers appear to define particular classes of stem cells, even across the plant and animal kingdoms. For example, the gene *piwi* is specifically expressed in *Drosophila* germinal stem cells. In a remarkable show of evolutionary conservation, *piwi* is structurally similar to a plant gene called *zwille*, which is seen in stem cells in the plant meristem, the equivalent of germinal tissue that generates flowers *(187,188)*. Hence, this family of related transcription factors, whose function remains to be elucidated, might help define the germ stem cell class and reveal evolutionarily conserved mechanisms of germ cell maintenance.

Neural stem cells, besides expressing Notch and various components of the EGF/FGF/BMP signaling pathways, have a number of cell-intrinsic markers. They possess the RNA binding protein Musashi, the mouse homolog of *Drosophila* Musashi. In the fly, Musashi is involved in neuron development *(189)*, and its presence in mouse neural stem cells indicates that it may also play an important role in these cells *(190,191)*. There is persuasive evidence that adult stem cells in the subventricular zone express the intermediate filament proteins Nestin *(96,192)* and GFAP *(96)*. Embryonic CNS progenitors also express green fluorescent protein (GFP) from the human promoter *(193)*. As yet, none of these markers appear to be exclusive to neural stem cells. For example, in the adult, Notch is also expressed on subpopulations of postmitotic neurons *(175)*, and Musashi and GFAP are expressed by astrocytes. Nevertheless, it is possible that particular combinations of these markers may define neural stem cells at the molecular level. TLX is expressed in embryonic and adult neural stem cells, and a GFP reporter allowed fluorescence-activated cell sorting (FACS) selection of stem cells *(194)*.

More information is needed regarding surface markers on neural stem cells, as these markers will greatly aid their live isolation and purification. Neural crest stem cells carry the low-affinity p75 neurotrophin receptor, which has allowed their retrieval, for example, from the sciatic nerve, suggesting that they may be available for longer periods than previously thought, for both for potential repair and potential tumor formation *(195)*. The surface marker CD133 enriches for human embryonic CNS stem cells *(45)*. For murine species, selection methods based on exclusion of cells expressing surface determinants characteristic of differentiated cells results in a remarkably pure population of adult SVZ stem cells, although only a subpopulation of the total stem cells present *(196)*. Adult murine stem cells express the carbohydrate moiety LewisX (LeX) or SSEA-1, which is also present on mouse embryonic stem cells where it might regulate FGF-2 mitogenicity *(197)* and adult bone marrow-derived stem cells *(198)*. LeX staining allows for enrichment of adult mouse SVZ cells from 1% up to 25% *(162)*.

Comparison of gene expression profiles are generating an abundance of data on genes expressed in stem cell populations. Cross-stem cell type comparisons have been used to indicate genes that might confer essential, common elements—so-called "stemness" markers. Different studies have yielded different sets of common stem cell genes, with unfortunately little overlap between them *(199–206)*, furthering our appreciation of diversity among stem cells. Gene array data for neural progenitor populations continue to emerge *(207–212)*. Methods of global gene analysis are highly likely to yield new markers that improve cell enrichment methods and to provide important novel insights into the biology of neural stem cells.

CONCLUSION

Stem cells are critically involved in the normal development and maintenance of a great variety of tissues, from plants to animals. It is interesting to consider why stem cells are used so prevalently to make tissues. Perhaps they provide a compact solution to disease prevention or to wear and tear: the information to generate a wide variety of cell types can be held in a succinct package, waiting for activating signals. Perhaps the embodiment of a variety of developmental possibilities within a single cell type allows effective integration of developmental and homeostatic signals to occur. Consistent with this idea, there is evidence that multipotent progenitors appear to integrate the input of combinations of factors that can act on them singly *(213,214)*. Thus information from different sources can play on a single cell, which reads the input and responds appropriately.

At this point, the best definition of neural stem cells is still probably the sparsest—cells that are able to self-renew and generate differentiated progeny. However, as research continues apace, we may soon be able to refine this definition, to subdivide it as distinct types of neural stem cells are revealed, and to add molecular signatures that will eventually allow a more complete understanding of this unique class of versatile cells.

ACKNOWLEDGMENTS

I thank Qin Shen, Yu Sun, Natalia Abramova, and Karen Kirchofer for their invaluable help and advice in preparing this manuscript.

REFERENCES

1. Altman, J. (1970) in *Developmental Neurobiology* (Himwich, W. A., ed.), Charles C Thomas, Springfield, IL, pp. 197–237.
2. Temple, S. (1989) Division and differentiation of isolated CNS blast cells in microculture. *Nature* **340,** 471–473.
3. Reynolds, B. A., Tetzlaff, W., and Weiss, S. (1992) A multipotent EGF-responsive striatal embryonic progenitor cell produces neurons and astrocytes. *J. Neurosci.* **12,** 4565–4574.
4. Davis, A. A. and Temple, S. (1994) A self-renewing multipotential stem cell in embryonic rat cerebral cortex. *Nature* **372,** 263–266.
5. Johe, K. K., Hazel, T. G., Muller, T., Dugich-Djordjevic, M. M., and McKay, R. D. (1996) Single factors direct the differentiation of stem cells from the fetal and adult central nervous system. *Genes Dev.* **10,** 3129–3140.
6. Kalyani, A., Hobson, K., and Rao, M. S. (1997) Neuroepithelial stem cells from the embryonic spinal cord: isolation, characterization, and clonal analysis. *Dev. Biol.* **186,** 202–223.
7. Stemple, D. L. and Anderson, D. J. (1992) Isolation of a stem cell for neurons and glia from the mammalian neural crest. *Cell* **71,** 973–985.
8. Walsh, C. and Cepko, C. L. (1993) Clonal dispersion in proliferative layers of developing cerebral cortex. *Nature* **362,** 632–635.
9. Leber, S. M. and Sanes, J. R. (1991) Lineage analysis with a recombinant retrovirus: application to chick spinal motor neurons. *Adv. Neurol.* **56,** 27–36.
10. Sanes, J. R. (1989) Analysing cell lineage with a recombinant retrovirus. *Trends Neurosci.* **12,** 21–28.
11. Temple, S. (1999) CNS development: the obscure origins of adult stem cells. *Curr. Biol.* **9,** R397–R399.

12. Weiss, S., Dunne, C., Hewson, J., et al. (1996) Multipotent CNS stem cells are present in the adult mammalian spinal cord and ventricular neuroaxis. *J. Neurosci.* **16,** 7599–7609.
13. Shihabuddin, L. S., Ray, J., and Gage, F. H. (1997) FGF-2 is sufficient to isolate progenitors found in the adult mammalian spinal cord. *Exp. Neurol.* **148,** 577–586.
14. Gould, E., Reeves, A. J., Graziano, M. S., and Gross, C. G. (1999) Neurogenesis in the neocortex of adult primates. *Science* **286,** 548–552.
15. Marmur, R., Mabie, P. C., Gokhan, S., Song, Q., Kessler, J. A., and Mehler, M. F. (1998) Isolation and developmental characterization of cerebral cortical multipotent progenitors. *Dev. Biol.* **204,** 577–591.
16. Morrison, S. J., Shah, N. M., and Anderson, D. J. (1997) Regulatory mechanisms in stem cell biology. *Cell* **88,** 287–298.
17. Morrison, S. J., Uchida, N., and Weissman, I. L. (1995) The biology of hematopoietic stem cells. *Annu. Rev. Cell Dev. Biol.* **11,** 35–71.
18. Okabe, S., Forsberg-Nilsson, K., Spiro, A. C., Segal, M., and McKay, R. D. (1996) Development of neuronal precursor cells and functional postmitotic neurons from embryonic stem cells in vitro. *Mech. Dev.* **59,** 89–102.
19. Dinsmore, J., Ratliff, J., Deacon, T., et al. (1996) Embryonic stem cells differentiated in vitro as a novel source of cells for transplantation. *Cell Transplant.* **5,** 131–143.
20. Renoncourt, Y., Carroll, P., Filippi, P., Arce, V., and Alonso, S. (1998) Neurons derived in vitro from ES cells express homeoproteins characteristic of motoneurons and interneurons. *Mech. Dev.* **79,** 185–197.
21. Brustle, O., Jones, K. N., Learish, R. D., et al. (1999) Embryonic stem cell-derived glial precursors: a source of myelinating transplants. *Science* **285,** 754–756.
22. Mujtaba, T., Piper, D. R., Kalyani, A., Groves, A. K., Lucero, M. T., and Rao, M. S. (1999) Lineage-restricted neural precursors can be isolated from both the mouse neural tube and cultured ES cells. *Dev. Biol.* **214,** 113–127.
23. Mujtaba, T., Mayer-Proschel, M., and Rao, M. S. (1998) A common neural progenitor for the CNS and PNS. *Dev. Biol.* **200,** 1–15.
24. Temple, S. and Alvarez-Buylla, A. (1999) Stem cells in the adult mammalian central nervous system. *Curr. Opin. Neurobiol.* **9,** 135–141.
25. Gage, F. H., Kempermann, G., Palmer, T. D., Peterson, D. A., and Ray, J. (1998) Multipotent progenitor cells in the adult dentate gyrus. *J. Neurobiol.* **36,** 249–266.
26. Gage, F. H., Coates, P. W., Palmer, T. D., et al. (1995) Survival and differentiation of adult neuronal progenitor cells transplanted to the adult brain. *Proc. Natl. Acad. Sci. USA* **92,** 11879–11883.
27. Cameron, H. A. and McKay, R. (1998) Stem cells and neurogenesis in the adult brain. *Curr. Opin. Neurobiol.* **8,** 677–680.
28. Kuhn, H. G. and Svendsen, C. N. (1999) Origins, functions, and potential of adult neural stem cells. *Bioessays* **21,** 625–630.
29. Rao, M. S. (1999) Multipotent and restricted precursors in the central nervous system. *Anat. Rec.* **257,** 137–148.
30. Tropepe, V., Sibilia, M., Ciruna, B. G., Rossant, J., Wagner, E. F., and van der Kooy, D. (1999) Distinct neural stem cells proliferate in response to EGF and FGF in the developing mouse telencephalon. *Dev. Biol.* **208,** 166–188.
31. Anderson, D. J. (1997) Cellular and molecular biology of neural crest cell lineage determination. *Trends Genet.* **13,** 276–280.
32. Anderson, D. J., Groves, A., Lo, L., et al. (1997) Cell lineage determination and the control of neuronal identity in the neural crest. *Cold Spring Harb. Symp. Quant. Biol.* **62,** 493–504.
33. LaBonne, C. and Bronner-Fraser, M. (1998) Induction and patterning of the neural crest, a stem cell-like precursor population. *J. Neurobiol.* **36,** 175–189.
34. Gaiano, N. and Fishell, G. (1998) Transplantation as a tool to study progenitors within the vertebrate nervous system. *J. Neurobiol.* **36,** 152–161.

35. Na, E., McCarthy, M., Neyt, C., Lai, E., and Fishell, G. (1998) Telencephalic progenitors maintain anteroposterior identities cell autonomously. *Curr. Biol.* **8,** 987–990.
36. Takahashi, M., Palmer, T. D., Takahashi, J., and Gage, F. H. (1998) Widespread integration and survival of adult-derived neural progenitor cells in the developing optic retina. *Mol. Cell Neurosci.* **12,** 340–348.
37. Campbell, K. and Bjorklund, A. (1995) Neurotransmitter-related gene expression in intrastriatal striatal transplants. III. Regulation by host cortical and dopaminergic afferents. *Brain Res. Mol. Brain Res.* **29,** 263–272.
38. Frantz, G. D. and McConnell, S. K. (1996) Restriction of late cerebral cortical progenitors to an upper-layer fate. *Neuron* **17,** 55–61.
39. Olsson, M., Campbell, K., and Turnbull, D. H. (1997) Specification of mouse telencephalic and mid-hindbrain progenitors following heterotopic ultrasound-guided embryonic transplantation. *Neuron* **19,** 761–772.
40. Suhonen, J. O., Peterson, D. A., Ray, J., and Gage, F. H. (1996) Differentiation of adult hippocampus-derived progenitors into olfactory neurons in vivo. *Nature* **383,** 624–627.
41. Herrera, D. G., Garcia-Verdugo, J. M., and Alvarez-Buylla, A. (1999) Adult-derived neural precursors transplanted into multiple regions in the adult brain. *Ann. Neurol.* **46,** 867–877.
42. Quinn, S. M., Walters, W. M., Vescovi, A. L., and Whittemore, S. R. (1999) Lineage restriction of neuroepithelial precursor cells from fetal human spinal cord. *J. Neurosci. Res.* **57,** 590–602.
43. Bjornson, C. R., Rietze, R. L., Reynolds, B. A., Magli, M. C., and Vescovi, A. L. (1999) Turning brain into blood: a hematopoietic fate adopted by adult neural stem cells in vivo. *Science* **283,** 534–537.
44. Clarke, D. L., Johansson, C. B., Wilbertz, J., et al. (2000) Generalized potential of adult neural stem cells. *Science* **288,** 1660–1663.
45. Uchida, N., Buck, D. W., He, D., et al. (2000) Direct isolation of human central nervous system stem cells. *Proc. Natl. Acad. Sci. USA* **97,** 14720–14725.
46. Alvarez-Buylla, A., Herrera, D. G., and Wichterle, H. (2000) The subventricular zone: source of neuronal precursors for brain repair. *Prog. Brain Res.* **127,** 1–11.
47. Lillien, L. and Raphael, H. (2000) BMP and FGF regulate the development of EGF-responsive neural progenitor cells. *Development* **127,** 4993–5005.
48. Anderson, D. J. (2001) Stem cells and pattern formation in the nervous system: the possible versus the actual. *Neuron* **30,** 19–35.
49. Qian, X., Shen, Q., Goderie, S. K., et al. (2000) Timing of CNS cell generation: a programmed sequence of neuron and glial cell production from isolated murine cortical stem cells. *Neuron* **28,** 69–80.
50. Temple, S. (2001) The development of neural stem cells. *Nature* **414,** 112–117.
51. Anderson, D. J. and Axel, R. (1985) Molecular probes for the development and plasticity of neural crest derivatives. *Cell* **42,** 649–662.
52. Hu, M., Krause, D., Greaves, M., et al. (1997) Multilineage gene expression precedes commitment in the hemopoietic system. *Genes Dev.* **11,** 774–785.
53. Cao, Y., Wilcox, K. S., Martin, C. E., Rachinsky, T. L., Eberwine, J., and Dichter, M. A. (1996) Presence of mRNA for glutamic acid decarboxylase in both excitatory and inhibitory neurons. *Proc. Natl. Acad. Sci. USA* **93,** 9844–9849.
54. Arber, S., Han, B., Mendelsohn, M., Smith, M., Jessell, T. M., and Sockanathan, S. (1999) Requirement for the homeobox gene *Hb9* in the consolidation of motor neuron identity. *Neuron* **23,** 659–674.
55. Thaler, J., Harrison, K., Sharma, K., Lettieri, K., Kehrl, J., and Pfaff, S. L. (1999) Active suppression of interneuron programs within developing motor neurons revealed by analysis of homeodomain factor HB9. *Neuron* **23,** 675–687.
56. Jan, Y. N. and Jan, L. Y. (1993) HLH proteins, fly neurogenesis, and vertebrate myogenesis. *Cell* **75,** 827–830.

57. Lo, L., Morin, X., Brunet, J. F., and Anderson, D. J. (1999) Specification of neurotransmitter identity by Phox2 proteins in neural crest stem cells. *Neuron* **22,** 693–705.
58. Lo, L., Tiveron, M. C., and Anderson, D. J. (1998) MASH1 activates expression of the paired homeodomain transcription factor Phox2a, and couples pan-neuronal and subtype-specific components of autonomic neuronal identity. *Development* **125,** 609–620.
59. Cau, E., Gradwohl, G., Fode, C., and Guillemot, F. (1997) Mash1 activates a cascade of bHLH regulators in olfactory neuron progenitors. *Development* **124,** 1611–1621.
60. Casarosa, S., Fode, C., and Guillemot, F. (1999) Mash1 regulates neurogenesis in the ventral telencephalon. *Development* **126,** 525–534.
61. Fode, C., Ma, Q., Casarosa, S., Ang, S. L., Anderson, D. J., and Guillemot, F. (2000) A role for neural determination genes in specifying the dorsoventral identity of telencephalic neurons. *Genes Dev.* **14,** 67–80.
62. Li, W. and LoTurco, J. J. (2000) Noggin is a negative regulator of neuronal differentiation in developing neocortex. *Dev. Neurosci.* **22,** 68–73.
63. Bonni, A., Sun, Y., Nadal-Vicens, M., et al. (1997) Regulation of gliogenesis in the central nervous system by the JAK-STAT signaling pathway. *Science* **278,** 477–483.
64. Rajan, P. and McKay, R. D. (1998) Multiple routes to astrocytic differentiation in the CNS. *J. Neurosci.* **18,** 3620–3629.
65. Gross, R. E., Mehler, M. F., Mabie, P. C., Zang, Z., Santschi, L., and Kessler, J. A. (1996) Bone morphogenetic proteins promote astroglial lineage commitment by mammalian subventricular zone progenitor cells. *Neuron* **17,** 595–606.
66. Nakashima, K. and Taga, T. (2002) Mechanisms underlying cytokine-mediated cell-fate regulation in the nervous system. *Mol. Neurobiol.* **25,** 233–244.
67. Nakashima, K., Yanagisawa, M., Arakawa, H., et al. (1999) Synergistic signaling in fetal brain by STAT3–Smad1 complex bridged by p300. *Science* **284,** 479–482.
68. Sun, Y., Nadal-Vicens, M., Misono, S., et al. (2001) Neurogenin promotes neurogenesis and inhibits glial differentiation by independent mechanisms. *Cell* **104,** 365–376.
69. Song, M. R. and Ghosh, A. (2004) FGF2-induced chromatin remodeling regulates CNTF-mediated gene expression and astrocyte differentiation. *Nat. Neurosci.* **7,** 229–235.
70. Chang, C. and Hemmati-Brivanlou, A. (1998) Cell fate determination in embryonic ectoderm. *J. Neurobiol.* **36,** 128–151.
71. Lemaitre, B., Nicolas, E., Michaut, L., Reichhart, J. M., and Hoffmann, J. A. (1996) The dorsoventral regulatory gene cassette spatzle/Toll/cactus controls the potent antifungal response in *Drosophila* adults. *Cell* **86,** 973–983.
72. Qian, X., Davis, A. A., Goderie, S. K., and Temple, S. (1997) FGF2 concentration regulates the generation of neurons and glia from multipotent cortical stem cells. *Neuron* **18,** 81–93.
73. Shen, Q., Qian, X., Capela, A., and Temple, S. (1998) Stem cells in the embryonic cerebral cortex: their role in histogenesis and patterning. *J. Neurobiol.* **36,** 162–174.
74. Doe, C. Q., Fuerstenberg, S., and Peng, C. Y. (1998) Neural stem cells: from fly to vertebrates. *J. Neurobiol.* **36,** 111–127.
75. Hall, P. A. and Watt, F. M. (1989) Stem cells: the generation and maintenance of cellular diversity. *Development* **106,** 619–633.
76. Potten, C. S. and Loeffler, M. (1990) Stem cells: attributes, cycles, spirals, pitfalls and uncertainties. Lessons for and from the crypt. *Development* **110,** 1001–1020.
77. Weiss, S., Reynolds, B. A., Vescovi, A. L., Morshead, C., Craig, C. G., and van der, K. D. (1996) Is there a neural stem cell in the mammalian forebrain? *Trends Neurosci.* **19,** 387–393.
78. Lansdorp, P. M., Dragowska, W., and Mayani, H. (1993) Ontogeny-related changes in proliferative potential of human hematopoietic cells. *J. Exp. Med.* **178,** 787–791.
79. Martin, K., Kirkwood, T. B., and Potten, C. S. (1998) Age changes in stem cells of murine small intestinal crypts. *Exp. Cell Res.* **241,** 316–323.

80. Kuhn, H. G., Dickinson-Anson, H., and Gage, F. H. (1996) Neurogenesis in the dentate gyrus of the adult rat: age-related decrease of neuronal progenitor proliferation. *J. Neurosci.* **16,** 2027–2033.
81. Lin, H. and Schagat, T. (1997) Neuroblasts: a model for the asymmetric division of stem cells. *Trends Genet.* **13,** 33–39.
82. Bryan, T. M. and Cech, T. R. (1999) Telomerase and the maintenance of chromosome ends. *Curr. Opin. Cell Biol.* **11,** 318–324.
83. Langford, L. A., Piatyszek, M. A., Xu, R., Schold, S. C., Jr., and Shay, J. W. (1995) Telomerase activity in human brain tumours. *Lancet* **346,** 1267–1268.
84. Le, S., Zhu, J. J., Anthony, D. C., Greider, C. W., and Black, P. M. (1998) Telomerase activity in human gliomas. *Neurosurgery* **42,** 1120–1124; discussion 1124–1125.
85. Weil, R. J., Wu, Y. Y., Vortmeyer, A. O., et al. (1999) Telomerase activity in micro-dissected human gliomas. *Mod. Pathol.* **12,** 41–46.
86. Counter, C. M., Hahn, W. C., Wei, W., et al. (1998) Dissociation among in vitro telomerase activity, telomere maintenance, and cellular immortalization. *Proc. Natl. Acad. Sci. USA* **95,** 14723–14728.
87. Roy, N. S., Nakano, T., Keyoung, H. M., et al. (2004) Telomerase immortalization of neuronally restricted progenitor cells derived from the human fetal spinal cord. *Nat. Biotechnol.* **22,** 297–305.
88. Blasco, M. A., Funk, W., Villeponteau, B., and Greider, C. W. (1995) Functional characterization and developmental regulation of mouse telomerase RNA. *Science* **269,** 1267–1270.
89. Blasco, M. A., Lee, H. W., Hande, M. P., et al. (1997) Telomere shortening and tumor formation by mouse cells lacking telomerase RNA. *Cell* **91,** 25–34.
90. Dye, C. A., Lee, J. K., Atkinson, R. C., Brewster, R., Han, P. L., and Bellen, H. J. (1998) The *Drosophila sanpodo* gene controls sibling cell fate and encodes a tropomodulin homolog, an actin/tropomyosin-associated protein. *Development* **125,** 1845–1856.
91. Bornemann, A., Maier, F., and Kuschel, R. (1999) Satellite cells as players and targets in normal and diseased muscle. *Neuropediatrics* **30,** 167–175.
92. Schultz, E. and McCormick, K. M. (1994) Skeletal muscle satellite cells. *Rev. Physiol. Biochem. Pharmacol.* **123,** 213–257.
93. Doerner, P. (1998) Root development: quiescent center not so mute after all. *Curr. Biol.* **8,** R42–44.
94. Morrison, S. J. and Weissman, I. L. (1994) The long-term repopulating subset of hematopoietic stem cells is deterministic and isolatable by phenotype. *Immunity* **1,** 661–673.
95. Doetsch, F. (2003) The glial identity of neural stem cells. *Nat. Neurosci.* **6,** 1127–1134.
96. Doetsch, F., Caille, I., Lim, D. A., Garcia-Verdugo, J. M., and Alvarez-Buylla, A. (1999) Subventricular zone astrocytes are neural stem cells in the adult mammalian brain. *Cell* **97,** 703–716.
97. Doetsch, F., Garcia-Verdugo, J. M., and Alvarez-Buylla, A. (1997) Cellular composition and three-dimensional organization of the subventricular germinal zone in the adult mammalian brain. *J. Neurosci.* **17,** 5046–5061.
98. Doetsch, F., Petreanu, L., Caille, I., Garcia-Verdugo, J. M., and Alvarez-Buylla, A. (2002) EGF converts transit-amplifying neurogenic precursors in the adult brain into multipotent stem cells. *Neuron* **36,** 1021–1034.
99. Potten, C. S. (1998) Stem cells in gastrointestinal epithelium: numbers, characteristics and death. *Philos. Trans. R. Soc. Lond. B Biol. Sci.* **353,** 821–830.
100. Whetton, A. D. and Graham, G. J. (1999) Homing and mobilization in the stem cell niche. *Trends Cell Biol.* **9,** 233–238.
101. Jacobson, M. (1991) *Developmental Neurobiology.* Plenum Press, New York.
102. Takahashi, T., Nowakowski, R. S., and Caviness, V. S., Jr. (1995) The cell cycle of the pseudostratified ventricular epithelium of the embryonic murine cerebral wall. *J. Neurosci.* **15,** 6046–6057.

103. Morshead, C. M., Craig, C. G., and van der Kooy, D. (1998) In vivo clonal analyses reveal the properties of endogenous neural stem cell proliferation in the adult mammalian forebrain. *Development* **125,** 2251–2261.
104. Garcia-Verdugo, J. M., Doetsch, F., Wichterle, H., Lim, D. A., and Alvarez-Buylla, A. (1998) Architecture and cell types of the adult subventricular zone: in search of the stem cells. *J. Neurobiol.* **36,** 234–248.
105. Weiss, S. and van der, K. D. (1998) CNS stem cells: where's the biology (a.k.a. beef)? *J. Neurobiol.* **36,** 307–314.
106. Knoblich, J. A., Jan, L. Y., and Jan, Y. N. (1995) Asymmetric segregation of Numb and Prospero during cell division. *Nature* **377,** 624–627.
107. Hirata, J., Nakagoshi, H., Nabeshima, Y., and Matsuzaki, F. (1995) Asymmetric segregation of the homeodomain protein Prospero during *Drosophila* development. *Nature* **377,** 627–630.
108. Doe, C. Q., Chu-LaGraff, Q., Wright, D. M., and Scott, M. P. (1991) The *prospero* gene specifies cell fates in the *Drosophila* central nervous system. *Cell* **65,** 451–464.
109. Li, L. and Vaessin, H. (2000) Pan-neural Prospero terminates cell proliferation during *Drosophila* neurogenesis. *Genes Dev.* **14,** 147–151.
110. Buescher, M., Yeo, S. L., Udolph, G., et al. (1998) Binary sibling neuronal cell fate decisions in the *Drosophila* embryonic central nervous system are nonstochastic and require inscuteable-mediated asymmetry of ganglion mother cells. *Genes Dev.* **12,** 1858–1870.
111. Wai, P., Truong, B., and Bhat, K. M. (1999) Cell division genes promote asymmetric interaction between Numb and Notch in the *Drosophila* CNS. *Development* **126,** 2759–2770.
112. Abdelilah-Seyfried, S., Chan, Y. M., Zeng, C., et al. (2000) A gain-of-function screen for genes that affect the development of the *Drosophila* adult external sensory organ. *Genetics* **155,** 733–752.
113. Berdnik, D., Torok, T., Gonzalez-Gaitan, M., and Knoblich, J. A. (2002) The endocytic protein alpha-Adaptin is required for numb-mediated asymmetric cell division in *Drosophila*. *Dev. Cell* **3,** 221–231.
114. Schober, M., Schaefer, M., and Knoblich, J. A. (1999) Bazooka recruits Inscuteable to orient asymmetric cell divisions in *Drosophila* neuroblasts. *Nature* **402,** 548–551.
115. Wodarz, A., Ramrath, A., Kuchinke, U., and Knust, E. (1999) Bazooka provides an apical cue for Inscuteable localization in *Drosophila* neuroblasts. *Nature* **402,** 544–547.
116. Chia, W., Kraut, R., Li, P., Yang, X., and Zavortink, M. (1997) On the roles of inscuteable in asymmetric cell divisions in Drosophila. *Cold Spring Harb. Symp. Quant. Biol.* **62,** 79–87.
117. Wodarz, A., Ramrath, A., Grimm, A., and Knust, E. (2000) *Drosophila* atypical protein kinase C associates with Bazooka and controls polarity of epithelia and neuroblasts. *J. Cell Biol.* **150,** 1361–1374.
118. Schaefer, M. and Knoblich, J. A. (2001) Protein localization during asymmetric cell division. *Exp. Cell Res.* **271,** 66–74.
119. Yu, F., Morin, X., Cai, Y., Yang, X., and Chia, W. (2000) Analysis of partner of inscuteable, a novel player of *Drosophila* asymmetric divisions, reveals two distinct steps in inscuteable apical localization. *Cell* **100,** 399–409.
120. Kraut, R., Chia, W., Jan, L. Y., Jan, Y. N., and Knoblich, J. A. (1996) Role of inscuteable in orienting asymmetric cell divisions in *Drosophila*. *Nature* **383,** 50–55.
121. Broadus, J., Fuerstenberg, S., and Doe, C. Q. (1998) Staufen-dependent localization of prospero mRNA contributes to neuroblast daughter-cell fate. *Nature* **391,** 792–795.
122. Schuldt, A. J., Adams, J. H., Davidson, C. M., et al. (1998) Miranda mediates asymmetric protein and RNA localization in the developing nervous system. *Genes Dev.* **12,** 1847–1857.
123. Shen, C. P., Knoblich, J. A., Chan, Y. M., Jiang, M. M., Jan, L. Y., and Jan, Y. N. (1998) Miranda as a multidomain adapter linking apically localized Inscuteable and basally localized Staufen and Prospero during asymmetric cell division in *Drosophila*. *Genes Dev.* **12,** 1837–1846.

124. Ikeshima-Kataoka, H., Skeath, J. B., Nabeshima, Y., Doe, C. Q., and Matsuzaki, F. (1997) Miranda directs Prospero to a daughter cell during *Drosophila* asymmetric divisions. *Nature* **390,** 625–629.

125. Lu, B., Rothenberg, M., Jan, L. Y., and Jan, Y. N. (1998) Partner of Numb colocalizes with Numb during mitosis and directs Numb asymmetric localization in *Drosophila* neural and muscle progenitors. *Cell* **95,** 225–235.

126. Wodarz, A. and Huttner, W. B. (2003) Asymmetric cell division during neurogenesis in *Drosophila* and vertebrates. *Mech. Dev.* **120,** 1297–1309.

127. Weigmann, A., Corbeil, D., Hellwig, A., and Huttner, W. B. (1997) Prominin, a novel microvilli-specific polytopic membrane protein of the apical surface of epithelial cells, is targeted to plasmalemmal protrusions of non-epithelial cells. *Proc. Natl. Acad. Sci. USA* **94,** 12425–12430.

128. Chenn, A., Zhang, Y. A., Chang, B. T., and McConnell, S. K. (1998) Intrinsic polarity of mammalian neuroepithelial cells. *Mol. Cell Neurosci.* **11,** 183–193.

129. Aaku-Saraste, E., Hellwig, A., and Huttner, W. B. (1996) Loss of occludin and functional tight junctions, but not ZO-1, during neural tube closure—remodeling of the neuroepithelium prior to neurogenesis. *Dev. Biol.* **180,** 664–679.

130. Zhadanov, A. B., Provance, D. W., Jr., Speer, C. A., et al. (1999) Absence of the tight junctional protein AF-6 disrupts epithelial cell-cell junctions and cell polarity during mouse development. *Curr. Biol.* **9,** 880–888.

131. Manabe, N., Hirai, S., Imai, F., Nakanishi, H., Takai, Y., and Ohno, S. (2002) Association of ASIP/mPAR-3 with adherens junctions of mouse neuroepithelial cells. *Dev. Dyn.* **225,** 61–69.

132. Stuckmann, I., Weigmann, A., Shevchenko, A., Mann, M., and Huttner, W. B. (2001) Ephrin B1 is expressed on neuroepithelial cells in correlation with neocortical neurogenesis. *J. Neurosci.* **21,** 2726–2737.

133. Takekuni, K., Ikeda, W., Fujito, T., et al. (2003) Direct binding of cell polarity protein PAR-3 to cell–cell adhesion molecule nectin at neuroepithelial cells of developing mouse. *J. Biol. Chem.* **278,** 5497–5500.

134. Zhong, W., Feder, J. N., Jiang, M. M., Jan, L. Y., and Jan, Y. N. (1996) Asymmetric localization of a mammalian numb homolog during mouse cortical neurogenesis. *Neuron* **17,** 43–53.

135. Wakamatsu, Y., Maynard, T. M., Jones, S. U., and Weston, J. A. (1999) NUMB localizes in the basal cortex of mitotic avian neuroepithelial cells and modulates neuronal differentiation by binding to NOTCH-1. *Neuron* **23,** 71–81.

136. Chenn, A. and McConnell, S. K. (1995) Cleavage orientation and the asymmetric inheritance of Notch1 immunoreactivity in mammalian neurogenesis. *Cell* **82,** 631–641.

137. Haydar, T. F., Ang, E., Jr., and Rakic, P. (2003) Mitotic spindle rotation and mode of cell division in the developing telencephalon. *Proc. Natl. Acad. Sci. USA* **100,** 2890–2895.

138. Kornack, D. R. and Rakic, P. (1995) Radial and horizontal deployment of clonally related cells in the primate neocortex: relationship to distinct mitotic lineages. *Neuron* **15,** 311–321.

139. Reid, C. B., Tavazoie, S. F., and Walsh, C. A. (1997) Clonal dispersion and evidence for asymmetric cell division in ferret cortex. *Development* **124,** 2441–2450.

140. Bhat, K. M. (1998) Cell–cell signaling during neurogenesis: some answers and many questions. *Int. J. Dev. Biol.* **42,** 127–139.

141. Ware, M. L., Tavazoie, S. F., Reid, C. B., and Walsh, C. A. (1999) Coexistence of widespread clones and large radial clones in early embryonic ferret cortex. *Cereb. Cortex* **9,** 636–645.

142. Noctor, S. C., Flint, A. C., Weissman, T. A., Dammerman, R. S., and Kriegstein, A. R. (2001) Neurons derived from radial glial cells establish radial units in neocortex. *Nature* **409,** 714–720.

143. Noctor, S. C., Martinez-Cerdeno, V., Ivic, L., and Kriegstein, A. R. (2004) Cortical neurons arise in symmetric and asymmetric division zones and migrate through specific phases. *Nat. Neurosci.* **7,** 136–144.

144. Miyata, T., Kawaguchi, A., Okano, H., and Ogawa, M. (2001) Asymmetric inheritance of radial glial fibers by cortical neurons. *Neuron* **31,** 727–741.

145. Qian, X., Goderie, S. K., Shen, Q., Stern, J. H., and Temple, S. (1998) Intrinsic programs of patterned cell lineages in isolated vertebrate CNS ventricular zone cells. *Development* **125,** 3143–3152.

146. Shen, Q., Zhong, W., Jan, Y. N., and Temple, S. (2002) Asymmetric Numb distribution is critical for asymmetric cell division of mouse cerebral cortical stem cells and neuroblasts. *Development* **129,** 4843–4853.

147. Li, H. S., Wang, D., Shen, Q., et al. (2003) Inactivation of Numb and Numblike in embryonic dorsal forebrain impairs neurogenesis and disrupts cortical morphogenesis. *Neuron* **40,** 1105–1118.

148. Cayouette, M., Whitmore, A. V., Jeffery, G., and Raff, M. (2001) Asymmetric segregation of Numb in retinal development and the influence of the pigmented epithelium. *J. Neurosci.* **21,** 5643–5651.

149. Seecof, R. L., Donady, J. J., and Teplitz, R. L. (1973) Differentiation of Drosophila neuroblasts to form ganglion-like clusters of neurons in vitro. *Cell Differ.* **2,** 143–149.

150. Huff, R., Furst, A., and Mahowald, A. P. (1989) *Drosophila* embryonic neuroblasts in culture: autonomous differentiation of specific neurotransmitters. *Dev. Biol.* **134,** 146–157.

151. Lu, B., Roegiers, F., Jan, L. Y., and Jan, Y. N. (2001) Adherens junctions inhibit asymmetric division in the *Drosophila* epithelium. *Nature* **409,** 522–525.

152. Fuchs, E. and Segre, J. A. (2000) Stem cells: a new lease on life. *Cell* **100,** 143–155.

153. Doetsch, F. (2003) A niche for adult neural stem cells. *Curr. Opin. Genet. Dev.* **13,** 543–550.

154. Steindler, D. A., Kadrie, T., Fillmore, H., and Thomas, L. B. (1996) The subependymal zone: "brain marrow." *Prog. Brain Res.* **108,** 349–363.

155. Murphy, M., Reid, K., Dutton, R., Brooker, G., and Bartlett, P. F. (1997) Neural stem cells. *J. Invest. Dermatol. Symp. Proc.* **2,** 8–13.

156. Lillien, L. (1997) Neural development: instructions for neural diversity. *Curr. Biol.* **7,** R168–R171.

157. Mehler, M. F. and Gokhan, S. (1999) Postnatal cerebral cortical multipotent progenitors: regulatory mechanisms and potential role in the development of novel neural regenerative strategies. *Brain Pathol.* **9,** 515–526.

158. Olsson, M., Bjerregaard, K., Winkler, C., Gates, M., Bjorklund, A., and Campbell, K. (1998) Incorporation of mouse neural progenitors transplanted into the rat embryonic forebrain is developmentally regulated and dependent on regional and adhesive properties. *Eur. J. Neurosci.* **10,** 71–85.

159. Gage, F. H. (2000) Mammalian neural stem cells. *Science* **287,** 1433–1438.

160. Chmielnicki, E., Benraiss, A., Economides, A. N., and Goldman, S. A. (2004) Adenovirally expressed noggin and brain-derived neurotrophic factor cooperate to induce new medium spiny neurons from resident progenitor cells in the adult striatal ventricular zone. *J. Neurosci.* **24,** 2133–2142.

161. Alvarez-Buylla, A. and Lim, D. A. (2004) For the long run; maintaining germinal niches in the adult brain. *Neuron* **41,** 683–686.

162. Capela, A. and Temple, S. (2002) LeX/ssea-1 is expressed by adult mouse CNS stem cells, identifying them as nonependymal. *Neuron* **35,** 865–875.

163. Louissaint, A., Jr., Rao, S., Leventhal, C., and Goldman, S. A. (2002) Coordinated interaction of neurogenesis and angiogenesis in the adult songbird brain. *Neuron* **34,** 945–960.

164. Palmer, T. D., Willhoite, A. R., and Gage, F. H. (2000) Vascular niche for adult hippocampal neurogenesis. *J. Comp. Neurol.* **425,** 479–494.

165. Shen, Q., Goderie, S. K., Jin, L., et al. (2004) Endothelial cells stimulate self-renewal and expand neurogenesis of neural stem cells. *Science* **304,** 1338–1340.
166. Milner, L. A., Kopan, R., Martin, D. I., and Bernstein, I. D. (1994) A human homologue of the *Drosophila* developmental gene, Notch, is expressed in CD34+ hematopoietic precursors. *Blood* **83,** 2057–2062.
167. Varnum-Finney, B., Purton, L. E., Yu, M., et al. (1998) The Notch ligand, Jagged-1, influences the development of primitive hematopoietic precursor cells. *Blood* **91,** 4084–4091.
168. Jones, P., May, G., Healy, L., et al. (1998) Stromal expression of Jagged 1 promotes colony formation by fetal hematopoietic progenitor cells. *Blood* **92,** 1505–1511.
169. Li, L., Milner, L. A., Deng, Y., et al. (1998) The human homolog of rat Jagged1 expressed by marrow stroma inhibits differentiation of 32D cells through interaction with Notch1. *Immunity* **8,** 43–55.
170. Walker, L., Lynch, M., Silverman, S., et al. (1999) The Notch/Jagged pathway inhibits proliferation of human hematopoietic progenitors in vitro. *Stem Cells* **17,** 162–171.
171. Lewis, J. (1998) Notch signalling and the control of cell fate choices in vertebrates. *Semin. Cell Dev. Biol.* **9,** 583–589.
172. Campos-Ortega, J. A. (1995) Genetic mechanisms of early neurogenesis in *Drosophila* melanogaster. *Mol. Neurobiol.* **10,** 75–89.
173. Skeath, J. B. and Doe, C. Q. (1998) Sanpodo and Notch act in opposition to Numb to distinguish sibling neuron fates in the *Drosophila* CNS. *Development* **125,** 1857–1865.
174. Gaiano, N., Nye, J. S., and Fishell, G. (2000) Radial glial identity is promoted by Notch1 signaling in the murine forebrain. *Neuron* **26,** 395–404.
175. Berezovska, O., Xia, M. Q., and Hyman, B. T. (1998) Notch is expressed in adult brain, is coexpressed with presenilin-1, and is altered in Alzheimer disease. *J. Neuropathol. Exp. Neurol.* **57,** 738–745.
176. Sestan, N., Artavanis-Tsakonas, S., and Rakic, P. (1999) Contact-dependent inhibition of cortical neurite growth mediated by notch signaling. *Science* **286,** 741–746.
177. Wang, S., Sdrulla, A. D., diSibio, G., et al. (1998) Notch receptor activation inhibits oligodendrocyte differentiation. *Neuron* **21,** 63–75.
178. Cameron, H. A., Hazel, T. G., and McKay, R. D. (1998) Regulation of neurogenesis by growth factors and neurotransmitters. *J. Neurobiol.* **36,** 287–306.
179. Shipley, G. D., Keeble, W. W., Hendrickson, J. E., Coffey, R. J., Jr., and Pittelkow, M. R. (1989) Growth of normal human keratinocytes and fibroblasts in serum-free medium is stimulated by acidic and basic fibroblast growth factor. *J. Cell Physiol.* **138,** 511–518.
180. Reddi, A. H. and Cunningham, N. S. (1990) Bone induction by osteogenin and bone morphogenetic proteins. *Biomaterials* **11,** 33–34.
181. Fuchs, E. and Byrne, C. (1994) The epidermis: rising to the surface. *Curr. Opin. Genet. Dev.* **4,** 725–736.
182. Donovan, P. J. (1994) Growth factor regulation of mouse primordial germ cell development. *Curr. Top. Dev. Biol.* **29,** 189–225.
183. Allouche, M. (1995) Basic fibroblast growth factor and hematopoiesis. *Leukemia* **9,** 937–942.
184. McKay, R. (1997) Stem cells in the central nervous system. *Science* **276,** 66–71.
185. Burgess, A. W. (1998) Growth control mechanisms in normal and transformed intestinal cells. *Philos. Trans. R. Soc. Lond. B Biol. Sci.* **353,** 903–909.
186. Murphy, M. S. (1998) Growth factors and the gastrointestinal tract. *Nutrition* **14,** 771–774.
187. Benfey, P. N. (1999) Stem cells: a tale of two kingdoms. *Curr. Biol.* **9,** R171–R172.
188. Cox, D. N., Chao, A., and Lin, H. (2000) piwi encodes a nucleoplasmic factor whose activity modulates the number and division rate of germline stem cells. *Development* **127,** 503–514.

189. Nakamura, M., Okano, H., Blendy, J. A., and Montell, C. (1994) Musashi, a neural RNA-binding protein required for *Drosophila* adult external sensory organ development. *Neuron* **13,** 67–81.

190. Good, P., Yoda, A., Sakakibara, S., et al. (1998) The human Musashi homolog 1 (MSI1) gene encoding the homologue of Musashi/Nrp-1, a neural RNA-binding protein putatively expressed in CNS stem cells and neural progenitor cells. *Genomics* **52,** 382–384.

191. Kaneko, Y., Sakakibara, S., Imai, T., et al. (2000) Musashi1: an evolutionarily conserved marker for CNS progenitor cells including neural stem cells. *Dev. Neurosci.* **22,** 139–153.

192. Lendahl, U., Zimmerman, L. B., and McKay, R. D. (1990) CNS stem cells express a new class of intermediate filament protein. *Cell* **60,** 585–595.

193. Malatesta, P., Hartfuss, E., and Gotz, M. (2000) Isolation of radial glial cells by fluorescent-activated cell sorting reveals a neuronal lineage. *Development* **127,** 5253–5263.

194. Shi, Y., Chichung Lie, D., Taupin, P., et al. (2004) Expression and function of orphan nuclear receptor TLX in adult neural stem cells. *Nature* **427,** 78–83.

195. Cheshier, S. H., Morrison, S. J., Liao, X., and Weissman, I. L. (1999) In vivo proliferation and cell cycle kinetics of long-term self-renewing hematopoietic stem cells. *Proc. Natl. Acad. Sci. USA* **96,** 3120–3125.

196. Rietze, R. L., Valcanis, H., Brooker, G. F., Thomas, T., Voss, A. K., and Bartlett, P. F. (2001) Purification of a pluripotent neural stem cell from the adult mouse brain. *Nature* **412,** 736–739.

197. Dvorak, P., Hampl, A., Jirmanova, L., Pacholikova, J., and Kusakabe, M. (1998) Embryoglycan ectodomains regulate biological activity of FGF-2 to embryonic stem cells. *J. Cell Sci.* **111(Pt 19),** 2945–2952.

198. Jiang, Y., Jahagirdar, B. N., Reinhardt, R. L., et al. (2002) Pluripotency of mesenchymal stem cells derived from adult marrow. *Nature* **418,** 41–49.

199. Ramalho-Santos, M., Yoon, S., Matsuzaki, Y., Mulligan, R. C., and Melton, D. A. (2002) "Stemness": transcriptional profiling of embryonic and adult stem cells. *Science* **298,** 597–600.

200. Ivanova, N. B., Dimos, J. T., Schaniel, C., Hackney, J. A., Moore, K. A., and Lemischka, I. R. (2002) A stem cell molecular signature. *Science* **298,** 601–604.

201. Burns, C. E. and Zon, L. I. (2002) Portrait of a stem cell. *Dev. Cell* **3,** 612–613.

202. Petkov, P. M., Zavadil, J., Goetz, D., et al. (2004) Gene expression pattern in hepatic stem/progenitor cells during rat fetal development using complementary DNA microarrays. *Hepatology* **39,** 617–627.

203. Ahn, J. I., Lee, K. H., Shin, D. M., et al. (2004) Comprehensive transcriptome analysis of differentiation of embryonic stem cells into midbrain and hindbrain neurons. *Dev. Biol.* **265,** 491–501.

204. Wieczorek, G., Steinhoff, C., Schulz, R., et al. (2003) Gene expression profile of mouse bone marrow stromal cells determined by cDNA microarray analysis. *Cell Tissue Res.* **311,** 227–237.

205. Bhattacharya, B., Miura, T., Brandenberg, R., et al. (2004) Gene expression in human embryonic stem cell lines: unique molecular signature. *Blood* **103,** 2956–2964.

206. Fortunel, N. O., Otu, H. H., Ng, H. H., et al. (2003) Comment on "'Stemness': transcriptional profiling of embryonic and adult stem cells" and "a stem cell molecular signature." *Science* **302,** 393; author reply 393.

207. Luo, Y., Cai, J., Liu, Y., Xue, H., Chrest, F. J., Wersto, R. P., and Rao, M. (2002) Microarray analysis of selected genes in neural stem and progenitor cells. *J. Neurochem.* **83,** 1481–1497.

208. Suslov, O. N., Kukekov, V. G., Ignatova, T. N., and Steindler, D. A. (2002) Neural stem cell heterogeneity demonstrated by molecular phenotyping of clonal neurospheres. *Proc. Natl. Acad. Sci. USA* **99,** 14506–14511.

209. Luo, Y., Cai, J., Ginis, I., et al. (2003) Designing, testing, and validating a focused stem cell microarray for characterization of neural stem cells and progenitor cells. *Stem Cells* **21,** 575–587.
210. Karsten, S. L., Kudo, L. C., Jackson, R., Sabatti, C., Kornblum, H. I., and Geschwind, D. H. (2003) Global analysis of gene expression in neural progenitors reveals specific cell-cycle, signaling, and metabolic networks. *Dev. Biol.* **261,** 165–182.
211. Oliver, T. G., Grasfeder, L. L., Carroll, A. L., et al. (2003) Transcriptional profiling of the Sonic hedgehog response: a critical role for N-myc in proliferation of neuronal precursors. *Proc. Natl. Acad. Sci. USA* **100,** 7331–7336.
212. Livesey, F. J., Young, T. L., and Cepko, C. L. (2004) An analysis of the gene expression program of mammalian neural progenitor cells. *Proc. Natl. Acad. Sci. USA* **101,** 1374–1379.
213. Shah, N. M. and Anderson, D. J. (1997) Integration of multiple instructive cues by neural crest stem cells reveals cell-intrinsic biases in relative growth factor responsiveness. *Proc. Natl. Acad. Sci. USA* **94,** 11369–11374.
214. Park, J. K., Williams, B. P., Alberta, J. A., and Stiles, C. D. (1999) Bipotent cortical progenitor cells process conflicting cues for neurons and glia in a hierarchical manner. *J. Neurosci.* **19,** 10383–10389.

2

Neural Stem Cells in the Adult Brain

Implications of Their Glial Characteristics

Daniel A. Lim and Arturo Alvarez-Buylla

INTRODUCTION

It is now widely accepted that new neurons are added continuously to some regions of the adult mammalian brain. More than 30 yr of reports describing neurogenesis in the adult brains of fish, frogs, reptiles, birds, and rodents *(1–6)* have recently culminated in studies demonstrating the birth of new central nervous system neurons in both primates *(7)* and humans *(8,9)*. Hence, the century-old, dogmatic proposition of a fixed, ended, immutable adult brain has been refuted, spurring new investigations into the regenerative capacity of the central nervous system.

The dentate gyrus of the hippocampus *(10)* and the lateral ventricle subventricular zone (SVZ) *(11)* are two brain regions in which neurons are born in the adult. The SVZ is the larger of these two germinal zones, and consists of a layer of cells adjacent to the ependyma along the entire length of the lateral ventricular wall. In postnatal *(12)* and adult rodents *(13)*, cells born in the SVZ migrate from the ventricular wall into the olfactory bulb (OB) where they differentiate into interneurons. In the monkey brain, the SVZ also generates neurons for the OB *(14,15)*; interestingly, it has been suggested that adult monkey SVZ cells also generate new neurons for the prefrontal, inferior temporal, and posterior parietal cortex *(16)*. These latter observations are a matter of debate *(17,18)*. The adult human SVZ also contains proliferating cells *(8,19)*, and, recently, astrocyte-like cells close to the walls of the human lateral ventricle have been shown to behave as stem cells in vitro *(9)*.

The proliferation of SVZ cells continues throughout life *(20,21)*. It has been estimated that at least 30,000 new OB neurons are born in the mouse every day to replace those that are dying *(13)*. This profound level of continuous neurogenesis argues for the presence of a self-renewing primary progenitor, or stem cell, within the SVZ. Self-renewing cells from the SVZ have been propagated in vitro in both adherent and nonadherent cultures, and these cells can differentiate into neurons, astrocytes, and oligodendrocytes *(22–24)*. Self-renewal and multilineage differentiation are two generic attributes of stem cells. A population of cells in the SVZ satisfies these two criteria and can thus be described as a neural stem cell. However, the precise definition of stem cells is a matter of debate *(25–27)*. The SVZ stem cell is perhaps most analogous

From: *Neural Development and Stem Cells, Second Edition*
Edited by: M. S. Rao © Humana Press Inc., Totowa, NJ

to stem cells found in the skin, intestine, and blood. Stem cells of the SVZ and these other regions generate new cells for their respective organ systems throughout the life of the animal. The constant production of new cells complements normal cell turnover, maintaining the tissue cell population. It is not clear how similar adult brain stem cells are to those of the embryo. We define the adult mouse SVZ stem cell as the self-renewing cell type responsible for maintaining the constant production of OB neurons in vivo.

Perhaps the most misleading notion about stem cells is that they should be undifferentiated or primitive, lacking expression of markers attributed to more mature cells. This perception has led many researchers to ignore the "mature-looking" cell as potential stem cells. However, it is becoming increasingly clear that stem cells can bear what were thought to be the biochemical and structural hallmarks of differentiated cells. For instance, skin stem cells express intermediate filament keratins found in mature keratinocytes *(28,29)*. Intestinal crypt stem cells, which continuously replace the epithelial lining of the digestive tract, have been described as being more epithelial than primitive *(30)*. Hematopoietic stem cells (HSCs), perhaps the best studied of all stem cells, express what have been considered to be lineage-restricted factors *(31)*.

In this chapter, we incorporate our understanding of the cellular composition of the SVZ with recent experimental results that identify the neural stem cell. Surprisingly, the stem cell candidate possesses attributes of mature glial cells. Given the prevailing view that glial cells represent an end point in neural development, a glial-like stem cell seems extraordinary. We therefore review the data concerning the SVZ stem cell identity. We then discuss the possibility that glial-like cells might be stem cells at other developmental times. Considering the accumulating evidence of glial-like stem cells, we propose a revision to our current understanding of developmental neural cell lineages.

CELLULAR COMPOSITION AND ORGANIZATION OF THE ADULT MOUSE SVZ

In the adult mouse, neuroblasts born along the entire length of the SVZ migrate anteriorly to the OB. The migratory neuroblasts (type A cells) move along each other forming elongated clusters of young neurons called chains *(32,33)*. The SVZ is organized as a network of interconnecting paths for chain migration widely distributed throughout the lateral ventricle wall *(34)*. These paths converge at the anterior SVZ, where the confluence of chains of type A cells continues along the rostral migratory stream (RMS), a restricted path that leads into the core of OB. In the OB, new neurons differentiate into local interneurons that become incorporated into local circuits *(35,36)*. It has been suggested that in neonatal rat brain, SVZ neuroblasts originate exclusively in the anterior SVZ, the so-called SVZa *(37)*. This is not observed in the adult *(34)*. The high concentration of neuroblasts that converge at the anterior SVZ may give the impression that this is the site of origin of these cells. Further work is required to describe potential differences between neonatal and adult SVZ and to determine the nature of cells in the neonatal caudal SVZ.

Chains of migrating type A cells in the adult mouse brain are ensheathed by the processes of slowly dividing SVZ astrocytes (type B cells) *(32,38)*. Scattered along the type A cell chains are clusters of rapidly dividing immature cells (type C cells). Type C cell clusters are often interposed between type B and A cells *(38)*. See Fig. 1 for a schematic cross section of the SVZ.

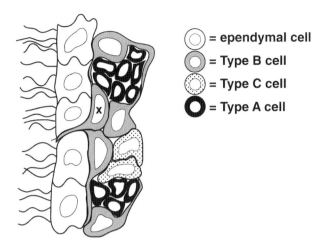

= ependymal cell

= Type B cell

= Type C cell

= Type A cell

Fig. 1. Schematic cross section of the adult SVZ. Ependymal cells (*white*) are multiciliated and are closely apposed to the underlying SVZ cells. The ventricular lumen is to the left. Type B cells (*gray*) are slowly dividing astrocyte-like cells that ensheath chains of migrating type A cells (*black*). In this cross section, type A cells would be migrating out of the plane of the paper. Type C cells (*stippled*) are highly mitotic and found as clusters along the chains of type A cells. See "Cellular Composition and Organization of the Adult Mouse SVZ" for details. Some type B cells (marked with "x") extend a cellular process between ependymal cells and contact the ventricle. Many of these ventricle-contacting type B cells have a short, single cilium lacking the central pair of microtubules (9+0 arrangement). Ventricle-contacting type B cells may be an actively dividing SVZ stem cell. See "The Ventricle-Contacting Type B Cell: Interkinetic Nuclear Movement?" for details.

SVZ cell types were identified based on morphological, immunocytochemical, and ultrastructural characteristics *(38)*. Type A cells are immunopositive for a neuron-specific β-tubulin revealed by monoclonal antibody Tuj1 and express a polysialylated form of neural cell adhesion molecule (PSA-NCAM). Type B cells contain intermediate filament bundles containing glial fibrillary acidic protein (GFAP), a marker assigned to mature astrocytes. Type C cells are ultrastructurally immature and do not stain for markers of mature brain cells. Both type A and C cells express the transcription factor Dlx2 *(39)*, which in development is involved in the production of cortical interneurons which migrate from the medial ganglionic eminences *(40,41)*. Adjacent to the SVZ is the layer of multiciliated ependymal cells. Interestingly, all SVZ cell types and the ependyma express nestin *(38)*, an intermediate filament protein found in neuroepithelial stem cells *(42)*.

Ependymal cells line the luminal surface of the brain ventricle and appear highly differentiated, bearing multiple beating cilia that move cerebrospinal fluid through the ventricular system. Ependymal cells express high levels of the cell surface marker CD24 (type A cells express lower levels of this antigen) *(43–45)*. The lateral ventricle ependyma is generally described as a layer of multiciliated epithelial cells that separate the SVZ from the ventricular lumen. However, on closer examination using electron microscopy (EM), the ependymal layer does not appear entirely contiguous. In normal mice, a small number of type B cells make direct contact with the ventricle *(39,46)*. Some of these type B cells contact the ventricle by extending a thin cellular process between ependymal cells while a few have a larger luminal surface (see "x"-marked cell in Fig. 1). Thus, the boundary between the ependymal layer and the SVZ is somewhat blurred by the small number of type B cells that are interdigitated with the ependymal cells. In addition to their unusual cellular location, some of the ventricle-contacting type B cells possess a single, thin cilium lacking the central pair of microtubules. Similar single cilia with this 9+0 microtubule arrangement have been described in embryonic neuroepithelial cells *(47,48)* and adult avian brain neuronal precursors *(49)*. As we discuss later, this cilium may be an indicator of stem cell progression through the cell cycle.

WHICH ARE THE SVZ STEM CELLS?

As mentioned in the introduction, stem cells can express markers of differentiated cells. Perhaps, then, it should not be surprising that candidates for the adult SVZ stem cell have been found to possess attributes of mature glia. Here, we review the recent accumulation of data indicating that the SVZ stem cell is an astrocyte-like, GFAP-positive cell.

The Label-Retaining Cell of the SVZ

A traditional view of adult stem cells is that they divide very slowly. For instance, to maintain hematopoiesis, HSCs enter the cell cycle every 1–3 mo *(50,51)*, and the slowest cycling cell in the skin has stem cell behavior *(52)*. Accordingly, data from two studies suggest that SVZ stem cells are the most slowly dividing cell of this region *(46,53)*. Owing to their slow cell cycle, stem cells are labeled infrequently by a single pulse of a nucleotide analog such as [^{3}H]thymidine or bromodeoxyuridine (BrdU). Efficient labeling of stem cells requires continuous or repeated administration of [^{3}H]thymidine or BrdU for a prolonged duration. Once having incorporated the label, the stem cells retain the mitotic marker for an extended period of time and can thus be identified as label-retaining cells (LRCs). Rapidly dividing progenitor cells dilute out the label and/or migrate from the region.

The label-retaining experiment has been performed in the SVZ *(44,54)*. BrdU was administered to animals for 2 wk in the drinking water, and 1 wk after the end of the BrdU administration, brain sections were processed with BrdU immunohistochemistry. Although the BrdU-positive nuclei are very clearly labeled, the resolution of the light microscope is not sufficient to distinguish ependymal cells from the closely apposed SVZ cells. Type B cells sometimes have their nuclei separated from the ventricular lumen by only a thin process of an adjacent ependymal cell, and such a nuclei could be easily mistaken as belonging to the ependymal layer *(38,39,46)*. In addition, some type B cells are interposed between ependymal cells and actually contact the ventricle. Double-immunohistochemistry for BrdU and the ependymal markers CD24 or S100 as well as EM analysis of [^{3}H]thymidine-treated brains did not reveal evidence of ependymal cell division.

Do ependymal cells ever divide in vivo? Previous reports are also conflicting. A survey of the literature reveals reports concluding that the lateral ventricle ependyma do not divide and others that claim to have evidence of ependymal proliferation in the same area *(55)*. It is difficult to come to any conclusion from the earlier reports as EM was not used to confirm ependymal cell identity in the lateral ventricle wall. There are also reports of ependymal cell proliferation in the fourth ventricle and central canal of the spinal cord *(56,57)*. However, more detailed EM analysis is required to confirm that the proliferating cells in these caudal regions correspond to multiciliated ependymal cells. Johannson et al. show by EM a ventricle-contacting cell in mitosis in the central canal; however, this cell appears unciliated. Perhaps the ependymal cells along the neuraxis are not all equivalent. In children, ependymal tumors occur most frequently in the fourth ventricle, and this may reflect such intrinsic differences *(58)*.

Epithelial layers with a stem cell component often display a remarkable regenerative capacity in pathological conditions. If the lateral ventricle ependyma contains a stem cell, then one might expect this epithelium to regenerate after injury. However, there is at present no convincing evidence that the lateral ventricle ependyma regenerates after injury. Interestingly, injury to the ependymal cells stimulates the subependymal astrocytes to proliferate and form a gliotic scar, which appears to substitute for the missing ependyma *(55,59)*. Again, ependyma of more caudal regions may behave differently and have some capacity to proliferate, and comparisons of the molecular characteristics of the ependyma throughout the neuraxis would be revealing.

Hence, the majority of SVZ LRCs are type B cells. LRCs, of course, are not necessarily stem cells. Labeled type B cells might simply represent endogenous local glial cell turnover. Furthermore, the SVZ stem cells may enter the cell cycle so rarely that a 2-wk period of labeling would not identify them.

Regeneration of SVZ From Slowly Dividing Type B Cells

Because they are believed to divide more slowly than other cell types, adult stem cells should be more resistant to antimitotic agents. Thus, treatment with certain types of antimitotic drugs should be able to eliminate rapidly dividing progenitor cells while sparing a population of stem cells capable of regenerating the killed cells. Infusion of the antimitotic cytosine-β-D-arabinofuranoside (Ara-C) into the SVZ for 6 d eliminates all type A and C cells *(46)*. The only cell types remaining are type B and ependyma. At the end of Ara-C treatment, no BrdU or [^{3}H]thymidine incorporation is observed in the SVZ. However, 12 h after Ara-C removal, type B cells begin incorporating BrdU. No ependymal cells incorporate the mitotic marker. Two days later, the first type C cells appear, and by 14 d, the entire cellular and architectural composition of the SVZ is regenerated. The appearance of type C cells followed by type A cells suggests a developmental lineage of B to C to A. See Fig. 2 for a lineage schematic.

Type B cells incorporate BrdU almost immediately after Ara-C removal. This rapid appearance of mitotic cells suggests that stem cells are recruited into cell division by the absence of progenitor cells (negative feedback loop). If this notion of stem cell induction were true, then one would predict the stem cells themselves to be slowly killed off with continued Ara-C administration. This appears to be the case. Increasing the duration of Ara-C treatment decreases the number of type B cells remaining in the SVZ (Doetsch and Alvarez-Buylla, *unpublished observations*). With continued Ara-C treatment or local irradiation *(60)*, it may be possible to deplete completely the SVZ of stem cells.

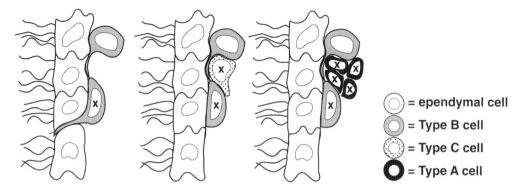

Fig. 2. Proposed SVZ cell lineage. In this model, a type B cell (*left*, marked with "x") divides asymmetrically to produce another type B cell and a type C cell (middle, marked with "x"). Type C cells are transit-amplifying cells that divide before generating type A cells (*right*, *black* cells marked with "x"). The remaining type B cell can later reenter the cell cycle to produce more neurons. Type B cells may also divide symmetrically.

Lineage Analysis of SVZ Stem Cells

To follow specifically the fate of type B cells, Doetsch et al. *(44)* injected an avian leukosis retroviral vector (RCAS) encoding alkaline phosphatase (AP) into the SVZ of transgenic mice. The transgene in the recipient mice directs expression of the avian retrovirus receptor to GFAP-positive cells *(61)*. Hence, the RCAS vector labels only mitotic type B cells. One day after injection, only type B cells express the RCAS marker AP gene, confirming the specificity of the initial infection. Three and one half days later, AP-positive cells are found en route to the OB, and by 14 d, many AP-positive neurons integrate into the OB. Although this experiment clearly demonstrates that type B cells can produce OB neurons, it does not exclude ependymal cells from this lineage. One could argue that ependymal cells produce OB neurons directly or through a type B cell intermediate. Nor do the data demonstrate that type B cells self-renew in vivo. However, the presence of AP-positive type B cells in the SVZ 14 d after infection suggests that stem cells were originally infected.

Tracing the Fate of Ependymal Cells In Vivo?

To determine if ependymal cells can give rise to OB neurons, Johannsen et al. performed experiments that were designed to follow the fate of ependymal cells in vivo. To label ependymal cells, they injected either the fluorescent lipophilic label DiI or adenovirus carrying the β-galactosidase marker into the lateral ventricular lumen. One day after injection, labeled cells appeared restricted to the ependymal layer. Ten days after injection, a large number of labeled cells were found either en route to the OB or in the OB. The interpretation of these data is difficult. Intraventricular injections of tracer substances label all cells that contact the ventricle. Because some type B cells contact the ventricle, it is possible that the DiI injection labeled B cells as well as the ciliated ependyma. Transfer of DiI from the ependyma to other cell types is also difficult to rule out. Johannsen et al. employed the adenoviral vector in an attempt to exclude these possibilities. They found that only ependymal cells express the adenovirus receptor CXADR and thus assumed that this would restrict adenoviral infection to the ependyma. This assumption is, however, not correct as adenoviral vectors have been reported to infect multiple brain cell types *(62)* including type B astrocytes and other SVZ cells *(63)*. Furthermore, the fact that type B cells contact the ventricle complicates the adenovirus result in the same way it renders the DiI experiment difficult to interpret. The present data support a more general conclusion that cells closely associated with the ependymal layer can generate OB neurons.

Neural Stem Cells In Vitro

Neural stem cells isolated from the adult brain SVZ can be propagated as nonadherent clusters of cells called neurospheres *(53,64,65)*. Cell proliferation is maintained by high concentrations of epidermal growth factor (EGF). On removal of EGF, these cultured cells are capable of differentiating into neurons, astrocytes, and oligodendrocytes.

Neurospheres can be grown from type B and C cells, making them both candidates for neural stem cells *(39)*. Given this finding, it seems that "stemness"—at least in vitro—may be more related to competence of a group of precursors early within a lineage rather than to a specific cell type. This notion is also supported by the finding that oligodendrocyte progenitors also show a similar potential to form neural stem cells in vitro when exposed to growth factors *(66,67)*. However, the aforementioned lineage tracing experiments as well as the AraC regeneration data indicate that type B cells are the primary precursors of the SVZ in vivo.

Two other groups have found that GFAP-positive astrocytes can behave as neural stem cells. Laywell et al. *(68)* found that postnatal GFAP-expressing cells from the multiple brain regions of the mouse can behave as neural stem cells in vitro. However, after 14 d, these astrocytes from the cortex, cerebellum, and spinal cord no longer display stem cell characteristics. SVZ GFAP-positive type B cells maintain stem cell behavior into adulthood *(44)*, and this finding was supported by data from Imura et al. *(69)*. In that study, the authors employed a mouse expressing the thymidine kinase gene under the control of the GFAP promoter. Gancyclovir selectively kills dividing cells expressing the thymidine kinase gene, and so by delivering gancyclovir to this GFAP-TK transgenic mouse, Imura et al. were able to eliminate GFAP-positive cells at various stages of development including adulthood. Very few neurospheres could be made from adult GFAP-TK animals treated with GCV, which can be explained by the selective loss of GFAP-positive type B cells as well as their type C cell descendants. Interestingly, neurospheres can be isolated from GCV-treated GFAP-TK embryos, indicating that neural stem cells earlier in development do not express GFAP.

It has been suggested that ependymal cells lining the lateral wall of the lateral ventricles can also give rise to neurospheres in cultures. However, recent data do not support this contention. Johanssen et al. grew neurospheres from putative ependymal cells based on their multiciliated morphologies or by injecting DiI into the lateral ventricles and selecting labeled cells. Rietze et al. *(70)* similarly labeled cells lining the lateral ventricle with DiI and used fluorescence-activated cell sorting (FACS) to identify the cell population capable of giving rise to neurospheres; the authors found that the neural stem cell-enriched population did not include ependymal cells but did include DiI-labeled cells. What is the explanation for these differences in experimental results? Some astrocytes make contact with the ventricle lumen, and, as mentioned earlier, DiI ventricular injections may label ependymal cells as well as this subpopulation of astrocytes; these astrocytes may be the cell type that gives rise to neurospheres. Other data from Chiasson et al. *(71)* and Laywell et al. *(68)* demonstrate that ependymal cells isolated from early postnatal or adult mouse brain are able to form neurosphere-like cell clusters; however, these cells are neither self-renewing nor multipotent. More recently, Capela and Temple *(45)* used the Lewis X cell surface marker, a carbohydrate in embryonic pluripotent stem cells as well as the adult SVZ, to separate SVZ cells by FACS for in vitro neurosphere assay analysis. The LeX-positive fraction was enriched for neurosphere-generating cells as compared to the LeX-negative fraction, which includes ependymal cells. Capela and Temple also isolated ependymal cells with the marker CD24 and negligible numbers of these cells produce neurospheres, leading to their conclusion that ependymal cells are not stem cells.

Although it is tempting to relate EGF-responsive cells in vitro to the in vivo stem cell behavior in vivo, a more conservative viewpoint is that the neurosphere assay reveals cell types that can self-renew and become multipotent in response to EGF signaling. The caveats of in vitro stem cell study are perhaps obvious but should be reiterated. Stem cells in vivo reside in niches that provide these primary progenitors with a microenvironment critical for their behavior. Cultured stem cells are removed from their normal cellular context. Furthermore, stem cells in culture are exposed to nonphysiological concentrations of mitogenic factors, which may alter their "normal" developmental potential. For example, hippocampal precursors grown in the presence of fibroblast growth factor-2 (FGF-2) can differentiate into neurons phenotypically distinct from those of the hippocampus *(72)*. In vitro cultures might remove transcriptional silencing and in such a way "deprogram" a cell, making the transcriptional profile more "generic," allowing a wider diversity of final cell fates.

Thus, any demonstration of stem cell behavior in vitro must be interpreted cautiously. In vitro manipulations may be necessary for stem cell behavior to be unveiled in a particular cell. While ciliated ependymal cells may divide in vitro in response to EGF, the evidence for ependymal cell division in vivo is not conclusive. Likewise, it is not clear that EGF is the primary mitogen for type B cells in vivo *(73)*, and so the multipotentiality of neurospheres may be a consequence of high levels of EGF signaling. Discovering the molecular signals present in the SVZ is critical for future in vitro studies.

Clues about the molecular signals critical for stem cell biology may come from the intercellular interactions observed in vivo. For instance, hematopoietic stem cells are best maintained in vitro on cultures of bone marrow stromal cells monolayers *(74)*. Skin stem cells are similarly clonogenic when cultured in contact with fibroblasts, their in vivo cellular neighbors *(75)*. In the SVZ, all cell types are in contact with astrocytes. Reconstituting the interaction between astrocytes and SVZ stem cells in vitro recapitulates the extensive production of young neurons observed in vivo *(76,77)*. Neurogenesis in these cultures is not dependent on exogenously added growth factors or serum. Understanding the molecular nature of the astrocyte–stem cell interaction may allow for the design of culture assays that fully reproduce in vivo stem cell behavior. Furthermore, the coculture in vitro assay may prove to more faithfully recapitulate the biology of SVZ stem cells than high concentrations of EGF or FGF-2.

The SVZ Stem Cell: A Particular Subtype of Astrocyte?

Type B cells produce OB neurons and can form multipotent neurospheres in vitro. Type B cells are also sufficient to regenerate the SVZ after the elimination of rapidly dividing cells. This body of evidence demonstrating stem cell behavior of type B cells should alter our perception of cells with glial characteristics in the brain. The expression of GFAP can no longer be ascribed only to cells committed to a glial lineage. Cells with morphological, ultrastructural, and antigenic features of astrocytes may very well have the ability to serve as stem cells. It remains to be determined if all brain astrocytes retain the ability to become stem cells. In the SVZ, only a small fraction of the GFAP-positive type B cells can form multipotent neurospheres. Given these data, it is likely that at any one time, only a subset of type B cells can serve as stem cells. If only a subset of type B cells are stem cells, markers specific to those cells would be useful for identification and isolation. Alternatively, a wider population of astrocytes in the adult brain may have stem cell potential, but at any one time only a small subpopulation may be competent to express this potential.

NEURAL STEM CELLS: FROM THE EMBRYO TO THE ADULT

The Ventricle-Contacting Type B Cell: Interkinetic Nuclear Movement?

As described and reviewed earlier, some type B cells contact the ventricle. In some of these ventricle-contacting type B cells the centriole projects a single 9+0 cilium similar to those on neuroepithelial cells and neuronal precursors of the avian brain *(49)*. In cultured cells, the appearance of a 9+0 cilium has been correlated with cell cycle progression *(78)*. About 6 h before S-phase, one of the interphase centrioles of fibroblasts become ciliated, differentiating them from quiescent cells. Perhaps, then, the 9+0 cilium on type B cells indicates their progression through the cell cycle. If this is correct, the ventricle-contacting type B cells could be activated SVZ stem cells just hours away from DNA replication.

Could it be that all dividing type B cells transiently contact the ventricle at some point during the cell cycle? Such a mechanism would be reminiscent of the interkinetic nuclear movement observed in the ventricular zone of embryos *(79,80)* and the adult avian brain *(49)*. In the ventricular zone, the nucleus of an actively dividing cell migrates to and from the ventricular lumen at different points in the cell cycle with mitosis occurring at the ventricular wall. Similarly, a dividing type B cell may actually push aside neighboring ependymal cells and contact the ventricle as it progresses through the cell cycle.

Nomenclature: Is There an Adult Ventricular Zone?

It is perhaps appropriate at this point to raise the problem of nomenclature and its inherent conceptual influences. First, the SVZ, sometimes called the subependymal layer (SEL) or zone (SEZ), suggests that this germinal center functions underneath the ependymal covering without contacting ventricular fluid. In fact, it is widely accepted that the so-called ventricular zone (VZ) *(81)* disappears during development and is no longer present in the adult. Notice that these influential statements are purely based on gross anatomical observations and have not been based on testing whether a VZ-like cell is present in the adult. Clearly, the recent finding that some type B cells may transiently come into contact with the cerebrospinal fluid both challenges this view and contradicts the prefix of "sub-" in SVZ, SEL, or SEZ. Second, using the terms SEL or SEZ may not only be inaccurate in terms of the localization of the germinal cells, but would also suggest that the adult cell genesis in this region is fundamentally different than that of the embryo. When is the SVZ is no longer a SVZ and become a SEZ? Based on the anatomical localization of the embryonic SVZ, and recent transplantation experiments *(82)*, it is evident that the SVZ of the lateral ganglionic eminence (LGE) has cells of similar properties to those present in the adult SVZ. Until an updated terminology becomes available, it is perhaps best to keep one term, SVZ, to describe both the developing and adult germinal zone that underlies the VZ and ependyma, respectively.

Do the Lineages of Neurons and Glia Separate Early in Development?

The recent identification of glial-like neural stem cells raises an important long-standing controversy concerning the developmental origin of neurons and glia in general. Do neurons and glia arise from a multipotential cell type, or are there specific types of cells devoted to one lineage or the other?

The controversy of multipotent stem cells vs lineage-restricted precursors can be traced back to the earliest studies of the neural tube *(83)*. The central nervous system arises from a sheet of cells called the neural epithelium. Early in development, the neural epithelium invaginates from the rest of the embryo, forming the neural tube. In 1887, Wilhelm His founded the concept of subclasses of neuroepithelial cells that are consigned to becoming either neurons or glia. His described two neural tube cell types based on their appearance. Germinal cells were the rounded cells near the lumen, and he proposed these to be precursors of neurons. He also described a columnar matrix of cells, known at that time as spongioblasts (today referred as radial glia), and proposed these to be committed to giving rise to glial cells. His was probably misled by artifacts of histology as he improperly described spongioblasts as a syncitium rather than as separate cells. The theories of His were countered by Schaper in 1894 and 1897. Schaper concluded that the germinal cells and spongioblasts are essentially the same cell type at different stages of cell cycle. However, it was not until 1935 that F. C. Sauer produced new evidence in favor of Schaper's theory. Later, more cell cycle studies confirmed that all neuroepithelial cells are the same, and that the differences in their location and appearance simply represent a different stage of the cell cycle. Nevertheless, the concept of a different origin for glial and neuronal cell types in the brain remained heavily ingrained in the neurosciences. The preceding description of a cell with glial characteristics challenges this view. Other recent work also suggests that the developmental predecessor of astrocytes, the radial glia, are also not committed glial progenitors, but the stem cells of the developing nervous system.

Radial Glial Cells as Neural Stem Cells

Radial glial cells arise during VZ development and are unique in that they extend processes from the ventricular lumen to the pial surface. Radial glial processes are commonly thought to serve as guides that neuroblasts migrate upon to reach their final destination *(84)*. After neuronal production ceases, radial glial are believed to retract from the ventricular and pial surfaces and differentiate into brain astrocytes *(85–88)*.

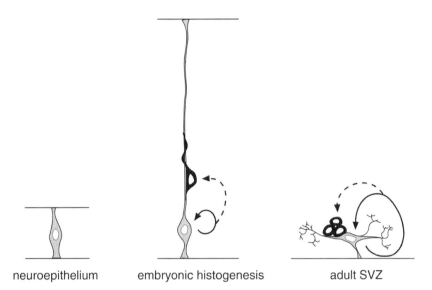

Fig. 3. Hypothetical relationship of neural stem cells from the early embryo to the adult SVZ. (**Left**) Neural stem cells (*gray*) in the early neuroepithelium extend from the ventricular lumen (*bottom*) to the pial (*top*) surfaces. (**Middle**) Like neuroepithelial stem cells, many radial glial cells (*gray*) also contact both the ventricular and pial surfaces. Radial glia behave as neural stem cells, perhaps an elongated form of the stem cell of the early neuroepithelium. Radial glia are known to divide and may self-renew (*solid arrow*) and produce neurons (*black*), possibly through intermediate cell types (*dotted arrow*). (**Right**) Radial glial give rise to astrocytes later in development. Cells derived from radial glial may come to reside in the adult SVZ where they are identified as type B cells (*gray*). Like radial glia and neuroepithelial cells, some SVZ type B cells contact the ventricle. These astrocyte-like cells behave as stem cells in that they self-renew (*solid arrow*) and produce neurons (*black*), possibly through intermediate cell types (*dotted arrow*).

It has previously been suggested that radial glia do not divide during the period of neurogenesis *(89)*.

It is interesting to compare the morphology of the neuroepithelial stem cell with that of radial glial cells. In the primitive neural tube, the neuroepithelial stem cells contact both the ventricular and pial surfaces (Fig. 3, left). As development progresses, the wall of the neural tube thickens as layers of cells are added. If multipotent neuroepithelial cells are to maintain their ventricular and pial contacts, then they must elongate to accommodate the thickening of the neural tube wall. Radial glial cells are elongated cells, many extending processes to both the ventricular and pial surfaces (Fig. 3, middle). Is it possible, then, that what we call radial glial cells are really just neuroepithelial stem cells with an elongated morphology?

There has been a gradual accumulation of data leading to a recent spurt of studies supporting the idea that radial glia are neural stem cells. Mammalian radial glial cells express nestin *(42,90)*, an intermediate filament that is found in neuroepithelial cells *(91)* as well as in cultured neural stem cells *(24)*. Radial glial cells are also found to be mitotic in vivo *(92,93)*, suggesting that radial glial cells have neuroepithelial characteristics *(94)*. In the avian brain, radial glia persist into adult life *(95)*. These cells continue to divide in the adult avian brain and their division correlates spatially and temporally with the appearance of new neurons, leading to the proposition that these radial cells are neuronal precursors *(96)*. Furthermore, the primary precursors in the adult avian brain undergo interkinetic nuclear migration *(49)*, a phenomenon typified by neuroepithelial cells. Earlier retroviral lineage analysis and in vitro studies demonstrate that at least some VZ cells are capable of producing both neurons and glia *(97–101)*. These earlier studies have been further bolstered by more recent studies *(102–106)*. Noctor et al. *(103)* showed in vivo with a green fluorescent protein (GFP)-retrovirus that the progeny of radial glia include neurons. Malatesta et al. *(106)* used a Cre-based fate map analysis to demonstrate that the majority of cortical projection neurons are derived from radial glia. Taken together, the data challenge the historical notions that neuroglia develop from a lineage separate from that of neurons and that radial glia are committed progenitors to astrocytes.

What Is the Origin and Nature of SVZ Type B Cells?

There is good evidence that radial glia become astrocytes late in development. Transitional forms between radial glia and astrocytes have been observed in vivo *(85–88)* and in vitro *(107)*. Furthermore, radial glial vitally labeled by injections of tracers onto the surface of the brain can differentiate into astrocytes in vitro *(108)*. It is interesting to consider that SVZ type B cells might be derived from radial glial cells and retain some neuroepithelial stem cell characteristics into adulthood (Fig. 3, right). There are, in fact, data supporting this consideration: Gaiano et al. *(109)* found that activated Notch signaling in embryonic neural progenitors instructed a radial glial fate, and later, these cells became astrocytes, many of which ended up in the SVZ. The microenvironment of the SVZ might provide signals that program type B cells for continuous OB neuron production. Astrocytes throughout the brain are also thought to be derived from radial glia, raising the intriguing possibility that some of these cells may also behave as neural stem cells under appropriate conditions. Compelling evidence in support of this idea comes from the demonstrations that in vitro stem cells can be propagated from regions other than the SVZ. Neurosphere-generating cells are found all along the entire ventricular neuraxis *(110)*. In addition, multipotent stem cells can also be isolated in vitro from the cortex, septum, hippocampus, and SVZ *(111,112)*. It will be interesting to determine if precursors similar to type B cells exist in these diverse brain regions. In the dentate gyrus of the hippocampus, astrocytes with characteristics similar to the SVZ type B cells have been found to function as primary progenitors in the generation of new neurons *(113–115)*. The origin of adult neural stem cells with glial characteristics in the SVZ and dentate gyrus is not known. The preceding arguments suggest that these adult stem cells may be derived from radial glia, but this hypothesis remains to be demonstrated.

Are Glial Tumors Neural Stem Cell Tumors?

Most brain tumors are glial. Based on the series of findings discussed earlier suggesting that adult neural stem cells have glial characteristics, we should consider the possibility that tumors may arise from stem cells. In fact, EGF receptor overexpression in nestin-positive postnatal brain cells lacking the INK4a-ARF locus leads to a high incidence of gliomas *(116)*, suggesting that a genetic alterations in a stem-like cell can generate a tumor that would be histologically classified as a glioma. Interestingly, the SVZ in some mammals is the most common site of gliomas induced by chemical carcinogens *(117)*. Although it is not a frequent site of tumors in humans, the SVZ is perhaps a site where stem cells acquire the initial genetic alterations in tumor cell progression. Certain mutations may enhance the migration of stem cells, leading to the subsequent formation of tumors at a distance from the SVZ. In fact, the overexpression of FGF2 in glial cells stimulates their migration *(61)*. Also, infusion of FGF2 or EGF into the lateral ventricle causes SVZ cells to migrate deeper into the striatum *(39,118,119)*.

THE PROBLEM WITH CALLING A CELL A GLIAL CELL

Some of the unavoidable, historical misconceptions about glial cells appear to have persisted to the present, and it is now important to reexamine the cells that we call glial in a new light. The concept of neuroglia, meaning "nerve glue," was originally based on an assumption by Rudolf Virchow in the mid-1800s that there must be a mesoderm-derived connective tissue-like component to the nervous system *(83)*. Virchow's theory has since been refuted; however, his ideas about the derivation and nature of glial cells seemingly instilled the field with the concept that glial cells should be distantly related to neurons. Perhaps the shadow of Virchow's conjectures extends to the present day, making it difficult to consider the possibility that glial-like cells are neural stem cells. As proposed in an earlier study, perhaps the radial glial cell should be called simply a radial cell to remove the influential connotation of the word "glial" *(96)*. Alternatively, some of the historical weight of the word "glial" needs to be lightened. In the brain, the term "glia" may be taken to encompass both fully differentiated supportive cells and others that are capable of behaving as neural stem cells. Neural stem cells may have roles often assigned to glia. The cellular anatomy of both the adult SVZ and developing VZ suggest that stem cells play important structural roles as the scaffold upon which neurogenesis and neuronal migration occur. Hence, it appears that in some cases, glial cells and stem cells are one in the same.

REFERENCES

1. Altman, J. (1970) Postnatal neurogenesis and the problem of neural plasticity, in *Developmental Neurobiology* (Himwich, W. A., ed.), C. C Thomas, Springfield, IL, pp. 197–237.
2. Lopez-Garcia, C., Molowny, A., Garcia-Verdugo, J. M., Martinez-Guijarro, F. J., and Bernabeu, A. (1990) Late generated neurons in the medial cortex of adult lizards send axons that reach the Timm-reactive zones. *Dev. Brain Res.* **57,** 249–254.
3. Straznicky, A. and Gaze, R. M. (1971) The growth of the retina in *Xenopus laevis*: an autoradiographic analysis. *J. Embryol. Exp. Morphol.* **26,** 67–79.
4. Birse, S. C., Leonard, R. B. and Coggeshall, R. E. (1980) Neuronal increase in various areas of the nervous system of the guppy, *Lebistes. J. Comp. Neurol.* **194,** 291–301.
5. Goldman, S. A. and Nottebohm, F. (1983) Neuronal production, migration, and differentiation in a vocal control nucleus of the adult female canary brain. *Proc. Natl. Acad. Sci. USA* **80,** 2390–2394.
6. Alvarez-Buylla, A. and Lois, C. (1995) Neuronal stem cells in the brain of adult vertebrates. *Stem Cells* **13,** 263–272.
7. Gould, E., Reeves, A. J., Graziano, M. S., and Gross, C. G. (1999) Neurogenesis in the neocortex of adult primates. *Science* **286,** 548–552.
8. Eriksson, P. S., Perfilieva, E., Bjork-Eriksson, T., et al. (1998) Neurogenesis in the adult human hippocampus. *Nat. Med.* **4,** 1313–1317.

9. Sanai, N., Tramontin, A. D., Quinones-Hinojosa, A., et al. (2004) Unique astrocyte ribbon in adult human brain contains neural stem cells but lacks chain migration. *Nature* **427,** 740–744.

10. Gage, F. H. (2002) Neurogenesis in the adult brain. *J. Neurosci.* **22,** 612–613.

11. Alvarez-Buylla, A. and Garcia-Verdugo, J. M. (2002) Neurogenesis in adult subventricular zone. *J. Neurosci.* **22,** 629–634.

12. Luskin, M. B. (1993) Restricted proliferation and migration of postnatally generated neurons derived from the forebrain subventricular zone. *Neuron* **11,** 173–189.

13. Lois, C. and Alvarez-Buylla, A. (1994) Long-distance neuronal migration in the adult mammalian brain. *Science* **264,** 1145–1148.

14. Pencea, V., Bingaman, K. D., Freedman, L. J., and Luskin, M. B. (2001) Neurogenesis in the subventricular zone and rostral migratory stream of the neonatal and adult primate forebrain. *Exp. Neurol.* **172,** 1–16.

15. Kornack, D. R. and Rakic, P. (2001) The generation, migration, and differentiation of olfactory neurons in the adult primate brain. *Proc. Natl. Acad. Sci. USA* **98,** 4752–4757.

16. Gould, E., Reeves, A. J., Graziano, M. S. A., and Gross, C. G. (1999) Neurogenesis in the neocortex of adult primates. *Science* **286,** 548–552.

17. Kornack, D. R. and Rakic, P. (2001) Cell proliferation without neurogenesis in adult primate neocortex. *Science* **294,** 2127–2130.

18. Koketsu, D., Mikami, A., Miyamoto, Y., and Hisatsune, T. (2003) Nonrenewal of neurons in the cerebral neocortex of adult macaque monkeys. *J. Neurosci.* **23,** 937–942.

19. Globus, J. H. and Kuhlenbeck, H. (1944) The subependymal cell plate (matrix) and its relationship to brain tumors of the ependymal type. *J. Neuropathol. Exp. Neurol.* **3,** 1–35.

20. Goldman, S. A., Kirschenbaum, B., Harrison-Restelli, C., and Thaler, H. T. (1997) Neuronal precursors of the adult rat subependymal zone persist into senescence, with no decline in spatial extent or response to BDNF. *J. Neurobiol.* **32,** 554–566.

21. Kuhn, H. G., Dickinson-Anson, H., and Gage, F. H. (1996) Neurogenesis in the dentate gyrus of the adult rat: age-related decrease of neuronal progenitor proliferation. *J. Neurosci.* **16,** 2027–2033.

22. Gage, F. H., Ray, J., and Fisher, L. J. (1995) Isolation, characterization, and use of stem cells from the CNS. *Annu. Rev. Neurosci.* **18,** 159–192.

23. Weiss, S., Reynolds, B. A., Vescovi, A. L., Morshead, C., Craig, C. G., and Van der Kooy, D. (1996) Is there a neural stem cell in the mammalian forebrain? *Trends Neurosci.* **19,** 387–393.

24. McKay, R. (1997) Stem cells in the central nervous system. *Science* **276,** 66–71.

25. Morrison, S. J., Shah, N. M., and Anderson, D. J. (1997) Regulatory mechanisms in stem cell biology. *Cell* **88,** 287–298.

26. Gage, F. H. (1998) Discussion point: stem cells of the central nervous system. *Curr. Opin. Neurobiol.* **8,** 671–675.

27. Alvarez-Buylla, A. and Temple, S. (1998) Stem cells in the developing and adult nervous system. *J. Neurobiol.* **36,** 105–110.

28. Coulombe, P. A., Kopan, R., and Fuchs, E. (1989) Expression of keratin K14 in the epidermis and hair follicle: insights into complex programs of differentiation. *J. Cell Biol.* **109,** 2295–2312.

29. Vasioukhin, V., Degenstein, L., Wise, B., and Fuchs, E. (1999) The magical touch: genome targeting in epidermal stem cells induced by tamoxifen application to mouse skin. *Proc. Natl. Acad. Sci. USA* **96,** 8551–8556.

30. Fuchs, E. and Segre, J. A. (2000) Stem cells: a new lease on life. *Cell* **100,** 143–155.

31. Hu, M., Krause, D., Greaves, M., et al. (1997) Multilineage gene expression precedes commitment in the hemopoietic system. *Genes Dev.* **11,** 774–785.

32. Lois, C., Garcia-Verdugo, J. M., and Alvarez-Buylla, A. (1996) Chain migration of neuronal precursors. *Science* **271,** 978–981.

33. Wichterle, H., Garcia-Verdugo, J. M., and Alvarez-Buylla, A. (1997) Direct evidence for homotypic, glia-independent neuronal migration. *Neuron* **18,** 779–791.
34. Doetsch, F. and Alvarez-Buylla, A. (1996) Network of tangential pathways for neuronal migration in adult mammalian brain. *Proc. Natl. Acad. Sci. USA* **93,** 14895–14900.
35. Petreanu, L. and Alvarez-Buylla, A. (2002) Maturation and death of adult-born olfactory bulb granule neurons: role of olfaction. *J. Neurosci.* **22,** 6106–6113.
36. Carleton, A., Petreanu, L. T., Lansford, R., Alvarez-Buylla, A., and Lledo, P. M. (2003) Becoming a new neuron in the adult olfactory bulb. *Nat. Neurosci.* **6,** 507–518.
37. Luskin, M. B. (1998) Neuroblasts of the postnatal mammalian forebrain: their phenotype and fate. *J. Neurobiol.* **36,** 221–233.
38. Doetsch, F., Garcia-Verdugo, J. M., and Alvarez-Buylla, A. (1997) Cellular composition and three-dimensional organization of the subventricular germinal zone in the adult mammalian brain. *J. Neurosci.* **17,** 5046–5061.
39. Doetsch, F., Petreanu, L., Caille, I., Garcia-Verdugo, J. M., and Alvarez-Buylla, A. (2002) EGF converts transit-amplifying neurogenic precursors in the adult brain into multipotent stem cells. *Neuron* **36,** 1021–1034.
40. Anderson, S. A., Qiu, M., Bulfone, A., et al. (1997) Mutations of the homebox genes *Dlx-1* and *Dlx-2* disrupt the striatal subventricular zone and differentiation of late born striatal neurons. *Neuron* **19,** 27–37.
41. Anderson, S. A., Eisenstat, D. D., Shi, L., and Rubenstein, J. L. R. (1997) Interneuron migration from basal forebrain to neocortex: dependence on *Dlx* genes. *Science* **278,** 474–476.
42. Lendahl, U., Zimmerman, L. B., and McKay, R. D. G. (1990) CNS stem cells express a new class of intermediate filament protein. *Cell* **60,** 585–595.
43. Calaora, V., Chazal, G., Nielsen, P. J., Rougon, G., and Moreau, H. (1996) mCD24 expression in the developing mouse brain and in zones of secondary neurogenesis in the adult. *Neuroscience* **73,** 581–594.
44. Doetsch, F., Caille, I., Lim, D. A., García-Verdugo, J. M., and Alvarez-Buylla, A. (1999) Subventricular zone astrocytes are neural stem cells in the adult mammalian brain. *Cell* **97,** 1–20.
45. Capela, A. and Temple, S. (2002) LeX/ssea-1 is expressed by adult mouse CNS stem cells, identifying them as nonependymal. *Neuron* **35,** 865–875.
46. Doetsch, F., Garcia-Verdugo, J. M., and Alvarez-Buylla, A. (1999) Regeneration of a germinal layer in the adult mammalian brain. *Proc. Natl. Acad. Sci. USA* **96,** 11619–11624.
47. Sotelo, J. R. and Trujillo-Cenóz, O. (1958) Electron microscope study on the development of ciliary components of the neural epithelium of the chick embryo. *Z. Zellforsch.* **49,** 1–12.
48. Stensaas, L. J. and Stensass, S. S. (1968) Light microscopy of glial cells in turtles and birds. *Z. Zellforsch.* **91,** 315–340.
49. Alvarez-Buylla, A., García-Verdugo, J. M., Mateo, A., and Merchant-Larios, H. (1998) Primary neural precursors and intermitotic nuclear migration in the ventricular zone of adult canaries. *J. Neurosci.* **18,** 1020–1037.
50. Bradford, G. B., Williams, B., Rossi, R., and Bertoncello, I. (1997) Quiescence, cycling, and turnover in the primitive hematopoietic stem cell compartment. *Exp. Hematol.* **25,** 445–453.
51. Cheshier, S. H., Morrison, S. J., Liao, X., and Weissman, I. L. (1999) In vivo proliferation and cell cycle kinetics of long-term self-renewing hematopoietic stem cells. *Proc. Natl. Acad. Sci. USA* **96,** 3120–3125.
52. Morris, R. J. and Potten, C. S. (1994) Slowly cycling (label-retaining) epidermal cells behave like clonogenic stem cells in vitro. *Cell Prolif.* **27,** 279–289.
53. Morshead, C. M., Reynolds, B. A., Craig, C. G., et al. (1994) Neural stem cells in the adult mammalian forebrain: a relatively quiescent subpopulation of subependymal cells. *Neuron* **13,** 1071–1082.

54. Johansson, C. B., Momma, S., Clarke, D. L., Risling, M., Lendahl, U., and Frisén, J. (1999) Identification of a neural stem cell in the adult mammalian central nervous system. *Cell* **96**, 25–34.
55. Bruni, J. E., Del Bigio, M. R., and Clattenburg, R. E. (1985) Ependyma: normal and pathological. A review of the literature. *Brain Res. Rev.* **9**, 1–19.
56. Namiki, J. and Tator, C. H. (1999) Cell proliferation and nestin expression in the ependyma of the adult rat spinal cord after injury. *J. Neuropathol. Exp. Neurol.* **58**, 489–498.
57. Liu, K., Wang, Z., Wang, H., and Zhang, Y. (2002) Nestin expression and proliferation of ependymal cells in adult rat spinal cord after injury. *Chin. Med. J. (Engl.)* **115**, 339–341.
58. Bigner, D. D., McLendon, R. E., and Bruner, J. M. (1998) *Russell & Rubinstein's Pathology of Tumors of the Nervous System.* Oxford University Press, New York.
59. Grondona, J. M., Pérez-Martín, M., Cifuentes, M., et al. (1996) Ependymal denudation, aqueductal obliteration and hydrocephalus after a single injection of neuraminidase into the lateral ventricle of adult rats. *J. Neuropathol. Exp. Neurol.* **55**, 999–1008.
60. Bellinzona, M., Gobbel, G. T., Shinohara, C., and Fike, J. R. (1996) Apoptosis is induced in the subependyma of young adult rats by ionizing irradiation. *Neurosci. Lett.* **208**, 163–166.
61. Holland, E. C. and Varmus, H. E. (1998) Basic fibroblast growth factor induces cell migration and proliferation after glia-specific gene transfer in mice. *Proc. Natl. Acad. Sci. USA* **95**, 1218–1223.
62. Davidson, B. L., Allen, E. D., Kozarsky, K. F., Wilson, J. M., and Roessler, B. J. (1993) A model system for in vivo gene transfer into the central nervous system using an adenoviral vector. *Nat. Genet.* **3**, 219–223.
63. Yoon, S. O., Lois, C., Alvirez, M., Alvarez-Buylla, A., Falck-Pederson, E., and Chao, M. V. (1996) Adenovirus-mediated gene delivery into neuronal precursors of the adult mouse brain. *Proc. Natl. Acad. Sci. USA* **93**, 11974–11979.
64. Reynolds, B. and Weiss, S. (1992) Generation of neurons and astrocytes from isolated cells of the adult mammalian central nervous system. *Science* **255**, 1707–1710.
65. Gritti, A., Parati, E. A., Cova, L., et al. (1996) Multipotential stem cells from the adult mouse brain proliferate and self-renew in response to basic fibroblast growth factor. *J. Neurosci.* **16**, 1091–1100.
66. Kondo, T. and Raff, M. (2000) Oligodendrocyte precursor cells reprogrammed to become multipotential CNS stem cells. *Science* **289**, 1754–1757.
67. Nunes, M. C., Roy, N. S., Keyoung, H. M., et al. (2003) Identification and isolation of multipotential neural progenitor cells from the subcortical white matter of the adult human brain. *Nat. Med.* **9**, 439–447.
68. Laywell, E. D., Rakic, P., Kukekov, V. G., Holland, E. C., and Steindler, D. A. (2000) Identification of a multipotent astrocytic stem cell in the immature and adult mouse brain. *Proc. Natl. Acad. Sci. USA* **97**, 13883–13888.
69. Imura, T., Kornblum, H. I., and Sofroniew, M. V. (2003) The predominant neural stem cell isolated from postnatal and adult forebrain but not early embryonic forebrain expresses GFAP. *J. Neurosci.* **23**, 2824–2832.
70. Rietze, R. L., Valcanis, H., Brooker, G. F., Thomas, T., Voss, A. K., and Bartlett, P. F. (2001) Purification of a pluripotent neural stem cell from the adult mouse brain. *Nature* **412**, 736–739.
71. Chiasson, B. J., Tropepe, V., Morshead, C. M., and Van der Kooy, D. (1999) Adult mammalian forebrain ependymal and subependymal cells demonstrate proliferative potential, but only subependymal cells have neural stem cell characteristics. *J. Neurosci.* **19**, 4462–4471.
72. Suhonen, J. O., Peterson, D. A., Ray, J., and Gage, F. H. (1996) Differentiation of adult hippocampus-derived progenitors into olfactory neurons *in vivo. Nature* **383**, 624–627.
73. Tropepe, V., Craig, C. G., Morshead, C. M., and Van der Kooy, D. (1997) Transforming growth factor-α null and senescent mice show decreased neural progenitor cell proliferation in the forebrain subependyma. *J. Neurosci.* **17**, 7850–7859.

74. Deryugina, E. I. and Muller-Sieburg, C. E. (1993) Stromal cells in long-term cultures: keys to the elucidation of hematopoietic development? *Crit. Rev. Immunol.* **13,** 115–150.
75. Rheinwald, J. G. and Green, H. (1975) Serial cultivation of strains of human epidermal keratinocytes: the formation of keratinizing colonies from single cells. *Cell* **6,** 331–337.
76. Lim, D. A. and Alvarez-Buylla, A. (1999) Interaction between astrocytes and adult subventricular zone precursors stimulates neurogenesis. *Proc. Natl. Acad. Sci. USA* **96,** 7526–7531.
77. Song, H., Stevens, C. F., and Gage, F. H. (2002) Astroglia induce neurogenesis from adult neural stem cells. *Nature* **417,** 39–44.
78. Ho, P. T. C. and Tucker, R. W. (1989) Centriole ciliation and cell cycle variability during G1 phase of BALB/c 3T3 cells. *J. Cell. Physiol.* **139,** 398–406.
79. Sauer, F. C. (1935) Mitosis in the neural tube. *J. Comp. Neurol.* **62,** 377–405.
80. Takahashi, T., Nowakowski, R. S., and Caviness, V. S., Jr. (1993) Cell cycle parameters and patterns of nuclear movement in the neocortical proliferative zone of the fetal mouse. *J. Neurosci.* **13,** 820–833.
81. T. B. Committee (1970) Embryonic vertebrate central nervous system: revised terminology. *Anat. Rec.* **166,** 257–262.
82. Wichterle, H., Garcia-Verdugo, J. M., Herrera, D. G., and Alvarez-Buylla, A. (1999) Young neurons from medial ganglionic eminence disperse in adult and embryonic brain. *Nat. Neurosci.* **2,** 461–466.
83. Jacobson, M. (1991) *Developmental Neurobiology.* Plenum Press, New York.
84. Rakic, P. (1972) Mode of cell migration to the superficial layers of fetal monkey neocortex. *J. Comp. Neurol.* **145,** 61–84.
85. Ramón y Cajal, S. (1911) *Histologie du Système Nerveux de l'Homme et des Vertébrés.* Maloine, Paris.
86. Schmechel, D. E. and Rakic, P. (1979) A Golgi study of radial glia cells in developing monkey telencephalon: morphogenesis and transformation into astrocytes. *Anat. Embryol.* **156,** 115–152.
87. Levitt, P. R., Cooper, M. L., and Rakic, P. (1981) Coexistence of neuronal and glial precursor cells in the cerebral ventricular zone of the fetal monkey: an ultrastructural immunoperoxidase analysis. *J. Neurosci.* **1,** 27–39.
88. Pixley, S. K. R. and De Vellis, J. (1984) Transition between immature radial glia and mature astrocytes studied with a monoclonal antibody to vimentin. *Dev. Brain Res.* **15,** 201–209.
89. Schmechel, D. E. and Rakic, P. (1979) Arrested proliferation of radial glial cells during midgestation in rhesus monkey. *Nature* **277,** 303–305.
90. Hockfield, S. and McKay, R. D. G. (1985) Identification of major cell classes in the developing mammalian nervous system. *J. Neurosci.* **5,** 3310–3328.
91. Zimmerman, L., Parr, B., Lendahl, U., et al. (1994) Independent regulatory elements in the nestin gene direct transgene expression to neural stem cells or muscle precursors. *Neuron* **12,** 11–24.
92. Misson, J. P., Edwards, M. A., Yamamoto, M., and Caviness, V. S., Jr. (1988) Mitotic cycling of radial glial cells of the fetal murine cerebral wall: a combined autoradiographic and immunohistochemical study. *Dev. Brain Res.* **38,** 183–190.
93. Frederiksen, K. and McKay, R. D. G. (1988) Proliferation and differentiation of rat neuroepithelial precursor cells in vivo. *J. Neurosci.* **8,** 1144–1151.
94. McKay, R. D. G. (1989) The origins of cellular diversity in the mammalian central nervous system. *Cell* **58,** 815–821.
95. Alvarez-Buylla, A., Theelen, M., and Nottebohm, F. (1988) Mapping of radial glia and of a new cell type in adult canary brain. *J. Neurosci.* **8,** 2707–2712.
96. Alvarez-Buylla, A., Theelen, M., and Nottebohm, F. (1990) Proliferation "hot spots" in adult avian ventricular zone reveal radial cell division. *Neuron* **5,** 101–109.

 97. Temple, S. (1989) Division and differentiation of isolated CNS blast cells in microculture. *Nature* **340,** 471–473.
 98. Gray, G. E. and Sanes, J. R. (1992) Lineage of radial glia in the chicken optic tectum. *Development* **114,** 271–283.
 99. Qian, X., Goderie, S. K., Shen, G., Stern, J. H., and Temple, S. (1998) Intrinsic programs of patterned cell lineages in isolated vertebrate CNS ventricular zone cells. *Development* **125,** 3143–3152.
100. Cepko, C. L., Austin, C. P., Walsh, C., Ryder, E. F., Halliday, A., and Fields-Berry, S. C. (1990) Studies of cortical development using retrovirus vectors. *Cold Spring Harb. Symp. Quant. Biol.* **LV,** 265–278.
101. Halliday, A. L. and Cepko, C. L. (1992) Generation and migration of cells in the developing striatum. *Neuron* **9,** 15–26.
102. Hartfuss, E., Galli, R., Heins, N., and Gotz, M. (2001) Characterization of CNS precursor subtypes and radial glia. *Dev. Biol.* **229,** 15–30.
103. Noctor, S. C., Flint, A. C., Weissman, T. A., Dammerman, R. S., and Kriegstein, A. R. (2001) Neurons derived from radial glial cells establish radial units in neocortex. *Nature* **409,** 714–720.
104. Gotz, M., Hartfuss, E., and Malatesta, P. (2002) Radial glial cells as neuronal precursors: a new perspective on the correlation of morphology and lineage restriction in the developing cerebral cortex of mice. *Brain Res. Bull.* **57,** 777–788.
105. Gregg, C. T., Chojnacki, A. K., and Weiss, S. (2002) Radial glial cells as neuronal precursors: the next generation? *J. Neurosci. Res.* **69,** 708–713.
106. Malatesta, P., Hack, M. A., Hartfuss, E., et al. (2003) Neuronal or glial progeny: regional differences in radial glia fate. *Neuron* **37,** 751–764.
107. Culican, S. M., Baumrind, N. L., Yamamoto, M., and Pearlman, A. L. (1990) Cortical radial glia: identification in tissue culture and evidence for their transformation to astrocytes. *J. Neurosci.* **10,** 684–692.
108. Voigt, T. (1989) Development of glial cells in the cerebral wall of ferrets: direct tracing of their transformation from radial glia into astrocytes. *J. Comp. Neurol.* **289,** 74–88.
109. Gaiano, N., Nye, J. S., and Fishell, G. (2000) Radial glial identity is promoted by Notch1 signaling in the murine forebrain. *Neuron* **26,** 395–404.
110. Weiss, S., Dunne, C., Hewson, J., et al. (1996) Multipotent CNS stem cells are present in the adult mammalian spinal cord and ventricular neuroaxis. *J. Neurosci.* **16,** 7599–7609.
111. Palmer, T. D., Ray, J., and Gage, F. H. (1995) FGF-2 responsive neuronal progenitors reside in proliferative and quiescent regions of the adult rodent brain. *Mol. Cell. Neurosci.* **6,** 474–486.
112. Palmer, T. D., Markakis, E. A., Willhoite, A. R., Safar, F., and Gage, F. H. (1999) Fibroblast growth factor-2 activates a latent neurogenic program in neural stem cells from diverse regions of the adult CNS. *J. Neurosci.* **19,** 8487–8497.
113. Seri, B., Garcia-Verdugo, J. M., McEwen, B. S., and Alvarez-Buylla, A. (2001) Astrocytes give rise to new neurons in the adult mammalian hippocampus. *J. Neurosci.* **21,** 7153–7160.
114. Filippov, V., Kronenberg, G., Pivneva, T., et al. (2003) Subpopulation of nestin-expressing progenitor cells in the adult murine hippocampus shows electrophysiological and morphological characteristics of astrocytes. *Mol. Cell. Neurosci.* **23,** 373–382.
115. Fukuda, S., Kato, F., Tozuka, Y., Yamaguchi, M., Miyamoto, Y., and Hisatsune, T. (2003) Two distinct subpopulations of nestin-positive cells in adult mouse dentate gyrus. *J. Neurosci.* **23,** 9357–9366.
116. Holland, E. C., Hively, W. P., DePinho, R., and Varmus, H. E. (1998) Constitutively active epidermal growth factor receptor cooperates with disruption of G1 cell-cycle arrest pathways to induce glioma-like lesions in mice. *Genes Dev.* **12,** 3675–3685.

117. Kleihues, P., Lantos, L., and Magee, P. N. (1976) Chemical carcinogenesis in the nervous system. *Int. Rev. Exp. Pathol.* **15,** 153–232.
118. Kuhn, H. G., Winkler, J., Kempermann, G., Thal, L. J., and Gage, F. H. (1997) Epidermal growth factor and fibroblast growth factor-2 have different effects on neural progenitors in the adult rat brain. *J. Neurosci.* **17,** 5820–5829.
119. Craig, C. G., Tropepe, V., Morshead, C. M., Reynolds, B. A., Weiss, S., and Van der Kooy, D. (1996) *In vivo* growth factor expansion of endogenous subependymal neural precursor cell populations in the adult mouse brain. *J. Neurosci.* **16,** 2649–2658.

3

Cellular and Molecular Properties of Multipotent Neural Stem Cells Throughout Ontogeny

Larysa Halyna Pevny

INTRODUCTION

Single cells isolated from the both the developing and the adult central nervous system (CNS) can give rise to neurons, astrocytes and oligodendrocytes and retain the ability to self-renew, in vitro. This observation has led to the conclusion that the CNS develops from multipotent, self-renewing stem cells (CNS stem cells) *(1–9)*. However, since the isolation of CNS stem cells from embryonic and adult CNS *(1,3,4,6,10,11)*, identification of their origin in vivo remains unclear *(12,13)*. Moreover, the cellular and molecular relationship between neural stem cell populations at different stages of ontogeny and different anatomical regions is unresolved. To understand exactly what characteristics define neural stem cell identity in vivo and in vitro it is first necessary to elucidate the lineage relationship between the various types of stem cells and how they contribute to the development, differentiation, maintenance, and function of the CNS *(14)*. To achieve this certain methodologies need to be developed for the direct isolation and characterization of neural stem cells from the embryonic and adult CNS.

In this chapter we summarize some of the shared and/or unique cellular and molecular characteristics of neural stem cells at different stages and regions of the developing and adult CNS and propose that these properties provide a means by which to distinguish between neural stem cell populations and thus to prospectively identify neural stem cells in vivo. We further discuss recently developed methods that provide a means to directly isolate cells with stem cell potential from mixed cultures of cells.

IN VITRO STEM CELL POTENTIAL OF EMBRYONIC AND ADULT CNS CELLS

Embryonic Neural Stem Cells

During early mammalian neurogenesis, cells with stem cell characteristics in vitro, including self-renewal ability, inhibition of overt differentiation, and maintenance of multipotency, initially comprise about 90% of the newly induced cells of the neural plate *(15)*. These cells, termed neuroepithelial (NEP) stem cells, are dependent on basic fibroblast growth factor (bFGF) *(10,16)* for their survival and proliferation.

From: *Neural Development and Stem Cells, Second Edition*
Edited by: M. S. Rao © Humana Press Inc., Totowa, NJ

Dissociated neuroepithelial cells undergo self-renewal, and single NEP cells can differentiate into neurons, astrocytes, and oligodendrocytes *(15,17,18)*. After neural induction the neural plate undergoes a series of morphogenetic movements to form a tube consisting of prominent vesicles anteriorly, which represent the anlage of the forebrain, midbrain, and hindbrain and a thin portion posteriorly that develops into the spinal cord. The initially homogeneous population of dividing cells in the neural tube is patterned over several days in a characteristic spatial and temporal profile with proliferating cells restricted to the inner ventricular and differentiated neurons, oligodendrocytes, and astrocytes migrating to outer mantle zone regions *(19–24)*. Clonal culture experiments in vitro have demonstrated that stem cells at this stage of development are located within the proliferative ventricular zone, and like the cells of the neural plate, require bFGF for their survival and proliferation in vitro as well as in vivo *(25–27)*.

By the second half of embryogenesis an additional stem cell population can be isolated *(11)*. The appearance of this population coincides with the formation of the subventricular zone (SVZ) in the forebrain (*see* Chapter 1). The SVZ is later called the subependymal zone as the ventricular zone diminishes in size to a single layer of ependymal cells. The proliferation of this second stem cell population is dependent on epidermal growth factor (EGF). These EGF-dependent stem cells grow in suspension culture as "neurospheres"; can be clonally propagated (undergo self-renewal); and differentiate into neurons, astrocytes, and oligodendrocytes in vitro *(5,28–30)*.

Several lines of evidence have recently proposed that radial glial cells in the embryonic CNS have stem cells characteristics. Radial glial cells appear to function as both neural progenitors *(31–37)* and as scaffolding on which neurons migrate *(38,39)*. As progenitors radial glia give rise to many, if not all, of the neurons generated within the cerebral cortex *(34,36)* and may also function as self-renewing multipotent population *(36,40–43)*. Furthermore, as discussed later, it has recently been proposed that adult SVZ cells are directly derived from embryonic radial glial cells that retain neuroepithelial stem cell characteristics into adulthood *(44,45)* (*see* Chapter 2).

Thus, during early neurogenesis a single population of stem cells is present that is localized to the VZ. At somewhat later developmental stages at least two additional populations of stem cells can be isolated one from the SVZ and a smaller population of cells (radial glia) localized to the diminishing ventricular zone. These populations appear display unique cellular characteristics such as their growth factor responsiveness, proliferation rates, and the subtypes of neurons they generate. In addition to these unique growth characteristics, stem/progenitor cells in the CNS are regionalized by patterning molecules. Patterning in the proliferating neuroepithelium is initiated at the time of neural induction and occurs along the rostrocaudal and dorsoventral axis *(46–49)*. The regional restriction of cell fate in vivo appears to be reflected and to a certain degree maintained in vitro. For example, it has been shown that positional markers that define rostrocaudal and dorsoventral identity of stem cells persist over multiple generations in vitro *(50–52)*. Specifically, neural stem cell colonies derived from the cortex and spinal cord of embryonic day (E14.5) differentially express regional marker genes along the anteroposterior axis *(52)* and this expression persists for at least 40 generations. What remains unclear is whether progenitor cells expressing particular regional transcription factors are committed in their fate (*see* later). For example, such cells may remain plastic until they have withdrawn from the cell cycle *(53–55)*. Support for plasticity of neural progenitor cells comes from recent data that illustrated that embryonic progenitors maintain expression of regional identity in vitro but can be respecified when grafted to heterologous sites in vivo (17). Moreover, exposure of regionally specified progenitor cells to growth factors can alter their regional fate in vitro (56) (see later).

Adult Neural Stem Cells

It is now commonly accepted that the adult mammalian brain is not simply a static postmitotic organ (9,57–61). In certain locations cells with in vitro stem cell potential persist into adulthood; these include the SVZ of the lateral ventricle (LV), the subgranular zone (SGZ) of the hippocampus, and the central canals of the spinal cord (61). Throughout life, cells born around the SVZ of the lateral ventricle cross a long distance anteriorly through the rostral migratory stream to the olfactory bulb (OB), where they differentiate into interneurons. New neuronal cells in the OB are generated from neural progenitors of the SVZ of the LV (62,63). SVZ cell types can be distinguished by their morphological and immunohistochemical characteristics (12). The exact origin of adult neural stem cells is still in question (62). One hypothesis suggests that adult neural stem cells are located in the ependymal layer of the lateral ventricle of the adult forebrain (13,59). These studies propose that this population of cells undergoes asymmetric cell division to generate a transient amplifying population of rapidly dividing subventricular zone cells (type C cells) that in turn generate migratory neuroblasts (type A cells). These cells then migrate along the rostral migratory stream to the OB. The location of neural stem cells along the ventricular system of the adult indicates that these cells might be related to their embryonic counterparts, which reside in the ventricular zone that lines the lumen of the neural tube. Ependymal cells are relatively quiescent in vivo but retain the ability to enter the cells cycle, and may respond to injury by proliferations. For example, infusion of either FGF or EGF will result in ependymal cell proliferation, and limited retroviral lineage analysis has suggested that individual ependymal cells can generate astrocytes and neurons in the brain (13,64). Moreover, ependymal tumors express both glial and neuronal markers, thus indicating that ependymal cells are multipotent. However, neurospheres derived from ependymal cells do not undergo significant self-renewal (65). The slowly dividing astrocytes (type B cells) found in the subventricular zone appear to serve as independent stem cells (see Chapter 2) (66,67). Recent compelling experiments, however, demonstrate that the majority of EGF-responsive cells in the adult SVZ that generate neurospheres are derived from the rapidly dividing transit-amplifying C cells (68) (see later). In addition to the germinal zone of the SVZ, continued neurogenesis is known to occur in the adult hippocampus: cell proliferation leading to neurogenesis has been described in the granular layer of the dentate gyrus (69,70). Progenitor cells are found along a thin strip of cells, referred to as the SGZ, located between the hilar region and the granule cell layer (71). Multipotent cells can also be isolated from other regions of the mammalian CNS such as the spinal cord and parenchyma of the adult brain throughout the rostrocaudal axis (11,13,59,72,73). For example, ependymal cells lining the central canal of the postnatal spinal cord can form multipotent neurospheres in vitro and thus have properties of neural stem cells (59).

Although it has been well established that neurogenesis continues in the adult CNS the fate and the role of the stem cell populations remains unclear. It has been demonstrated that stem cells such as those found in the SVZ of the LV or the SGZ of the hippocampus generate progenitor cells that replenish the pool of olfactory interneurons and neuronal and glial cells in the granular layer of the dentate gyrus (DG) *(74)*, respectively. Retrograde tracing studies have shown that the newly generated neuronal cells extend axons *(75,76)* receive synaptic input *(77)* and participate in functional synaptic circuitry *(78)*. In addition, it has been hypothesized that these cells have diverse functions such as memory *(79–81)*, learning *(82–84)*, and cell replacement *(85)*. For example there is now growing evidence that injury or disease lead to elevated levels of neurogenesis and cell survival. Ischemic insults have been shown to trigger neurogenesis from neural stem or progenitor cells in the SVZ of the LV, the DG of the hippocampus, and even in the spinal cord (reviewed in ref. *85*). Although the transcriptional and cellular events that maintain neural stem cell identity in the adult remain unclear, evidence suggests that the underlying mechanisms probably share a common, early embryonic lineage gene expression program (*see* later).

IDENTITY OF NEURAL STEM CELLS IN VIVO

As discussed previously, many candidates have been proposed as the cell in the embryo and the adult in vivo that possesses the ability to generate neurosphere forming cells in vitro, including NEP cells, radial glial cells, SVZ cells, and ependymal cells. To date, the existence of cells that clonogenically generate neurons, astrocytes, and oligodendrocytes in vivo remains unclear. Despite a large body of lineage tracing experiments performed on the CNS, there are yet no reported examples of a single progenitor cell that generates neurons, astrocytes, and oligodendrocytes in vivo *(86,87)*. It is therefore important to consider whether the cells that form neurospheres in vitro actually represent transformed cells that do not possess stem cell characteristics in vivo. Recent results have suggested that the ability to form a sphere and grow in nonadherent cell culture conditions is not a property that is unique to stem cells. Ependymal cells, astrocytes, oligodendrocyte precursors, and neuronal progenitor cells can form neurosphere like aggregates that can be passaged for a limited time period. Moreover, a number of experiments with both embryonic and adult neural progenitor cells provide evidence that support the observation that manipulation of differentiated neural cells in culture can reprogram progenitor cell characteristics *(56,68,76,88,89)*. For example, Brewer and colleagues *(89)* described how postmitotic neurons could be induced to dedifferentiate into dividing progenitors; further, Kondo and Raff *(88)* showed that glial progenitors can be dedifferentiated and then induced to differentiate into neurons. Doetsch et al. *(68)* have provided compelling evidence that progenitor cells retain stem cell properties. Specifically, they showed that after exposure to high concentrations of EGF, type C amplifying progenitors of the adult SVZ function as stem cells in vitro.

More recently, a molecular mechanism by which progenitor cell reprogramming can occur has been put forward. Gabay et al. propose that tripotent progenitors (give rise to neurons, astrocytes, and oligodendrocytes) can be generated in vitro by deregulation of normal dorsoventral positional cues *(56)*. Such deregulation can be achieved by the exposure of cells to mitogenic growth factors such as EGF or FGF, both of which are components of the neurosphere assay. Specifically, the authors used a mutant mouse in which *Olig2*, a bHLH transcription factor, is disrupted by gene targeting and replace by the jellyfish green fluorescent protein (GFP). The authors isolated *Olig2*-positive ventral spinal cord cells, and a separate population of *Olig2* negative dorsal spinal cord cells by cell sorting for GFP. Neurospheres were then generated from these two distinct spinal cord populations. Because *Olig2* is required for oligodendrocyte development and is not expressed in the dorsal spinal cord, it was anticipated that dorsal neurospheres would not give rise to oligodendrocytes. However, both dorsal and ventral neurospheres were tripotent. In a parallel set of experiments, the authors went on to demonstrate that exposure of monolayer cultures of neuroepithelial cells isolated from the dorsal rat embryonic spinal cord to FGF induced a Sonic Hedgehog–dependent ventralization and onset of *Olig2* expression.

Taken together, these studies illustrate the importance of identifying the origin of the neurosphere-forming cell, to distinguish one population of neurosphere forming cell from another and to identify those neurosphere forming stem cells that are truly stem cell in character.

SHARED MOLECULAR CHARACTERISTICS
OF EMBRYONIC AND ADULT NEURAL STEM CELLS

The relationship between "stem cell" populations at different stages of ontogeny and various rostrocaudal and dorsoventral locations remains unclear. Neural stem cells isolated from embryonic and adult CNS are defined by common cellular characteristics. First, cells isolated from the embryonic ventricular zone VZ and SVZ surrounding the adult LV and SGZ of the DG in the hippocampus and cells from the central canal of the adult spinal cord all share the ability to form neurospheres, to self-renew, and to differentiate into neurons astrocytes and oligodendrocytes in vitro *(3,4,90)*. Second, both embryonic and adult neural stem cells of the CNS can differentiate appropriately after transplantation into a new host *(91–94)*. For example, adult hippocampal stem cells can give rise to specific and region appropriate cell types not only in the hippocampus but also in the OB, cerebellum, and retina *(95,96)*.

These common cellular characteristics correlate with the expression of common/ generic molecular markers. Universal markers of cells with stem cell potential in the CNS include members of a number of transcription factors, such as members of the *SOX*, *PAX*, *HES*, and *BFAP* gene families, members of the Notch and Wnt signaling pathway, the RNA binding proteins Musashi1 and Musashi2, the intermediate filament protein Nestin, and others (Table 1). The expression of the majority of these markers is activated during the initial phases of neural induction *(13,59,97–102)* and is then maintained in stem/progenitor cell populations throughout development. Moreover, proliferating cell population in the adult CNS share the expression of a number of these universal markers, including Nestin, Notch1, Sox1-3 (Fig. 1), *Musashi*, and so forth, with embryonic ventricular zone stem cells, raising the possibility that molecules involved in the consolidation of neural fate during primary neural induction also play a role in adult neurogenesis. The maintenance of embryonic in adult neural progenitors is further supported by the conservation of expression of molecules responsible for embryonic neural induction in regions of adult neurogenesis. For example, the neural

Table 1
Molecular Markers (Including Antigens) that Mark Neural Stem/Progenitor Cells

Stem cell marker	Comments
Nestin	All dividing neural stem cells and progenitor cells, immature astrocytes
Msi1 (homolog of *Drosophila* musachi/Nrp-1)	Dividing neural stem cells and progenitor cells, some astrocytes
Nucleostemnin	Specific to dividing populations
Sox1	Dividing neural stem cells and progenitor cells
Sox2	All dividing neural stem cells and progenitor cells
Notch1	Dividing neural stem cells and progenitor cells, immature astrocytes
Telomerase activity/TERT	Neural stem cells and subset of progenitors
ABCG2 (BCRP1)	Subset of neural stem cells
Lex1(SSEA1)	Embryonic and adult neural stem cells.
CD133/CD34	Neural stem cells
TLX	Dividing neural stem cells and progenitor cells
Low Hoescht/ Rhodamine staining	Marks quiescent stem cell populations but not rapidly dividing stem cell populations
Aldeflour labeling	General method to identify stem cell populations

Adapted from Pevny, L. H. and Rao, M. S. (2003), *Trends Neurosci.* **26**, 351–359.

inducing signaling molecule Noggin is expressed in adult LV ependymal cells, suggesting that it may function to promote neurogenesis. In support of this hypothesis overexpression of BMP, a Noggin antagonist, in the ependyma leads to a reduction in SVZ cell proliferation and abolishes neuroblast regeneration in the SVZ *(103)*.

The expression profiles of universal stem cells markers support the likelihood of common/generic molecular mechanisms shared by neural stem cells throughout their ontogeny. These molecular mechanisms are key regulatory components that define the "stem cell state," including self-renewal, symmetric vs asymmetric cell division, maintenance of progenitor/stem cell morphological identity, and multilineage differentiation. Many of the markers universally expressed in neural stem cell populations throughout ontogeny e.g. members of the *SOXB1* gene family *(104,105)*, the Wnt and Notch signaling pathway, the orphan receptor TLX *(106)*, and the RNA binding protein Musashi *(107)*, among others are also required to maintain neural stem/progenitor cells in an undifferentiated, proliferative state. Specifically, TLX mutant mice show a loss of cell proliferation and reduced labeling of Nestin in neurogenic areas of the adult brain *(106)* inhibition of *SOXB1* signaling in chick neural progenitors results in their premature exit and differentiation cells *(104,105)*; and targeted ablation of Musashi1/Musashi2 results in a reduced proliferative activity of CNS progenitor cells *(107)*. The Notch pathway appears to play an essential role in the maintenance of a stem/progenitor cell pool as well as play a role in regulating asymmetric vs symmetric division. Both during embryogenesis *(108–112)* and in adulthood, expression of Notch1 or one of its downstream regulators such as HES-1 inhibits neuronal differentiation and results in the maintenance of a progenitor state. However, the exact mechanism by which Notch

A EGFP Expression in the Lateral Ventricle

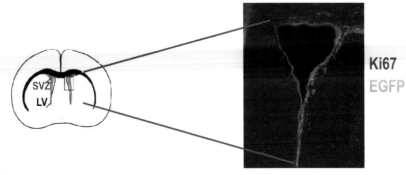

B EGFP Expression in the Subgranular Zone of the Hippocampus

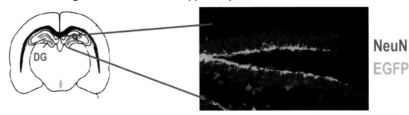

C EGFP Expression in the Central Canal of the Spinal Cord

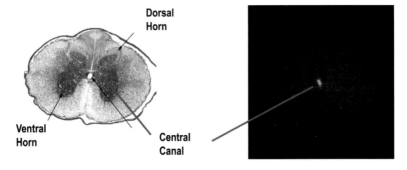

D SOX2-EGFP universally marks multipotential neurosphere forming cells.

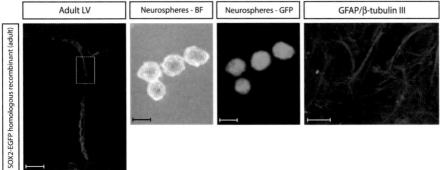

Fig. 1. (A) EGFP expression in the lateral ventricle. (B) EGFP expression in the subgranular zone of the hippocampus. (C) EGFP expression in the central canal of the spinal cord. (D) *SOX2–EGFP* universally marks multipotential neurosphere-forming cells.

signaling regulates cell fate is not completely understood. Recently, for example, numerous studies in vertebrates have suggested that rather than simply inhibiting neuronal differentiation and maintaining a neural progenitor state, Notch may in some contexts promote the acquisition of glial identity *(109,113–117)*. This is consistent with the possibility that, as discussed earlier, certain glial cell types (radial glia, astrocytes) maybe multipotent progenitors. The role of some of these universal markers is restricted to only certain characteristics of neural stem cells. For example, Bmi-1, a polycomb family transcriptional repressor, is required for the self-renewal of CNS stem cells but not for their survival or differentiation *(118,119)*. Thus Bmi-1 dependence distinguishes stem cell self-renewal from restricted progenitor proliferation in the CNS. Taken together, these data are beginning to reveal that the molecules encoding for universal stem cells markers may not only serve to identify stem cells but also function to maintain the stem cell state *(14)*.

The function of a number of these universal neural stem cell markers, however, is not restricted to CNS stem cells. For example, Bmi-1 transcriptional repressor plays an analogous role in the maintenance of self-renewal of hematopoietic stem cells, as demonstrated for neural stem cells *(120–122)*. These studies, thus raise the possibility that stem cells from different tissues may be more closely related than previously assumed and may share common molecular regulators. Several investigators have therefore proposed a concept of "stemness" or a molecular signature that may be universal to stem cell populations irrespective of the tissue source from which they are identified. By analyzing gene expression in different stem cells populations these experiments set out to identify true markers of stem cells in general, specifically addressing whether stem cells share a similar transcriptional profile. To begin to address this question several groups have used DNA microarrays *(123,124)* and subtractive hybridization *(125,126)* comparing stem cells containing populations of different origin such as hematopoietic, neural, and embryonic stem cells with differentiated tissues. These studies concluded that embryonic, hematopoietic and neural stem cells share many similarities at the transcriptional level. These results indicate that it may be possible to identify markers that are shared by multiple types of stem cells present in the nervous system as well as shared among stem cells isolated from distinct tissue types. In contrast, D'Amour and Gage took a more targeted approach to directly compare genetic and functional differences between multipotent neural stem cells and pluripotent embryonic stem cells. Specifically, D'Amour and Gage, directly compared neural progenitor cells isolated from the embryonic CNS with embryonic stem cells, using the *Sox2* promoter for isolation of purified populations by fluorescence-activated cell sorting (FACS) *(127)*. Their studies revealed substantial differences in expression profile and cellular potency between these two stem cell populations. Such direct comparisons have begun to reveal the molecular basis for the functional differences in pluripotent embryonic stem cells vs multipotent neural stem/progenitor cells.

These results raise the possibility that it may be feasible to identify markers that are shared by multiple types of stem cells present in the nervous system as well as unique that distinguish diverse stem cell populations or stem cells from proliferating progenitor cells.

IDENTIFICATION OF NEURAL STEM CELLS
USING A COMBINATION OF UNIVERSAL MARKERS
AND STEM CELL SUBTYPE MARKERS

Universal Markers Tools to Isolate Prospectively Pure Populations of Neural Stem/Progenitor Cell Populations

The cellular properties used to define a neural stem cell, specifically, the ability to form neurospheres, the ability to self-renew, and the ability to undergo multipotent differentiation correlates with the expression of a number of general or "universal" molecular markers (see Table 1). Taking advantage of the shared expression among different neural stem cells, several laboratories have developed approaches to isolate, characterize, and manipulate neural stem cells by both prospective positive and negative selection strategies. Several groups have proposed a "negative" selection criterion that is based on the observation that stem cells do not express markers characteristic of differentiated cells. For example, Rao and colleagues have used the absence of expression of neuronal, astrocytic, and oligodendroglial markers to enrich samples from stem cells from late fetal stages *(15,128)*. Using a similar negative selection strategy, Maric et al. used surface ganglioside epitopes emerging on differentiated CNS cells to isolate neural progenitors from E13 rat telencephalon by FACS *(129)*. Similarly, Bartlett and colleagues have suggested two potential markers that can be used to enrich for neural stem cells in adults. The authors showed that low levels of staining for peanut agglutinin (PNA) and heat stable antigen (HAS) can, when combined with size selection, be used to select for stem cell populations from neurospheres cultures *(130)*.

Parallel approaches have identified positive selection markers that may be used to distinguish neural stem cells. Recently, it has been demonstrated that the LeX/SSEA-1 antigen is expressed by a subset of cells in the adult SVZ, providing one of the first examples of a cell surface molecule expressed on CNS stem cells. Using this cell-surface antigen for FACS sorting, Capella and colleagues were able to isolated cells that formed multipotent neurospheres from the adult brain *(131)*. However, the prospective isolation of CNS stem cells has, unlike the isolation of hematopoietic stem cells, been seriously impeded owing to the lack of CNS specific surface stem cells markers. Nonetheless, parallel approaches have identified a small subset of positive selection markers that can be used to identify neural stem cells directly or by the generation of mouse lines in which the expression of a drug-selection marker of GFP is driven by regulatory elements of a universal stem cells marker. Quesenberry and colleagues have shown that within a neurosphere derived from adult tissue, populations of cells that display low levels of staining with Hoechst and Rhodamine 123 are enriched for self-renewing stem cells *(132,133)*. The efflux is likely to be mediated by ABCG2, a member of the multidrug resistance family of transporters that is present on neural stem cells during development and is down-regulated in differentiated cells *(15,134)*. To provide a means by which to isolate prospectively neural stem/progenitor cells, a number of mouse line have been generated in which the expression of the live marker GFP is driven by the regulatory domain of a universal stem cell marker. For example, transgenic lines have been generated that carry EGFP under the control of the neural specific enhancer for the *Nestin* gene *(135–138)* and by the introduction via homologous recombination of EGFP in the genomic loci of the neuron-specific *SOX1* and

SOX2 genes *(127,139,140)*. These mouse lines have provide a means by which to
isolate neural stem/progenitor cells directly from the developing and adult CNS.
For example, prospective clonal analysis of *SOX2-EGFP*–positive cells demonstrated
that multipotent stem cells isolated from both the embryonic CNS and the adult CNS
all express *SOX2–EGFP* (Fig. 1; *139*). Moreover, Li et al., using the *Sox2* promoter
driving the drug resistance gene neomycin, have been able to isolate 90% pure populations of neural progenitor cells from differentiating embryonic stem cells *(141)*.
An additional use of such mouse lines is for the discovery of identification and analysis of genetic and functional differences between stem cell populations. For example,
as discussed earlier, D'Amour et al. have used neural stem cells isolated by FACS
based on *SOX2* expression to compare expression profiles of neural and embryonic
stem cells *(127)*. Along the same lines, Aubert et al. have taken advantage of the neural
specific *SOX1–EGFP* reporter to purify neuroepithelial cells by FACS sorting from
E10.5 for differential screening of microarrays *(140)*. These studies have led to the
identification of a number of novel neural progenitor specific factors. Thus, positive
and negative selection criteria can be used to define populations of stem cells at various
stages of development. These markers, either singly or in concert, will help localize
stem cells in vivo and their expression in neurospheres may help determine whether a
particular neurosphere contains multipotent neural stem cells.

REFERENCES

1. Davis, A. A. and Temple, S. (1994) A self renewing multipotential stem cell in embryonic rat cerebral cortex. *Neuron* **372,** 263–266.
2. Morshead, C. M., Reynolds, B. A., Craig, C. G., et al. (1994) Neural stem cells in the
   adult mammalian forebrain: a relatively quiescent subpopulation of subependymal cells.
   Neuron **13,** 1071–1082.
3. Gritti, A., Parati, E. A., Cova, L., et al. (1996) Multipotential stem cells from the adult
   mouse brain proliferate and self-renew in response to basic fibroblast growth factor.
   J. Neurosci. **16,** 1091–1100.
4. Johe, K. K., Hazel, T. G., Muller, T., Dugich-Djordjevic, M. M., and McKay, R. D. G.
   (1996) Single factors direct the differentiation of stem cells from the fetal and adult central nervous system. *Genes Dev.* **10,** 3129–3140.
5. Reynolds, B. A. and Weiss, S. (1996) Clonal and population analyses demonstrate that an
   EGF-responsive mammalian embryonic CNS precursor is a stem cell. *Dev. Biol.* **175,** 1–13.
6. Palmer, T. D., Takahashi, J., and Gage, F. H. (1997) The adult rat hippocampus contains
   primordial neural stem cells. *Mol. Cell. Neurosci.* **8,** 389–404.
7. Gage, F. (2000) Mammalian neural stem cells. *Science* **28,** 1433–1438.
8. Temple, S. and Buylla-Alvarez, A. (1999) Stem cells in the adult mammalian central
   nervous system. *Curr. Opin. Neurobiol.* **9,** 135–141.
9. Seaberg, R. M. and van der Kooy, D. (2003) Stem and progenitor cells: the premature
   desertion of rigorous definitions. *Trends Neurosci.* **26,** 125–131.
10. Kilpatrick, T. J. and Barlett, B. F. (1995) Cloned multipotential precursors from the mouse
    cerebrum require FGF-2 whereas glial restricted precursors are stimulated by either
    FGF-2 or EGF. *J. Neurosci.* **15,** 3653–3661.
11. Weiss, S., Dunne, C., Hewson, J., et al. (1996) Multipotent CNS stem cells are present in
    the adult mammalian spinal cord and ventricular neuroaxis. *J. Neurosci.* **16,** 7599–7609.
12. Doetsch, F., Caille, I., Lim, D. A., Garcia-Verdugo, J. M., and Alvarez-Buylla, A. (1999)
    Subventricular zone astrocytes are neural stem cells in the adult mammalian brain. *Cell* **97,**
    703–716.

13. Johansson, C. B., Momma, S., Clarke, D. L., Risling, M., Lendahl, U., and Frisen, J. (1999) Identification of a neural stem cell in the adult mammalian central nervous system. *Cell* **96,** 25–34.
14. Pevny, L. and Rao, M. S. (2003) The stem-cell menagerie. *Trends Neurosci.* **26,** 351–359.
15. Cai, J., Wu, Y., Mirua, T., et al. (2002) Properties of a fetal multipotent neural stem cell (NEP cell). *Dev. Biol.* **251,** 221–240.
16. Qian, X., Davis, A. A., Goderie, S. K., and Temple, S. (1997) FGF2 concentration regulates the generation of neurons and glia from multipotent cortical stem cells. *Neuron* **18,** 81–93.
17. Kalyani, A., Hobson, K., and Rao, M. S. (1997) Neuroepithelial stem cells from the embryonic spinal cord: isolation, characterisation, and clonal analysis. *Dev. Biol.* **186,** 202–223.
18. Mujtaba, T., Piper, D. R., Kalyani, A., Groves, A. K., Lucero, M. T., and Rao, M. S. (1999) Lineage-restricted neural precursors can be isolated from both the mouse neural tube and cultured ES cells. *Dev. Biol.* **214,** 113–127.
19. Altman, J. and Bayer, S. A. (1984) *The Development of the Rat Spinal Cord.* Springer-Verlag, Berlin.
20. Bayer, S. A. and Altman, J. (1991) *Neocortical Development.* Raven, New York.
21. Lillien, L. (1998) Neural progenitors and stem cells: mechanisms of progenitor heterogeneity. *Curr. Opin. Neurobiol.* **8,** 37–44.
22. McConnell, S. K. (1995) Constructing the cerebral cortex: neurogenesis and fate determination. *Neuron* **15,** 791–803.
23. Rakic, P. (1988) Specification of cerebral cortical areas. *Science* **241,** 170–176.
24. Wentworth, L. E. (1984) The development of the cervical spinal cord of the mouse embryo. II. A Golgi analysis of sensory, commissural, and association cell differentiation. *J. Comp. Neurol.* **222,** 96–115.
25. Ortega, S., Ittmann, M., Tsang, S. H., Ehrlich, M., and Basilico, C. (1998) Neuronal defects and delayed wound healing in mice lacking fibroblast growth factor 2. *Proc. Natl. Acad. Sci. USA* **95,** 5672–5677.
26. Raballo, R., Rhee, J., Lyn-Cook, R., Leckman, J. F., Schwartz, M. L., and Vaccarino, F. M. (2000) Basic fibroblast growth factor (Fgf2) is necessary for cell proliferation and neurogenesis in the developing cerebral cortex. *J. Neurosci.* **20,** 12–23.
27. Vaccarino, F. M., Schwartz, M. L., Raballo, R., et al. (1999) Changes in cerebral cortex size are governed by fibroblast growth factor during embryogenesis. *Nat. Neurosci.* **2,** 246–253.
28. Reynolds, B. A. and Weiss, S. (1992) Generation of neurons and astrocytes from isolated cells of the adult mammalian central nervous system. *Science* **255,** 1707–1710.
29. Reynolds, B. A., Tetzlaff, W., and Weiss, S. A. (1992) Multipotent EGF-responsive striatal embryonic progenitor cell produces neurons and astrocytes. *J. Neurosci.* **12,** 4565–4574.
30. Nakamura, N., Mitamura, T., Takahashi, T., Kobayashi, T., and Mekada, E. (2000) Importance of the major extracellular domain of CD9 and the epidermal growth factor (EGF)-like domain of heparin-binding EGF-like growth factor for up-regulation of binding and activity. *J. Biol. Chem.* **275,** 18284–18290.
31. Gotz, M., Hartfuss, E., and Malatesta, P. (2002) Radial glial cells as neuronal precursors: a new perspective on the correlation of morphology and lineage restriction in the developing cerebral cortex of mice. *Brain Res. Bull.* **57,** 777–788.
32. Heins, N., Malatesta, P., Cecconi, F., et al. (2002) Glial cells generate neurons: the role of the transcription factor Pax6. *Nat. Neurosci.* **5,** 308–315.
33. Hall, A. C., Mira, H., Wagner, J., and Arenas, E. (2003) Region-specific effects of glia on neuronal induction and differentiation with a focus on dopaminergic neurons. *Glia* **43,** 47–51.

34. Malatesta, P., Hack, M. A., Hartfuss, E., et al. (2003) Neuronal or glial progeny: regional differences in radial glia fate. *Neuron* **37,** 751–764.

35. Johnson, M. W., Miyata, H., and Vinters, H. V. (2002) Ezrin and moesin expression within the developing human cerebrum and tuberous sclerosis-associated cortical tubers. *Acta Neuropathol. (Berl.)* **104,** 188–196.

36. Noctor, S. C., Flint, A. C., Weissman, T. A., Wong, W. S., Clinton, B. K., and Kreigstein, A. R. (2002) Dividing precursor cells of the embryonic cortical ventricular zone have morphological and molecular characteristics of radial glia. *J. Neurosci.* **15,** 3161–3173.

37. Miyata, T., Kawaguchi, A., Okano, H., and Ogawa, M. (2001) Asymmetric inheritance of radial glial fibers by cortical neurons. *Neuron* **31,** 727–741.

38. Rakic, P. (1971) Neuron-glia relationship during granule cell migration in developing cerebellar cortex. A Golgi and electronmicroscopic study in *Macacus Rhesus*. *J. Comp. Neurol.* **141,** 283–312.

39. Sidman, R. L. and Rakic, P. (1973) Neuronal migration, with special reference to developing human brain: a review. *Brain Res.* **62,** 1–35.

40. Gray, G. E. and Sanes, J. R. (1992) Lineage of radial glia in the chicken optic tectum. *Development* **114,** 271–283.

41. Hartfuss, E., Forster, E., Bock, H. H., et al. (2003) Reelin signaling directly affects radial glia morphology and biochemical maturation. *Development* **130,** 4597–4609.

42. Malatesta, P., Hartfuss, E., and Gotz, M. (2000) Isolation of radial glial cells by fluorescent-activated cell sorting reveals a neuronal lineage. *Development* **127,** 5253–5263.

43. Noctor, S. C., Flint, A. C., Weissman, T. A., Dammerman, R. S., and Kreigstein, A. R. (2001) Neurons derived from radial glial cells establish radial units in neocortex. *Nature* **409,** 714–720.

44. Alvarez-Buylla, A., Seri, B., and Doetsch, F. (2002) Identification of neural stem cells in the adult vertebrate brain. *Brain Res. Bull.* **57,** 737–749.

45. Tramontin, A. D., Garcia-Verdugo, J. M., Lim, D. A., and Alvarez-Buylla, A. (2003) Postnatal development of radial glia and the ventricular zone (VZ): a continuum of the neural stem cell compartment. *Cereb. Cortex* **13,** 580–587.

46. Lumsden, A. and Krumlauf, R. (1996) Patterning the vertebrate neuraxis. *Science* **274,** 1009–1115.

47. Wilson, S. I. and Rubenstein, J. L. (2000) Induction and dorsoventral patterning of the telencephalon. *Neuron* **28,** 641–651.

48. Jessell, T. M. (2000) Neuronal specification in the spinal cord: inductive signals and transcriptional codes. *Nat. Rev. Genet.* **1,** 20–29.

49. Briscoe, J., Pierani, A., Jessell, T. M., and Ericson, J. (2000) A homeodomain protein code specifies progenitor cell identity and neuronal fate in the ventral neural tube. *Cell* **101,** 435–445.

50. Hitoshi, S., Tropepe, V., Ekker, M., and van der Kooy, D. (2002) Neural stem cell lineages are regionally specified, but not committed, within distinct compartments of the developing brain. *Development* **129,** 233–244.

51. Nakagawa, Y., Kaneko, T., Ogura, T., et al. (1996) Roles of cell-autonomous mechanisms for differential expression of region-specific transcription factors in neuroepithelial cells. *Development* **122,** 2449–2464.

52. Zappone, M. S., Galli, R., Catena, R., et al. (2000) Sox2 regulatory sequences direct expression of a (beta)-geo transgene to telencephalic neural stem cells and precursors of the mouse embryo, revealing regionalization of gene expression in CNS stem cells. *Development* **127,** 2367–2382.

53. McConnell, S. K. and Kaznowski, C. E. (1991) Cell cycle dependence of laminar determination in developing neocortex. *Science* **254,** 282–285.

54. Anderson, C. W. (2001) Anatomical evidence for brainstem circuits mediating feeding motor programs in the leopard frog, *Rana pipiens*. *Exp. Brain Res.* **140,** 12–19.

55. Edlund, T. and Jessell, T. M. (1999) Progression from extrinsic to intrinsic signaling in cell fate specification: a view from the nervous system. *Cell* **96,** 211–224.

56. Gabay, L., Lowell, S., Rubin, L. L., and Anderson, D. J. (2003) Deregulation of dorsoventral patterning by FGF confers trilineage differentiation capacity on CNS stem cells in vitro. *Neuron* **40,** 485–499.

57. Alvarez-Buylla, A. and Garcia Verdugo, J. M. (2002) Neurogenesis in the adult subventricular zone. *J. Neurosci.* **22,** 629–634.

58. Gage, F. H. (2000) Mammalian neural stem cells. *Science* **287,** 1433–1438.

59. Johansson, C. B., Svensson, M., Wallstedt, L., Janson, A. M., and Frisen, J. (1999) Neural stem cells in the adult human brain. *Exp. Cell Res.* **253,** 733–736.

60. Seaberg, R. M. and van der Kooy, D. (2002) Adult rodent neurogenic regions: the ventricular subependyma contains neural stem cells, but the dentate gyrus contains restricted progenitors. *J. Neurosci.* **22,** 1784–1793.

61. Taupin, P. and Gage, F. (2002) Adult neurogenesis and neural stem cells of the central nervous system in mammals. *J. Neurosci. Res.* **69,** 745–749.

62. Barres, B. A. (1999) A new role for glia: generation of neurons. *Cell* **97,** 667–670.

63. Momma, S., Johansson, C. B., and Frisen, J. (2000) Get to know your stem cells. *Curr. Opin. Neurobiol.* **10,** 45–49.

64. Josephson, R., Muller, T., Pickel, J., et al. (1998) POU transcription factors control expression of CNS stem cell-specific genes. *Development* **125,** 3087–3100.

65. Chiasson, B. J., Tropepe, V., Morshead, C. M., and van der Kooy, D. (1999) Adult mammalian forebrain ependymal and subependymal cells demonstrate proliferative potential, but only subependymal cells have neural stem cell characteristics. *J. Neurosci.* **19,** 4462–4471.

66. Alvarez-Buylla, A., Herrara, D. G., and Wichterle, H. (2000) The subventricular zone: source of neuronal precursors for brain repair. *Prog. Brain Res.* **127,** 1–11.

67. Garcia-Verdugo, J. M., Doetsch, F., Wichterle, H., Lim, D. A., and Alvarez-Buylla, A. (1998) Architecture and cell types of the adult subventricular zone: in search of stem cells. *J. Neurobiol.* **36,** 234–248.

68. Doetsch, F., Petreanu, L., Caille, I., Garcia-Verdugo, J. M., and Alvarez-Buylla, A. (2002) EGF converts transit-amplifying neurogenic precursors in the adult brain into multipotent stem cells. *Neuron* **36,** 1021–1034.

69. Altman, J. and Das, G. D. (1965) Autoradiographic and histological evidence of postnatal neurogenesis in rats. *J. Comp. Neurol.* **124,** 319–335.

70. Kuhn, H. G., Dickinson-Anson, H., and Gage, F. H. (1996) Neurogenesis in the dentate gyrus of the adult rat: age related decrease of neuronal progenitor proliferation. *J. Neurosci.* **16,** 2027–2033.

71. Gage, F. H. (1998) Stem cells of the central nervous system. *Curr. Opin. Neurobiol.* **8,** 671–676.

72. Shihabuddin, L. S., Horner, P. J., Ray, J., and Gage, F. H. (2000) Adult spinal cord stem cells generate neurons after transplantation in the adult dentate gyrus. *J. Neurosci.* **20,** 8727–8735.

73. Marmur, R., Mabie, P. C., Gokhan, S., Song, Q., Kessler, J. A., and Mehler, M. F. (1998) Isolation and developmental characterization of cerebral cortical multipotent progenitors. *Dev. Biol.* **204,** 577–591.

74. Cameron, H. A. and McKay, R. (1998) Stem cells and neurogenesis in the adult brain. *Curr. Opin. Neurobiol.* **8,** 677–680.

75. Stanfield, B. B. and Trice, J. E. (1988) Evidence that granule cells generated in the dentate gyrus of adult rats extend axonal projections. *Exp. Brain Res.* **72,** 399–406.

76. Palmer, T. D., Markakis, E. A., Willhoite, A. R., Safar, F., and Gage, F. H. (1999) Fibro-blast growth factor-2 activates a latent neurogenic program in neural stem cells from diverse regions of the adult CNS. *J. Neurosci.* **19,** 8487–8497.

77. Markakis, E. A., Palmer, T. D., Randolph-Moore, L., Rakic, P., and Gage, F. H. (2004) Novel neuronal phenotypes from neural progenitor cells. *J. Neurosci.* **24,** 2886–2897.

78. Carlen, M., Cassidy, R. M., Brismar, H., Smith, G. A., Enquist, L. W., and Frisen, J. (2002) Functional integration of adult-born neurons. *Curr. Biol.* **12,** 606–608.

79. Feng, R., Rampon, C., Tang, Y. P., et al. (2001) Deficient neurogenesis in forebrain-specific presenilin-1 knockout mice is associated with reduced clearance of hippocampal memory traces. *Neuron* **32,** 911–926 (Erratum **33,** 313).

80. Macklis, J. D. (2001) New memories from new neurons. *Nature* **410,** 314–415.

81. Shors, T. J., Miesefaes, G., Beylin, A., Zhao, M., Rydel, T., and Gould, E. (2001) Neurogenesis in the adult is involved in the formation of trace memories. *Nature* **410,** 372–375.

82. Gould, E. and Gross, C. G. (2002) Neurogenesis in adult mammals: some progress and problems. *J. Neurosci.* **22,** 619–623.

83. Kempermann, G., Kuhn, H. G., and Gage, F. (1997) More hippocampal neurons in adult mice living in an enriched environment. *Nature* **386,** 493–495.

84. Kempermann, G. and Gage, F. (2002) Genetic influence on phenotypic differentiation of adult hippocampal neurogenesis. *Brain Res. Dev. Brain Res.* **134,** 1–12.

85. Kokaia, Z. and Lindvall, O. (2003) Neurogenesis after ischaemic brain insults. *Curr. Opin. Neurobiol.* **13,** 127–132.

86. Leber, S. M., Breedlove, S. M., and Sanes, J. R. (1990) Lineage, arrangement and death of clonally related motoneurons in chick spinal cord. *J. Neurosci.* **10,** 2451–2462.

87. Luskin, M. B., Parnavelas, J. G., and Barfield, J. A. (1993) Neurons, astrocytes and oligo-dendrocytes of the rat cerebral cortex originate from separate progenitor cells: an ultra-structural analysis of clonally related cells. *J. Neurosci.* **13,** 1730–1750.

88. Kondo, T. and Raff, M. C. (2000) Oligodendrocyte precursor cells reprogrammed to become multipotential CNS stem cells. *Science* **289,** 1754–1757.

89. Brewer, G. J. (1999) Regeneration and proliferation of embryonic and adult rat hippoc-ampal neurons in culture. *Exp. Neurol.* **159,** 237–247.

90. Shihabuddin, L. S., Ray, J., and Gage, F. H. (1997) FGF-2 is sufficient to isolate progeni-tors found in the adult mammalian spinal cord. *Exp. Neurol.* **148,** 577–586.

91. Brustle, O., Maskos, U., and McKay, R. D. G. (1995) Host-guided migration allows tar-geted introduction of neurons into the embryonic brain. *Neuron* **15,** 1275–1285.

92. Campbell, K., Olsson, M., and Bjorklund, A. (1995) Regional incorporation and site-specific differentiation of striatal precursors transplanted to the embryonic forebrain ven-tricle. *Neuron* **15,** 1259–1273.

93. Fishell, G. (1995) Striatial precursors adopt cortical identities in response to local cues. *Development* **121,** 803–812.

94. Vicario-Abejon, C., Johe, K. K., Hazel, T. G., Collazo, D., and McKay, R. (1995) Func-tions of basic fibroblast growth factor and neurotrophins in the differentiation of hippoc-ampal neurons. *Neuron* **15,** 105–114.

95. Gage, F. H., Ray, J., and Fisher, L. J. (1995) Isolation, characterisation and use of stem cells from the CNS. *Annu. Rev. Neurosci.* **18,** 159–192.

96. Takahashi, M., Palmer, T. D., Takahashi, J., and Gage, F. H. (1998) Widespread intergration and survival of adult-derived neural progenitor cells in the developing optic retina. *Mol. Cell. Neurosci.* **12,** 340–348.

97. Frederiksen, K. and McKay, R. D. (1998) Proliferation and differentiation of rat neuro-epithelial precursor cells *in vivo*. *J. Neurosci.* **9,** 1144–1151.

98. Lendahl, U., Zimmerman, L. B., and McKay, R. D. G. (1990) CNS stem cells express a new class of intermediate filament protein. *Cell* **60,** 585–595.

99. Pevny, L. H., Sockanathan, S., Placzek, M., and Lovell-Badge, R. (1998) A role for SOX1 in neural determination. *Development* **125**, 1967–1978.
100. Sakakibara, S., Imai, T., Hamaguchi, K., et al. (1996) Mouse Musashi-1, a neural RNA-1 binding protein highly enriched in the mammalian CNS stem cell. *Dev. Biol.* **176**, 230–242.
101. Sakakibara, S. and Okano, H. (1997) Expression of neural RNA-binding proteins in the postnatal CNS: implications of their roles in neuronal and glial cell development. *J. Neurosci.* **17**, 8300–8312.
102. Weinmaster, G., Roberts, V. J., and Lemke, G. (1991) A homolog of *Drosophila* Notch expressed during mammalian development. *Development* **113**, 199–205.
103. Lim, D. A., Tramontin, A. D., Trevejo, J. M., Herrera, D. G., Garcia-Verdugo, J. M., and Alvarez-Buylla, A. (2000) Noggin antagonizes BMP signaling to create a niche for adult neurogenesis. *Neuron* **28**, 713–726.
104. Graham, V., Khudyakov, J., Ellis, P., and Pevny, L. (2003) SOX2 Functions to maintain neural progenitor identity. *Neuron* **39**, 749–765.
105. Bylund, M., Andersson, E., Novitch, B. G., and Muhr, J. (2003) Vertebrate neurogenesis is counteracted by Sox1-3 activity. *Nat. Neurosci.* **6**, 1162–1168.
106. Shi, Y., Chichung Lie, D., Taupin, P., et al. (2004) Expression and function of orphan nuclear receptor TLX in adult neural stem cells. *Nature* **427**, 78–83.
107. Sakakibara, S., Nakamura, Y., Yoshida, T., et al. (2002) RNA-binding protein Musashi family: roles for CNS stem cells and a subpopulation of ependymal cells revealed by targeted disruption and antisense ablation. *Proc. Natl. Acad. Sci. USA* **99**, 15194–15199.
108. Chambers, C. B., Peng, Y., Nguyen, H., Gaiano, N., Fishell, G., and Nye, J. S. (2001) Spatiotemporal selectivity of response to Notch1 signals in mammalian forebrain precursors. *Development* **128**, 689–702.
109. Gaiano, N., Nye, J. S., and Fishell, G. (2000) Radial glial identity is promoted by Notch1 signaling in the murine forebrain. *Neuron* **26**, 395–404.
110. Gaiano, N. and Fishell, G. (2002) The role of notch in promoting glial and neural stem cell fates. *Annu. Rev. Neurosci.* **25**, 471–490.
111. Ishibashi, M., Moriyoshi, K., Sasai, Y., Shiota, K., Nakanishi, S., and Kageyama, R. (1994) Persistent expression of helix–loop–helix factor HES-1 prevents mammalian neural differentiation in the central nervous system. *EMBO J.* **13**, 1799–1805.
112. Ishibashi, M., Ang, S. L., Shiota, K., Nakanishi, S., Kageyama, R., and Guillemot, F. (1995) Targeted disruption of mammalian hairy and Enhancer of split homolog-1 (HES-1) leads to up-regulation of neural helix-loop-helix factors, premature neurogenesis, and severe neural tube defects. *Genes Dev.* **9**, 3136–3148.
113. Furukawa, T., Morrow, E. M., and Cepko, C. L. (1997) Crx, a novel otx-like homeobox gene, shows photoreceptor-specific expression and regulates photoreceptor differentiation. *Cell* **91**, 531–541.
114. Akita, J., Takahashi, M., Hojo, M., Nishida, A., Haruta, M., and Honda, Y. (2002) Neuronal differentiation of adult rat hippocampus-derived neural stem cells transplanted into embryonic rat explanted retinas with retinoic acid pretreatment. *Brain Res.* **954**, 286–293.
115. Morrison, S. J., Csete, M., Groves, A. K., Melega, W., Wold, B., and Anderson, D. J. (2000) Culture in reduced levels of oxygen promotes clonogenic sympathoadrenal differentiation by isolated neural crest stem cells. *J. Neurosci.* **20**, 7370–7376.
116. Scheer, N., Groth, A., Hans, S., and Campos-Ortega, J. A. (2001) An instructive function for Notch in promoting gliogenesis in the zebrafish retina. *Development* **128**, 1099–1107.
117. Hojo, M., Ohtsuka, T., Hashimoto, N., Gradwohl, G., Guillemot, F., and Kageyama, R. (2000) Glial cell fate specification modulated by the bHLH gene *Hes5* in mouse retina. *Development* **127**, 2515–2522.
118. Park, I. K., Morrison, S. J., and Clarke, M. F. (2004) Bmi1, stem cells, and senescence regulation. *J. Clin. Invest.* **113**, 175–179.

119. Molofsky, A. V., Pardal, R., Iwashita, T., Park, I. K., Clarke, M. F., and Morrison, S. J. (2003) Bmi-1 dependence distinguishes neural stem cell self-renewal from progenitor proliferation. *Nature* **425,** 962–967.

120. Ezoe, S., Matsumura, I., Satoh, Y., Tanaka, H., and Kanakura, Y. (2004) Cell cycle regulation in hematopoietic stem/progenitor cells. *Cell Cycle* **3,** 314–318.

121. Raaphorst, F. M. (2003) Self-renewal of hematopoietic and leukemic stem cells: a central role for the Polycomb-group gene *Bmi-1. Trends Immunol.* **24,** 522–524.

122. Akasaka, T., Tsuji, K., Kawahira, H., et al. (1997) The role of *mel-18*, a mammalian Polycomb group gene, during IL-7-dependent proliferation of lymphocyte precursors. *Immunity* **7,** 135–146.

123. Ivanova, N. B., Dimos, J. T., Schaniel, C., Hackney, J. A., Moore, K. A., and Lemischka, I. R. (2002) A stem cell molecular signature. *Science* **298,** 601–604.

124. Ramalho-Santos, M., Yoon, S., Matsuzaki, Y., Mulligan, R. C., and Melton, D. A. (2002) "Stemness": transcriptional profiling of embryonic and adult stem cells. *Science* **298,** 597–600.

125. Terskikh, A. V., Easterday, M. C., Li, L., Hood, L., Kornblum, H. I., and Geschwind, D. (2001) From hematopoiesis to neuropoiesis: evidence of overlapping genetic programs. *Proc. Natl. Acad. Sci. USA* **98,** 7934–7939.

126. Geschwind, D., Ou, J., Easterday, M. C., et al. (2001) A genetic analysis of neural progenitor differentiation. *Neuron* **29,** 325–339.

127. D'Amour, K. A. and Gage, F. H. (2003) Genetic and functional differences between multipotent neural and pluripotent embryonic stem cells. *Proc. Natl. Acad. Sci. USA* **100(Suppl 1),** 11866–11872.

128. Rao, M. (1999) Multipotent and restricted precursors in the central nervous system. *Anat. Rec.* **257,** 137–148.

129. Maric, D., Maric, I., Chang, Y. H., and Barker, J. L. (2003) Prospective cell sorting of embryonic rat neural stem cells and neuronal and glial progenitors reveals effects of basic fibroblast growth factor and epidermal growth factor on self-renewal and differentiation. *J. Neurosci.* **23,** 240–251.

130. Bartlett, P. F., Brooker, G. J., Faux, C. H., et al. (1998) Regulation of neural stem cell differentiation in the forebrain. *Immunol. Cell Biol.* **76,** 414–418.

131. Capela, A. and Temple, S. (2002) LeX/SSEA-1 is expressed by adult mouse CNS stem cells, identifying them as non-ependymal. *Neuron* **35,** 865–875.

132. Quesenberry, P. J., Hulspas, R., Joly, C., et al. (1999) Correlates between hematopoiesis and neuropoiesis: neural stem cells. *J. Neurotrauma* **16,** 661–666.

133. Hulspas, R. and Quesenberry, P. J. (2000) Characterization of neurosphere cell phenotypes by flow cytometry. *Cytometry* **40,** 245–250.

134. Goodell, M. A., Brose, K., Paradis, G., Conner, A. S., and Mulligan, R. C. (1996) Isolation and functional properties of murine hematopoietic stem cells that are replicating in vivo. *J. Exp. Med.* **183,** 1797.

135. Yamaguchi, M., Saito, H., Suzuki, M., and Mori, K. (2000) Visualization of neurogenesis in the central nervous system using nestin promoter-GFP transgenic mice. *Dev. Neurosci.* **11,** 1991–1996.

136. Roy, N. S., Benraiss, A., Wang, S., et al. (2000) Promoter-targeted selection and isolation of neural progenitor cells from the adult ventricular zone. *J. Neurosci. Res.* **59,** 321–331.

137. Sawamoto, K., Nakao, N., Kakishita, K., et al. (2001) Generation of dopaminergic neurons in the adult brain from mesencephalic precursor cells labeled with nestin-GFP transgene. *J. Neurosci.* **21,** 3895–3903.

138. Mignone, J. L., Kukekov, V., Chiang, A. S., Steindler, D., and Enikolopov, G. (2004) Neural stem and progenitor cells in nestin-GFP transgenic mice. *J. Comp. Neurol.* **469,** 311–324.

139. Ellis, P., Fagan, M., Taranova, O., et al. *SOX2*, a persistent marker for neural stem cells derived from ES cells, the embryo or the adult. *Dev. Neurosci.*, in press.
140. Aubert, J., Stavridis, M. P., Tweedie, S., et al. (2003) Screening for mammalian neural genes via fluorescence-activated cell sorter purification of neural precursors from Sox1-gfp knock-in mice. *Proc. Natl. Acad. Sci. USA* **100(Suppl 1),** 11836–11841.
141. Li, M., Pevny, L., Lovell-Badge, R., and Smith, A. (1998) Generation of purified neural precursors from embryonic stem cells by lineage selection. *Curr. Biol.* **8,** 971–974.

4

Multipotent Stem Cells
in the Embryonic Nervous System

Ali Jalali, Michael Bonaguidi,
Caitilin Hamill, and John A. Kessler

INTRODUCTION

Neural stem cells are multipotent stem cells that have an unlimited capacity to proliferate and self-renew but whose progeny are restricted to the neural lineages. Neural stem cells can generate large numbers of mature neuronal and glial progeny, often through transient amplification of intermediate progenitor pools, similar to the pattern observed in other organ systems (1). Although self-renewal can occur through symmetric cell divisions that generate two identical daughter cells, asymmetric cell divisions that generate a renewable stem cell and a more lineage-restricted daughter cell are a hallmark of stem cells. Cells that do not self-renew indefinitely but that nevertheless proliferate and have the capacity to generate multiple phenotypes are often referred to as multipotential progenitor cells, but they will be included in a broad definition of stem cells for the purposes of this review. Other stem cell–derived precursor populations that are able to proliferate but that have more restricted lineage potential (e.g., glial restricted or neuronal restricted cells) are discussed elsewhere in this volume.

At present there are no generally accepted markers that allow the unambiguous identification of stem cells in the embryonic nervous system in vivo. The intermediate filament protein Nestin is the most commonly used marker of neural stem cells (2). Other proteins that are expressed in brain primarily by neural stem and more restricted progenitor cells include Musashi1, Sox1, Sox2, and Vimentin (3–5, see also ref. 6 for an extensive study of various progenitor and mature neural markers). In addition to the aforementioned intracellular antigens, neural stem cells express (or lack) a number of surface proteins that allow the use of fluorescence-activated cell sorting (FACS) for enrichment of these cells among more differentiated cells in culture (7–10).

Embryonic neural stem cells arise from neuroepithelial cells in the neural plate region of the embryonic ectoderm, which, by the end of neurulation, develops into the neural tube, crest, and placodes. For the purposes of this chapter, we may suppose that all of the neurons, astroglial, oligodendroglial, and ependymal cells of the central nervous system (CNS) develop from the undifferentiated neuroepithelial cells that line the

From: *Neural Development and Stem Cells, Second Edition*
Edited by: M. S. Rao © Humana Press Inc., Totowa, NJ

inside of the entire neural tube *(11)*. These "primitive neuroepithelial cells" are elongated cells extending from the ventricular (apical) to the pial (basal) surface of the early neural tube. As these proliferating cells progress through their asynchronous cell cycles, their nuclei move between the ventricular and pial aspects (interkinetic nuclear migration) yielding the pseudostratified appearance of the neuroepithelial cells. As the neural tube wall thickens, neuroepithelial cells retain their position subjacent to the ventricular surface (ventricular zone) and many extend radial processes to the pial surface *(12)*. While many of these radially elongated neuroepithelial cells maintain their multipotential progenitor capacity, they are often referred to as radial glia, in part due to their expression of some traditional glial markers such as glial fibrillary acidic protein (GFAP) and astrocyte-specific glutamate transporter (GLAST) as well as emergence of certain cytoskeletal, cytoplasmic, and junctional features of glia *(13,14; see also* refs. *15* and *16* for review). It has been suggested that radial glia constitute the majority of the progenitor population in the ventricular zone *(12,17)*, and little direct evidence for ventricular zone precursors with short or no radial process exists *(18)*. During late embryonic life, the ventricular zone (VZ) gives rise to deeper regional subventricular zones (SVZs) that persist in an attenuated form into the adult state. Neurons and radial glia are generated predominantly within the early embryonic VZ, whereas oligodendrocytes and astrocytes are largely generated during perinatal and early postnatal periods within regional and cortical SVZs. This topic is discussed further later in this chapter.

Patterns of labeling and growth of putative stem cells within the early neural tube suggest that the earliest cell divisions are symmetric, with the elaboration of equivalent daughter cells *(19,20)*. In slice cultures of developing ferret brain, early cell divisions are oriented primarily in a plane vertical to the ventricular surface and generate two apparently similar daughter cells. This process presumably allows exponential expansion of the resident progenitor population. By contrast, later cell divisions occur predominantly in a horizontal or oblique plane and generate two different daughter cells by asymmetric cell division *(21; see also* refs. *22* and *23* for review). A similar pattern of asymmetric division is also observed in rat telencephalic slice cultures where a radial glial progenitor often gives rise to another radial glial cell and an intermediate neuronal progenitor cell which will subsequently divide symmetrically in the SVZ and migrate, in distinct phases, to its cortical destination *(24)*. These asymmetric divisions during later embryonic life result in elaboration of the neuronal and glial cell populations as well as renewal of neural progenitors. In their final division, radial glia often give rise to neuronal and/or glial committed daughter cells, both of which migrate away from the ventricular surface and mature as they reach their cortical destination *(24)*.

CULTURE OF EMBRYONIC NEURAL STEM CELLS

Neural stem cells can be obtained for in vitro studies from embryonic CNS by dissecting and dissociating the VZ/SVZ tissue followed by culture in a defined, serum-free medium with a supplemental mitogen such as basic fibroblast growth factor-2 (bFGF-2 also known as FGF2) or epidermal growth factor (EGF) *(25–28)*. In the presence of an adhesive substrate such as polylysine or fibronectin, neural stem cells grow as a monolayer which, at a moderate plating density, allows relatively simple clonal analysis of the resulting population of stem and/or differentiated cells *(29–31)*. Isolated neural stem cells proliferate faster on a nonadhesive substrate, where the cells grow as float-ing, clonal aggregates (neurospheres) composed of a heterogeneous mixture of stem and more differentiated cells *(32)*. To analyze the composition of neurospheres, which contain from a few to thousands of cells, the aggregates are dissociated and plated on an adhesive substrate in the absence or presence of mitogen at clonal density to pro-mote the differentiation of these cells into neuronal, astroglial, or oligodendroglial lin-eages *(26,33,34)*. Studies using these neurosphere assays have allowed examination of the developmental potential of single mitotic stem cells and the effects of defined epi-genetic signals in altering cell fate *(3,35,36)*. However, the presence of exogenous mitogens and the absence of many tissue signaling and structural cues are inherent limitations to these studies in vitro, necessitating in vivo verification of culture results.

STUDY OF EMBRYONIC NEURAL STEM CELLS IN VIVO

Depending on the animal and the accessibility of its embryos, in vivo studies of embryonic neural stem cells can be moderately simple to very difficult. Tracking the progeny of individual neural stem cells is typically accomplished through labeling of these proliferating cells using viral or electroporation delivery of reporter constructs, requiring access to the lumen of neural tube. This can be accomplished by microinjec-tion of reporter constructs into the embryo using naked eye or visual guidance such as with an ultrasound biomicroscope for early mouse embryos *(37)*. The great advantage of these approaches is that they allow study of stem cells within their normal environ-mental context, but the interpretation of such studies done in vivo is also limited by the lack of unambiguous markers for the stem cells and their various progeny.

An elegant in vivo approach for lineage analysis uses a library of heterogeneous retroviral vectors with numerous genetic tags. Any daughter cells containing precisely the same mixture of tags are presumed to arise from the same progenitor, even if the progeny are scattered widely. Injection of this retroviral library into E15–17 rat embryos generated some spread clones with different cell types and an equivalent num-ber of smaller clones of a single cell type *(38,39)*. This is the pattern that would be expected if the retrovirus infected asymmetrically dividing cells since one daughter cell would display the multipotent stem cell phenotype, and the other would display the phenotype of a committed cell. In turn, this suggests that most cells generated by the VZ during this time period arise from multipotent progenitor cells undergoing active asymmetric division, a conclusion consistent with studies of stem cells in cul-ture *(40,41)*. However, the precise proportions of stem cells, multipotent progenitors, and committed progenitors at differing developmental stages and in different regions of the generative zones are unknown.

DEVELOPMENTAL CHANGES IN NEURAL STEM CELLS

Although neural stem cells retain the ability to generate neurons, oligodendroglia, and astrocytes throughout the embryonic and postnatal periods (and even in the adult; *see* Chapter 2), there are clearly developmental changes both in their bias toward dif-ferentiation into specific cell types and in their responses to epigenetic signals. Early VZ stem cells in culture are predisposed to become neurons and to a lesser extent oligodendroglia, whereas SVZ stem cells are biased toward astrocytic differentiation.

This sequence is similarly recapitulated in vivo, where the majority of neurons are born soon after neurulation followed by glia (astrocytes and oligodendrocytes, respectively) in perinatal and early postnatal periods. The onset of neuro- and gliogenesis is earlier in the caudal neural tube (future spinal cord) while certain parts of the CNS such as cerebellum have later onset neurogenesis that continues postnatally (*see* ref. *23* for review). Epidermal growth factor receptors (EGFRs) are not expressed by VZ stem cells but are expressed by later progenitors in the SVZ. Neural stem cells thus become progressively more biased toward a glial fate during development coincident with an increase in expression of EGFRs. Retroviral introduction of extra EGFRs into VZ progenitor cells results in premature expression of traits characteristic of later SVZ progenitors including the bias toward astrocytic differentiation *(42)*.

The role of EGF signaling in the change in stem cell glial propensity is at least partly mediated by making the neural stem cells more susceptible to the astrocyte-inducing effects of leukemia inhibitory factor (LIF) via an increase is STAT3 signaling *(43)*. Therefore, developmental increases in levels of EGFRs expressed by progenitor cells mediate some changes in cellular responses to environmental signals and the tendency to differentiate into astrocytes. However, similar experiments involving introduction of extra copies of the EGFR into early embryonic retinal progenitor cells did not bias the cells toward a glial fate *(44)*. Also, pharmacologic blockade of EGFR signaling does not alter the developmentally increased bias of cultured progenitor cells to undergo astrocytic differentiation *(45)*, suggesting that the competence to generate glia is also temporally regulated by other mechanisms. There are also striking differences between VZ and SVZ stem cell responses to differentiating signals such as the BMPs *(46)* or LIF *(43,47)*, so that the same signals may induce different phenotypes at different developmental stages. Thus analysis of the factors regulating stem cell differentiation requires knowledge of the history of the cell and the intrinsic milieu of the cell at that particular developmental stage. Further discussion of the extrinsic and intrinsic signaling pathways involved in neural stem cell proliferation and differentiation is provided in later sections of this chapter.

REGIONAL DIFFERENCES IN EMBRYONIC NEURAL STEM CELLS

Throughout development, different regions of the neural tube come under the influence of various signaling molecules secreted by a number of embryonic tissues and organizing centers. In the caudal neural tube, for instance, neural stem cells are under the influence of sonic hedgehog (Shh) from notochord and floor plate and bone morphogenic proteins (BMPs) from dorsal ectoderm and roof plate, as well as retinoic acid (RA), fibroblast growth factors (FGFs), and orthologs of *Drosophila* wingless (Wnts). In the mammalian cortex, FGF8 is produced by the anterior neural ridge (ANR), while some Wnts and BMPs are secreted by the cortical hem (dorsomedial telencephalon). There are also sources of Shh and RA around the rostral neural tube (*see* refs. *48–50* for review). As a result of these regional differences in the signaling environment of neural progenitors, different parts of the neural tube develop distinct neuronal and glial biases, and their neural progeny undergo different migration and differentiation patterns. For example, practically all neocortical projection neurons are derived from dorsal cortical VZ and migrate along radial glial processes to their proper layer position in the cortex. However, some neocortical interneurons are born in the ventral VZ (in the ganglionic eminences) and migrate tangentially in a ventricle-directed manner to reach their neocortical targets while some others are derived from dorsal VZ and take a branching cell migration pattern to reach their final neocortical position *(51)*. In the spinal cord, the dorsoventral gradient of signaling molecules results in precise regions where neural stem cells give rise to distinct populations of interneurons, motor neurons, and oligodendrocytes (*see* refs. *52* and *53* for review), which migrate radially and/or tangentially to reach their destinations in the adult spinal cord. Alteration of signaling gradients in the spinal cord and other regions of the CNS results in misspecification of neural stem cells under the influence of those signaling centers.

REGULATION OF NEURAL STEMS CELL BY EXTRINSIC CUES

Neural stem cells receive spatial patterning cues along the dorsalventral (DV) *(54)* and anterior–posterior (AP) axes of the neural tube *(55)* and from other signaling centers as mentioned previously. These patterning cues regulate the internal transcriptional environment of stem cells which, in turn, regulate their responses to extrinsic cues, resulting in a wide variety of neural stem cells with different regional biases that can vary throughout the embryonic life (temporal differences). Neurosphere assays and in vitro clonal analyses of embryonic neural stem cells demonstrate that all the various stem cell populations conserve the capacity to proliferate and maintain their self-renewal ability and multipotentiality. The degree to which expansion of neural progenitor cells *ex vivo* causes developmental reprogramming remains to be determined. Nevertheless, individual or combinations of extrinsic signals influence the proliferation rate, fate bias, and cell cycle characteristics of embryonic neural stem cells in a variety of ways which are discussed in the following sections.

Regulation of Embryonic Neural Stem Cell Proliferation by Extrinsic Factors

Proliferation of stem cells is regulated by a variety of factors. The best characterized mitogens include the FGF and EGF families *(25–28)*. Stem cells can be expanded in culture by growth factors either as neurosphere clonal aggregates or as a monolayer of cells plated onto an adherent substratum. As mentioned previously, stem cells exhibit differing requirements for EGF and FGF2 during neural development. The preponderance of evidence suggests that proliferation of early embryonic progenitor species is regulated by FGF2 *(25,28,56)*, while later embryonic progenitors proliferate in either EGF or FGF *(46)*. Substantial evidence exists that FGF and EGF receptor activation regulates stem cell proliferation and survival in vivo. Mice lacking functional FGF2 have reduced tissue mass and reduced numbers of both neurons and glia in the cerebral cortex *(57,58)*, and injection of neonates with neutralizing antibodies to FGF2 reduces DNA synthesis in several areas of brain *(58)*. Conversely, injection of FGF2 into the cerebral ventricles of rat embryos increases the volume of cerebral cortex and the number of neurons generated *(59)*, and subcutaneous administration of FGF2 to neonatal rats increases neuroblast proliferation in regions still undergoing neurogenesis *(60)*. Finally, ligands of the FGF family including FGF2 are expressed contiguous to generative zones in the developing brain in vivo from early embryogenesis into adulthood *(61,62)*. Similarly, targeted deletion of the EGF receptor leads to defects in cortical neurogenesis *(63)*, and deletion of functional transforming growth factor-α (TGF-α) (which activates EGF receptors) leads to diminished proliferation of precursors in the SVZ of mature animals. Additional evidence involving injection of EGF receptor ligands into brains of mature rats supports a role for these ligands in stem cell proliferation in adults. Finally, TGF-α is expressed in close proximity to EGFR in several parts of the developing brain in vivo from E13 into adulthood *(64)*.

A number of other secreted factors have been demonstrated to promote stem cell proliferation. *Shh* is a member of the hedgehog *(hh)* multigene family that encodes signaling proteins involved in induction and patterning processes in vertebrate and invertebrate embryos *(see* refs. *62* and *65* for review). However, in addition to its effects on axial patterning and cellular differentiation, Shh directly regulates proliferation of neural stem cells. Ectopic overexpression of Shh in the mouse dorsal neural tube increases the rate of proliferation of embryonic spinal cord progenitor cells *(66)*, and Shh treatment increases proliferation of spinal cord stem cells in vitro *(67)*. Further, the N-terminal signaling domain of Shh increases proliferation of cultured SVZ stem cells *(68)*. In addition, this factor is a potent mitogen for cerebellar granule cell precursors *(69)*, neuronal restricted precursors in the spinal cord *(70)*, cultured retinal progenitor cells, and skeletal muscle cells, and overexpression of Shh leads to basal cell carcinoma *(see* refs. *65* and *66* for review). Wingless-int (Wnt) proteins have also been implicated in proliferation of neural stem cells. Dorsal midline Wnts, Wnt1 and Wnt3a, have mitogenic activity when overexpressed in the neural tube, while ventral Wnts Wnt3, Wnt4, Wnt7a, and Wnt7b do not effect proliferation in that system *(71,72)*. Wnts 3, 7a, and 7b stimulate the proliferation of cortex explant progenitors and increase the number of cells that can generate primary neurospheres in vitro *(73)*. Further, disruption of both Wnt1 and Wnt3a leads to deficits in expansion of dorsal neural progenitor cells *(74)*. The mitogenic effects of Wnt remain when Shh or FGF2 signaling is inhibited, although it has not been demonstrated whether Wnt signaling *per se* can act as a mitogen. However, overexpression of β-catenin, a transducer of Wnt signaling, maintains neural stem cells in cell cycle leading to excessive rounds of cell division *(75)*.

Other factors that positively regulate cell cycle include vasoactive intestinal peptide (VIP) and insulin-like growth factor 1 (IGF-1). Injection of pregnant mice from E9 to E11 with a VIP antagonist reduces bromodeoxyuridine (BrdU) labeling in germinal zones in the developing embryonic brains and reduces the subsequent size of the ventricular and intermediate zones *(76)*. Further, IGF1 is necessary for either EGF or FGF2-mediated proliferation of cultured neural stem cells, and neurosphere generation is dependent on IGF1 in a dose-dependent manner *(77)*. Similarly, IGF1 is a mitogen for purified granule cell precursors *(78)* and retinal precursors *(79)*. Other types of regulatory signals decrease stem cell proliferation, often by promoting exit from cell cycle and differentiation. Examples include cytokines such as the BMP family and stem cell factor (SCF), peptides such as pituitary adenylate cyclase-activating peptide (PACAP) and opioids, neurotrophins such as brain-derived neurotrophic factor (BDNF) and neurotrophin-3 (NT-3), and neurotransmitters including glutamate, γ-aminobutyric acid (GABA), and dopamine. These factors are discussed in more depth when the issue of lineage commitment is addressed later in this chapter.

Neural Stem Cell Survival and Programmed Cell Death

Many of the same factors that promote proliferation of stem cells also enhance their survival. Embryonic and postnatal stem cells do not survive well in culture in the absence of added growth factors, but they survive when cultured in the presence of mitogens such as FGF2 or EGF along with IGF and/or insulin *(80)*. FGF2 is an essential survival and proliferation factor for cortical progenitors both in vivo *(59,81)* and in vitro *(82,83)*. Other FGF family members such as FGF4 and FGF8b can also promote survival, but not proliferation, of cortical precursor cells as demonstrated by clonal analysis using retroviral tagging *(84)*. EGF/TNF-α can also promote the survival of late (SVZ) embryonic stem cells by activating either EGFR or ErbB3 *(85)*. EGFR is necessary for progenitor survival along the dorsal midline *(86)*, where ErbB3 expression is limited. However some neural stem cells express ErbB3 in vitro, and both EGF and the Neuregulins increase cell survival by signaling through Erb pathways *(87)*. Neurotrophins also modulate survival of some neural stem cell and progenitor populations. Cultured cortical progenitors express BDNF, NT-3, and their receptors TrkB and TrkC. Inhibition of endogenous neurotrophins decreases the survival of cortical progenitors by decreasing phosphatidyl inositol-3-kinase (PI3-kinase) signaling, and also decreases both proliferation and neurogenesis by inhibiting activation of the MEK/ERK pathway *(88)*. Erythropoietin also promotes survival and proliferation of neural progenitor cells, and loss of the erythropoietin receptor in mice affects brain development as early as E10.5, resulting in a reduction in the number of progenitor cells and increased apoptosis *(89)*.

Stem cell numbers are primarily regulated by the balance between proliferation and reentry into cell cycle and the rate of exit from cell cycle into a differentiated or quiescent state *(20,90)*. However, stem cell numbers may also be influenced by apoptotic cell death within periventricular generative zones. Targeted disruption of either apoptotic intermediaries Caspase-9 or Caspase-3 leads to decreased programmed cell death (PCD) of cortical precursors, causing expansion and exencephaly of the forebrain as well as supernumerary neurons in the cerebral cortex *(91)*. Further, Caspase-3 activation leads to PCD indicating that neural progenitors possess a Caspase-dependent apoptotic pathway *(92)*. By contrast, disruption of either Bcl-X or Bax does not alter the size of the VZ *(93,94)*, demonstrating that not all apoptotic pathways are involved in PCD of neural stem cells. Similarly, the Fas "death receptor" is unlikely to play a role in PCD of early neural stem cells since Fas expression during nervous system development occurs relatively late and not in the VZ *(95)*. By contrast, disruption of the c-Jun N-terminal kinase signaling pathway leads to precocious degeneration of cerebral precursors *(91)*. Removal of cell survival and/or proliferation cues also leads to PCD. In the developing chick neural tube, removal of the ventral source of Shh causes massive cell death, which is rescued by expression of a dominant-negative form of Ptc1 that interferes with a C-terminal apoptotic domain exposed by cleavage of Ptc1 by Caspase-3. Transfection of cultured stem cells with the C-terminal region of Ptc1 is sufficient to induce cell death. Further, overexpression of Ptc1 in cultured stem cells induces apoptosis, which is blocked by addition of Shh *(96)*. These observations suggest that Ptc1 expression is proapoptotic and induces PCD in the absence of Shh.

Maintenance of the Neural Stem Cell Fate

In early embryos, the neural stem cell phenotype is maintained by both daughter cells during the period of symmetric cell divisions and rapid expansion of the stem cell pool, and during later asymmetric cell divisions it is maintained by one daughter cell of each pair. A number of extrinsic cues have been identified as factors that promote self-renewal, but in some stem cells they simultaneously seem to bias commitment. The most extensively studied example of such inhibitory signaling involves the Notch pathway. Notch and its ligands Delta and Serrate are integral membrane proteins that generally transmit signals only between cells in direct contact. Overexpression of Delta1 (i.e., activation of Notch on neighboring cells) suppresses neurogenesis, whereas overexpression of a dominant negative inhibitor of Delta1 leads to premature commitment of stem cells to the neuronal fate *(97)*. Activation of Notch also regulates transcription of its downstream targets, including inhibition of production of Notch ligands by that cell. Through a process termed lateral inhibition, cells that produce ligand force neighboring cells to produce less ligand, thereby enabling the ligand-producing cells to increase production even further. The effect of such a feedback loop is to amplify small differences between neighboring cells and to drive them into different developmental pathways. Delta1 is expressed by a scattered subset of cells (nascent neurons *[98]*) in the outer part of the VZ, whereas Notch1 is expressed throughout the VZ *(99)*. Delta production by daughter cells undergoing neuronal differentiation activates Notch in their dividing partners, thereby inhibiting their neuronal differentiation and maintaining a cohort of stem cells so that neurogenesis can continue. Some of these effects are mediated through activation of genes of the *Hes* family such as *Hes1* and *Hes5*, as discussed later in this chapter (*see also* ref. *100* for review). Notch1 signaling also inhibits differentiation into alternative fates such as oligodendroglial differentiation *(101)*. Further studies suggest that notch signaling promotes the generation of radial glia *(102)* and can even bias cells toward a glial fate rather than promoting self-renewal *(103)*. However, because both embryonic radial glia *(104,105)* and later adult SVZ "astrocytes" *(106)* possess stem cell properties, the reported bias toward a glial fate (in part defined by expression of GFAP) may be equivalent to maintaining the stem cell fate.

More recent studies demonstrate that extrinsic factors signaling through the leukemia inhibitory factor receptor (LIFR)/glycoprotein130 (gp130) complex including ciliary neurotrophic factor (CNTF) and LIF promote self-renewal *(107)*. In *LIFR* null mice, adult neural stem cell numbers are reduced. Further, intraventricular infusion of CNTF into the adult mouse forebrain, in the absence or presence of EGF, enhances neural stem cell self-renewal in vivo. CNTF inhibits lineage restriction of EGF-responsive neural stem cells to glial progenitors in vitro, which in turn results in enhanced expansion of stem cell number without disturbing cell proliferation. Further, a link between gp130 regulation and Notch activity has been identified. CNTF increases Notch1 activity in forebrain EGF-responsive neural stem cells. Infusion of EGF plus CNTF into adult forebrain lateral ventricles also increases periventricular Notch1 activity compared with EGF alone. Interestingly, the gp130-enhanced Notch1 signaling that regulates neural stem cell maintenance appears to be *Hes1/5* independent *(108)*. Wnts may also play a role in neural stem cell maintenance in addition to their proliferative role. Wnt7a and 7b increase the number of cells that can generate primary neurospheres in vitro *(73)*. Further, overexpression of the Wnt signaling mediator β-catenin in developing brain increases stem cell reentry into cell cycle within the VZ *(75)*. However, the effects of β-catenin on reentry of cultured stem cells into the cell cycle depend on the presence of concurrent FGF signaling *(109)*.

Exit From Cell Cycle and Lineage Commitment

Many extrinsic signals promote exit from the cell cycle by neural stem cells, often by activating cyclin-dependent kinase inhibitors (CKIs) *(110–112)*. Bone morphogenetic proteins (BMPs) promote rapid exit of stem cells from the cell cycle via CKI p19INK4d *(113)* even in the presence of mitogens such as FGF2, EGF, or Shh *(68,114)*. PACAP is an antimitogenic signal in the developing cerebral cortex *(115)* and in cortical precursor cells cultured in the presence of mitogens such as EGF, FGF2, and IGF1 *(116)*. The effects of PACAP are mediated by p57Kip2 protein, but not other CKIs such as p21Cip1 or p27Kip1 *(117)*. Intriguingly, PACAP conversely stimulates proliferation during oligodendrocyte (OL) development and delays maturation and/or myelinogenesis *(118)*. Furthermore, proliferation of cortical stem cells cultured in the presence of FGF2 is diminished by cotreatment with the prodifferentiation factor Neurotrophin 3 (NT-3) *(82,83)*.

Neurotransmitters also regulate cell cycle in neural stem cells (*see* ref. *119* for review). Depending upon the developmental stage of the stem cell, GABA may either increase *(120,121)* or decrease *(122)* proliferation and partially blocks the mitogenic actions of FGF2 on cortical progenitors *(123)*. Similar to GABA, glutamate may also increase or decrease cell proliferation in the cortex by changing the cell cycle time, and both glutamate and GABA increase the size of cortical VZ clones but decrease SVZ clone size *(121)*. In contrast, dopamine D1-like receptor activation reduces G_1- to S-phase entry in VZ stem cells, whereas D2-like receptor activation promotes reentry in SVZ stem cells *(124)*. In striatal progenitor cells, *N*-methyl-D-aspartate (NMDA) receptor activation promotes and is required for proliferation *(125)*, while receptor blockade inhibits it *(126)*. In sum, these studies suggest that the effects of amino acid neurotransmitters on the proliferative behavior of neural stem cells are dependent on and contribute to the regional and temporal differences among different populations of stem cells *(127,128)*.

Substantial overlap exists among the extrinsic factors involved in proliferation and survival and those that regulate lineage commitment and cellular differentiation (*see* ref. *129* for review). For example, withdrawal of FGF2 from cultured stem cells promotes generation of neurons and glia, suggesting that the factor represses intrinsic programs of stem cell differentiation. However, exposure of stem cells to FGF2 also alters their subsequent developmental bias. Treatment of cultured stem cells with FGF2 promotes expression of the EGF receptor *(56,130)* and enhances expression of differentiated traits such as the catecholamine biosynthetic enzyme tyrosine hydroxylase *(131)*. Moreover, the concentrations of FGF2 to which neural stem cells are exposed in vitro influence cell fate; low concentrations of FGF2 favor neuronal differentiation, whereas higher concentrations favor oligodendroglial differentiation *(28)*. This may reflect preferential activation of different subtypes of FGF receptors by different concentrations of the factor, a conclusion supported by observations of the differential neurogenic effects of other FGF family members. For example, treatment of cultured stem cells with FGF1 in the presence of heparan sulfate proteoglycan preferentially promotes neuronal differentiation, whereas FGF2 treatment of sister cultures preferentially promotes proliferation *(132)*. FGF8 collaborates with Shh to induce dopaminergic neurons in the mid/hindbrain, whereas FGF4 in association with Shh induces a serotonergic cell fate *(133)*.

Shh is another important factor in the regulation of lineage commitment by neural stem cells (*see* ref. *65* for review). Treatment of cultured neural stem cells with Shh promotes the elaboration of both neuronal and oligodendroglial lineage species *(68)*, suggesting direct differentiating actions of Shh on neural stem cells. Furthermore, neural stem cells express Smoothened *(68)*, the signaling component of the Shh receptor, and constitutively active forms of Smoothened reproduce inductive effects of Shh *(134)*, suggesting that Shh exerts its inductive effects directly on stem cells. As noted above, interactions between the effects of Shh and other growth factors including Wnt, FGF4, and FGF8, are critical for specifying alternate cellular phenotypes in the brain *(133)*. Interactions between Shh and members of the BMP family are important for the specification of dorsal and intermediate dorsoventral cell types in the neural tube (*see* refs. *135* and *136* for review), and Shh inhibits BMP signaling, in part by inducing the endogenous BMP inhibitor noggin *(137)*. Shh and BMP signaling exert directly opposing effects on both proliferation and differentiation of cultured neural stem cells *(68)*.

Other extrinsic neuronal differentiation factors include BMP family members *(36,66,68)*, Wnt family members *(138)*, retinoid-activated pathways *(139,140)*, platelet-derived growth factor (PDGF) *(27,141,142)*, cell adhesion molecule L1 *(143)*, paracrine nitric oxide *(144)*, and other signaling molecules (*see* refs. *127* and *145* for review). The existence of so many pathways for neuronal lineage commitment and differentiation presumably reflects the diversity of neuronal phenotypes that must be generated. Clearly, there is diversity among stem/progenitor cell populations even at early developmental stages (*see* refs. *25* and *146* for review), and there are developmental changes in stem cells that lead to markedly different cell fate decisions in response to the same factors at different developmental stages *(46)*. Commitment and differentiation of stem cells to specific neuronal lineages, thus, reflect complex patterns of developmental events and numerous pathways for neurogenesis.

Just as multiple extrinsic cues induce neuronal differentiation, several different pathways lead neural stem cells toward astrocytic lineage commitment. Gliogenesis peaks during late embryonic and early perinatal cerebral cortical development, and SVZ stem cells are biased toward astrocytic differentiation compared with VZ stem cells. BMP treatment promotes the elaboration of mature astrocytes from both late embryonic SVZ-derived stem cells and early postnatal cerebral cortical multipotent progenitors and bipotent oligodendroglial-type 2 astroglial (O-2A) progenitor cells in culture *(114,147)*, and transgenic overexpression of BMP4 increases the number of astrocytes in the brain *(148)*. Ciliary neurotrophic factor (CNTF) and LIF also potentiate the generation of astrocytes from embryonic neural stem cells. Genetic and developmental analyses confirm that a CNTF/LIF subgroup of factors that interacts with gp130/LIF-β receptors participates in astrogliogenesis *(149,150)*. However, BMP-2 treatment of progenitor cells cultured from animals that are deficient in the LIF-β receptor induces astrocytic lineage commitment, indicating that astrocytic differentiation does not require signaling through gp130/LIFRs *(150)*. CNTF and LIF signal through the

JAK/STAT signaling pathway, whereas the BMPs signal through Smad-mediated pathways. Formation of a complex between STAT3 and Smad1, bridged by the transcriptional coactivator p300, may mediate cooperative effects of these two classes of factors on stem cell commitment to the astrocytic lineage *(151)*. However, the astrocyte inducing effects of CNTF/LIF are dependent on the EGFR. Premature elevation of EGFRs confers premature competence to interpret LIF as an astrocyte-inducing signal whereas EGFR-null progenitors from late embryonic cortex do not interpret LIF as an astrocyte-inducing signal. LIF responsiveness in EGFR-null cells is rescued by the addition of EGFRs but not FGFRs. Further, EGFRs regulate an increase both in STAT3 levels and STAT3 phosphorylation in response to LIF. Increasing STAT3 also increases the phosphorylation of STAT3 by LIF, but, in contrast to overexpressing EGFRs, increasing STAT3 does not augment the astrocyte-inducing effect of LIF. These observations suggest that EGFRs also regulate LIF responsiveness downstream of STAT3 *(43)*. Other astrocyte inducing extrinsic cues have been recently described. Studies in both the cortex and retina have provided evidence that Notch, or its downstream transcriptional effectors such as *Hes* genes, can promote CNS astrocytic differentiation in vivo *(102,152; see also* ref. *103* for review), as well as in vitro *(153)*. PACAP promotes SVZ progenitor exit from cell cycle and an astrocyte fate similar to BMP induction but through cAMP and CREB signaling instead of Smad *(154)*. Neuregulin1 (Nrg1), also known as glial growth factor (GGF), promotes astrocyte differentiation at the expense of oligodendrocyte differentiation *(87,155)*. Taken together, various pathways exist for astrocyte differentiation, which may produce different astrocyte populations similar to the diversity of neurogenic pathways.

In view of the foregoing observations regarding multiple pathways of neuronal and astrocytic lineage commitment, it is not surprising that oligodendroglia (OLs) also appear to be generated from multiple lineages in response to a number of different epigenetic signals (*see* refs. *156* and *157* for review). During embryonic spinal cord development the expression of Jagged, a Notch ligand, coincides with the elaboration of foci of OL precursors from paramedian generative zones. Shh, a notochord-derived signal, was originally described to support the generation of mature OL lineage species from caudal regions of the neuraxis (spinal cord), but has more recently been confirmed to function similarly in anterior regions (telencephalon) *(158,159)*. Oligodendroglia are first generated in the embryonic spinal cord in response to signals derived from the floor plate and notochord including but not limited to Shh *(160,161)*. Treatment of spinal cord explants with Shh induces both OLs and neurons *(161)*, and antibodies that neutralize Shh prevent OL lineage commitment *(160)*. Shh treatment of embryonic neural stem cells cultured as neurospheres also induces both oligodendroglial and neuronal differentiation *(68)*, suggesting that OL lineage commitment reflects direct effects of Shh on stem cells. Other factors are also capable of promoting OL lineage commitment by cultured neural stem cells. For example, increased concentrations of FGF2 or brief exposure to thyroid hormone foster OL differentiation *(27,28,162)*. Conversely OL commitment by neural stem cells is inhibited by the BMPs both in culture *(68,163)* and in vivo *(148)*, and by Notch1 *(101)* and neuregulins *(87)* in culture. The regulation of later stages of OL differentiation from glial restricted precursors is described elsewhere in this volume.

INTRINSIC FACTORS REGULATING NEURAL STEM CELL FATE

While extrinsic cues play a role in determining the rate of neural stem cell proliferation as well as the timing of differentiation and the fate of the cell and its progeny, they are not sufficient to explain all of the complex decisions made by neural stem cells. When a clonal population of neural stem cells is exposed to an extrinsic factor in vitro, there is variability in the response of the cells to the factor and the ultimate effects on differentiation. One reason for this variability is that proteins and other molecules expressed within each cell, or intrinsic factors, vary within populations of neural stem cells and alter cellular responses to extrinsic cues. Intrinsic regulators include the cellular machinery necessary for asymmetric cell divisions, transcription factors and chromosomal modifications controlling gene expression. It is not clearly understood how differences in levels of intrinsic factors arise across a clonal population of cells. The two predominant theories are that extrinsic factors modulate levels of intrinsic molecules over time such that slight differences in the level and combination of signaling molecules encountered accumulate to give each cell a unique identity and/or there is an inherent mechanism that may be linked to the number of times the cell has divided. Intrinsic factors in turn alter the amount of signaling molecules secreted; thus there exists a dynamic relationship between intrinsic and extrinsic cues.

Positive and Negative bHLH Factors

One of the most studied groups of intrinsic factors influencing cell cycle exit and fate determination by embryonic neural stem cells are the basic helix–loop–helix (bHLH) transcription factors. bHLH proteins are critical for all phases of neural development: proliferation, neurogenesis, astrogliogenesis and oligodendrogenesis. In general, negative bHLH factors promote cell cycle continuation and prevent differentiation while positive bHLH factors promote differentiation into specific cell types. Astrocyte formation seems to be an exception and is discussed later in this chapter. Levels of bHLH factors vary across a population of neural stem cells and contribute to the complexity of responses to extrinsic cues observed both in culture and in a developing embryo.

The major negative bHLH transcription factors expressed by neural stem cells are the Hes and Herp (Hes related protein, also known as Hey) families. Hes family proteins were originally isolated as mammalian orthologs of *hairy* and *enhancer of split*, which negatively regulate neurogenesis in *Drosophila (164,165)*. Until recently, Hes proteins were largely viewed as mediators of Notch signaling. While it is clear that Notch receptor activation directly leads to increased levels of Hes proteins, new evidence indicates that other signaling pathways also promote their expression. For example, TGF-β signaling positively regulates *Hes1 (166)*. Furthermore, there are Hes-independent effects of Notch activation. For instance, the Notch intracellular domain associates with the transcription factor LEF1 to control a range of target genes *(167)*. Therefore, activation of Notch signaling and increasing levels of Hes proteins are not exactly functionally equivalent, although the effects of expressing a constitutively active form of the Notch receptor and over expressing Hes proteins are similar.

Of the seven murine Hes family members, Hes1, Hes3, and Hes5 have been most extensively studied in the central nervous system. Hes1 and Hes5 expression in the CNS is largely confined to cells in the periventricular proliferative zones, although

Hes1 continues to be expressed by mature astrocytes *(165,168)*. Hes3 is expressed exclusively by cerebellar purkinje cells *(165)*. Overexpression of Hes1 prevents both migration of neural stem cells out of the VZ and expression of neuronal markers *(169)*, whereas null mutation of Hes1 or Hes5 leads to premature expression of neuronal traits *(170,171)*. Hes1 negatively regulates transcriptional activation mediated by proneural bHLH genes and thus normally functions to repress the commitment of stem cells to the neuronal lineage, thereby maintaining their self-renewing state *(172)*. Interestingly, one member of the Hes family, Hes6, represses the actions of other Hes proteins through multiple mechanisms and promotes neuronal differentiation when overexpressed in neural stem cell cultures *(173)*. Finally, the related Herp family in mouse consists of three members that are expressed in only partially overlapping domains, and it is hypothesized that the Herp proteins functionally replace the Hes proteins in cells lacking Hes expression.

Stem cell fate may also be maintained by the four members of the ID (*i*nhibitor of *d*ifferentiation) family of proteins that resemble bHLH factors but that lack a basic region necessary for DNA binding. The ID proteins act as dominant negative inhibitors by preferentially dimerizing with a subset of bHLH factors to form inactive complexes, thereby decreasing bHLH-mediated transcriptional activity *(174)*. In one well-described example, IDs sequester E proteins, inhibiting the function of bHLH proteins that require E proteins for their activity. For example, the proneural bHLH protein Neurogenin2 must bind to E12 in order to bind to DNA and activate target gene transcription in stem cells. In the presence of IDs, E12 is effectively sequestered and Neurogenin2 target genes (including the neuronal differentiation gene *NeuroD*) are indirectly repressed, inhibiting neuronal differentiation *(175)*. IDs also actively promote proliferation of neural stem cells by binding to Retinoblastoma family members and inhibiting their ability to interfere with cell cycle progression *(176)*. Members of the ID family are expressed throughout the nervous system during neurogenesis with localization of ID transcripts within putative neural stem cells *(177,178)*. Targeted disruption of both ID1 and ID3 in the same animals results in premature withdrawal of neuroblasts from cell cycle and expression of neuron-specific differentiation markers *(179)*. These observations suggest that expression of ID proteins is necessary to maintain stem cells in the undifferentiated, proliferative state.

In addition to HLH transcription factors, recent work has demonstrated that β-catenin regulates neural stem cell proliferation and ultimately cortical size. β-catenin serves both a mechanical function as a component of adherens junctions and a signal transduction function upon translocation to the nucleus. In adherens junctions, β-catenin is among the complex of molecules that link cadherins to the actin cytoskeleton *(180,181)*. The cytoplasmic pool of β-catenin is regulated by phosphorylation by GSK-3β leading to ubiquitination and degradation in proteasomes *(182)*. Under certain conditions, particularly in response to Wnt/Wingless signaling, GSK-3β activity is inhibited and free β-catenin is able to translocate to the nucleus and mediate transcription, for instance by binding to LEF/TCF to activate Wnt target-genes *(182)*. β-Catenin is highly expressed in neural stem cells and is enriched at adherens junctions surrounding the ventricles *(75)*. Transgenic mice expressing stabilized β-catenin in neural precursor cells have dramatically increased brain size with the proliferative zone expanded laterally to such an extent that the brain appears to be convoluted. Immunohistochemical analysis revealed that the neural stem cell population is greatly increased owing to enhanced reentry of cells into cell cycle *(183)*. However, the effects of β-catenin on stem cell fate in vitro are dependent upon the presence or absence of concurrent FGF signaling. In the presence of FGF signaling, β-catenin maintains cells in cell cycle whereas in the absence of FGF signaling it biases stem cells toward neuronal differentiation *(109)*.

The observation that maintenance of the stem cell phenotype requires inhibition of positive bHLH factors by ID proteins and/or Hes family members suggests that positive bHLH factors are involved in directing stem cell differentiation. There is, in fact, a large body of evidence that regulatory cascades of bHLH and other transcription factors play essential roles in mammalian neurogenesis and oligodendrogenesis. Positive bHLH factors include neuron-promoting factors (proneural genes) and oligodendrocyte-promoting factors. Proneural bHLH proteins are a family of transcriptional transactivators that have been shown to be crucial for neuron formation. They are expressed in progenitor cells in the ventricular zone and at low levels in the intermediate zone, but they are not found in the differentiating neurons in the cortical plate *(184–186)*. Proneural proteins are expressed in progenitors that give rise to both neurons and astrocytes *(187)*. Recently, some mammalian orthologs of *Drosophila atonal* (*NeuroD*, *Nex/NeuroD2*) have been referred to as neuron-differentiation genes because they act downstream of proneural Neurogenins, are expressed later in the course of differentiation, and seem to direct a cell toward a more terminal neuron fate *(188)*. These proteins are expressed only in cells destined to become neurons and in immature neurons in the cortical plate and are maintained as neuronal differentiation proceeds *(189)*. Proneural and neuron-differentiation proteins are sufficient to induce exit from cell cycle and neuronal differentiation when they are expressed in cultured neural stem cells *(190)*. These proteins act as transcriptional activators and form heterodimers with E proteins to bind DNA at hexameric E-box sites (CANNTG) to activate the transcription of target genes *(190)*.

In the telencephalon, proneural genes *Neurogenin1* (*Ngn1*) and *Ngn2* are expressed dorsally in developing neocortex while *Mash1* (mouse *achaete-scute* homolog) is expressed ventrally in the ganglionic eminences *(184–186)*. Loss of *Mash1* results in a significant loss of GABAergic interneurons of the cortex, which mostly originate in the ganglionic eminences *(191)*. Double knockout of *Mash1* and *Ngn2* drastically reduces the number of cortical neurons formed. When stem cells are cultured from these double mutant mice they produce far more astrocytes and fewer neurons than control cultures *(192)*. These observations are consistent with the ability of proneural proteins to up-regulate panneuronal proteins such as β-tubulin III and neurofilament M. Interestingly, there is evidence that proneural proteins specify the regional identity of neurons as well. In mice lacking *Ngn2*, *Mash1* is expressed ectopically in dorsal cortical progenitors. The number of neurons formed in these mice is unchanged, but their identity is changed from a glutamatergic pyramidal neuron phenotype to a GABAergic interneuron phenotype *(192)*. This phenotype is also seen when the *Ngn2* coding sequence is replaced by the *Mash1* coding sequence *(193)*. However, when the reverse experiment is performed (*Ngn2* is knocked into the *Mash1* locus), the ventral telencephalon forms normally *(194)*. Thus, the proneural genes clearly promote neuronal differentiation of stem cells and their additional role in subtype identity depends on other factors within the cells.

As mentioned before, a dynamic relationship exists between the intrinsic and extrinsic cues, an elegant example of which seen in the mechanism by which proneural genes actively inhibit astrocytic differentiation of stem cells in addition to promoting neuronal differentiation. The active inhibition of the astrocyte fate was demonstrated in a series of in vitro studies. Ngn1 overexpression in neural stem cells extracted from E14 mouse cortex led to increased neuronal differentiation and suppressed astrocyte formation. BrdU labeling showed no change in the rate of proliferation of neural progenitors indicating that the effect was not due to selective proliferation of neuronal committed precursors. As mentioned previously, gp130 signaling by LIF/CNTF has been shown to promote astrocyte formation (as determined by immunoreactivity to anti-GFAP antibody). In cultures of neural stem cells overexpressing Ngn1, the number of astrocytes formed on addition of LIF/CNTF is greatly reduced. Finally, expression of Ngn1 in astrocyte cultures results in severe disruption of cell morphology and cell adhesion *(195)*. A molecular mechanism for this active suppression of gliogenesis has been proposed. As mentioned earlier, LIF and CNTF signaling converge with BMP signaling by the formation of a highly gliogenic STAT–p300–SMAD complex in cells with little or no Ngn expression *(151)*. When Ngn is expressed in neural stem cells, it binds to and effectively sequesters p300, preventing the formation of the STAT–p300–SMAD complex. This mechanism is further supported by the observation that a mutant of Ngn1 that cannot bind DNA is still capable of suppressing gliogenesis *(195)*.

Thus far, only one family of positive bHLH factors has been shown to be pro-oligodendroglial, the *Olig* gene family. *Olig1* and *Olig2* are expressed in ventral regions of the developing brain and spinal cord in a pattern that covers, but is not limited to, the area from which oligodendrocytes arise *(196–198)*. *Olig1* and *Olig2* double mutant mice lack all oligodendrocytes and oligodendrocyte precursor cells in the entire central nervous system *(199)*. Misexpression of *Olig1* in the embryonic rat brain results in an increased number of oligodendrocytes *(196)*. These results demonstrate that *Olig* genes function to specify oligodendrocytes. However, *Olig* genes are expressed in stem cells destined to become neurons as well. In the spinal cord, they are expressed in progenitor cells that will give rise to motor neurons, although *Olig* expression is lost as these cells mature *(197,200,201)*. *Ngn2* is also expressed in motor neuron precursor cells and is necessary for the formation of neurons from these *Olig* expressing cells *(200,201)*. In the brain, *Olig2* is expressed rather broadly throughout the ventral telencephalon and therefore may be involved in GABAergic neuron specification in addition to its role in oligodendrogenesis.

The transcription factors responsible for astrogliogenesis are still unknown. It appears that the astrocyte fate is determined in part by a lack of proneural and pro-oligodendroglial transcription factors, although recent evidence suggests that Notch activation or over expression of Hes proteins actively promotes astrocyte differentiation under certain conditions. When Hes1, Hes5, Herp1, or Herp2 is expressed early in brain development, the population of neural stem cells increases at the expense of early-born neurons (although if the expression is transient there is an increase in late-born neurons) but when expressed later in development there is an increase in the number of astrocytes *(152,164,165,169–172,202–205)*. Hes proteins have also been shown to promote astrocytic fate in glial restricted progenitor cells (GRPs) isolated from rat spinal cords *(168)*. (For more information on GRPs, see Chapter 7 in this volume). As mentioned previously, neural stem cells proceed through rather distinct phases of symmetric division, neurogenesis, and astrogliogenesis. This pattern is observed both in vivo and in culture. The timing of these phases is correlated with the levels of Hes and proneural bHLH proteins in the stem cell population as a whole. During the proliferative phase, Hes levels are high and proneural levels are low. During the neuron differentiation phase, proneural levels increase significantly and Hes levels decrease. During the astrocyte differentiation phase, Hes predominates and proneural proteins decrease to very low levels *(188)*.

Homeodomain Genes in Fate Commitment

Homeodomain genes have long been regarded as patterning genes that are expressed in distinct domains to define cellular positions along the dorsal–ventral, anterior–posterior, and medial–lateral axes of the developing nervous system. All neural stem cells express a region-specific combination of homeodomain genes. When grown in culture, some studies have shown continuous expression of region-specific genes while others show that they are dysregulated when the cells are removed from signaling centers and grown in the presence of mitogens. In the developing embryo, homeodomain gene expression is necessary for the maintenance of patterning. For example, *Pax6* expression is necessary to maintain dorsal–ventral patterning in the central nervous system. *Pax6* is expressed in the developing eye, olfactory epithelium, telencephalon, diencephalon, hindbrain, and spinal cord (although expression in each of these tissues varies with the age of the embryo) *(206)*. In the telencephalon, *Pax6* is expressed only in the dorsal (pallial) region. Loss of *Pax6* leads to ectopic dorsal expression of genes ordinarily confined to the ventral ganglionic eminences such as the *Dlx* genes *(207,208)*. However, a new role for homeodomain genes in the direct control of lineage commitment is emerging, and a model is gaining support in which the specification of a generic neuron occurs concomitantly with the specification of a specific subtype of neuron with appropriate regional identity. This is illustrated by studies of the function of *Pax6* in the developing brain in which *Pax6* is expressed exclusively by radial glial cells *(207)*. In the *Sey* (small eye) mouse, which carries a mutation in the *Pax6* gene, the morphology, gene expression and neurogenic potential of radial glia are altered *(207,209)*. In vitro, radial glia derived from *Sey* mice give rise to significantly fewer neuronal clones and more glial clones *(209)*. Furthermore, expression of *Pax6* in mature astrocyte cultures leads to positive immunoreactivity to antibodies against neuron-specific proteins *(209)*. This is consistent with previous studies demonstrating that loss of *Pax6* from the dorsal forebrain results in loss of expression of *Ngn2 (210)*. Moreover, in the ventral spinal cord, the enhancer elements that drive *Ngn2* expression are dependent on *Pax6* function *(210)*. However, the difference in phenotype between the *Ngn2* mutant mouse and the *Sey* mouse indicate that the effects of Pax6 mutation on neurogenic potential are mediated through mechanisms beyond the control of *Ngn2*.

In addition to regulating the patterning of the nervous system and the neurogenic potential of neural stem cells, homeodomain genes are also well described as regulators of neuron subtype identity. For example, *Dlx*, the vertebrate ortholog of *Drosophila Distal-less*, is a family of homeodomain genes expressed in the ventral telencephalic ganglionic eminence stem cells. *Dlx1* and *Dlx2* are expressed in cells that give rise to virtually all GABAergic neurons in the forebrain *(211–214)*. *Dlx1/2* double mutants show a dramatic reduction in late-born projection neurons (GABAergic) of the basal ganglia and of several types of interneurons (GABAergic, dopaminergic and cholinergic) in the cerebral cortex *(212)*. These data indicate that *Dlx* genes are important for development of late-born neurons from the ganglionic eminence generative zone. Dlx proteins may actively promote a GABAergic phenotype by positively regulating the GABA synthesis enzyme glutamic acid decarboxylase (*see* ref. *215* for review).

Homeodomain proteins and positive bHLH factors act together in fate determination. A striking example is the *Lim* homeodomain gene family during motor neuron development. In the spinal cord, combinatorial actions of proneural bHLH and Lim homeodomain proteins in developing motor neurons brings the two classes of transcription factors together literally on the same enhancer sequence for a motor neuron-specific gene. Lim homeodomain proteins Isl1 and Lhx3 act with proneural/neuron-differentiation bHLH proteins NeuroM and Ngn2 in specification of spinal cord motor neurons. Isl1, Lhx3, NeuroM, or Ngn1 can each weakly activate the Hb9 promoter, a motor neuron specific promoter, when acting alone. When all four proteins are expressed together they act synergistically to strongly activate the Hb9 promoter. This synergy arises from a conformational change that occurs when the two Lim homeodomain proteins bind the promoter. This conformational change in the DNA facilitates concurrent binding of the bHLH factors to the promoter, resulting in strong activation of the *Hb9* gene *(216,217)*. Such cooperation is not limited to neuron formation: Olig2 associates directly with homeodomain protein Nkx2.2 to mediate oligodendrogenesis *(218)*.

In summary, lineage commitment and progressive differentiation involve the coordinated interplay of positive and negative regulatory signals, including cascades of transcription factors that regulate lineage-specific gene expression. Furthermore, multiple signaling cascades are involved in the generation of different populations of neurons, oligodendrocytes, and astrocytes, and activation of these cascades reflects the effects of both cell intrinsic as well as extrinsic factors that promote cell differentiation.

Cell Cycle Exit and Cell Differentiation

The discovery that there is overlap between factors regulating cell cycle progression and those regulating cell fate decisions sheds light on the mechanism by which cell cycle exit is coordinated with fate determination. Patterning genes *BF1*, *Emx2*, and *Pax6* regulate the rate of proliferation of cortical progenitor cells *(219–222)*. In the developing retina, patterning genes *Rx1*, *Six3*, and *XOptx2* promote proliferation of progenitor cells, although this effect is seen only in the regions in which they are usually expressed *(223–226)*. Cell cycle control protein p21 has been implicated in the oligodendrocyte lineage since its buildup in the cell is necessary for oligodendrogenesis, where it serves a function independent of its ability to promote exit from cell cycle *(227)*.

There is also evidence that the level of proneural genes may be coordinated with the stage of the cell cycle in vivo. As discussed previously, neural stem cells undergo interkinetic nuclear migration as they progress through the cell cycle such that S phase occurs when the nucleus is located furthest from the ventricle, and G_2, M, and G_1 phases occur when the nucleus is close to the ventricular surface. *In situ* analysis and BrDU labeling revealed that the expression of Ngn1, Ngn2, Notch1, and Delta1 is much higher when the cell body is near the ventricular surface during G_2, M and G_1, and that expression is greatly reduced during S phase when the cell body is further from the ventricle *(228)*. In a population of neural stem cells, either in vivo or in culture, cell cycle stages are asynchronous; therefore the neurogenic potential also fluctuates asynchronously. This may contribute to the variation in response to extrinsic factors observed in clonal cultures of neural stem cells and may partially explain how the cellular complexity of the nervous system is achieved.

REFERENCES

1. Potten, C. S. and Loeffler, M. (1990) Stem cells: attributes, cycles, spirals, pitfalls and uncertainties. Lessons for and from the crypt. *Development* **110,** 1001–1020.
2. Lendahl, U., Zimmerman, L. B., and McKay, R. D. (1990) CNS stem cells express a new class of intermediate filament protein. *Cell* **60,** 585–595.
3. Sakakibara, S., Imai, T., Hamaguchi, K., et al. (1996) Mouse-Musashi-1, a neural RNA-binding protein highly enriched in the mammalian CNS stem cell. *Dev. Biol.* **176,** 230–242.
4. Pevny, L. H., Sockanathan, S., Placzek, M., and Lovell-Badge, R. (1998) A role for SOX1 in neural determination. *Development* **125,** 1967–1978.
5. Graham, V., Khudyakov, J., Ellis, P., and Pevny, L. (2003) SOX2 functions to maintain neural progenitor identity. *Neuron* **39,** 749–765.
6. Liu, Y., Wu, Y., Lee, J. C., et al. (2002) Oligodendrocyte and astrocyte development in rodents: an in situ and immunohistological analysis during embryonic development. *Glia* **40,** 25–43.
7. Morrison, S. J., White, P. M., Zock, C., and Anderson, D. J. (1999) Prospective identification, isolation by flow cytometry, and in vivo self-renewal of multipotent mammalian neural crest stem cells. *Cell* **96,** 737–749.
8. Uchida, N., Buck, D. W., He, D., et al. (2000) Direct isolation of human central nervous system stem cells. *Proc. Natl. Acad. Sci. USA* **97,** 14720–14725.
9. Rietze, R. L., Valcanis, H., Brooker, G. F., Thomas, T., Voss, A. K., and Bartlett, P. F. (2001) Purification of a pluripotent neural stem cell from the adult mouse brain. *Nature* **412,** 736–739.
10. Maric, D., Maric, I., Chang, Y. H., and Barker, J. L. (2003) Prospective cell sorting of embryonic rat neural stem cells and neuronal and glial progenitors reveals selective effects of basic fibroblast growth factor and epidermal growth factor on self-renewal and differentiation. *J. Neurosci.* **23,** 240–251.
11. Rakic, P. (1995) Radial versus tangential migration of neuronal clones in the developing cerebral cortex. *Proc. Natl. Acad. Sci. USA* **92,** 11323–11327.
12. Noctor, S. C., Flint, A. C., Weissman, T. A., Wong, W. S., Clinton, B. K., and Kriegstein, A. R. (2002) Dividing precursor cells of the embryonic cortical ventricular zone have morphological and molecular characteristics of radial glia. *J. Neurosci.* **22,** 3161–3173.
13. Parnavelas, J. G. and Nadarajah, B. (2001) Radial glial cells: Are they really glia? *Neuron* **31,** 881–884.
14. Rakic, P. (2003) Developmental and evolutionary adaptations of cortical radial glia. *Cereb. Cortex* **13,** 541–549.
15. Morest, D. K. and Silver, J. (2003) Precursors of neurons, neuroglia, and ependymal cells in the CNS: What are they? Where are they from? How do they get where they are going? *Glia* **43,** 6–18.
16. Kriegstein, A. R. and Gotz, M. (2003) Radial glia diversity: a matter of cell fate. *Glia* **43,** 37–43.
17. Hartfuss, E. (2003) *Characterization of Subtypes of Precursor Cells in the Developing Central Nervous System.* Fakultät für Biologie, Ludwig-Maximilians Universität München. (Ph.D. thesis)

18. Gotz, M., Hartfuss, E., and Malatesta, P. (2002) Radial glial cells as neuronal precursors: a new perspective on the correlation of morphology and lineage restriction in the developing cerebral cortex of mice. *Brain Res. Bull.* **57,** 777–788.
19. Rakic, P. (1995) A small step for the cell, a giant leap for mankind: a hypothesis of neocortical expansion during evolution. *Trends Neurosci.* **18,** 383–388.
20. Caviness, V. S., Jr. and Takahashi, T. (1995) Proliferative events in the cerebral ventricular zone. *Brain Dev.* **17,** 159–163.
21. Chenn, A. and McConnell, S. K. (1995) Cleavage orientation and the asymmetric inheritance of Notch1 immunoreactivity in mammalian neurogenesis. *Cell* **82,** 631–641.
22. Lu, B., Jan, L., and Jan, Y. N. (2000) Control of cell divisions in the nervous system: symmetry and asymmetry. *Annu. Rev. Neurosci.* **23,** 531–556.
23. Temple, S. (2001) The development of neural stem cells. *Nature* **414,** 112–117.
24. Noctor, S. C., Martinez-Cerdeno, V., Ivic, L., and Kriegstein, A. R. (2004) Cortical neurons arise in symmetric and asymmetric division zones and migrate through specific phases. *Nat. Neurosci.* **7,** 136–144.
25. Kilpatrick, T. J. and Bartlett, P. F. (1995) Cloned multipotential precursors from the mouse cerebrum require FGF-2, whereas glial restricted precursors are stimulated with either FGF-2 or EGF. *J. Neurosci.* **15,** 3653–3661.
26. Weiss, S., Reynolds, B. A., Vescovi, A. L., Morshead, C., Craig, C. G., and van der Kooy, D. (1996) Is there a neural stem cell in the mammalian forebrain? *Trends Neurosci.* **19,** 387–393.
27. Johe, K. K., Hazel, T. G., Muller, T., Dugich-Djordjevic, M. M., and McKay, R. D. (1996) Single factors direct the differentiation of stem cells from the fetal and adult central nervous system. *Genes Dev.* **10,** 3129–3140.
28. Qian, X., Davis, A. A., Goderie, S. K., and Temple, S. (1997) FGF2 concentration regulates the generation of neurons and glia from multipotent cortical stem cells. *Neuron* **18,** 81–93.
29. Gage, F. H., Coates, P. W., Palmer, T. D., et al. (1995) Survival and differentiation of adult neuronal progenitor cells transplanted to the adult brain. *Proc. Natl. Acad. Sci. USA* **92,** 11879–11883.
30. Palmer, T. D., Ray, J., and Gage, F. H. (1995) FGF-2-responsive neuronal progenitors reside in proliferative and quiescent regions of the adult rodent brain. *Mol. Cell Neurosci.* **6,** 474–486.
31. Palmer, T. D., Takahashi, J., and Gage, F. H. (1997) The adult rat hippocampus contains primordial neural stem cells. *Mol. Cell Neurosci.* **8,** 389–404.
32. Reynolds, B. A. and Weiss, S. (1996) Clonal and population analyses demonstrate that an EGF-responsive mammalian embryonic CNS precursor is a stem cell. *Dev. Biol.* **175,** 1–13.
33. Reynolds, B. A., Tetzlaff, W., and Weiss, S. (1992) A multipotent EGF-responsive striatal embryonic progenitor cell produces neurons and astrocytes. *J. Neurosci.* **12,** 4565–4574.
34. Vescovi, A. L., Reynolds, B. A., Fraser, D. D., and Weiss, S. (1993) bFGF regulates the proliferative fate of unipotent (neuronal) and bipotent (neuronal/astroglial) EGF-generated CNS progenitor cells. *Neuron* **11,** 951–966.
35. Temple, S. (1989) Division and differentiation of isolated CNS blast cells in microculture. *Nature* **340,** 471–473.
36. Mabie, P. C., Mehler, M. F., and Kessler, J. A. (1999) Multiple roles of bone morphogenetic protein signaling in the regulation of cortical cell number and phenotype. *J. Neurosci.* **19,** 7077–7088.
37. Gaiano, N., Kohtz, J. D., Turnbull, D. H., and Fishell, G. (1999) A method for rapid gain-of-function studies in the mouse embryonic nervous system. *Nat. Neurosci.* **2,** 812–819.
38. Walsh, C. and Cepko, C. L. (1992) Widespread dispersion of neuronal clones across functional regions of the cerebral cortex. *Science* **255,** 434–440.

39. Reid, C. B., Liang, I., and Walsh, C. (1995) Systematic widespread clonal organization in cerebral cortex. *Neuron* **15,** 299–310.
40. Davis, A. A. and Temple, S. (1994) A self-renewing multipotential stem cell in embryonic rat cerebral cortex. *Nature* **372,** 263–266.
41. Williams, B. P. and Price, J. (1995) Evidence for multiple precursor cell types in the embryonic rat cerebral cortex. *Neuron* **14,** 1181–1188.
42. Burrows, R. C., Wancio, D., Levitt, P., and Lillien, L. (1997) Response diversity and the timing of progenitor cell maturation are regulated by developmental changes in EGFR expression in the cortex. *Neuron* **19,** 251–267.
43. Viti, J., Feathers, A., Phillips, J., and Lillien, L. (2003) Epidermal growth factor receptors control competence to interpret leukemia inhibitory factor as an astrocyte inducer in developing cortex. *J. Neurosci.* **23,** 3385–3393.
44. Lillien, L. and Wancio, D. (1998) Changes in epidermal growth factor receptor expression and competence to generate glia regulate timing and choice of differentiation in the retina. *Mol. Cell Neurosci.* **10,** 296–308.
45. Zhu, G., Mehler, M. F., Mabie, P. C., and Kessler, J. A. (2000) Developmental changes in neural progenitor cell lineage commitment do not depend on epidermal growth factor receptor signaling. *J. Neurosci. Res.* **59,** 312–320.
46. Zhu, G., Mehler, M. F., Mabie, P. C., and Kessler, J. A. (1999) Developmental changes in progenitor cell responsiveness to cytokines. *J. Neurosci. Res.* **56,** 131–145.
47. Molne, M., Studer, L., Tabar, V., Ting, Y. T., Eiden, M. V., and McKay, R. D. (2000) Early cortical precursors do not undergo LIF-mediated astrocytic differentiation. *J. Neurosci. Res.* **59,** 301–311.
48. Monuki, E. S. and Walsh, C. A. (2001) Mechanisms of cerebral cortical patterning in mice and humans. *Nat. Neurosci.* **4(Suppl),** 1199–1206.
49. O'Leary, D. D. and Nakagawa, Y. (2002) Patterning centers, regulatory genes and extrinsic mechanisms controlling arealization of the neocortex. *Curr. Opin. Neurobiol.* **12,** 14–25.
50. Campbell, K. (2003) Dorsal-ventral patterning in the mammalian telencephalon. *Curr. Opin. Neurobiol.* **13,** 50–56.
51. Nadarajah, B., Alifragis, P., Wong, R. O., and Parnavelas, J. G. (2003) Neuronal migration in the developing cerebral cortex: observations based on real-time imaging. *Cereb. Cortex* **13,** 607–611.
52. Jessell, T. M. (2000) Neuronal specification in the spinal cord: inductive signals and transcriptional codes. *Nat. Rev. Genet.* **1,** 20–29.
53. Osterfield, M., Kirschner, M. W., and Flanagan, J. G. (2003) Graded positional information: interpretation for both fate and guidance. *Cell* **113,** 425–428.
54. Parmar, M., Skogh, C., Bjorklund, A., and Campbell, K. (2002) Regional specification of neurosphere cultures derived from subregions of the embryonic telencephalon. *Mol. Cell. Neurosci.* **21,** 645–656.
55. Hitoshi, S., Tropepe, V., Ekker, M., and van der Kooy, D. (2002) Neural stem cell lineages are regionally specified, but not committed, within distinct compartments of the developing brain. *Development* **129,** 233–244.
56. Ciccolini, F. and Svendsen, C. N. (1998) Fibroblast growth factor 2 (FGF-2) promotes acquisition of epidermal growth factor (EGF) responsiveness in mouse striatal precursor cells: identification of neural precursors responding to both EGF and FGF-2. *J. Neurosci.* **18,** 7869–7880.
57. Ortega, S., Ittmann, M., Tsang, S. H., Ehrlich, M., and Basilico, C. (1998) Neuronal defects and delayed wound healing in mice lacking fibroblast growth factor 2. *Proc. Natl. Acad. Sci. USA* **95,** 5672–5677.
58. Tao, Y., Black, I. B., and DiCicco-Bloom, E. (1997) In vivo neurogenesis is inhibited by neutralizing antibodies to basic fibroblast growth factor. *J. Neurobiol.* **33,** 289–296.

59. Vaccarino, F. M., Schwartz, M. L., Raballo, R., et al. (1999) Changes in cerebral cortex size are governed by fibroblast growth factor during embryogenesis. *Nat. Neurosci.* **2,** 246–253.

60. Tao, Y., Black, I. B., and DiCicco-Bloom, E. (1996) Neurogenesis in neonatal rat brain is regulated by peripheral injection of basic fibroblast growth factor (bFGF). *J. Comp Neurol.* **376,** 653–663.

61. Emoto, N., Gonzalez, A. M., Walicke, P. A., et al. (1989) Basic fibroblast growth factor (FGF) in the central nervous system: identification of specific loci of basic FGF expression in the rat brain. *Growth Factors* **2,** 21–29.

62. Goodrich, L. V. and Scott, M. P. (1998) Hedgehog and patched in neural development and disease. *Neuron* **21,** 1243–1257.

63. Kornblum, H. I., Hussain, R., Wiesen, J., et al. (1998) Abnormal astrocyte development and neuronal death in mice lacking the epidermal growth factor receptor. *J. Neurosci. Res.* **53,** 697–717.

64. Kornblum, H. I., Hussain, R. J., Bronstein, J. M., Gall, C. M., Lee, D. C., and Seroogy, K. B. (1997) Prenatal ontogeny of the epidermal growth factor receptor and its ligand, transforming growth factor alpha, in the rat brain. *J. Comp. Neurol.* **380,** 243–261.

65. Marti, E. and Bovolenta, P. (2002) Sonic hedgehog in CNS development: one signal, multiple outputs. *Trends Neurosci.* **25,** 89–96.

66. Rowitch, D. H., S-Jacques, B., Lee, S. M., Flax, J. D., Snyder, E. Y., and McMahon, A. P. (1999) Sonic hedgehog regulates proliferation and inhibits differentiation of CNS precursor cells. *J. Neurosci.* **19,** 8954–8965.

67. Gabay, L., Lowell, S., Rubin, L. L., and Anderson, D. J. (2003) Deregulation of dorsoventral patterning by FGF confers trilineage differentiation capacity on CNS stem cells in vitro. *Neuron* **40,** 485–499.

68. Zhu, G., Mehler, M. F., Zhao, J., Yu Yung, S., and Kessler, J. A. (1999) Sonic hedgehog and BMP2 exert opposing actions on proliferation and differentiation of embryonic neural progenitor cells. *Dev. Biol.* **215,** 118–129.

69. Wechsler-Reya, R. J. and Scott, M. P. (1999) Control of neuronal precursor proliferation in the cerebellum by Sonic Hedgehog. *Neuron* **22,** 103–114.

70. Kalyani, A. J., Piper, D., Mujtaba, T., Lucero, M. T., and Rao, M. S. (1998) Spinal cord neuronal precursors generate multiple neuronal phenotypes in culture. *J. Neurosci.* **18,** 7856–7868.

71. Lee, S. M., Tole, S., Grove, E., and McMahon, A. P. (2000) A local Wnt-3a signal is required for development of the mammalian hippocampus. *Development* **127,** 457–467.

72. Megason, S. G. and McMahon, A. P. (2002) A mitogen gradient of dorsal midline Wnts organizes growth in the CNS. *Development* **129,** 2087–2098.

73. Viti, J., Gulacsi, A., and Lillien, L. (2003) Wnt regulation of progenitor maturation in the cortex depends on Shh or fibroblast growth factor 2. *J. Neurosci.* **23,** 5919–5927.

74. Ikeya, M., Lee, S. M., Johnson, J. E., McMahon, A. P., and Takada, S. (1997) Wnt signalling required for expansion of neural crest and CNS progenitors. *Nature* **389,** 966–970.

75. Chenn, A. and Walsh, C. A. (2002) Regulation of cerebral cortical size by control of cell cycle exit in neural precursors. *Science* **297,** 365–369.

76. Gressens, P., Hill, J. M., Paindaveine, B., Gozes, I., Fridkin, M., and Brenneman, D. E. (1994) Severe microcephaly induced by blockade of vasoactive intestinal peptide function in the primitive neuroepithelium of the mouse. *J. Clin. Invest* **94,** 2020–2027.

77. Arsenijevic, Y., Weiss, S., Schneider, B., and Aebischer, P. (2001) Insulin-like growth factor-I is necessary for neural stem cell proliferation and demonstrates distinct actions of epidermal growth factor and fibroblast growth factor-2. *J. Neurosci.* **21,** 7194–7202.

78. Lin, X. and Bulleit, R. F. (1997) Insulin-like growth factor I (IGF-I) is a critical trophic factor for developing cerebellar granule cells. *Brain Res. Dev. Brain Res.* **99,** 234–242.

79. Frade, J. M., Marti, E., Bovolenta, P., et al. (1996) Insulin-like growth factor-I stimulates neurogenesis in chick retina by regulating expression of the alpha 6 integrin subunit. *Development* **122**, 2497–2506.

80. Drago, J., Murphy, M., Carroll, S. M., Harvey, R. P., and Bartlett, P. F. (1991) Fibroblast growth factor-mediated proliferation of central nervous system precursors depends on endogenous production of insulin-like growth factor I. *Proc. Natl. Acad. Sci. USA* **88**, 2199–2203.

81. Raballo, R., Rhee, J., Lyn-Cook, R., Leckman, J. F., Schwartz, M. L., and Vaccarino, F. M. (2000) Basic fibroblast growth factor (Fgf2) is necessary for cell proliferation and neurogenesis in the developing cerebral cortex. *J. Neurosci.* **20**, 5012–5023.

82. Ghosh, A. and Greenberg, M. E. (1995) Distinct roles for bFGF and NT-3 in the regulation of cortical neurogenesis. *Neuron* **15**, 89–103.

83. Lukaszewicz, A., Savatier, P., Cortay, V., Kennedy, H., and Dehay, C. (2002) Contrasting effects of basic fibroblast growth factor and neurotrophin 3 on cell cycle kinetics of mouse cortical stem cells. *J. Neurosci.* **22**, 6610–6622.

84. Hajihosseini, M. K. and Dickson, C. (1999) A subset of fibroblast growth factors (Fgfs) promote survival, but Fgf-8b specifically promotes astroglial differentiation of rat cortical precursor cells. *Mol. Cell. Neurosci.* **14**, 468–485.

85. Riese, D. J., Kim, E. D., Elenius, K., et al. (1996) The epidermal growth factor receptor couples transforming growth factor-alpha, heparin-binding epidermal growth factor-like factor, and amphiregulin to Neu, ErbB-3, and ErbB-4. *J. Biol. Chem.* **271**, 20047–20052.

86. Dumstrei, K., Nassif, C., Abboud, G., Aryai, A., and Hartenstein, V. (1998) EGFR signaling is required for the differentiation and maintenance of neural progenitors along the dorsal midline of the *Drosophila* embryonic head. *Development* **125**, 3417–3426.

87. Calaora, V., Rogister, B., Bismuth, K., et al. (2001) Neuregulin signaling regulates neural precursor growth and the generation of oligodendrocytes in vitro. *J. Neurosci.* **21**, 4740–4751.

88. Barnabe-Heider, F. and Miller, F. D. (2003) Endogenously produced neurotrophins regulate survival and differentiation of cortical progenitors via distinct signaling pathways. *J. Neurosci.* **23**, 5149–5160.

89. Yu, X., Shacka, J. J., Eells, J. B., et al. (2002) Erythropoietin receptor signalling is required for normal brain development. *Development* **129**, 505–516.

90. Sommer, L. and Rao, M. (2002) Neural stem cells and regulation of cell number. *Prog. Neurobiol.* **66**, 1–18.

91. Haydar, T. F., Kuan, C. Y., Flavell, R. A., and Rakic, P. (1999) The role of cell death in regulating the size and shape of the mammalian forebrain. *Cereb. Cortex* **9**, 621–626.

92. D'Sa-Eipper, C. and Roth, K. A. (2000) Caspase regulation of neuronal progenitor cell apoptosis. *Dev. Neurosci.* **22**, 116–124.

93. Motoyama, N., Wang, F., Roth, K. A., et al. (1995) Massive cell death of immature hematopoietic cells and neurons in Bcl-x-deficient mice. *Science* **267**, 1506–1510.

94. Roth, K. A., Kuan, C., Haydar, T. F., et al. (2000) Epistatic and independent functions of caspase-3 and Bcl-X(L) in developmental programmed cell death. *Proc. Natl. Acad. Sci. USA* **97**, 466–471.

95. Cheema, Z. F., Wade, S. B., Sata, M., Walsh, K., Sohrabji, F., and Miranda, R. C. (1999) Fas/Apo [apoptosis]-1 and associated proteins in the differentiating cerebral cortex: induction of caspase-dependent cell death and activation of NF-kappaB. *J. Neurosci.* **19**, 1754–1770.

96. Thibert, C., Teillet, M. A., Lapointe, F., Mazelin, L., Le Douarin, N. M., and Mehlen, P. (2003) Inhibition of neuroepithelial patched-induced apoptosis by sonic hedgehog. *Science* **301**, 843–846.

97. Austin, C. P., Feldman, D. E., Ida, J. A., Jr., and Cepko, C. L. (1995) Vertebrate retinal ganglion cells are selected from competent progenitors by the action of Notch. *Development* **121**, 3637–3650.

98. Henrique, D., Adam, J., Myat, A., Chitnis, A., Lewis, J., and Ish-Horowicz, D. (1995) Expression of a Delta homologue in prospective neurons in the chick. *Nature* **375,** 787–790.

99. Myat, A., Henrique, D., Ish-Horowicz, D., and Lewis, J. (1996) A chick homologue of Serrate and its relationship with Notch and Delta homologues during central neurogenesis. *Dev. Biol.* **174,** 233–247.

100. Artavanis-Tsakonas, S., Rand, M. D., and Lake, R. J. (1999) Notch signaling: cell fate control and signal integration in development. *Science* **284,** 770–776.

101. Wang, S., Sdrulla, A. D., diSibio, G., et al. (1998) Notch receptor activation inhibits oligodendrocyte differentiation. *Neuron* **21,** 63–75.

102. Gaiano, N., Nye, J. S., and Fishell, G. (2000) Radial glial identity is promoted by Notch1 signaling in the murine forebrain. *Neuron* **26,** 395–404.

103. Wang, S. and Barres, B. A. (2000) Up a notch: instructing gliogenesis. *Neuron* **27,** 197–200.

104. Malatesta, P., Hartfuss, E., and Gotz, M. (2000) Isolation of radial glial cells by fluorescent-activated cell sorting reveals a neuronal lineage. *Development* **127,** 5253–5263.

105. Noctor, S. C., Flint, A. C., Weissman, T. A., Dammerman, R. S., and Kriegstein, A. R. (2001) Neurons derived from radial glial cells establish radial units in neocortex. *Nature* **409,** 714–720.

106. Doetsch, F., Caille, I., Lim, D. A., Garcia-Verdugo, J. M., and Alvarez-Buylla, A. (1999) Subventricular zone astrocytes are neural stem cells in the adult mammalian brain. *Cell* **97,** 703–716.

107. Shimazaki, T., Shingo, T., and Weiss, S. (2001) The ciliary neurotrophic factor/leukemia inhibitory factor/gp130 receptor complex operates in the maintenance of mammalian forebrain neural stem cells. *J. Neurosci.* **21,** 7642–7653.

108. Chojnacki, A., Shimazaki, T., Gregg, C., Weinmaster, G., and Weiss, S. (2003) Glycoprotein 130 signaling regulates Notch1 expression and activation in the self-renewal of mammalian forebrain neural stem cells. *J. Neurosci.* **23,** 1730–1741.

109. Israsena, N., Hu, M., Fu, W., Kan, L., and Kessler, J. A. (2004) The presence of FGF2 signaling determines whether β-catenin exerts effects on proliferation or neuronal differentiation of neural stem cells. *Dev. Biol.* **268,** 220–231.

110. Zindy, F., Soares, H., Herzog, K. H., Morgan, J., Sherr, C. J., and Roussel, M. F. (1997) Expression of INK4 inhibitors of cyclin D-dependent kinases during mouse brain development. *Cell Growth Differ.* **8,** 1139–1150.

111. van Lookeren Campagne, M. and Gill, R. (1998) Tumor-suppressor p53 is expressed in proliferating and newly formed neurons of the embryonic and postnatal rat brain: comparison with expression of the cell cycle regulators p21Waf1/Cip1, p27Kip1, p57Kip2, p16Ink4a, cyclin G1, and the proto-oncogene Bax. *J. Comp. Neurol.* **397,** 181–198.

112. Watanabe, G., Pena, P., Shambaugh, G. E., 3rd, Haines, G. K., 3rd, and Pestell, R. G. (1998) Regulation of cyclin dependent kinase inhibitor proteins during neonatal cerebella development. *Brain Res. Dev. Brain Res.* **108,** 77–87.

113. Coskun, V., Venkatraman, G., Yang, H., Rao, M. S., and Luskin, M. B. (2001) Retroviral manipulation of the expression of bone morphogenetic protein receptor Ia by SVZa progenitor cells leads to changes in their p19(INK4d) expression but not in their neuronal commitment. *Int. J. Dev. Neurosci.* **19,** 219–227.

114. Gross, R. E., Mehler, M. F., Mabie, P. C., Zang, Z., Santschi, L., and Kessler, J. A. (1996) Bone morphogenetic proteins promote astroglial lineage commitment by mammalian subventricular zone progenitor cells. *Neuron* **17,** 595–606.

115. Suh, J., Lu, N., Nicot, A., Tatsuno, I., and DiCicco-Bloom, E. (2001) PACAP is an antimitogenic signal in developing cerebral cortex. *Nat. Neurosci.* **4,** 123–124.

116. Lu, N., Zhou, R., and DiCicco-Bloom, E. (1998) Opposing mitogenic regulation by PACAP in sympathetic and cerebral cortical precursors correlates with differential expression of PACAP receptor (PAC1-R) isoforms. *J. Neurosci. Res.* **53,** 651–662.

117. Carey, R. G., Li, B., and DiCicco-Bloom, E. (2002) Pituitary adenylate cyclase activating polypeptide anti-mitogenic signaling in cerebral cortical progenitors is regulated by p57Kip2-dependent CDK2 activity. *J. Neurosci.* **22,** 1583–1591.

118. Lee, M., Lelievre, V., Zhao, P., et al. (2001) Pituitary adenylyl cyclase-activating polypeptide stimulates DNA synthesis but delays maturation of oligodendrocyte progenitors. *J. Neurosci.* **21,** 3849–3859.

119. Nguyen, L., Rigo, J. M., Rocher, V., et al. (2001) Neurotransmitters as early signals for central nervous system development. *Cell Tissue Res.* **305,** 187–202.

120. Fiszman, M. L., Borodinsky, L. N., and Neale, J. H. (1999) GABA induces proliferation of immature cerebellar granule cells grown in vitro. *Brain Res. Dev. Brain Res.* **115,** 1–8.

121. Haydar, T. F., Wang, F., Schwartz, M. L., and Rakic, P. (2000) Differential modulation of proliferation in the neocortical ventricular and subventricular zones. *J. Neurosci.* **20,** 5764–5774.

122. LoTurco, J. J., Owens, D. F., Heath, M. J., Davis, M. B., and Kriegstein, A. R. (1995) GABA and glutamate depolarize cortical progenitor cells and inhibit DNA synthesis. *Neuron* **15,** 1287–1298.

123. Antonopoulos, J., Pappas, I. S., and Parnavelas, J. G. (1997) Activation of the GABAA receptor inhibits the proliferative effects of bFGF in cortical progenitor cells. *Eur. J. Neurosci.* **9,** 291–298.

124. Ohtani, N., Goto, T., Waeber, C., and Bhide, P. G. (2003) Dopamine modulates cell cycle in the lateral ganglionic eminence. *J. Neurosci.* **23,** 2840–2850.

125. Luk, K. C., Kennedy, T. E., and Sadikot, A. F. (2003) Glutamate promotes proliferation of striatal neuronal progenitors by an NMDA receptor-mediated mechanism. *J. Neurosci.* **23,** 2239–2250.

126. Sadikot, A. F., Burhan, A. M., Belanger, M. C., and Sasseville, R. (1998) NMDA receptor antagonists influence early development of GABAergic interneurons in the mammalian striatum. *Brain Res. Dev. Brain Res.* **105,** 35–42.

127. Cameron, H. A., Hazel, T. G., and McKay, R. D. (1998) Regulation of neurogenesis by growth factors and neurotransmitters. *J. Neurobiol.* **36,** 287–306.

128. Contestabile, A. (2000) Roles of NMDA receptor activity and nitric oxide production in brain development. *Brain Res. Brain Res. Rev.* **32,** 476–509.

129. Ferguson, K. L. and Slack, R. S. (2003) Growth factors: Can they promote neurogenesis? *Trends Neurosci.* **26,** 283–285.

130. Santa-Olalla, J. and Covarrubias, L. (1999) Basic fibroblast growth factor promotes epidermal growth factor responsiveness and survival of mesencephalic neural precursor cells. *J. Neurobiol.* **40,** 14–27.

131. Daadi, M. M. and Weiss, S. (1999) Generation of tyrosine hydroxylase-producing neurons from precursors of the embryonic and adult forebrain. *J. Neurosci.* **19,** 4484–4497.

132. Bartlett, P. F., Brooker, G. J., Faux, C. H., et al. (1998) Regulation of neural stem cell differentiation in the forebrain. *Immunol. Cell Biol.* **76,** 414–418.

133. Ye, W., Shimamura, K., Rubenstein, J. L., Hynes, M. A., and Rosenthal, A. (1998) FGF and Shh signals control dopaminergic and serotonergic cell fate in the anterior neural plate. *Cell* **93,** 755–766.

134. Hynes, M., Ye, W., Wang, K., et al. (2000) The seven-transmembrane receptor smoothened cell-autonomously induces multiple ventral cell types. *Nat. Neurosci.* **3,** 41–46.

135. Ruiz, I. A. A., Palma, V., and Dahmane, N. (2002) Hedgehog-Gli signalling and the growth of the brain. *Nat. Rev. Neurosci.* **3,** 24–33.

136. Roelink, H. (1996) Tripartite signaling of pattern: interactions between Hedgehogs, BMPs and Wnts in the control of vertebrate development. *Curr. Opin. Neurobiol.* **6,** 33–40.

137. Hirsinger, E., Duprez, D., Jouve, C., Malapert, P., Cooke, J., and Pourquie, O. (1997) Noggin acts downstream of Wnt and Sonic Hedgehog to antagonize BMP4 in avian somite patterning. *Development* **124,** 4605–4614.

138. Lumsden, A. and Krumlauf, R. (1996) Patterning the vertebrate neuraxis. *Science* **274,** 1109–1115.
139. Toresson, H., Mata de Urquiza, A., Fagerstrom, C., Perlmann, T., and Campbell, K. (1999) Retinoids are produced by glia in the lateral ganglionic eminence and regulate striatal neuron differentiation. *Development* **126,** 1317–1326.
140. Pierani, A., Brenner-Morton, S., Chiang, C., and Jessell, T. M. (1999) A sonic hedgehog-independent, retinoid-activated pathway of neurogenesis in the ventral spinal cord. *Cell* **97,** 903–915.
141. Williams, B. P., Park, J. K., Alberta, J. A., et al. (1997) A PDGF-regulated immediate early gene response initiates neuronal differentiation in ventricular zone progenitor cells. *Neuron* **18,** 553–562.
142. Park, J. K., Williams, B. P., Alberta, J. A., and Stiles, C. D. (1999) Bipotent cortical progenitor cells process conflicting cues for neurons and glia in a hierarchical manner. *J. Neurosci.* **19,** 10383–10389.
143. Dihne, M., Bernreuther, C., Sibbe, M., Paulus, W., and Schachner, M. (2003) A new role for the cell adhesion molecule L1 in neural precursor cell proliferation, differentiation, and transmitter-specific subtype generation. *J. Neurosci.* **23,** 6638–6650.
144. Cheng, A., Wang, S., Cai, J., Rao, M. S., and Mattson, M. P. (2003) Nitric oxide acts in a positive feedback loop with BDNF to regulate neural progenitor cell proliferation and differentiation in the mammalian brain. *Dev. Biol.* **258,** 319–333.
145. Sun, Y. E., Martinowich, K., and Ge, W. (2003) Making and repairing the mammalian brain—signaling toward neurogenesis and gliogenesis. *Semin. Cell Dev. Biol.* **14,** 161–168.
146. Temple, S. and Qian, X. (1996) Vertebrate neural progenitor cells: subtypes and regulation. *Curr. Opin. Neurobiol.* **6,** 11–17.
147. Mabie, P. C., Mehler, M. F., Marmur, R., Papavasiliou, A., Song, Q., and Kessler, J. A. (1997) Bone morphogenetic proteins induce astroglial differentiation of oligodendroglial-astroglial progenitor cells. *J. Neurosci.* **17,** 4112–4120.
148. Gomes, W. A., Mehler, M. F., and Kessler, J. A. (2003) Transgenic overexpression of BMP4 increases astroglial and decreases oligodendroglial lineage commitment. *Dev. Biol.* **255,** 164–177.
149. McKay, R. (1997) Stem cells in the central nervous system. *Science* **276,** 66–71.
150. Koblar, S. A., Turnley, A. M., Classon, B. J., et al. (1998) Neural precursor differentiation into astrocytes requires signaling through the leukemia inhibitory factor receptor. *Proc. Natl. Acad. Sci. USA* **95,** 3178–3181.
151. Nakashima, K., Yanagisawa, M., Arakawa, H., et al. (1999) Synergistic signaling in fetal brain by STAT3–Smad1 complex bridged by p300. *Science* **284,** 479–482.
152. Hojo, M., Ohtsuka, T., Hashimoto, N., Gradwohl, G., Guillemot, F., and Kageyama, R. (2000) Glial cell fate specification modulated by the bHLH gene Hes5 in mouse retina. *Development* **127,** 2515–2522.
153. Tanigaki, K., Nogaki, F., Takahashi, J., Tashiro, K., Kurooka, H., and Honjo, T. (2001) Notch1 and Notch3 instructively restrict bFGF-responsive multipotent neural progenitor cells to an astroglial fate. *Neuron* **29,** 45–55.
154. Vallejo, I. and Vallejo, M. (2002) Pituitary adenylate cyclase-activating polypeptide induces astrocyte differentiation of precursor cells from developing cerebral cortex. *Mol. Cell Neurosci.* **21,** 671–683.
155. Canoll, P. D., Musacchio, J. M., Hardy, R., Reynolds, R., Marchionni, M. A., and Salzer, J. L. (1996) GGF/neuregulin is a neuronal signal that promotes the proliferation and survival and inhibits the differentiation of oligodendrocyte progenitors. *Neuron* **17,** 229–243.
156. Qi, Y., Stapp, D., and Qiu, M. (2002) Origin and molecular specification of oligodendrocytes in the telencephalon. *Trends Neurosci.* **25,** 223–225.

157. Rogister, B., Ben-Hur, T., and Dubois-Dalcq, M. (1999) From neural stem cells to myelinating oligodendrocytes. *Mol. Cell Neurosci.* **14,** 287–300.
158. Nery, S., Wichterle, H., and Fishell, G. (2001) Sonic hedgehog contributes to oligodendrocyte specification in the mammalian forebrain. *Development* **128,** 527–540.
159. Murray, K., Calaora, V., Rottkamp, C., Guicherit, O., and Dubois-Dalcq, M. (2002) Sonic hedgehog is a potent inducer of rat oligodendrocyte development from cortical precursors in vitro. *Mol. Cell. Neurosci.* **19,** 320–332.
160. Orentas, D. M. and Miller, R. H. (1996) The origin of spinal cord oligodendrocytes is dependent on local influences from the notochord. *Dev. Biol.* **177,** 43–53.
161. Pringle, N. P., Yu, W. P., Guthrie, S., et al. (1996) Determination of neuroepithelial cell fate: induction of the oligodendrocyte lineage by ventral midline cells and sonic hedgehog. *Dev. Biol.* **177,** 30–42.
162. Chandran, S., Kato, H., Gerreli, D., Compston, A., Svendsen, C. N., and Allen, N. D. (2003) FGF-dependent generation of oligodendrocytes by a hedgehog-independent pathway. *Development* **130,** 6599–6609.
163. Mekki-Dauriac, S., Agius, E., Kan, P., and Cochard, P. (2002) Bone morphogenetic proteins negatively control oligodendrocyte precursor specification in the chick spinal cord. *Development* **129,** 5117–5130.
164. Akazawa, C., Sasai, Y., Nakanishi, S., and Kageyama, R. (1992) Molecular characterization of a rat negative regulator with a basic helix–loop–helix structure predominantly expressed in the developing nervous system. *J. Biol. Chem.* **267,** 21879–21885.
165. Sasai, Y., Kageyama, R., Tagawa, Y., Shigemoto, R., and Nakanishi, S. (1992) Two mammalian helix–loop–helix factors structurally related to *Drosophila hairy* and *Enhancer of split*. *Genes Dev.* **6,** 2620–2634.
166. Blokzijl, A., Dahlqvist, C., Reissmann, E., et al. (2003) Cross-talk between the Notch and TGF-β signaling pathways mediated by interaction of the Notch intracellular domain with Smad3. *J. Cell. Biol.* **163,** 723–728.
167. Ross, D. A. and Kadesch, T. (2001) The notch intracellular domain can function as a coactivator for LEF-1. *Mol. Cell Biol.* **21,** 7537–7544.
168. Wu, Y., Liu, Y., Levine, E. M., and Rao, M. S. (2003) Hes1 but not Hes5 regulates an astrocyte versus oligodendrocyte fate choice in glial restricted precursors. *Dev. Dyn.* **226,** 675–689.
169. Ishibashi, M., Moriyoshi, K., Sasai, Y., Shiota, K., Nakanishi, S., and Kageyama, R. (1994) Persistent expression of helix-loop-helix factor HES-1 prevents mammalian neural differentiation in the central nervous system. *EMBO J.* **13,** 1799–1805.
170. Ishibashi, M., Ang, S. L., Shiota, K., Nakanishi, S., Kageyama, R., and Guillemot, F. (1995) Targeted disruption of mammalian *hairy* and *Enhancer of split* homolog-1 (HES-1) leads to up-regulation of neural helix–loop–helix factors, premature neurogenesis, and severe neural tube defects. *Genes Dev.* **9,** 3136–3148.
171. Ohtsuka, T., Sakamoto, M., Guillemot, F., and Kageyama, R. (2001) Roles of the basic helix-loop-helix genes *Hes1* and *Hes5* in expansion of neural stem cells of the developing brain. *J. Biol. Chem.* **276,** 30467–30474.
172. Nakamura, Y., Sakakibara, S., Miyata, T., et al. (2000) The bHLH gene *hes1* as a repressor of the neuronal commitment of CNS stem cells. *J. Neurosci.* **20,** 283–293.
173. Gratton, M. O., Torban, E., Jasmin, S. B., Theriault, F. M., German, M. S., and Stifani, S. (2003) *Hes6* promotes cortical neurogenesis and inhibits *Hes1* transcription repression activity by multiple mechanisms. *Mol. Cell Biol.* **23,** 6922–6935.
174. Norton, J. D., Deed, R. W., Craggs, G., and Sablitzky, F. (1998) Id helix–loop–helix proteins in cell growth and differentiation. *Trends Cell Biol.* **8,** 58–65.
175. Norton, J. D. (2000) ID helix–loop–helix proteins in cell growth, differentiation and tumorigenesis. *J. Cell Sci.* **113(Pt 22),** 3897–3905.

176. Toma, J. G., El-Bizri, H., Barnabe-Heider, F., Aloyz, R., and Miller, F. D. (2000) Evidence that helix–loop–helix proteins collaborate with retinoblastoma tumor suppressor protein to regulate cortical neurogenesis. *J. Neurosci.* **20,** 7648–7656.

177. Jen, Y., Manova, K., and Benezra, R. (1997) Each member of the Id gene family exhibits a unique expression pattern in mouse gastrulation and neurogenesis. *Dev. Dyn.* **208,** 92–106.

178. Riechmann, V. and Sablitzky, F. (1995) Mutually exclusive expression of two dominant-negative helix–loop–helix (dnHLH) genes, Id4 and Id3, in the developing brain of the mouse suggests distinct regulatory roles of these dnHLH proteins during cellular proliferation and differentiation of the nervous system. *Cell Growth Differ.* **6,** 837–843.

179. Lyden, D., Young, A. Z., Zagzag, D., et al. (1999) Id1 and Id3 are required for neurogenesis, angiogenesis and vascularization of tumour xenografts. *Nature* **401,** 670–677.

180. Hinck, L., Nathke, I. S., Papkoff, J., and Nelson, W. J. (1994) Dynamics of cadherin/catenin complex formation: novel protein interactions and pathways of complex assembly. *J. Cell Biol.* **125,** 1327–1340.

181. Nathke, I. S., Hinck, L., Swedlow, J. R., Papkoff, J., and Nelson, W. J. (1994) Defining interactions and distributions of cadherin and catenin complexes in polarized epithelial cells. *J. Cell Biol.* **125,** 1341–1352.

182. Kikuchi, A. (2000) Regulation of beta-catenin signaling in the Wnt pathway. *Biochem. Biophys. Res. Commun.* **268,** 243–248.

183. Chenn, A. and Walsh, C. A. (2003) Increased neuronal production, enlarged forebrains and cytoarchitectural distortions in beta-catenin overexpressing transgenic mice. *Cereb. Cortex* **13,** 599–606.

184. Sommer, L., Ma, Q., and Anderson, D. J. (1996) neurogenins, a novel family of atonal-related bHLH transcription factors, are putative mammalian neuronal determination genes that reveal progenitor cell heterogeneity in the developing CNS and PNS. *Mol. Cell Neurosci.* **8,** 221–241.

185. Lo, L. C., Johnson, J. E., Wuenschell, C. W., Saito, T., and Anderson, D. J. (1991) Mammalian achaete-scute homolog 1 is transiently expressed by spatially restricted subsets of early neuroepithelial and neural crest cells. *Genes Dev.* **5,** 1524–1537.

186. Guillemot, F., Lo, L. C., Johnson, J. E., Auerbach, A., Anderson, D. J., and Joyner, A. L. (1993) Mammalian *achaete-scute* homolog 1 is required for the early development of olfactory and autonomic neurons. *Cell* **75,** 463–476.

187. Nieto, M., Schuurmans, C., Britz, O., and Guillemot, F. (2001) Neural bHLH genes control the neuronal versus glial fate decision in cortical progenitors. *Neuron* **29,** 401–413.

188. Ross, S. E., Greenberg, M. E., and Stiles, C. D. (2003) Basic helix–loop–helix factors in cortical development. *Neuron* **39,** 13–25.

189. Lee, J. K., Cho, J. H., Hwang, W. S., Lee, Y. D., Reu, D. S., and Suh-Kim, H. (2000) Expression of neuroD/BETA2 in mitotic and postmitotic neuronal cells during the development of nervous system. *Dev. Dyn.* **217,** 361–367.

190. Farah, M. H., Olson, J. M., Sucic, H. B., Hume, R. I., Tapscott, S. J., and Turner, D. L. (2000) Generation of neurons by transient expression of neural bHLH proteins in mammalian cells. *Development* **127,** 693–702.

191. Casarosa, S., Fode, C., and Guillemot, F. (1999) *Mash1* regulates neurogenesis in the ventral telencephalon. *Development* **126,** 525–534.

192. Fode, C., Ma, Q., Casarosa, S., Ang, S. L., Anderson, D. J., and Guillemot, F. (2000) A role for neural determination genes in specifying the dorsoventral identity of telencephalic neurons. *Genes Dev.* **14,** 67–80.

193. Chapouton, P., Schuurmans, C., Guillemot, F., and Gotz, M. (2001) The transcription factor *neurogenin 2* restricts cell migration from the cortex to the striatum. *Development* **128,** 5149–5159.

194. Parras, C. M., Schuurmans, C., Scardigli, R., Kim, J., Anderson, D. J., and Guillemot, F. (2002) Divergent functions of the proneural genes *Mash1* and *Ngn2* in the specification of neuronal subtype identity. *Genes Dev.* **16,** 324–338.

195. Sun, Y., Nadal-Vicens, M., Misono, S., et al. (2001) Neurogenin promotes neurogenesis and inhibits glial differentiation by independent mechanisms. *Cell* **104,** 365–376.

196. Lu, Q. R., Yuk, D., Alberta, J. A., et al. (2000) Sonic hedgehog—regulated oligodendrocyte lineage genes encoding bHLH proteins in the mammalian central nervous system. *Neuron* **25,** 317–329.

197. Takebayashi, H., Yoshida, S., Sugimori, M., et al. (2000) Dynamic expression of basic helix–loop–helix *Olig* family members: implication of *Olig2* in neuron and oligodendrocyte differentiation and identification of a new member, *Olig3. Mech. Dev.* **99,** 143–148.

198. Zhou, Q., Wang, S., and Anderson, D. J. (2000) Identification of a novel family of oligodendrocyte lineage-specific basic helix–loop–helix transcription factors. *Neuron* **25,** 331–343.

199. Zhou, Q. and Anderson, D. J. (2002) The bHLH transcription factors OLIG2 and OLIG1 couple neuronal and glial subtype specification. *Cell* **109,** 61–73.

200. Mizuguchi, R., Sugimori, M., Takebayashi, H., et al. (2001) Combinatorial roles of olig2 and neurogenin2 in the coordinated induction of pan-neuronal and subtype-specific properties of motoneurons. *Neuron* **31,** 757–771.

201. Novitch, B. G., Chen, A. I., and Jessell, T. M. (2001) Coordinate regulation of motor neuron subtype identity and pan-neuronal properties by the bHLH repressor Olig2. *Neuron* **31,** 773–789.

202. Sakamoto, M., Hirata, H., Ohtsuka, T., Bessho, Y., and Kageyama, R. (2003) The basic helix–loop–helix genes *Hesr1/Hey1* and *Hesr2/Hey2* regulate maintenance of neural precursor cells in the brain. *J. Biol. Chem.* **278,** 44808–44815.

203. Tomita, K., Ishibashi, M., Nakahara, K., et al. (1996) Mammalian *hairy* and *Enhancer of split* homolog 1 regulates differentiation of retinal neurons and is essential for eye morphogenesis. *Neuron* **16,** 723–734.

204. Castella, P., Wagner, J. A., and Caudy, M. (1999) Regulation of hippocampal neuronal differentiation by the basic helix–loop–helix transcription factors *HES-1* and *MASH-1. J. Neurosci. Res.* **56,** 229–240.

205. Furukawa, T., Mukherjee, S., Bao, Z. Z., Morrow, E. M., and Cepko, C. L. (2000) rax, Hes1, and notch1 promote the formation of Müller glia by postnatal retinal progenitor cells. *Neuron* **26,** 383–394.

206. Walther, C. and Gruss, P. (1991) *Pax-6,* a murine paired box gene, is expressed in the developing CNS. *Development* **113,** 1435–1449.

207. Gotz, M., Stoykova, A., and Gruss, P. (1998) *Pax6* controls radial glia differentiation in the cerebral cortex. *Neuron* **21,** 1031–1044.

208. Stoykova, A., Gotz, M., Gruss, P., and Price, J. (1997) *Pax6*-dependent regulation of adhesive patterning, R-cadherin expression and boundary formation in developing forebrain. *Development* **124,** 3765–3777.

209. Heins, N., Malatesta, P., Cecconi, F., et al. (2002) Glial cells generate neurons: the role of the transcription factor *Pax6. Nat. Neurosci.* **5,** 308–315.

210. Scardigli, R., Schuurmans, C., Gradwohl, G., and Guillemot, F. (2001) Crossregulation between *Neurogenin2* and pathways specifying neuronal identity in the spinal cord. *Neuron* **31,** 203–217.

211. Anderson, S. A., Eisenstat, D. D., Shi, L., and Rubenstein, J. L. (1997) Interneuron migration from basal forebrain to neocortex: dependence on *Dlx* genes. *Science* **278,** 474–476.

212. Anderson, S. A., Qiu, M., Bulfone, A., et al. (1997) Mutations of the homeobox genes *Dlx-1* and *Dlx-2* disrupt the striatal subventricular zone and differentiation of late born striatal neurons. *Neuron* **19,** 27–37.

213. Stuhmer, T., Anderson, S. A., Ekker, M., and Rubenstein, J. L. (2002) Ectopic expression of the *Dlx* genes induces glutamic acid decarboxylase and *Dlx* expression. *Development* **129,** 245–252.
214. Stuhmer, T., Puelles, L., Ekker, M., and Rubenstein, J. L. (2002) Expression from a Dlx gene enhancer marks adult mouse cortical GABAergic neurons. *Cereb. Cortex* **12,** 75–85.
215. Panganiban, G. and Rubenstein, J. L. (2002) Developmental functions of the *Distal-less/Dlx* homeobox genes. *Development* **129,** 4371–4386.
216. Allan, D. W. and Thor, S. (2003) Together at last: bHLH and LIM-HD regulators cooperate to specify motor neurons. *Neuron* **38,** 675–677.
217. Lee, S. K. and Pfaff, S. L. (2003) Synchronization of neurogenesis and motor neuron specification by direct coupling of bHLH and homeodomain transcription factors. *Neuron* **38,** 731–745.
218. Sun, T., Dong, H., Wu, L., Kane, M., Rowitch, D. H., and Stiles, C. D. (2003) Cross-repressive interaction of the Olig2 and Nkx2.2 transcription factors in developing neural tube associated with formation of a specific physical complex. *J. Neurosci.* **23,** 9547–9556.
219. Hardcastle, Z. and Papalopulu, N. (2000) Distinct effects of XBF-1 in regulating the cell cycle inhibitor p27(XIC1) and imparting a neural fate. *Development* **127,** 1303–1314.
220. Dou, C. L., Li, S., and Lai, E. (1999) Dual role of brain factor-1 in regulating growth and patterning of the cerebral hemispheres. *Cereb. Cortex* **9,** 543–550.
221. Heins, N., Cremisi, F., Malatesta, P., et al. (2001) *Emx2* promotes symmetric cell divisions and a multipotential fate in precursors from the cerebral cortex. *Mol. Cell Neurosci.* **18,** 485–502.
222. Estivill-Torrus, G., Pearson, H., van Heyningen, V., Price, D. J., and Rashbass, P. (2002) *Pax6* is required to regulate the cell cycle and the rate of progression from symmetrical to asymmetrical division in mammalian cortical progenitors. *Development* **129,** 455–466.
223. Loosli, F., Winkler, S., Burgtorf, C., et al. (2001) Medaka eyeless is the key factor linking retinal determination and eye growth. *Development* **128,** 4035–4044.
224. Andreazzoli, M., Gestri, G., Angeloni, D., Menna, E., and Barsacchi, G. (1999) Role of *Xrx1* in *Xenopus* eye and anterior brain development. *Development* **126,** 2451–2460.
225. Carl, M., Loosli, F., and Wittbrodt, J. (2002) *Six3* inactivation reveals its essential role for the formation and patterning of the vertebrate eye. *Development* **129,** 4057–4063.
226. Zuber, M. E., Perron, M., Philpott, A., Bang, A., and Harris, W. A. (1999) Giant eyes in *Xenopus laevis* by overexpression of *XOptx2*. *Cell* **98,** 341–352.
227. Zezula, J., Casaccia-Bonnefil, P., Ezhevsky, S. A., et al. (2001) p21cip1 is required for the differentiation of oligodendrocytes independently of cell cycle withdrawal. *EMBO Rep.* **2,** 27–34.
228. Murciano, A., Zamora, J., Lopez-Sanchez, J., and Frade, J. M. (2002) Interkinetic nuclear movement may provide spatial clues to the regulation of neurogenesis. *Mol. Cell Neurosci.* **21,** 285–300.

5

Regulation of Neural Stem Cell Death

Rizwan S. Akhtar and Kevin A. Roth

INTRODUCTION

Nervous system development is a complex process that begins with a small number of cells and ends with a highly organized and specialized organ. Neural stem cells play a critical role in this process. These cells have the capacity to self-renew, proliferate, and give rise to lineage-restricted neuronal and/or glial progenitor cells and postmitotic specialized daughter cells. The number of neural stem cells contributing to neural development depends on the balance between proliferation, self-renewal, differentiation, and cell death. Studies of apoptosis-associated molecules have indicated significant cell death in neural precursor cells, defined as neural stem cells and lineage restricted progenitors, and immature neurons prior to the generation of synaptic contacts. These studies complement the extensive body of work dedicated to cell death regulation in mature neurons, where competition for limited amounts of target-derived neurotrophic factors plays a direct role in activating cell death pathways during neuronal histogenesis and cell injury. The striking neurodevelopmental abnormalities observed in mice with targeted disruptions in genes regulating cell death emphasizes the importance of programmed cell death during development. Studies of these animals further reveal that cell death regulation is remarkably specific to cell type and stage of neural differentiation.

Recently, neural stem cells have been identified in and isolated from the adult brain, where they contribute to active neurogenesis in select brain regions. Dysregulated proliferation and/or cell death of adult neural stem cells has been postulated to contribute to psychiatric and neurological diseases. The transplantation of neural stem cells into injured areas of the adult brain, such as those damaged by hypoxic–ischemic insult or neurodegenerative diseases, is being studied in animal models and may soon become feasible in humans. For these reasons, a comprehensive understanding of the molecular signals that control neural stem cell death is of great interest.

In this chapter, we review the forms of cell death seen in the developing and adult nervous systems and consider the molecular requirements for cell death in neural precursor cells and immature neurons. Estimates of the magnitude of cell death occurring during mammalian nervous development have varied widely, and we discuss this interesting controversy. Finally, we review recent evidence for neural stem cell death in the adult nervous system.

From: *Neural Development and Stem Cells, Second Edition*
Edited by: M. S. Rao © Humana Press Inc., Totowa, NJ

OVERVIEW OF FORMS OF CELL DEATH IN THE NERVOUS SYSTEM

Several morphologically distinct forms of cell death can be seen in the nervous system in response to physiological or pathological stimuli. The term "programmed cell death" refers to cell death occurring normally during development, which is distinct from pathological cell death following toxic stimuli *(1)*. By definition, programmed cell death is both spatially and temporally reproducible. For example, in the nematode *Caenorhabditis elegans*, programmed cell death selectively removes 131 of the 1090 somatic cells generated during development *(2)*. In mammals, programmed cell death is seen during the regression of vestigial organs, the folding, fusion, and maturation of the neural tube and neural plate, and the elimination of newly generated neurons during neural histogenesis *(3,4)*. A great deal of attention has been focused on determining the molecules and key regulatory steps that initiate and execute programmed cell death. It is useful to classify types of programmed cell death based on morphological criteria, although in some cases, multiple morphological forms of death can be visualized in the same cell or following the same death stimulus.

Apoptosis

The most common morphological type of programmed cell death in the nervous system is apoptosis *(5)*. First formally described by Kerr, Wyllie, and Currie in 1972, apoptosis is evidenced by condensation of nuclear chromatin followed by nuclear fragmentation *(6)*. Similarly, the cytoplasm of the apoptotic cell condenses and forms cytoplasmic membrane protrusions, or "blebs." These fragments form apoptotic bodies, or membrane-bound vesicles that contain a heterogeneous mix of intracellular materials. Apoptotic bodies are rapidly removed by neighboring cells or phagocytes, making apoptosis a remarkably efficient method of disposing dysfunctional or redundant cells without producing significant inflammation. Other hallmark signs of apoptosis include cell rounding following cytoskeletal collapse and exposure of phosphatidylserine on the outer cell membrane surface. A combination of light microscopy and ultrastructural examination provides the best evidence for apoptotic processes *(7,8)*.

Like many aspects of our understanding of cell death regulation, early discoveries of the molecular requirements for apoptosis were made in simpler nematode systems. In *C. elegans*, the *ced-3* gene is required for the execution of programmed cell death *(9,10)*. Successful cloning of *ced-3* revealed its similarity to human interleukin-1 β converting enzyme, which was later renamed caspase-1 *(10–12)*. Since that time, approx 15 mammalian homologs have been identified that are collectively termed caspases. Caspases are cysteine proteases that are synthesized as inactive zymogens and are cleaved at specific sequences containing aspartate to form the active enzyme. In turn, a wide variety of intracellular proteins are substrates for caspases, including structural proteins, protein kinases, DNA metabolism and repair enzymes, a number of signaling molecules, and other caspases *(13,14)*.

As we will discuss, caspases are critical for most, but not all, forms of programmed cell death. Specific initiator caspases are activated based on the nature of the apoptotic stimulus and the particular intracellular pathway activated. On receipt of a pro-death stimulus, upstream initiator caspases catalyze the cleavage and activation of downstream effector caspases. Initiator caspases include caspase-2, -8, -9, and -10, and effector caspases include caspase-3, -6, and -7. The cleavage events triggered by effector caspase activation are commonly considered indicators of apoptosis, although caspase-mediated cleavage events are not necessarily required for cell death. Furthermore, under some circumstances, caspase-cleaved products are found unassociated with cell death.

Given the wide number of caspase substrates, the enzymatic activity of caspases is under tight regulation. A major portion of this regulation is accomplished by members of the Bcl-2 family of proteins. While caspases are more involved in the execution phase of cell death, the Bcl-2 family is positioned to regulate entry into these death pathways. In 1984, the oncogene *bcl-2* was found linked to the immunoglobulin heavy chain in the 14;18 chromosome translocation known to be responsible for follicular lymphoma *(15,16)*. Since that time, a large number of Bcl-2–related molecules have been identified *(17,18)*, and recent studies indicate that several Bcl-2 family members contribute to regulation of programmed cell death in neuronal cell populations.

Bcl-2 family members can be divided into three subfamilies based on the number of conserved Bcl-2 homology (BH) domains present on each molecule and by whether the activated molecule inhibits or promotes cell death. The first subfamily is composed of anti-death molecules that express four conserved BH domains, such as Bcl-2 and Bcl-x_L. The second subfamily consists of pro-death molecules that express multiple BH domains, typically BH1, 2, and 3, and includes Bax and Bak. The remaining pro-death Bcl-2 family members comprise the BH3-domain only subfamily, which contain a BH3 domain, but not BH1 or BH2 domains. This structurally diverse subfamily includes Bid, Bad, Noxa, Puma, and Hrk/Dp5. As a family, these molecules exhibit developmentally regulated, tissue-specific expression patterns. Bcl-2 family members are also regulated by phosphorylation, subcellular localization, proteolysis, and other posttranslational modifications.

An elegant "suicide rheostat" model was proposed to explain the roles of Bcl-2 family members in the regulation of cell death *(19)*. The BH domains expressed by these molecules allow homo- and heterodimerization between pro- and anti-death members. According to this model, in the "living state," pro-death Bcl-2 family members are prevented from inducing death pathways by being bound to anti-death molecules. The presence of an apoptotic stimulus tips the balance toward the pro-death molecules, either by decreasing the activation of anti-death molecules or by increasing the effectiveness of pro-death molecules. Several roles for Bcl-2 family members have been described, many of which involve upstream signal transduction processes that converge on mitochondrial function and the activation of effector caspases.

Intrinsic Pathway of Apoptosis

A number of key cell death regulators reside and/or act at the mitochondria and are critical components of the intrinsic apoptotic pathway (Fig. 1). Ultimately, the intrinsic apoptotic pathway results in mitochondrial dysfunction and activation of caspase-3. Caspase-3 is the predominant effector caspase in the nervous system, and its activation is responsible for producing cytological features of apoptosis. Caspase-3 resides in an inactive zymogen form and becomes activated by cleavage by initiator caspases. This cleavage event generates an 18-kDa large subunit and a 12-kDa small subunit from a 32-kDa precursor *(20)*. Several cytosolic factors capable of inducing caspase-3

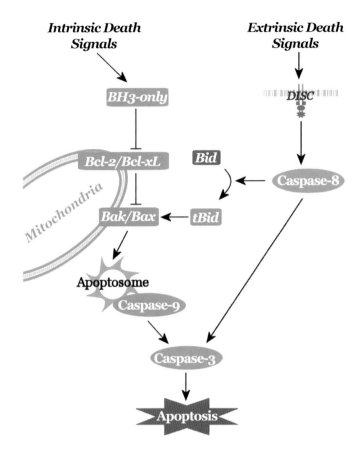

Fig. 1. Apoptosis is regulated by the intrinsic and extrinsic pathways. Intrinsic death stimuli signal through pro-death BH3-domain only molecules. These molecules influence anti-death Bcl-2 family members (Bcl-2, Bcl-x$_L$) and pro-death multidomain members (Bax, Bak). Once activated, pro-death members Bax and Bak stimulate mitochondrial release of cytochrome *c* and the formation of the apoptosome. This complex activates caspase-9 and -3, which ultimately leads to apoptosis. The extrinsic death pathway is activated by binding of extracellular death ligands and the formation of the death inducing signaling complex (DISC). The DISC directly activates caspase-8, which can activate caspase-3. In addition, the DISC catalyzes the activation of Bid, which modulates mitochondrial cytochrome *c* release. See text for details.

cleavage were isolated in cell free experiments and called apoptotic protease activating factor-1 (Apaf-1) and Apaf-2 *(21,22)*. Two additional factors, dATP and Apaf-3 (later identified as caspase-9), were also necessary *(23)*. Apaf-1 was characterized as a 130-kDa cytosolic protein *(21,23)*. The identification of Apaf-2 as cytochrome *c* indicated a critical role for mitochondrial function in apoptosis initiation. Caspase-9 is a 45-kDa cytosolic protein that is synthesized as an inactive proenzyme *(23–25)*. Using active site mutations of caspase-9 to prevent caspase-3 activation, a linear relationship between caspase-9 and caspase-3 activation was identified *(23)*. Therefore, Apaf-1, caspase-9, cytochrome *c*, and dATP critically regulate caspase-3 activation.

In the unstimulated state, Apaf-1 is a compact molecule with its N-terminal caspase recruitment domain (CARD) internally sequestered *(23)*. Upon binding of cytosolic cytochrome *c* and dATP, Apaf-1 is linearized and the CARD becomes exposed, which recruits pro-caspase-9 *(22)*. The "apoptosome," a 1.4 MDa ATP-dependent complex formed by cytochrome *c*, Apaf-1, and pro-caspase-9, has been reported to consist of seven activated Apaf-1 molecules arranged as a seven spoked wheel *(26)*. Each Apaf-1 molecule is bound to one cytochrome *c* molecule and a dimer of caspase-9. Once formed, the apoptosome transduces intrinsic apoptotic signaling by catalyzing the further activation of caspase-9. Ultimately, activated caspase-9 cleaves and activates caspase-3. In this manner, mitochondrial release of cytochrome *c* directly influences caspase activation. The formation of the apoptosome is a highly regulated event in the intrinsic apoptotic pathway. Another small molecule, apoptosis-inducing factor (AIF), is also released by mitochondria during apoptosis signaling. AIF is capable of inducing nuclear condensation and DNA fragmentation independently of effector caspases, and can induce other downstream markers of apoptosis.

The release of mitochondrial cytochrome *c* during apoptosis is due to alterations of mitochondrial membrane permeability, and at the molecular level, one of the primary functions of Bcl-2 family members is the regulation of mitochondrial membrane integrity *(27,28)*. Two pro-apoptotic members of the Bcl-2 family, Bax and Bak, are clearly involved in the release of cytochrome *c* from the mitochondrial membrane. A great number of apoptotic stimuli, both during development and in the context of pathological insults, affect Bax and/or Bak function. It has been proposed that Bax and Bak form homo- and hetero-oligomeric pores through which cytochrome *c*, AIF, and other small intermembrane proteins are released. Alternatively, Bax and Bak may induce the formation of the membrane permeability transition pore and a loss of membrane potential.

In the unactivated state, Bax is predominantly cytoplasmic, where it may be complexed with anti-apoptotic members of the Bcl-2 family. An apoptotic stimulus may induce conformational changes in BH3-domain only proteins, the anti-apoptotic molecules Bcl-2 or Bcl-x$_L$, or Bax itself *(29–32)*. These changes liberate Bax, allowing it to translocate to the outer mitochondrial membrane. In contrast to Bax, Bak resides at the mitochondrial surface at baseline, where it may undergo conformational changes in apoptotic conditions.

Bcl-x plays a critical role in modulating Bax and Bak-dependent apoptosis and can be alternatively spliced to form a pro-apoptotic molecule, Bcl-x$_S$, or an anti-apoptotic form, Bcl-x$_L$. Bcl-x$_S$ is expressed only weakly or not at all in the nervous system *(33,34)*. Bcl-x$_L$ is highly expressed in the embryonic nervous system and persists in the adult brain at high levels *(34,35)*. Consistent with the hypothesis that pro- and anti-death Bcl-2 family members interact to control apoptosis, Bcl-x$_L$ is able to hetero-dimerize with Bax and Bak and prevent their channel forming activity at the mitochondrial surface *(19,34,36–39)*. Similarly, Bax is able to bind Bcl-x$_L$ and attenuate the latter molecule's ability to suppress apoptosis *(38)*. The contributions of these and other molecules to neural stem cell death are discussed in the following paragraphs.

Extrinsic Pathway of Apoptosis

The extrinsic pathway of apoptosis initiation couples extracellular death signals with intracellular death effectors (Fig. 1). Whereas the intrinsic apoptotic pathway is thought to begin with activation of BH3-domain only proteins, the extrinsic pathway is initiated by extracellular death cytokines, such as Fas ligand (CD95L) and tumor necrosis factor (TNF). This pathway allows signals from neighboring cells or the extracellular milieu to induce apoptosis by interacting with cell surface "death receptors" *(40,41)*. By recruiting intracellular molecules, ligand-bound death receptors can directly activate initiator caspases and apoptosis. Upon cytokine binding, the intracellular domains of death receptors oligomerize and recruit intracellular proteins that express death domains. The complex formed is referred to as the death inducing signaling complex (DISC). The DISC actively recruits the inactive zymogen form of caspase-8 and catalyzes its cleavage *(42,43)*. Caspase-8 is an initiator caspase that activates effector caspases such as caspase-3 and -7.

Caspase-8 activation, in some cell types, also triggers the intrinsic death pathway through Bcl-2 family intermediaries, which may serve to amplify the death receptor signal *(43,44)*. Activated caspase-8 has been shown to cleave Bid, a BH3-domain only member of the Bcl-2 protein family. Truncated Bid (tBid) translocates to the mitochondrial surface and engages the intrinsic apoptotic pathway by inducing the release of mitochondrial cytochrome *c (44)*. Several cytokines signal via the extrinsic apoptotic death pathway, and evidence for extrinsic death signaling during neural stem cell death is reviewed in the following paragraphs.

Autophagy

The second major morphological type of programmed cell death is autophagic cell death *(5)*. Autophagy has been investigated in yeast as a catabolic survival mechanism following nutrient starvation. Autophagic cell death is characterized by the presence of large numbers of autophagosomes in a cell displaying additional cytological evidence of degeneration. Although the precise molecular mechanism of autophagy is currently being pursued, autophagy plays a significant role in programmed cell death in some lower animals and possibly in mammals *(13,45)*. Autophagy is mediated in part by lysosomal enzymes and autophagic cell death may involve lysosomal dysfunction. The specific and nonspecific catabolic enzymes harbored within lysosomes are routinely used in recycling of damaged or redundant organelles and other cytoplasmic components. On activation of autophagic cell death, numerous vacuoles containing intracellular material begin to form, which ultimately fuse with the lysosomal compartment and are degraded *(45)*. These characteristic double membrane-bound vesicles can be positively identified by ultrastructural examination. In addition, some instances of autophagic cell death show nuclear pyknosis and other cytological features of apoptosis. The role of autophagy in neural programmed cell death, although far from clear, is currently under investigation. A large number of cells are able to efficiently die and dispose of their cellular content via autophagy, making this death mechanism a good candidate for bulk degradation of supernumerary cells. In this respect, disposal of apoptotic bodies from a large number of dying cells would require a large number of phagocytes or a great phagocytic capacity of neighboring cells, two features that may not be present in the developing nervous system.

Necrosis

While the majority of programmed cell death in the nervous system has been described as apoptotic, autophagic, or a combination of both, a minority displays necrotic features *(5)*. Necrosis is often described as a chaotic, passive death process that arises when cells are exposed to extreme stress, such as the lack of oxygen and essential nutrients or the exposure to toxic compounds, elevated or decreased tempera-ture, or excessive mechanical strain. However, recent evidence suggests that necrosis may follow predictable patterns and be regulated in some fashion *(46)*. Our under-standing of the regulation of necrosis remains incomplete. Some preliminary evidence suggests that loss of mitochondrial membrane potential or the accumulation of reactive oxygen species following "apoptotic stimuli" may lead to necrosis. Furthermore, mutations in several genes named degenerins in *C. elegans* can induce necrosis *(47)*. Necrosis has extensively been studied in models of neuronal excitotoxic death, but the role of necrosis in neural stem cell death is unclear.

MOLECULAR REGULATION
OF NEURAL STEM CELL DEATH DURING DEVELOPMENT

The molecules and regulatory steps controlling programmed cell death during development have received considerable scientific interest over the last few decades. In the nervous system, the molecular requirements for death vary based on the specific cell type in question, the differentiation state of the cell, and the functional synaptic connections made by the cell. During development, specific molecules are required for cell death as neural precursor cells become mature neurons, and will be reviewed here.

Caspase Regulation of Developmental Cell Death

Caspase-3 is expressed in the brain throughout embryonic development, including in the cortical plate and ventricular zone where neural precursors are known to reside *(48,49)*. Caspase-3 plays an important role in affecting programmed cell death of neu-ral precursor cell populations. These founder cells initially reside in the ventricular zone, and give rise to immature neurons during development. Programmed cell death, in addition to differentiation, removes individual cells from this neural precursor cell population. Apaf-1 and caspase-9 are also expressed in the brain and spinal cord during prenatal development and in adult tissues, indicating that the necessary regulators of apoptotic cell death are present and capable of triggering neural stem cell death *(50–53)*.

If caspases are critical for programmed cell death of neural stem cells, early neural progenitors, and newly born immature neurons, the deficiency of these molecules would be predicted to cause significant abnormalities in brain development. This hypothesis was proven correct by the generation of caspase-3-, caspase-9-, and Apaf-1-deficient mice.

Caspase-3 knockout mice show extensive perinatal lethality and are smaller than their wild-type littermates *(50)*. These mice have significant ventricular zone hyperpla-sia, resulting from a defect in programmed cell death in neural precursor cells, and show prominent exencephaly and cranial defects (Fig. 2). Surviving animals show multiple indentations and ectopic neuronal masses in the cortex and persistent germi-nal layers in the developing cerebellum. Importantly, there is a striking decrease in the number of cells undergoing apoptosis during development in caspase-3-deficient embryos as compared to wild-type embryos *(50)*. Caspase-3 deficiency does not sig-nificantly alter proliferation in the ventricular zone, consistent with the thought that decreased programmed cell death, and not increased proliferation, of caspase-3-defi-cient neural precursor cells leads to the neurodevelopmental phenotype *(49)*.

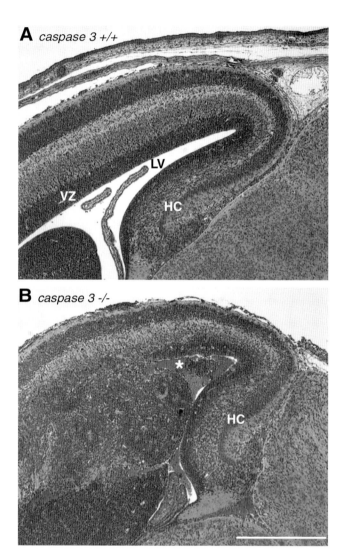

Fig. 2. Deficiency of caspase-3 induces neurodevelopmental abnormalities. **(A,B)** Sagittal sections from mouse embryonic forebrain stained with hematoxylin and eosin. **(A)** *Caspase-3* +/+ mouse embryo shows normal brain development, including well-demarcated ventricular zone (VZ), cortical lamination, patent lateral ventricle (LV), and developing hippocampus (HC). **(B)** *Caspase-3* -/- mouse shows expansion of neural precursor cells in the ventricular zone, intraventricular hemorrhage (marked with an asterisk), and neural precursor cells growing into and filling the ventricular lumen. Scale bar = 500 μm.

Interestingly, we have found that mouse-strain specific genetic modifiers alter the neurodevelopmental phenotype and perinatal lethality caused by caspase-3 deficiency. Caspase-3-deficient 129X1/SvJ mice showed exencephaly, neural precursor cell expansion, and perinatal lethality; in contrast, caspase-3-deficient C57BL/6J mice were normal *(54)*. Intercrosses of C57BL/6J and 129X1/SvJ mice have indicated the presence of one or more incompletely penetrant autosomal dominant modifiers in the

129X1/SvJ genome that affect the severity of the caspase-3-deficient neuronal phenotype *(54)*. Future studies of the variable caspase-3 developmental phenotype will shed light on these modifiers, and these observations serve as an important reminder of the importance of genetic background when considering data and conclusions derived from gene-disrupted mice.

As mentioned earlier, both caspase-8 and caspase-9 are able to activate caspase-3, resulting from activation of the extrinsic and intrinsic apoptotic pathways, respectively. Caspase-9-dependent activation of caspase-3 has been directly demonstrated in the developing nervous system. No caspase-3 activation is detected in the caspase-9-deficient brain, suggesting that caspase-9 and -3 participate in a linear signaling pathway *(51,55–57)*. Furthermore, gene disruption of *caspase-9* in mice produces a neurodevelopmental phenotype similar to that seen in caspase-3-deficient mice. Caspase-8 expression can be detected in the mid- and hind-brains of E9.5–10.5 mice embryos, and caspase-8-deficient embryos show aberrant neural tube formation, hepatic erythrocytosis, and developmental heart abnormalities *(58–62)*. Given the embryonic lethality before E12.5, it is unclear whether caspase-8 deficiency has any effects on nervous system development occurring at later times. However, alterations in other components of the extrinsic death pathways, such as CD95 and CD95L, fail to affect nervous system development and mice deficient in these molecules show no abnormalities in neural precursor cell death *(63–65)*. Additional studies of genes associated with the extrinsic death pathway are required before conclusions can be drawn about this pathway's regulation of neural stem cell death.

Gene disruption of either *caspase-9* or *apaf-1* in mice produces severe brain abnormalities resulting from dysregulation in programmed cell death of neural precursor cells *(51–53,55)*. Both caspase-9 and Apaf-1-deficient mice are perinatal lethal and demonstrate exencephaly, cerebral ventricular stenosis, neural precursor cell hyperplasia, and ectopic neural masses (Fig. 3). These changes result from a marked hyperplasia of proliferative zones in the forebrain and midbrain. These mice also have defects in neural tube closure and frequently exhibit intracerebral hemorrhage. There are no gross malformations in the spinal cord or other nonneural organs in caspase-9-deficient mice *(51,55)*. Importantly, the Apaf-1-deficient phenotype can have several additional abnormalities not seen in caspase-9- or caspase-3-deficient animals. Apaf-1-deficient mice display a midline facial cleft, absence of cranial bones, imperfect palatal fusion, persistent interdigital webs, retinal hyperplasia, and alterations of the lens and ocular vasculature *(52,53)*. These results suggest that Apaf-1 may have caspase-9-independent roles in regulating apoptosis in the primordial palate, and provide additional evidence for the remarkable cell-type specificity of regulatory death molecules.

The neuropathological findings in caspase-9- and Apaf-1-deficient mice are due to a striking reduction in apoptosis of neural precursor cell populations. There is a significant reduction in Tdt-mediated dUTP nick-end labeling (TUNEL) staining, activated caspase-3 immunoreactivity, and morphological features of apoptosis in both caspase-9- and Apaf-1-deficient mice *(51–53,55)*. Concomitantly, there is an increase in the number of neural precursor cells in the ventricular zone, as would be expected from reduced apoptosis of these cells *(51)*.

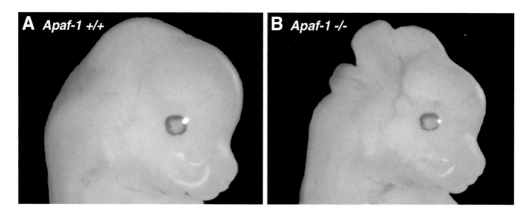

Fig. 3. Abnormal brain development is associated with Apaf-1 deficiency. (**A**) An *Apaf-1* +/+ mouse is developmentally normal at embryonic day 13. (**B**) In comparison, Apaf-1 deficiency causes exencephaly and abnormal craniofacial development.

Bcl-2 Family Regulation of Developmental Cell Death

Upstream regulators of caspase function, notably members of the Bcl-2 family, influence cell death during neural development in a cell-type-specific manner. Of the anti-apoptotic Bcl-2 family, *bcl-x* has been shown to critically regulate programmed cell death of newly born immature neurons. A great deal of interest has been focused on individual pro-death Bcl-2 molecules in a variety of neuronal cell death paradigms; however, programmed cell death in neural precursor cells appears to depend on the expression of both Bax and Bak. In neural precursor cells, a balance exists between Bcl-x_L, Bax, and Bak, and may be the primary global mechanism by which cell death is regulated in these populations during development.

Bcl-2 Family Molecules in Neural Precursor Cells

Expression of *bcl-x* is significant during brain development, and *bcl-x* disruption induces pronounced cell death in the rostral spinal cord, brain stem, dorsal root ganglia, lamina terminalis, and intermediate zone of the brain *(66–68)*. However, there is no effect of *bcl-x* disruption in the embryonic mouse ventricular zone, and neural precursor cells do not show increased apoptosis in *bcl-x* disrupted mice. This finding is not surprising since the expression of Bcl-x_L is very low in the ventricular zone *(48)*. Also, *bcl-x* disruption does not prevent the caspase-9- or caspase-3-deficient neurodevelopmental phenotype *(48,68,69)*. Based on these observations, the endogenous stimuli that control neural precursor cell death and survival appear not to depend on Bcl-x_L expression alone. The upstream factors that control programmed cell death in these cells remain under investigation.

Bax is expressed at high levels in both the embryonic and adult brain and a number of reports have described the role of Bax in controlling neuron death in response to diminished target-derived survival signals, making it a candidate for regulation of cell death in neural precursor cells *(19,38,70)*. Bak, a second multidomain pro-apoptotic Bcl-2 family member, is also expressed during mouse brain development and may also regulate neural stem cell death *(71–74)*. Alone, gene disruptions in *bax* or *bak* have little effect on programmed cell death in neural precursor cells. There is no exencephaly,

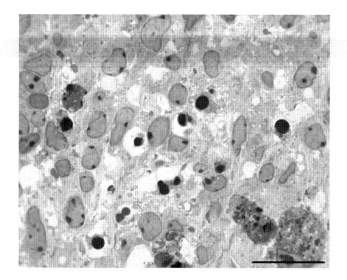

Fig. 4. Bcl-x$_L$ deficiency results in extensive death of newly generated neurons. Many apoptotic nuclei with condensed nuclei can be appreciated in the intermediate zone of a gestational day 12 *bcl-x -/-* mouse (1 μm thick plastic section stained with toluidine blue). Phagocytic cells filled with debris can be seen in lower right. Scale bar = 20 μm.

hyperplasia of the ventricular zone, ectopic neuronal structures, or telencephalic expansion in Bax or Bak-deficient embryos, as seen with disruptions of *caspase-3*, *caspase-9*, or *Apaf-1 (57,75)*. These findings suggest that either neural precursor cell death during embryonic development is independent of Bax and Bak, or that multidomain pro-apoptotic Bcl-2 family members act in concert to regulate neural precursor cell death. The generation of Bax/Bak double-deficient mice provided strong support for the latter hypothesis.

Bax/Bak double-deficient embryos demonstrate altered neural precursor cell death *(75,76)*. Double deficiency in both Bax and Bak is perinatal lethal; a small percentage of affected animals survived to adulthood and have persistent interdigital webs, imperforate vaginal introitus, and abnormal responses to auditory stimulation *(75)*. However, Bax/Bak double-deficient embryos do not have as severe a neurodevelopmental phenotype as caspase-9-, Apaf-1-, or caspase-3-deficient mice. Instead, a generalized increase in the number of periventricular neural precursor cells is evident primarily in the postnatal nervous system *(76)*. These results suggest that Bax and Bak play a role in controlling the number of neural precursor cells, but that other still to be defined molecules must contribute to the regulation of neural stem cell death during development.

Bcl-2 Family Molecules in Immature Neurons

Although *bcl-x* expression alone is not critically involved in neural precursor cell death, the same cannot be said for immature neuron death. Bcl-x$_L$ deficiency results in extensive cell death of newly generated neurons (Fig. 4). As these cells differentiate and migrate into the intermediate and marginal zones, Bcl-x$_L$ expression is up-regulated and necessary to prevent programmed cell death. In vitro preparation of telencephalic cultures from *bcl-x* disrupted E12.5 embryos confirms that newly generated immature neurons require *bcl-x* for survival *(68,77)*.

Bcl-x_L-deficient embryos show activation of caspase-3 throughout the developing brain, anterior spinal cord, and dorsal root ganglia *(48,78)*. This activation was especially intense in the marginal zone where post-mitotic immature neurons were present, suggesting that Bcl-x_L acts by inhibiting a caspase-3-dependent death program in neurons *(48)*. Accordingly, *bcl-x/caspase-3* double-deficient mice do not show ectopic pyknotic clusters in the cerebrum or an increase in apoptotic cells in the spinal cord or dorsal root ganglia *(48)*. *Bcl-x/caspase-9* double-deficient mice, as well as *bcl-x/Apaf-1* double-deficient mice, also show attenuated immature neuron apoptosis *(69,79,80)*.

The primary method by which Bcl-x_L prevents caspase-3 activation and apoptosis in immature neurons may be by binding to Bax and preventing Bax insertion into the mitochondrial membrane. This fact was demonstrated in *bcl-x/bax* double disrupted mice, as Bax deficiency completely prevented *bcl-x* disruption-induced apoptosis in the marginal zone, brain stem, and spinal cord *(81)*. This finding indicates that Bcl-x_L and Bax critically interact to regulate survival of newly generated neurons.

Summary

These studies implicate the Bcl-2 family, caspases, and other components of the intrinsic apoptotic death pathway as the primary molecules responsible for cell death regulation in neural precursor cells and immature neurons. It is clear that disruption of apoptosome formation, either by inoperation of Apaf-1 or caspase-9, or by modulation of Bax, Bak, or Bcl-x_L, significantly alters programmed cell death during brain development. In addition, the primary downstream target of the apoptosome, caspase-3, plays an important role in neurodevelopment. The analysis of gene-disrupted mice has afforded much insight into the role of neural precursor cell death in nervous system development.

NEURAL STEM CELL DEATH IN RESPONSE TO PATHOLOGICAL CONDITIONS

Injury to the developing brain has serious consequences for brain structure and function, and it is possible that injury of adult neural stem cells may lead to neurological and psychiatric disorders. Neural precursor cells in the developing and mature brain may be exposed to pathological stimuli including infectious agents, hypoxic–ischemic injury, and DNA damage. Neural precursor cells are exquisitely sensitive to DNA damage, suggesting that dysregulation of DNA repair mechanisms may affect survival and death of neural precursor cells or immature neurons. Specifically, p53, retinoblastoma (Rb), XRCC4, and DNA ligase IV have been implicated in regulating cell death in both neural precursor cells and immature neurons. For these reasons, we have investigated the regulation of apoptosis in neural precursor cells in vitro in response to a number of death stimuli.

Pathological Insults to Neural Precursor Cells

Neural precursor cells can be readily isolated from the embryonic telencephalon, and such cells are useful for defining the molecular requirements for neural stem cell death following exposure to various stimuli. In neural precursor cells, caspase-3 activation and cell death is readily seen following in vitro or in vivo exposure to cytosine arabinoside (AraC), γ-irradiation, and staurosporine *(82–84)* (Fig. 5). By isolating neu-

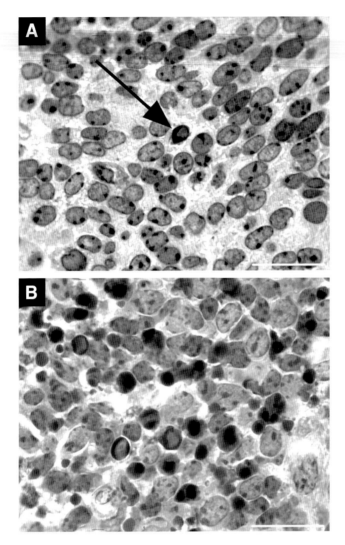

Fig. 5. DNA damage induces cell death in neural precursor cells. **(A,B)** Plastic sections of ventricular zone stained with toluidine blue. **(A)** Untreated embryos display rare apoptotic cells in the ventricular zone (arrow, center). **(B)** *In utero* exposure to cytosine arabinoside (AraC) induces widespread apoptosis, as evidenced by condensed pyknotic nuclei, in neural precursor cells of the ventricular zone. Scale bars = 20 µm.

ral precursor cells from caspase-3-deficient mice, we have found that caspase-3 is required for the generation of apoptotic features in neural precursor cells exposed to DNA-damaging agents *(83)*. However, caspase-3-deficient neural precursor cells are not protected from the death promoting effects of these stimuli *(83)*. This result, although surprising, may be explained in several ways.

First, caspase-3 may have functional overlap with other effector caspases in the developing nervous system. Caspase-6 and -7 are structurally homologous to caspase-3 and share similar substrate specificities. In certain cell types, caspase-6 and -7 make significant contributions to effector caspase activity in the absence of caspase-3 *(85)*, and it is possible that caspase-6 or -7 may subserve the function of caspase-3 in caspase-3-deficient neural precursor cells. However, caspase-6-deficient neural precursor cells and caspase-3/caspase-6 double-deficient cells are similarly sensitive to DNA damage in in vitro systems *(84)*. Similarly, minimal caspase-3 like activity is detected in caspase-3-deficient neural precursor cells, as evidenced by in vitro biochemical assays for DEVD cleavage. This result suggests that caspase-7, which shares substrate specificity with caspase-3, may not compensate for caspase-3 deficiency in neural precursor cells exposed to DNA-damaging agents *(84)*.

Second, activation of initiator caspases, upstream of caspase-3, may represent the commitment point to death. This commitment point is independent of the presence of caspase-3, which is required only for producing the morphological features of apoptosis and not death *per se*. Data strongly suggest that activation of caspase-9 may be this commitment point in neural precursor cells. Several apoptotic stimuli induce caspase-9 activation in neural precursor cells *(84)*. Activation of caspase-9 by γ-irradiation in freshly isolated neural precursor cells occurs independently of caspase-3, concordant with an upstream location of caspase-9 in the intrinsic apoptotic pathway *(84)*. Broad-spectrum caspase inhibition in freshly isolated neural precursor cells prevents caspase-3 activation and loss in cell viability following AraC treatment *(82)*. In vivo, AraC-induced DNA damage causes increased caspase-3 activation, pyknotic nuclei, and increased karyorrhectic debris in telencephalic structures of embryonic day 13 (E13) mice. These pathological findings are prevented in caspase-9-deficient embryos, indicating that caspase-9 is critical for caspase-3 activation, apoptotic morphological features, and cell death in neural precursor cells *(83)*.

Much like the in vivo results of Apaf-1 deficiency, the in vitro responses of Apaf-1-deficient cell cultures are similar to caspase-9-deficient cultures. A number of Apaf-1-deficient nonneural cell types are resistant to apoptotic stimuli, including DNA-damaging agents and staurosporine *(52,53,86)*. Transplacental exposure to AraC causes caspase-3 activation and apoptotic morphological features in the telencephalic ventricular zone of wild-type, but not Apaf-1-deficient, mouse embryos. In addition, freshly isolated Apaf-1-deficient neural precursor cells are resistant to AraC treatment as compared to wild-type cultures *(84)*.

Bax- or Bak-deficient neural precursor cells derived from the embryonic telencephalon show little protection from apoptosis following pathological insult. For example, DNA damage in neural precursor cells causes marked pyknosis, TUNEL positivity, and activation of caspase-3. Bax deficiency does not alter this response *(83)*. Although Bax-deficient neural precursor cells are not resistant to DNA damage-induced death, Bax/Bak double-deficient cells are markedly protected and show attenuated caspase-3 activation and death *(83,84)*. Double-deficient neural precursor cells derived from the cerebellum are also resistant to thapsigargin, a disruptor of Ca^{2+} trafficking at the endoplasmic reticulum *(76)*. Therefore, the functional overlap of Bax and Bak seen during development is conserved in the response to pathological insults.

The tumor suppressor protein p53 has a wide range of functions in cell cycle arrest and cell death *(87–89)*. A large number of genes, including members of the Bcl-2 family, are transcriptional targets for p53. p53-dependent up-regulation of Bax and the BH3-domain only molecules Noxa and Puma may be critical for death in neural precursor cells following specific apoptotic stimuli. p53 is highly expressed in the ventricular zone during development, and a small subset of p53-deficient mice show neural tube defects and hindbrain exencephaly without ventricular expansion *(90–93)*. This phenotype is not as severe as that seen in Apaf-1 or caspase-9 deficiency, and does not seem to arise from decreased death of neural precursor cells. p53-deficient neural precursors, both in vivo and in vitro, show decreased pyknosis, TUNEL positivity, and activated caspase-3 in response to DNA damage *(83)*.

In short, the molecular requirements for neural precursor cell apoptosis following DNA damage are not identical to the requirements for programmed cell death during brain development, although components of the intrinsic apoptotic pathway are utilized in both situations.

Pathological Insults to Immature Neurons

Several in vitro studies have confirmed the caspase dependence of *bcl-x* disruption induced death in immature telencephalic neurons. *Bcl-x* disrupted primary telencephalic neurons are markedly sensitive to trophic factor withdrawal induced death *(94,95)*. This death is prevented by concomitant caspase-9 or caspase-3 deficiency *(48,77,94,95)*. *p53* disruption, however, fails to affect the extent of *bcl-x* disruption induced-death in vivo or in vitro *(96)*.

The tumor suppressor retinoblastoma (Rb) has been implicated in terminal mitosis of newly born neurons, and interestingly, Rb-deficient mice show extensive immature neuron death similar to that observed in Bcl-x_L-deficient embryos *(97–99)*. It appears that Rb expression is required during the transition between a neural progenitor cell and an immature neuron, when cells become postmitotic and adopt a neuronal fate *(100)*. Rb-deficient mice are embryonic lethal at E14.5 as a result of hematopoietic and neurological deficits. Cell death in Rb-deficient neurons is positive for TUNEL and activated caspase-3 *(101,102)*. This latter finding suggests a role for caspase-3 in mediating Rb deficiency-induced cell death. Concomitant p53 deficiency prevents the appearance of TUNEL positivity in the CNS of Rb mutants *(101)*. However, increased apoptosis in the Rb mutant CNS is not prevented by caspase-3 deficiency, suggesting that caspase-3 activation *per se* is not required for cell death in this paradigm *(102)*.

DNA repair enzymes XRCC4 and DNA ligase IV may regulate survival and cell death of immature neurons. These enzymes are activated by double stranded DNA breaks, a stimulus that also activates p53. An unexpected consequence of gene disruption in XRCC4 or DNA ligase IV, two molecules required following DNA recombination or DNA damage, was that migrating and differentiating cortical neurons in deficient mice undergo massive apoptosis during development *(103–105)*. XRCC4-deficient immature neurons undergo apoptosis immediately after they enter the cortical plate. This death was prevented by concomitant p53 deficiency *(106,107)*. The precise role of double-stranded DNA breaks during brain development is still largely unknown, and has contributed to the debate on the relative magnitude of cell death during nervous system development.

Summary

Although not identical to stimuli that induce programmed cell death, pathological insults to neural precursor cell populations may have significant effects on normal brain function. During embryogenesis, the developing brain may be particularly susceptible to DNA damage that may have long-term functional consequences. Furthermore, the appreciation of neural stem cells in the adult has steadily grown, and it is likely that alterations in neural stem cell physiology underlie the effect of pathological insults seen in neurogenic regions of the adult brain. Pathological injury induced death in neural precursor cells and immature neurons depends on many of the same molecules and critical regulatory steps that control entry to programmed cell death during brain development. The further study of both programmed and pathological cell death in these cell populations in tandem will undoubtedly help to fill in the gaps of our understanding of death regulation in these important cell types.

MAGNITUDE OF CELL DEATH
IN THE DEVELOPING NERVOUS SYSTEM

It is clear that perturbation of programmed cell death pathways alters normal brain development. However, the relative magnitude of death during nervous system development is not agreed upon, despite considerable study. In fact, estimates of programmed cell death in the brain vary widely. Much of this controversy stems from disparate results obtained using different apoptosis detection methods.

Overview of Cell Death Indicators

Apoptotic cells have classically been identified by cytological examination. The appearance of condensed, pyknotic nuclei, nuclear membrane blebbing, and the production of apoptotic bodies can be appreciated by light and/or electron microscopy. The extensive DNA laddering seen in apoptotic cells produces DNA fragments with free 3'-OH ends. These nick ends can be labeled by terminal deoxynucleotidyl transferase (TdT) with dUTP-conjugates. This technique, named TdT-mediated dUTP nick-end labeling (TUNEL) has been widely used for the presumptive determination of apoptosis *in situ (8)*. However, TUNEL does not indicate which regulated death pathway is activated in the labeled cells, nor is it always specific for apoptotic cell death. A related technique, *in situ* end labeling plus (ISEL+), has generated relatively high estimates of programmed cell death during development, whereas TUNEL-based estimates have been significantly lower.

During the generation of apoptotic bodies, there is a detectable loss in plasma membrane polarity leading to the exposure of phosphatidylserine on the apoptotic cell surface. Phosphatidylserine receptor (PSR), located on the surface of phagocytic cells, mediates clearance of apoptotic bodies without the inflammatory response associated with necrosis *(108,109)*. Exposed phosphatidylserine is bound by the protein annexin V and can be detected using annexin V conjugates in flow cytometry and immunocytochemical applications. Interestingly, a fraction of PSR-deficient mice demonstrate exencephaly, expanded proliferative zones, and other findings reminiscent of the Apaf-1 or caspase-9-deficient phenotype *(110)*. Although it is clear that apoptotic clearance has a role in proper neural development, it remains to be determined how PSR-dependent removal of apoptotic bodies influences death in neural precursor cells.

In contrast to the previously described methods, activated caspase detection can help determine which specific regulated cell death pathway is engaged by apoptotic stimuli. Many specific antibodies are commercially available and detect epitopes generated on the cleavage and activation of a number of caspases. For example, antibodies have been generated that recognize specific epitopes on the p18 large subunit of cleaved caspase-3 *(78)*. These antibodies have greatly aided the visualization of apoptosis both in vitro and in vivo. Since the caspase family is homologous, it is possible that certain antibodies that claim specificity to single caspases are in fact immunoreactive to several closely related enzymes. Although there are caveats to their use, the detection of activated caspases is perhaps the most sensitive and specific *in situ* apoptosis detection method available.

Experimental Evidence for the Magnitude of Cell Death During Development

Many reports have suggested that the magnitude of cell death in neural precursor cells is relatively low. Biotin-conjugated annexin V staining of embryonic telencephalon shows only a limited number of dispersed cells undergoing apoptosis, and activated caspase-3 immunoreactivity is rare in the ventricular zone of mouse embryos *(48,111)*. A small number of pyknotic cells are seen in the mouse E12.5 ventricular zone, and TUNEL staining of paraffin sections of embryonic E14–19 rat brain show less than 0.3–0.9% of total cells are positive in the ventricular zone *(48,112)*. These numbers are equivalent to results obtained by counting pyknotic nuclei in these sections, although the lack of pyknotic nuclei does not conclusively indicate a low magnitude of cell death *(113)*. The sensitivity and specificity of nick end-labeling techniques varies widely and has resulted in quite disparate estimates of neural precursor cell death. Using the ISEL+ technique, Chun and colleagues have suggested that a large percentage of proliferating cells in the developing brain undergo apoptosis *(114)*. With a careful validation of the ISEL+ technique, this and subsequent studies reported that 45–75% of cells in the ventricular zone undergo apoptosis. Cells detected by this technique were not simply undergoing DNA synthesis, since apoptotic cells were more widespread than the cells undergoing proliferation, as determined by pulse BrdU incorporation *(114,115)*. Such a high fraction of programmed cell death challenges previous conclusions about the magnitude of death during development.

Several alternate explanations for the results obtained with ISEL+ have been postulated. ISEL+ may label transient DNA breaks in cells that have not entered apoptotic pathways, as would be seen during DNA rearrangement. It has been hypothesized that DNA recombination events may be required for some, currently unknown, process during neurogenesis, akin to that seen during development of the immune system *(116–118)*. However, this theory is unproven, since a candidate molecule generated by recombination, similar to T-cell receptors or immunoglobulins, has not been identified in the nervous system. Furthermore, a locus of recombination is not obvious in the developing brain, and gene products that generate neural recombination events have not been isolated. It is possible that the ISEL+ technique may be greatly sensitive to early apoptotic DNA breaks, thereby identifying a larger temporal window of cell death. Alternatively, ISEL+ may label DNA rearrangement and/or double-stranded DNA repair in neural precursor cells that are shortly becoming immature neurons. Without functional end-joining proteins, such as XRCC4 or DNA ligase IV, the double-stranded DNA breaks in these cells would not be repaired, and these cells would undergo apoptosis shortly after maturation *(103–105,118)*.

In total, the evidence suggests that the magnitude of cell death of neural precursor cells is significantly less than that estimated by ISEL+ staining alone but that the death that does occur is extremely important for normal nervous system development. In addition, as rapidly proliferating cell populations may be susceptible to genotoxic injury, it is possible that programmed cell death of neural stem cells may prevent the survival of neural precursor cells with oncogenic potential.

NEURAL STEM CELL DEATH IN THE ADULT

With the recent identification of neural stem cells in the adult brain, consideration of regulated cell death pathways in these cells is warranted. The molecules that regulate neural stem cell death in the embryo may not have similar functions in adult stem cell populations for several reasons, making the studies of adult neural stem cell death pathways particularly exciting. First, the expression patterns of many regulatory death molecules change during neurogenesis in the embryo. The expression levels of apoptosis-associated molecules in adult neural stem cells are unknown but will surely influence cell death responsiveness. Second, the microenvironment of the adult brain is markedly different from that of the embryo, and extrinsic regulators of neural stem cell death that are present in the embryo may be absent or altered in the adult. Furthermore, adult neural stem cells, given their multipotency and proliferative potential, may become oncogenic if cell death pathways are dysregulated. Finally, recent attempts at transplantation of neural stem cells into injured or degenerating adult brain have been hampered by a significant amount of cell death of neural stem cell grafts.

There is clear evidence for adult neurogenesis in the dentate gyrus of the hippocampus and in the olfactory bulb *(119–121)*. These neurons arise from neural stem cells in the subgranular zone of the hippocampus and the subventricular zone of the lateral ventricle. Recently, claims for neurogenesis in the adult neocortex have challenged the long accepted hypothesis that cortical neurogenesis in the adult mammalian brain is minor *(122,123)*.

Cell Death of Newly Generated Neurons in the Dentate Gyrus

New neurons in the dentate gyrus originate in the subgranular zone, located between the dentate gyrus and the hippocampal hilus *(120)*. These neurons attain both morphological and functional characteristics of dentate granule neurons, and may have roles in hippocampal memory formation or mood homeostasis. Many of these cells seem to die soon after birth *(122,124,125)*. In the rodent, strain-dependent factors may influence survival of newly generated neurons in the dentate gyrus *(126)*. The number of newly generated neurons may be increased by cognitive tasks, but it is not entirely clear whether this effect is due to prevention of programmed cell death or to a generalized increase in hippocampal neurogenesis *(122,127)*. A percentage of newly generated neurons in the adult dentate gyrus do appear pyknotic and exposure to alcohol or nicotine increases pyknosis, TUNEL positivity, and activated caspase-3 immunoreactivity in the dentate gyrus *(128,129)*.

A significant number of reports indicate that newly generated neurons in the dentate gyrus decrease in number over time. Many authors have suggested that this decline may be due to death of neural stem cells. However, an analysis of the particular program of cell death engaged by these dying cells has not, to our knowledge, been completed. It will be interesting to determine the molecular requirements for adult hippocampal neural precursor death in both the rodent and primate.

Cell Death of Newly Generated Neurons in the Olfactory Bulb

In the rodent, newly generated granule and periglomerular neurons in the olfactory bulb originate in the rostral region of the lateral ventricle and migrate to the olfactory bulb *(119)*. This rostral migratory stream provides newly generated neurons to the olfactory bulb, where they play roles in odor discrimination and odor memory. The ultimate fate of these neurons is thought to be cell death, although the precise mechanism of death is unclear *(130,131)*. In untreated adolescent rats, apoptotic figures and TUNEL positivity have been demonstrated along the rostral migratory stream and in laminar regions of the olfactory bulb *(132,133)*. Significant numbers of TUNEL positive cells are also seen in the adult subventricular zone, rostral migratory stream, and olfactory bulb *(134,135)*.

Neurons in the rodent olfactory bulb are dependent on sensory input for survival. Deafferation of the olfactory receptor neurons induces a reduction of epithelial thickness and cell death in the olfactory epithelium *(136)*. This apoptotic stimulus results in increased pyknosis in the olfactory bulb and increased TUNEL positivity in lateral ventricle, rostral migratory stream, and the olfactory bulb, suggesting that sensory withdrawal-induced death in these populations is apoptotic *(133,137–139)*. Similar results have been shown using anosmic mice, which express mutated cyclic nucleotide-gated channels in olfactory receptor neurons *(140,141)*. In these mice, an increase in TUNEL positivity can be seen in the granule cell layer of the olfactory bulb *(142)*. It is not clear whether cell death in the olfactory bulb occurs solely in postmitotic olfactory receptor neurons or whether neural precursor cells are also subjected to cell death in the adult.

CONCLUSIONS

The regulation of cell death in the nervous system has a great impact on many aspects of both normal homeostasis and pathophysiology. The underutilization of cell death may lead to developmental abnormalities or to cancer, while exacerbated cell death may result in neurodegeneration or the loss of function following traumatic injury. The Bcl-2 and caspase families are important for the regulation of cell death, and the striking effect of gene disruptions in members of these families illustrate the significant role apoptosis plays during nervous system development. A number of questions about neural stem cell death remain, including its magnitude. It is possible that certain neural stem cells are selected for death while others are not, but the basis of such a selective process is unknown. Finally, the molecular regulation of neural stem cell death is still incompletely defined and it will be critical to identify both the stimuli inducing neural stem cell death and the intrinsic molecules involved in its execution.

ACKNOWLEDGMENTS

We thank Angela Schmeckebier for help in preparing this manuscript. K. A. R. is supported by NIH Grants 35107 and 41962. R. S. A. received support from the UAB Medical Scientist Training Program (NIH Grant 08361).

REFERENCES

1. Burek, M. J. and Oppenheim, R. W. (1996) Programmed cell death in the developing nervous system. *Brain Pathol.* **6,** 427–446.
2. Sulston, J. E. and Horvitz, H. R. (1977) Post-embryonic cell lineages of the nematode, *Caenorhabditis elegans. Dev. Biol.* **56,** 110–156.

3. Ernst, M. (1926) Über untergang von Zellen während der normalen Entwicklung bei Wirbeltieren. *Z. Anat. Entwickl. Gesch.* **79,** 228–262.
4. Glücksmann, A. (1951) Cell deaths in normal vertebrate ontogeny. *Biol. Rev.* **26,** 59–86.
5. Clarke, P. G. (1990) Developmental cell death: morphological diversity and multiple mechanisms. *Anat. Embryol. (Berl.)* **181,** 195–213.
6. Kerr, J. F., Wyllie, A. H., and Currie, A. R. (1972) Apoptosis: a basic biological phenomenon with wide-ranging implications in tissue kinetics. *Br. J. Cancer* **26,** 239–257.
7. Hacker, G. (2000) The morphology of apoptosis. *Cell Tissue Res.* **301,** 5–17.
8. Roth, K. A. (2002) *In situ* detection of apoptotic neurons. In Neuromethods, Vol. 37: *Apoptosis Techniques and Protocols* (LeBlanc, A. C., ed.), Humana Press, Totowa, NJ, pp. 205–224.
9. Ellis, H. M. and Horvitz, H. R. (1986) Genetic control of programmed cell death in the nematode *C. elegans. Cell* **44,** 817–829.
10. Yuan, J., Shaham, S., Ledoux, S., Ellis, H. M., and Horvitz, H. R. (1993) The C. elegans cell death gene ced-3 encodes a protein similar to mammalian interleukin-1 beta-converting enzyme. *Cell* **75,** 641–652.
11. Cerretti, D. P., Kozlosky, C. J., Mosley, B., et al. (1992) Molecular cloning of the interleukin-1 beta converting enzyme. *Science* **256,** 97–100.
12. Thornberry, N. A., Bull, H. G., Calaycay, J. R., et al. (1992) A novel heterodimeric cysteine protease is required for interleukin-1 beta processing in monocytes. *Nature* **356,** 768–774.
13. Degterev, A., Boyce, M., and Yuan, J. (2003) A decade of caspases. *Oncogene* **22,** 8543–8567.
14. Boatright, K. M., Renatus, M., Scott, F. L., et al. (2003) A unified model for apical caspase activation. *Mol. Cell* **11,** 529–541.
15. Tsujimoto, Y., Finger, L. R., Yunis, J., Nowell, P. C., and Croce, C. M. (1984) Cloning of the chromosome breakpoint of neoplastic B cells with the t(14;18) chromosome translocation. *Science* **226,** 1097–1099.
16. Bakhshi, A., Jensen, J. P., Goldman, P., et al. (1985) Cloning the chromosomal breakpoint of t(14;18) human lymphomas: clustering around JH on chromosome 14 and near a transcriptional unit on 18. *Cell* **41,** 899–906.
17. Cory, S., Huang, D. C., and Adams, J. M. (2003) The Bcl-2 family: roles in cell survival and oncogenesis. *Oncogene* **22,** 8590–8607.
18. Akhtar, R. S., Ness, J. M., and Roth, K. A. (2004) Bcl-2 family regulation of neuronal development and neurodegeneration. *Biochim. Biophys. Acta* **1644,** 189–203.
19. Oltvai, Z. N., Milliman, C. L., and Korsmeyer, S. J. (1993) Bcl-2 heterodimerizes in vivo with a conserved homolog, Bax, that accelerates programmed cell death. *Cell* **74,** 609–619.
20. Armstrong, R. C., Aja, T. J., Hoang, K. D., et al. (1997) Activation of the CED3/ICE-related protease CPP32 in cerebellar granule neurons undergoing apoptosis but not necrosis. *J. Neurosci.* **17,** 553–562.
21. Liu, X., Kim, C. N., Yang, J., Jemmerson, R., and Wang, X. (1996) Induction of apoptotic program in cell-free extracts: requirement for dATP and cytochrome c. *Cell* **86,** 147–157.
22. Zou, H., Henzel, W. J., Liu, X., Lutschg, A., and Wang, X. (1997) Apaf-1, a human protein homologous to *C. elegans* CED-4, participates in cytochrome c-dependent activation of caspase-3. *Cell* **90,** 405–413.
23. Li, P., Nijhawan, D., Budihardjo, I., et al. (1997) Cytochrome *c* and dATP-dependent formation of Apaf-1/caspase-9 complex initiates an apoptotic protease cascade. *Cell* **91,** 479–489.
24. Duan, H., Orth, K., Chinnaiyan, A. M., et al. (1996) ICE-LAP6, a novel member of the ICE/Ced-3 gene family, is activated by the cytotoxic T cell protease granzyme B. *J. Biol. Chem.* **271,** 16720–16724.

25. Srinivasula, S. M., Fernandes-Alnemri, T., Zangrilli, J., et al. (1996) The Ced-3/interleukin 1beta converting enzyme-like homolog Mch6 and the lamin-cleaving enzyme Mch2alpha are substrates for the apoptotic mediator CPP32. *J. Biol. Chem.* **271,** 27099–27106.

26. Acehan, D., Jiang, X., Morgan, D. G., Heuser, J. E., Wang, X., and Akey, C. W. (2002) Three-dimensional structure of the apoptosome: implications for assembly, procaspase-9 binding, and activation. *Mol. Cell* **9,** 423–432.

27. Scorrano, L. and Korsmeyer, S. J. (2003) Mechanisms of cytochrome *c* release by proapoptotic BCL-2 family members. *Biochem. Biophys. Res. Commun.* **304,** 437–444.

28. Mattson, M. P. and Kroemer, G. (2003) Mitochondria in cell death: novel targets for neuroprotection and cardioprotection. *Trends Mol. Med.* **9,** 196–205.

29. Yang, E., Zha, J., Jockel, J., Boise, L. H., Thompson, C. B., and Korsmeyer, S. J. (1995) Bad, a heterodimeric partner for Bcl-XL and Bcl-2, displaces Bax and promotes cell death. *Cell* **80,** 285–291.

30. Zha, J., Harada, H., Osipov, K., Jockel, J., Waksman, G., and Korsmeyer, S. J. (1997) BH3 domain of BAD is required for heterodimerization with BCL-XL and pro-apoptotic activity. *J. Biol. Chem.* **272,** 24101–24104.

31. Kelekar, A., Chang, B. S., Harlan, J. E., Fesik, S. W., and Thompson, C. B. (1997) Bad is a BH3 domain-containing protein that forms an inactivating dimer with Bcl-XL. *Mol. Cell Biol.* **17,** 7040–7046.

32. Oda, E., Ohki, R., Murasawa, H., et al. (2000) Noxa, a BH3-only member of the Bcl-2 family and candidate mediator of p53-induced apoptosis. *Science* **288,** 1053–1058.

33. Boise, L. H., Gonzalez-Garcia, M., Postema, C. E., et al. (1993) bcl-x, a bcl-2-related gene that functions as a dominant regulator of apoptotic cell death. *Cell* **74,** 597–608.

34. Gonzalez-Garcia, M., Perez-Ballestero, R., Ding, L., et al. (1994) bcl-XL is the major bcl-x mRNA form expressed during murine development and its product localizes to mitochondria. *Development* **120,** 3033–3042.

35. Gonzalez-Garcia, M., Garcia, I., Ding, L., et al. (1995) bcl-x is expressed in embryonic and postnatal neural tissues and functions to prevent neuronal cell death. *Proc. Natl. Acad. Sci. USA* **92,** 4304–4308.

36. Yin, X. M., Oltvai, Z. N., and Korsmeyer, S. J. (1994) BH1 and BH2 domains of Bcl-2 are required for inhibition of apoptosis and heterodimerization with Bax. *Nature* **369,** 321–323.

37. Sato, T., Hanada, M., Bodrug, S., et al. (1994) Interactions among members of the Bcl-2 protein family analyzed with a yeast two-hybrid system. *Proc. Natl. Acad. Sci. USA* **91,** 9238–9242.

38. Sedlak, T. W., Oltvai, Z. N., Yang, E., et al. (1995) Multiple Bcl-2 family members demonstrate selective dimerizations with Bax. *Proc. Natl. Acad. Sci. USA* **92,** 7834–7838.

39. Chittenden, T., Flemington, C., Houghton, A. B., et al. (1995) A conserved domain in Bak, distinct from BH1 and BH2, mediates cell death and protein binding functions. *EMBO J.* **14,** 5589–5596.

40. Wang, S. and El Deiry, W. S. (2003) TRAIL and apoptosis induction by TNF-family death receptors. *Oncogene* **22,** 8628–8633.

41. Barnhart, B. C., Lee, J. C., Alappat, E. C., and Peter, M. E. (2003) The death effector domain protein family. *Oncogene* **22,** 8634–8644.

42. Scaffidi, C., Medema, J. P., Krammer, P. H., and Peter, M. E. (1997) FLICE is predominantly expressed as two functionally active isoforms, caspase-8/a and caspase-8/b. *J. Biol. Chem.* **272,** 26953–26958.

43. Muzio, M., Stockwell, B. R., Stennicke, H. R., Salvesen, G. S., and Dixit, V. M. (1998) An induced proximity model for caspase-8 activation. *J. Biol. Chem.* **273,** 2926–2930.

44. Luo, X., Budihardjo, I., Zou, H., Slaughter, C., and Wang, X. (1998) Bid, a Bcl2 interacting protein, mediates cytochrome c release from mitochondria in response to activation of cell surface death receptors. *Cell* **94,** 481–490.

45. Kim, J. and Klionsky, D. J. (2000) Autophagy, cytoplasm-to-vacuole targeting pathway, and pexophagy in yeast and mammalian cells. *Annu. Rev. Biochem.* **69,** 303–342.

46. Syntichaki, P. and Tavernarakis, N. (2003) The biochemistry of neuronal necrosis: rogue biology? *Nat. Rev. Neurosci.* **4,** 672–684.

47. Hall, D. H., Gu, G., Garcia-Anoveros, J., Gong, L., Chalfie, M., and Driscoll, M. (1997) Neuropathology of degenerative cell death in Caenorhabditis elegans. *J. Neurosci.* **17,** 1033–1045.

48. Roth, K. A., Kuan, C., Haydar, T. F., et al. (2000) Epistatic and independent functions of caspase-3 and Bcl-X(L) in developmental programmed cell death. *Proc. Natl. Acad. Sci. USA* **97,** 466–471.

49. Pompeiano, M., Blaschke, A. J., Flavell, R. A., Srinivasan, A., and Chun, J. (2000) Decreased apoptosis in proliferative and postmitotic regions of the caspase 3-deficient embryonic central nervous system. *J. Comp Neurol.* **423,** 1–12.

50. Kuida, K., Zheng, T. S., Na, S., et al. (1996) Decreased apoptosis in the brain and premature lethality in CPP32-deficient mice. *Nature* **384,** 368–372.

51. Hakem, R., Hakem, A., Duncan, G. S., et al. (1998) Differential requirement for caspase 9 in apoptotic pathways in vivo. *Cell* **94,** 339–352.

52. Cecconi, F., Alvarez-Bolado, G., Meyer, B. I., Roth, K. A., and Gruss, P. (1998) Apaf1 (CED-4 homolog) regulates programmed cell death in mammalian development. *Cell* **94,** 727–737.

53. Yoshida, H., Kong, Y. Y., Yoshida, R., et al. (1998) Apaf1 is required for mitochondrial pathways of apoptosis and brain development. *Cell* **94,** 739–750.

54. Leonard, J. R., Klocke, B. J., D'Sa, C., Flavell, R. A., and Roth, K. A. (2002) Strain-dependent neurodevelopmental abnormalities in caspase-3-deficient mice. *J. Neuropathol. Exp. Neurol.* **61,** 673–677.

55. Kuida, K., Haydar, T. F., Kuan, C. Y., et al. (1998) Reduced apoptosis and cytochrome c-mediated caspase activation in mice lacking caspase 9. *Cell* **94,** 325–337.

56. Kuan, C. Y., Roth, K. A., Flavell, R. A., and Rakic, P. (2000) Mechanisms of programmed cell death in the developing brain. *Trends Neurosci.* **23,** 291–297.

57. Roth, K. A. and D'Sa, C. (2001) Apoptosis and brain development. *Ment. Retard. Dev. Disabil. Res. Rev.* **7,** 261–266.

58. Chinnaiyan, A. M., O'Rourke, K., Yu, G. L., et al. (1996) Signal transduction by DR3, a death domain-containing receptor related to TNFR-1 and CD95. *Science* **274,** 990–992.

59. Sakamaki, K., Tsukumo, S., and Yonehara, S. (1998) Molecular cloning and characterization of mouse caspase-8. *Eur. J. Biochem.* **253,** 399–405.

60. Varfolomeev, E. E., Schuchmann, M., Luria, V., et al. (1998) Targeted disruption of the mouse caspase 8 gene ablates cell death induction by the TNF receptors, Fas/Apo1, and DR3 and is lethal prenatally. *Immunity* **9,** 267–276.

61. Sanchez, I., Xu, C. J., Juo, P., Kakizaka, A., Blenis, J., and Yuan, J. (1999) Caspase-8 is required for cell death induced by expanded polyglutamine repeats. *Neuron* **22,** 623–633.

62. Sakamaki, K., Inoue, T., Asano, M., et al. (2002) Ex vivo whole-embryo culture of caspase-8-deficient embryos normalize their aberrant phenotypes in the developing neural tube and heart. *Cell Death. Differ.* **9,** 1196–1206.

63. Watanabe-Fukunaga, R., Brannan, C. I., Itoh, N., et al. (1992) The cDNA structure, expression, and chromosomal assignment of the mouse Fas antigen. *J. Immunol.* **148,** 1274–1279.

64. Takahashi, T., Tanaka, M., Brannan, C. I., et al. (1994) Generalized lymphoproliferative disease in mice, caused by a point mutation in the Fas ligand. *Cell* **76,** 969–976.

65. Adachi, M., Suematsu, S., Kondo, T., et al. (1995) Targeted mutation in the Fas gene causes hyperplasia in peripheral lymphoid organs and liver. *Nat. Genet.* **11,** 294–300.

66. Veis, D. J., Sorenson, C. M., Shutter, J. R., and Korsmeyer, S. J. (1993) Bcl-2-deficient mice demonstrate fulminant lymphoid apoptosis, polycystic kidneys, and hypopigmented hair. *Cell* **75,** 229–240.

67. Nakayama, K., Nakayama, K., Negishi, I., Kuida, K., Sawa, H., and Loh, D. Y. (1994) Targeted disruption of Bcl-2 alpha beta in mice: occurrence of gray hair, polycystic kidney disease, and lymphocytopenia. *Proc. Natl. Acad. Sci. USA* **91,** 3700–3704.

68. Motoyama, N., Wang, F., Roth, K. A., et al. (1995) Massive cell death of immature hematopoietic cells and neurons in Bcl-x-deficient mice. *Science* **267,** 1506–1510.

69. Zaidi, A. U., D'Sa-Eipper, C., Brenner, J., et al. (2001) Bcl-X(L)-caspase-9 interactions in the developing nervous system: evidence for multiple death pathways. *J. Neurosci.* **21,** 169–175.

70. Krajewski, S., Krajewska, M., Shabaik, A., Miyashita, T., Wang, H. G., and Reed, J. C. (1994) Immunohistochemical determination of in vivo distribution of Bax, a dominant inhibitor of Bcl-2. *Am. J. Pathol.* **145,** 1323–1336.

71. Farrow, S. N., White, J. H., Martinou, I., et al. (1995) Cloning of a bcl-2 homologue by interaction with adenovirus E1B 19K. *Nature* **374,** 731–733.

72. Chittenden, T., Harrington, E. A., O'Connor, R., et al. (1995) Induction of apoptosis by the Bcl-2 homologue Bak. *Nature* **374,** 733–736.

73. Kiefer, M. C., Brauer, M. J., Powers, V. C., et al. (1995) Modulation of apoptosis by the widely distributed Bcl-2 homologue Bak. *Nature* **374,** 736–739.

74. Krajewska, M., Mai, J. K., Zapata, J. M., et al. (2002) Dynamics of expression of apoptosis-regulatory proteins Bid, Bcl-2, Bcl-X, Bax and Bak during development of murine nervous system. *Cell Death. Differ.* **9,** 145–157.

75. Lindsten, T., Ross, A. J., King, A., et al. (2000) The combined functions of proapoptotic Bcl-2 family members bak and bax are essential for normal development of multiple tissues. *Mol. Cell* **6,** 1389–1399.

76. Lindsten, T., Golden, J. A., Zong, W. X., Minarcik, J., Harris, M. H., and Thompson, C. B. (2003) The proapoptotic activities of Bax and Bak limit the size of the neural stem cell pool. *J. Neurosci.* **23,** 11112–11119.

77. Roth, K. A., Motoyama, N., and Loh, D. Y. (1996) Apoptosis of bcl-x-deficient telencephalic cells in vitro. *J. Neurosci.* **16,** 1753–1758.

78. Srinivasan, A., Roth, K. A., Sayers, R. O., et al. (1998) In situ immunodetection of activated caspase-3 in apoptotic neurons in the developing nervous system. *Cell Death. Differ.* **5,** 1004–1016.

79. Yoshida, H., Okada, Y., Kinoshita, N., et al. (2002) Differential requirement for Apaf1 and Bcl-X(L) in the regulation of programmed cell death during development. *Cell Death. Differ.* **9,** 1273–1276.

80. Cecconi, F., Roth, K. A., Dolgov, O., et al. (2004) Apaf1-dependent programmed cell death is required for inner ear morphogenesis and growth. *Development* **131,** 2125–2135.

81. Shindler, K. S., Latham, C. B., and Roth, K. A. (1997) Bax deficiency prevents the increased cell death of immature neurons in bcl-x-deficient mice. *J. Neurosci.* **17,** 3112–3119.

82. D'Sa-Eipper, C. and Roth, K. A. (2000) Caspase regulation of neuronal progenitor cell apoptosis. *Dev. Neurosci.* **22,** 116–124.

83. D'Sa-Eipper, C., Leonard, J. R., Putcha, G., et al. (2001) DNA damage-induced neural precursor cell apoptosis requires p53 and caspase 9 but neither Bax nor caspase 3. *Development* **128,** 137–146.

84. D'Sa, C., Klocke, B. J., Cecconi, F., et al. (2003) Caspase regulation of genotoxin-induced neural precursor cell death. *J. Neurosci. Res.* **74,** 435–445.

85. Zheng, T. S., Hunot, S., Kuida, K., et al. (2000) Deficiency in caspase-9 or caspase-3 induces compensatory caspase activation. *Nat. Med.* **6,** 1241–1247.

86. Honarpour, N., Du, C., Richardson, J. A., Hammer, R. E., Wang, X., and Herz, J. (2000) Adult Apaf-1-deficient mice exhibit male infertility. *Dev. Biol.* **218,** 248–258.

87. Vousden, K. H. and Lu, X. (2002) Live or let die: the cell's response to p53. *Nat. Rev. Cancer* **2,** 594–604.

88. Fei, P. and El Deiry, W. S. (2003) P53 and radiation responses. *Oncogene* **22,** 5774–5783.

89. Fridman, J. S. and Lowe, S. W. (2003) Control of apoptosis by p53. *Oncogene* **22,** 9030–9040.

90. Schmid, P., Lorenz, A., Hameister, H., and Montenarh, M. (1991) Expression of p53 during mouse embryogenesis. *Development* **113,** 857–865.

91. Sah, V. P., Attardi, L. D., Mulligan, G. J., Williams, B. O., Bronson, R. T., and Jacks, T. (1995) A subset of p53-deficient embryos exhibit exencephaly. *Nat. Genet.* **10,** 175–180.

92. Armstrong, J. F., Kaufman, M. H., Harrison, D. J., and Clarke, A. R. (1995) High-frequency developmental abnormalities in p53-deficient mice. *Curr. Biol.* **5,** 931–936.

93. Komarova, E. A., Chernov, M. V., Franks, R., et al. (1997) Transgenic mice with p53-responsive lacZ: p53 activity varies dramatically during normal development and determines radiation and drug sensitivity in vivo. *EMBO J.* **16,** 1391–1400.

94. Shindler, K. S., Yunker, A. M., Cahn, R., Zha, J., Korsmeyer, S. J., and Roth, K. A. (1998) Trophic support promotes survival of bcl-x-deficient telencephalic cells in vitro. *Cell Death. Differ.* **5,** 901–910.

95. Zaidi, A. U., McDonough, J. S., Klocke, B. J., et al. (2001) Chloroquine-induced neuronal cell death is p53 and Bcl-2 family-dependent but caspase-independent. *J. Neuropathol. Exp. Neurol.* **60,** 937–945.

96. Klocke, B. J., Latham, C. B., D'Sa, C., and Roth, K. A. (2002) p53 deficiency fails to prevent increased programmed cell death in the Bcl-X(L)-deficient nervous system. *Cell Death. Differ.* **9,** 1063–1068.

97. Lee, E. Y., Chang, C. Y., Hu, N., et al. (1992) Mice deficient for Rb are nonviable and show defects in neurogenesis and haematopoiesis. *Nature* **359,** 288–294.

98. Jacks, T., Fazeli, A., Schmitt, E. M., Bronson, R. T., Goodell, M. A., and Weinberg, R. A. (1992) Effects of an Rb mutation in the mouse. *Nature* **359,** 295–300.

99. Clarke, A. R., Maandag, E. R., van Roon, M., et al. (1992) Requirement for a functional Rb-1 gene in murine development. *Nature* **359,** 328–330.

100. Slack, R. S., El Bizri, H., Wong, J., Belliveau, D. J., and Miller, F. D. (1998) A critical temporal requirement for the retinoblastoma protein family during neuronal determination. *J. Cell Biol.* **140,** 1497–1509.

101. Macleod, K. F., Hu, Y., and Jacks, T. (1996) Loss of Rb activates both p53-dependent and independent cell death pathways in the developing mouse nervous system. *EMBO J.* **15,** 6178–6188.

102. Simpson, M. T., MacLaurin, J. G., Xu, D., et al. (2001) Caspase 3 deficiency rescues peripheral nervous system defect in retinoblastoma nullizygous mice. *J. Neurosci.* **21,** 7089–7098.

103. Frank, K. M., Sekiguchi, J. M., Seidl, K. J., et al. (1998) Late embryonic lethality and impaired V(D)J recombination in mice lacking DNA ligase IV. *Nature* **396,** 173–177.

104. Barnes, D. E., Stamp, G., Rosewell, I., Denzel, A., and Lindahl, T. (1998) Targeted disruption of the gene encoding DNA ligase IV leads to lethality in embryonic mice. *Curr. Biol.* **8,** 1395–1398.

105. Gao, Y., Sun, Y., Frank, K. M., et al. (1998) A critical role for DNA end-joining proteins in both lymphogenesis and neurogenesis. *Cell* **95,** 891–902.

106. Gao, Y., Ferguson, D. O., Xie, W., et al. (2000) Interplay of p53 and DNA-repair protein XRCC4 in tumorigenesis, genomic stability and development. *Nature* **404,** 897–900.

107. Frank, K. M., Sharpless, N. E., Gao, Y., et al. (2000) DNA ligase IV deficiency in mice leads to defective neurogenesis and embryonic lethality via the p53 pathway. *Mol. Cell* **5,** 993–1002.

108. Fadok, V. A., Bratton, D. L., Rose, D. M., Pearson, A., Ezekewitz, R. A., and Henson, P. M. (2000) A receptor for phosphatidylserine-specific clearance of apoptotic cells. *Nature* **405,** 85–90.

109. Savill, J. and Fadok, V. (2000) Corpse clearance defines the meaning of cell death. *Nature* **407,** 784–788.
110. Li, M. O., Sarkisian, M. R., Mehal, W. Z., Rakic, P., and Flavell, R. A. (2003) Phosphatidylserine receptor is required for clearance of apoptotic cells. *Science* **302,** 1560–1563.
111. van den Eijnde, S. M., Lips, J., Boshart, L., et al. (1999) Spatiotemporal distribution of dying neurons during early mouse development. *Eur. J. Neurosci.* **11,** 712–724.
112. Thomaidou, D., Mione, M. C., Cavanagh, J. F., and Parnavelas, J. G. (1997) Apoptosis and its relation to the cell cycle in the developing cerebral cortex. *J. Neurosci.* **17,** 1075–1085.
113. Chun, J. (2000) Cell death, DNA breaks and possible rearrangements: an alternative view. *Trends Neurosci.* **23,** 407–409.
114. Blaschke, A. J., Staley, K., and Chun, J. (1996) Widespread programmed cell death in proliferative and postmitotic regions of the fetal cerebral cortex. *Development* **122,** 1165–1174.
115. Blaschke, A. J., Weiner, J. A., and Chun, J. (1998) Programmed cell death is a universal feature of embryonic and postnatal neuroproliferative regions throughout the central nervous system. *J. Comp Neurol.* **396,** 39–50.
116. Schatz, D. G. (1997) V(D)J recombination moves in vitro. *Semin. Immunol.* **9,** 149–159.
117. Chun, J. and Schatz, D. G. (1999) Rearranging views on neurogenesis: neuronal death in the absence of DNA end-joining proteins. *Neuron* **22,** 7–10.
118. Gilmore, E. C., Nowakowski, R. S., Caviness, V. S., Jr., and Herrup, K. (2000) Cell birth, cell death, cell diversity and DNA breaks: how do they all fit together? *Trends Neurosci.* **23,** 100–105.
119. Alvarez-Buylla, A. and Garcia-Verdugo, J. M. (2002) Neurogenesis in adult subventricular zone. *J. Neurosci.* **22,** 629–634.
120. Kempermann, G. (2002) Why new neurons? Possible functions for adult hippocampal neurogenesis. *J. Neurosci.* **22,** 635–638.
121. Taupin, P. and Gage, F. H. (2002) Adult neurogenesis and neural stem cells of the central nervous system in mammals. *J. Neurosci. Res.* **69,** 745–749.
122. Gould, E., Beylin, A., Tanapat, P., Reeves, A., and Shors, T. J. (1999) Learning enhances adult neurogenesis in the hippocampal formation. *Nat. Neurosci.* **2,** 260–265.
123. Rakic, P. (2002) Neurogenesis in adult primate neocortex: an evaluation of the evidence. *Nat. Rev. Neurosci.* **3,** 65–71.
124. Cameron, H. A., Woolley, C. S., McEwen, B. S., and Gould, E. (1993) Differentiation of newly born neurons and glia in the dentate gyrus of the adult rat. *Neuroscience* **56,** 337–344.
125. Eriksson, P. S., Perfilieva, E., Bjork-Eriksson, T., et al. (1998) Neurogenesis in the adult human hippocampus. *Nat. Med.* **4,** 1313–1317.
126. Kempermann, G., Kuhn, H. G., and Gage, F. H. (1997) Genetic influence on neurogenesis in the dentate gyrus of adult mice. *Proc. Natl. Acad. Sci. USA* **94,** 10409–10414.
127. Kempermann, G., Brandon, E. P., and Gage, F. H. (1998) Environmental stimulation of 129/SvJ mice causes increased cell proliferation and neurogenesis in the adult dentate gyrus. *Curr. Biol.* **8,** 939–942.
128. Gould, E., Vail, N., Wagers, M., and Gross, C. G. (2001) Adult-generated hippocampal and neocortical neurons in macaques have a transient existence. *Proc. Natl. Acad. Sci. USA* **98,** 10910–10917.
129. Jang, M. H., Shin, M. C., Jung, S. B., et al. (2002) Alcohol and nicotine reduce cell proliferation and enhance apoptosis in dentate gyrus. *NeuroReport* **13,** 1509–1513.
130. Morshead, C. M. and van der Kooy, D. (1992) Postmitotic death is the fate of constitutively proliferating cells in the subependymal layer of the adult mouse brain. *J. Neurosci.* **12,** 249–256.

131. Morshead, C. M., Craig, C. G., and van der Kooy, D. (1998) In vivo clonal analyses reveal the properties of endogenous neural stem cell proliferation in the adult mammalian forebrain. *Development* **125,** 2251–2261.
132. Brunjes, P. C. and Armstrong, A. M. (1996) Apoptosis in the rostral migratory stream of the developing rat. *Brain Res. Dev. Brain Res.* **92,** 219–222.
133. Fiske, B. K. and Brunjes, P. C. (2001) Cell death in the developing and sensory-deprived rat olfactory bulb. *J. Comp Neurol.* **431,** 311–319.
134. Biebl, M., Cooper, C. M., Winkler, J., and Kuhn, H. G. (2000) Analysis of neurogenesis and programmed cell death reveals a self-renewing capacity in the adult rat brain. *Neurosci. Lett.* **291,** 17–20.
135. Moreno-Lopez, B., Romero-Grimaldi, C., Noval, J. A., Murillo-Carretero, M., Matarredona, E. R., and Estrada, C. (2004) Nitric oxide is a physiological inhibitor of neurogenesis in the adult mouse subventricular zone and olfactory bulb. *J. Neurosci.* **24,** 85–95.
136. Brunjes, P. C. (1994) Unilateral naris closure and olfactory system development. *Brain Res. Brain Res. Rev.* **19,** 146–160.
137. Corotto, F. S., Henegar, J. R., and Maruniak, J. A. (1994) Odor deprivation leads to reduced neurogenesis and reduced neuronal survival in the olfactory bulb of the adult mouse. *Neuroscience* **61,** 739–744.
138. Najbauer, J. and Leon, M. (1995) Olfactory experience modulated apoptosis in the developing olfactory bulb. *Brain Res.* **674,** 245–251.
139. Mandairon, N., Jourdan, F., and Didier, A. (2003) Deprivation of sensory inputs to the olfactory bulb up-regulates cell death and proliferation in the subventricular zone of adult mice. *Neuroscience* **119,** 507–516.
140. Brunet, L. J., Gold, G. H., and Ngai, J. (1996) General anosmia caused by a targeted disruption of the mouse olfactory cyclic nucleotide-gated cation channel. *Neuron* **17,** 681–693.
141. Zhao, H. and Reed, R. R. (2001) X inactivation of the OCNC1 channel gene reveals a role for activity-dependent competition in the olfactory system. *Cell* **104,** 651–660.
142. Petreanu, L. and Alvarez-Buylla, A. (2002) Maturation and death of adult-born olfactory bulb granule neurons: role of olfaction. *J. Neurosci.* **22,** 6106–6113.

6

Neuronal Progenitor Cells of the Mammalian Neonatal Anterior Subventricular Zone

Douglas L. Falls and Marla B. Luskin

INTRODUCTION

The identification of progenitor cell populations capable of producing neurons and defining the intrinsic and extrinsic factors that regulate neuronal progenitor cell proliferation have been subjects of increasing interest over the last decade. Two major reasons for this emphasis are the gradual acceptance that at least some regions of the brain generate neurons throughout life and the growing appreciation that neuronal progenitor cells could be used to therapeutically treat disorders and injuries of the central nervous system (CNS) (1). Despite early studies by Altman and Das (2) demonstrating ongoing neurogenesis in the adult rodent hippocampus and olfactory bulb, it was widely believed until recently that in primates the generation of neurons ceases in the late embryonic or early postnatal period (e.g., ref. 3). Although it is certainly true that a large majority of neurons are generated prenatally or in the early postnatal period, strong evidence that new olfactory bulb neurons are produced throughout life in primates, as well as lower mammals, is discussed below, and there is also evidence of ongoing neurogenesis in the primate hippocampus (4,5). In addition, olfactory receptor neurons, the first-order neurons in the olfactory system, have been found to regenerate throughout life in all vertebrates examined (6,7). Thus, the capacity, and indeed, the fact of neurogenesis continuing throughout life in the CNS of higher, as well as lower, mammals is now well established.

Experimentally, neurogenesis is commonly assessed by injecting a proliferation marker—such as [3H]thymidine or the thymidine analog bromodeoxyuridine (BrdU)—which is incorporated into genomic DNA during the S phase of mitosis, and then after some period of time (hours to years) determining by autoradiography (for [3H]thymidine) or immunohistochemistry (for BrdU) the number of cells in which the proliferation marker is co-localized with a neuron-specific marker protein such as type III β-tubulin (often referred to as"TuJ1"). The demonstration by this method of ongoing neurogenesis producing new neurons for the olfactory bulb, hippocampus, and olfactory epithelium raises the question of what the characteristics are of the progenitor cell populations that give rise to these new neurons. Populations of neural progenitor cells that postnatally generate olfactory bulb, hippocampal, and olfactory epithelial neurons

From: *Neural Development and Stem Cells, Second Edition*
Edited by: M. S. Rao © Humana Press Inc., Totowa, NJ

have now been identified *(8–14)*. Furthermore, though under normal circumstances neurogenesis in the adult mammalian brain appears to be limited to the generation of hippocampal and olfactory bulb neurons, brain injury (primarily in the form of seizures or stroke) or the administration of neurotrophic factors has also been shown to induce production of new neurons (e.g., refs. *15–19*), raising the possibility that latent, as yet unidentified, progenitor populations capable of generating neurons exist in the mature brain. Thus, most neurons are born prenatally, but several progenitor cell populations are active postnatally, and in addition there may be latent progenitors called into action by injury or other stressors.

Differences among progenitor cell populations in the CNS are revealed by the range of cell-types each population produces. In addition to neurons, there are two classes of macroglia in the CNS: astrocytes and oligodendrocytes. While the neuroepithelial cells that form the walls of the neural tube and their derivatives that reside in the ventricular zone are believed to be multipotent stem cells—that is, cells capable of self-renewal and of generating both neurons and the two classes of macroglia—their progeny can be progenitors with a more restricted potential. Here we refer to progenitors capable of producing only neurons as "neuronal restricted progenitors" and to progenitors capable of producing only glia as "glial restricted progenitors." Others have used the similar terms "neuronal restricted precursors" (NRPs) and "glial restricted precursors" (GRPs) *(20)*. To be classified as a neuronal restricted progenitor, a cell must satisfy the following criteria: (1) it is capable of proliferating; (2) it has an absolute commitment to the neuronal lineage—that is, even in conditions favorable for glial differentiation, after heterotypic transplantation to a nonnative environment, or when grown in culture, it gives rise only to neurons; and (3) it expresses a subset of neuron-specific markers (e.g., type III β-tubulin and microtubule-associated protein-2 [MAP-2]). The neuronal progenitors identified to date also typically express the embryonic isoform of the neural cell adhesion molecule E-NCAM, which is also known as polysialated or PSA-NCAM. It is important to emphasize that not all neurons arise from neuronal restricted progenitors. For example, the embryonic precursors of glutamatergic cortical neurons are believed to express neuron-specific markers only after they have become postmitotic *(21–24)*, whereas, by definition "neuronal restricted progenitors" must be capable of proliferating and at the same time express neuron-specific markers. It is of great interest, but as yet entirely unknown, why some neurons develop via a pathway that appears to obligatorily involve neuronal restricted progenitors whereas others develop via a pathway that does not involve neuronal restricted progenitors.

The two best characterized populations of neuronal restricted progenitors are the cells that give rise to olfactory bulb interneurons in the neonate and the spinal cord neuronal restricted precursors (SC-NRPs) *(20,25,26)*. This chapter focuses on the cells of the neonatal forebrain anterior subventricular zone (SVZa), which give rise to the olfactory bulb interneurons and which we argue constitute a pure population of neuronal restricted progenitors. These cells are of interest both because they serve as a model for understanding the mechanisms controlling generation of neurons that will be integrated into already established, functional circuits postnatally and because they themselves might be a useful source of neuronal progenitor cell transplants for use in the treatment of neurological diseases and injury.

In this chapter, we first provide a general description of the features of the neuronal progenitor cells of the SVZa, which are intermediate progenitors in the lineage from neural stem cells to differentiated neurons. We continue with a more detailed examination of the neuronal characteristics of these cells and the maintenance of these properties when the cells are transplanted. We next discuss the developmental origins and evolution throughout life of this localized collection of neuronal restricted progenitors. While most of the research we present utilizes a rodent model system, we then discuss data demonstrating similar neurogenesis in primates. For the remainder of the chapter we consider a central issue in the study of neurogenesis: the extrinsic and intrinsic factors that regulate the cell cycle of neuronal progenitor cells. We conclude with thoughts about future research directions for understanding how the proliferation of SVZa neuronal progenitor cells is regulated.

THE NEONATAL SVZa CONSTITUTES
A DISCRETE NEUROGENIC REGION

While early studies concluded that the postnatal subventricular zone (SVZ) is primarily gliogenic, a lineage analysis using retroviruses capable of expressing bacterial β-galactosidase revealed that a specialized region of the neonatal SVZ surrounding the anterior dorsolateral tip of the lateral ventricle—the SVZa—is composed exclusively of neuronal progenitor cells *(10)*. Without exception, the cells emanating from the neonatal SVZa were found to generate olfactory bulb neurons *(10)*. These SVZa-derived neuronal progenitor cells migrate along a pathway, known as the rostral migratory stream (RMS). The SVZa is the most posterior portion of the RMS. Conversely, the cell dense RMS may be considered an extension of the SVZ. The RMS is a continuous band of cells which, for the purposes of discussion, can be subdivided into five parts (listed posterior to anterior): (a) the *SVZa,* which overlies the anterior horn of the lateral ventricle and is the most expansive portion of the RMS; (b) the vertical limb (*RMSvl*), a short, curved segment partially underlying the genu of the corpus callosum; (c) the elbow (*RMSe*), where the RMS changes direction from vertical to horizontal; (d) the horizontal limb (*RMShl*), a thinner, linear portion; and (e) the subependymal zone (*sez*), the elongated globe-shaped termination of the RMS within the core of the olfactory bulb. From the sez, the SVZa-derived cells migrate radially into more superficial regions of the olfactory bulb to become granule and periglomerular interneurons *(27)*.

The granule and periglomerular interneurons of the olfactory bulb principally develop postnatally. Large numbers of these neurons are generated during the first 2 wk of life *(28–30)*. It stands to reason, therefore, that progenitors for these interneurons—the SVZa cells and their progeny along the RMS—are also present in large numbers during this period and that there are fewer of these progenitors at earlier and later times. The data support this inference. In the early neonatal period, large numbers of SVZa cells and their progeny migrate toward the olfactory bulb *(10,31)*. After the neonatal period the SVZa and other parts of the migratory pathway are substantially smaller *(10)*.

In contrast to the neurogenic SVZa, retroviral lineage analysis revealed that virtually all the progenitor cells within the neonatal SVZ posterior to the SVZa give rise to glia (mainly astrocytes) of the cerebral cortex and other forebrain structures *(32; see also* refs. *33–37)*. We refer to this region of the subventricular zone as the SVZp. Therefore, the neonatal SVZ can be divided into the posterior SVZ (SVZp) containing primarily glial progenitors of the cerebral cortex and the SVZa, which contains exclusively neuronal progenitors. While there are no known neuroanatomic planes or barriers between the neonatal SVZa and SVZp, in the neonate the diameter of the neurogenic SVZa is several times larger than the diameter of the gliogenic SVZp *(38)*, and this difference in diameter can be used to guide dissection of SVZa tissue free of SVZp tissue (e.g., ref. *38*). SVZa cells isolated by such dissections have been analyzed by reverse transcriptase-polymerase chain reaction (RT-PCR) and immunocytochemistry for the expression of glial markers (e.g., glial fibrillary acidic protein [GFAP]). These analyses, as well as examination of brain sections for glial markers by *in situ* hybridization and immuno-histochemistry, have further substantiated the conclusion derived from lineage studies that glial cells are virtually absent in the neonatal SVZa *(38,39)*.

After ≈P7 in the rat, the SVZa and other parts of the RMS begin to include cells that express glial markers *(39)*. As the animal ages, GFAP immunoreactivity increases along the entire rostrocaudal extent of the RMS, including the SVZa, and reaches nearly stable expression by P21. The source of the GFAP-positive cells present after P7 is unknown. Despite the presence of glial cells, neuronal progenitors continue to predominate in all parts of the RMS and continue to migrate to the olfactory bulb throughout adulthood (e.g., *40,41)*.

The interpretation that there is a sharp division between an anterior neurogenic region of the SVZ and a posterior gliogenic region in the neonate has been challenged by a study of the neonatal SVZ that combined injection of high dosages of retroviral lineage markers with videomicroscopy *(42,43)*. The image sequences were interpreted as showing a population of tangentially migrating cells throughout the SVZ, both anterior and posterior. Although some of these tangentially migrating cells moved in a posterior direction for a time, the ultimate fate of all was to become olfactory bulb interneurons.

There is also not a consensus regarding the composition of the adult SVZa. Some investigators contend that a discrete neurogenic SVZa and gliogenic SVZp do not exist in the adult *(44–46)*. Immunohistochemical and electron microscopic study of the adult rodent forebrain has suggested that there is an anterior[high]-posterior[low] gradient of neurogenesis in the adult SVZ and that there is some neurogenesis in even quite posterior regions. Furthermore, as discussed above, GFAP(+) cells can be detected in the SVZa within 1–2 wk after birth. In the adult these astrocyte-like cells appear to serve two roles: they form "glial tubes" through which SVZa-derived neuronal progenitors migrate *(45,47)* and, they may be stem cells from which derive the neuronally restricted progenitors that generate the olfactory bulb interneurons born past the neonatal period. The potential role of these glial cells as stem cells is considered further below.

In summary, olfactory bulb interneurons are produced throughout life, making the olfactory bulb a highly plastic region in the CNS. The progenitors of these neurons continuously migrate into the bulb along a pathway referred to as the rostral migratory stream (RMS). In the neonate, the "headwaters" of the RMS is a distinct region of the SVZ opposed to the anterior-lateral wall of the telencephalic lateral ventricles referred to as the SVZa. Glial markers are absent from the neonatal RMS, but after the neonatal period glial cells, of unknown origin, appear within the RMS and may contribute to later olfactory bulb neurogenesis. The available evidence supports the idea that the cells of the neonatal RMS are a pure population of neuronal progenitors. Data discussed below demonstrate that they fulfill all of the criteria for classification as "neuronally restricted progenitors."

CHARACTERISTICS OF THE SVZa-DERIVED NEURONAL PROGENITOR CELLS IN VIVO AND IN VITRO

Two of the three criteria for "neuronal restricted progenitor" cells described in the introduction are that candidate cells proliferate and that they express neuron-specific markers while proliferating. The immature neurons arising in the telencephalic ventricular zone destined for the cerebral cortex do not fulfill the second of these criteria—they are postmitotic before expressing neuronal cell type-specific markers—and thus they are not neuronal restricted progenitor cells. However, the neuronal progenitor cells of the SVZa and their progeny migrating along the RMS do express neuron-specific markers despite being mitotically active. One such marker protein is type III β-tubulin. Virtually all the cells in the neonatal RMS express type III β-tubulin; and following administration of BrdU to label proliferating cells, virtually all BrdU(+) cells in the pathway are also type III β-tubulin(+) *(48,49)*. Other markers characteristic of neurons that are expressed by the SVZa progenitors include, for example, MAP-2 *(50)*, PSA-NCAM *(51)*, p75 (the low-affinity nerve growth factor receptor; S. Wiegand, T. Zigova, and M.B. Luskin, *unpublished data*), and a novel cell surface marker mAb-2F7, which labels neurons and neuronal progenitor cells exclusively *(52)*. Therefore, although type III β-tubulin is routinely used to assess neuronal differentiation of SVZa-derived neuronal progenitors, it is only one of several neuron-specific markers that these cells express, and expression of this protein by SVZa-derived cells that incorporate BrdU supports their classification as "neuronal restricted progenitor" cells.

The migration of SVZa-derived neuronal progenitor cells is the subject of active research *(53)* but beyond the scope of this chapter. However, brief mention is warranted. After leaving the SVZa, the SVZa-derived neuronal progenitor cells almost never deviate from the RMS until, after reaching the sez, they migrate radially into the neuronal layers of the olfactory bulb. Most of the migrating SVZa-derived cells exhibit an elongated morphology with a relative long leading process and a short tail *(10,54)* strikingly similar to the processes of postmitotic immature neurons migrating to the developing cerebral cortex along radial glia *(55)*. However, unlike these immature cortical neurons, the SVZa progenitors do not migrate along radial glia *(31,39)*. The neonatal SVZa-derived cells seem to provide their own substrate for migration and appear to successively leapfrog over one another in a process called chain migration *(40,56)* by which one progenitor cell serves as a stepping stone for the adjacent cells. The rate of migration of SVZa-derived cells in the neonatal as well as the adult RMS is significantly faster than that of neurons migrating along radial glia *(10,40; for review see 57)*.

The signals that confine the SVZa-derived progenitors to the RMS and direct their migration toward the olfactory bulb may include both chemoattractant and chemorepellant molecules and both diffusible and membrane- and ECM-bound molecules. Some of the candidate signals under investigation are proteoglycans *(58–60)*, PSA-NCAM *(61–63)*, and slit *(64,65)*. Like SVZa-derived neuronal progenitor cells, γ-amino-butyric acid-ergic (GABAergic) cortical neurons migrate unguided by radial glia (for review, *see* refs. *53, 66,* and *67*). It is intriguing that SVZa neuronal progenitor cells are also GABAergic and that they may share with cortical GABAergic neurons a subpallial origin (discussed later), unlike the radial glia-guided glutamatergic neurons of the cerebral cortex which derive from the pallial ventricular zone. These similarities suggest the possibility that the underlying mechanisms guiding SVZa-derived neuronal progenitor cell migration and cortical GABAergic neurons may also be similar. However, with respect to the current review, which focuses on cell cycle regulation of neuronal progenitors, the most pertinent aspect of migration behavior is the fact that the SVZa-derived progenitors exhibit a leading and trailing process, much like immature postmitotic cortical neurons. Cortical glutamatergic neuron precursors do not exhibit these morphological features until they are postmitotic. This raises the question of how SVZa-derived progenitors coordinate the formation of processes with cell cycle progression.

The development of methods for preparing pure cultures of SVZa-derived neuronal progenitors has facilitated conducting additional analyses of these cells in vitro. Luskin and her associates have taken advantage of the clearly identifiable neonatal SVZa to microdissect and culture the SVZa progenitor cells for up to 1 wk *(38)*. Characterization of the cultures demonstrated that essentially all cells have neuronal characteristics (e.g., type III β-tubulin+, MAP-2+, and PSA-NCAM+) at early (1 d) times in culture and a large majority expressed these characteristics at late times in culture (8 d), though at late times GFAP+ cells were also detected. The cultured SVZa cells incorporated BrdU, and cells labeled for both BrdU and type III β-tubulin were detected at both early and late times *(38)*. Furthermore, although they continued to undergo division, the cells in culture formed neuronal-like processes, which after approximately the initial day in culture were often more elaborate than the processes exhibited in vivo.

It is not simply sufficient to determine which neuron-specific markers SVZa cells express. Deciphering the functional properties of these immature neurons is also necessary. To date it has been shown that they express voltage-gated potassium and sodium channels and GABA-activated chloride channels *(68–70)*, further supporting the idea that although they are mitotically active they have distinct neuronal characteristics. In part these functional properties are shared with immature but postmitotic granule neurons migrating from the external to the internal granule cell layer of the cerebellum.

All of the in vitro experiments just described were done using a culture medium containing fetal bovine or horse serum. Experiments are being conducted in our laboratory now to find the optimum conditions for propagating cultured SVZa cells in serum-free media for extended periods. The ability to grow these neuronal progenitors in defined medium will facilitate study of the signaling proteins ("growth factors") that regulate their cell cycle and differentiation.

CHARACTERISTICS OF TRANSPLANTED SVZa-DERIVED NEURONAL PROGENITOR CELLS

Data presented above demonstrates that SVZa-derived neuronal progenitors satisfy two of the criteria for neuronal restricted progenitor cells—that is, that the cells are proliferative and they express neuronal characteristics. The third criterion is that the candidate cells are committed to a neuronal phenotype. Homotypic and heterotypic transplantation experiments *(27,71)* using microdissected and dissociated SVZa progenitors confirm that the SVZa cells are indeed committed to a neuronal phenotype. After homotypic transplantation into the SVZa, the phenotype and proliferative characteristics of the transplanted cells (labeled with PKH26, a lipophilic dye, or with BrdU) were identical to those of endogenous SVZa progenitors. The transplanted cells did not express GFAP but they did proliferate, expressed neuronal cell type-specific markers in the migratory pathway, and generated granule and periglomerular cells. To investigate whether the cells maintain a neuronal phenotype in a foreign environment, SVZa cells were transplanted into the neonatal and adult striatum *(71,72)*. The cells migrated away from the transplant site, dispersed widely in the striatum, and uniformly continued to express a neuronal phenotype even several weeks after transplantation. Preliminary analysis of their phenotype showed that the transplanted cells morphologically resembled the granule cells of the olfactory bulb and some of the cells expressed GABA (T. Zigova and M.B. Luskin, *unpublished data*), the neurotransmitter primarily expressed by the SVZa-derived cells and their progeny in the olfactory bulb. It remains to be determined whether a subset of the transplanted SVZa cells in the striatum synthesize dopamine in addition to GABA, as is the normal fate of some SVZa-derived neurons in the olfactory bulb *(73)*. These transplantation data complete the argument for classifying SVZa cells as "neuronal restricted progenitors": they proliferate while expressing neuronal markers and are uniformly committed to a neuronal fate regardless of the environment. Furthermore, these transplantation experiments show that SVZa cells are capable of migrating and differentiating in a foreign environment, characteristics that may suit them for use as therapeutic transplants for treatment of neurological disease.

THE PRENATAL EMERGENCE OF THE ROSTRAL MIGRATORY STREAM

As described later, there is evidence that the progenitors of the RMS arise from stem cells originally located in the lateral ganglionic eminence (LGE). To determine when and where cells comprising the RMS initially exhibit their characteristic neuronal phenotype and mitotic capacity, Pencea and Luskin *(74)* analyzed the cells of the rat forebrain between E14 and P2. At E14, cells with a neuronal phenotype [type III β-tubulin(+)] were detected within the ventricular zone in close proximity to the mantle layer (outer cellular layer) of the future olfactory bulb. By E15, cells in this location expressing neuronal markers were also PSA-NCAM–immunoreactive *(56,75)* and had become aligned in chains of similarly oriented cells, a hallmark of the postnatal RMS *(44,51)*. The cells that form chains organize into a patch that enlarges in the anterior–posterior and medial–lateral dimensions from E16 to E22 (birth). By comparing the forebrain cytoarchitecture to the pattern of cell-type specific staining, it was determined that the patch constitutes only the central part of the proximal RMS. The part of the RMS surrounding the patch expresses PSA-NCAM and neuron-specific markers at a level lower than the patch but still distinctly above background.

The proliferative activity of cells comprising the patch versus non-patch regions of the RMS was analyzed using BrdU *(74)*. From E15 to E22 the region of the patch incorporates less BrdU than nonpatch portions of the developing RMS, indicating that the cells of the patch have a relatively lower mitotic activity. However, around the time of birth (P0–P1) there is some inductive activity that dramatically increases the proliferative activity of the cells within the patch such that the patch and nonpatch regions can no longer be distinguished. Thus, the embryonic RMS consists of two parts, a "patch" region and a surrounding "nonpatch" region, which is distinguishable from the patch by its higher proliferative activity and somewhat lower expression of neural marker proteins. However, by around the time of birth the patch/nonpatch organization is replaced by homogeneous high-level expression of neuronal marker proteins throughout the RMS and a posterior[high]-anterior[low] gradient of BrdU incorporation. The quite unanticipated implication of this study is that the RMS, including the SVZa, develops independent of the cortical SVZ, which begins to form several days later than the SVZa.

THE STEM CELLS THAT GIVES RISE
TO THE NEURONAL PROGENITOR CELLS OF THE RMS

The progenitor cells of the RMS constitute a distinct population of cells in the neonatal brain separable from the SVZp (see earlier) and the overlying corpus callosum. There is evidence that in the adult subventricular zone the stem cell that gives rise to RMS progenitor cells is a GFAP-expressing cell referred to as a "B-type" cell *(46)*. However, the neonatal SVZa and the adult SVZ have significant differences with respect to the expression and distribution of GFAP. In brief, a cell comparable to the B-type cell has not been identified in the neonatal SVZa and in fact GFAP(+) cells have not been detected in the neonatal RMS (discussed earlier). Thus, while in the adult there may be multipotent [GFAP(+)] stem cells resident in the SVZ, such cells do not appear to be present in the neonatal SVZa.

Several studies now suggest that the stem cells from which the RMS progenitor cells initially arise reside in the LGE (for review, see *53* and *67*). Using ultrasound guided injection of retroviral lineage markers, Wichterle et al. *(76)* showed that at mid-embryonic stages (E12.5–14.5), LGE-derived cells migrate profusely to the olfactory bulb. The stem cells in the LGE are likely to be radial glia or radial glia-derived since in vitro ablation of GFAP+ cells eliminates stem cells in SVZ cultures *(77)* and since a cre/lox-based lineage tracing technique for marking radial glia and their descendants indicated that all forebrain neurons derive from radial glia *(78*; note, however, that a specific assessment of olfactory bulb neurogenesis was not reported in this article). It has been proposed that "while radial glia serve as progenitors for all neuronal classes, generation of interneuron populations throughout the brain may require the establishment of secondary proliferative zones as a necessary step in their development" *(78)*. Thus, the possibility that radial glia of the LGE are the ultimate source of the RMS progenitors cannot be excluded.

THE PRIMATE RMS IS ANALOGOUS TO THE RODENT RMS

Most studies of the postnatal production of olfactory bulb interneurons have examined this process in rodents. Investigators have designed studies to determine whether the SVZ of the postnatal primate forebrain, like the rodent, also harbors a specialized population of neuronal progenitor cells surrounding the lateral ventricles with the capacity to divide while they migrate. Olfactory bulb neurogenesis has now been examined in rhesus monkeys ranging in age from 2 d to 8 yr *(50)*, adult Rhesus monkeys *(79)*, and adult squirrel monkeys *(80)*. As is typically done in rodent studies, the living primates were injected with BrdU to label newly born cells and the tissue was later harvested and double- or triple-labeled using antibodies to BrdU and to neuron- or glial-specific proteins—for example, anti-neuron-specific type III β-tubulin (TuJ1) or anti-MAP-2 to identify neurons and anti-GFAP to identify glia. From birth onward the distribution of BrdU(+) cells with a neuronal phenotype in primates is largely overlapping and highly analogous with that of the rodent *(50)*. Similar to the rodent RMS, the neuronal progenitors are most numerous in neonates. The cytoarchitectonic arrangement and appearance of the neuronal progenitor cells is quite varied in the primate compared to the rodent; but, like the rodent, in some locations the cells are aligned in parallel arrays resembling the neuronal chains of the adult rodent RMS *(45,51,81)*. Much as in the rodent brain, the chains are progressively more pervasive in older primates. Furthermore, akin to the RMS of the adult rodent *(45,47)*, in the primate RMS, including the region that is analogous to the rodent SVZa, astrocytes form long tubes enveloping the chains of neuronal progenitors and there are clusters of proliferating neurons at all ages *(50)*. Thus, throughout life, a distinct part of the primate SVZ, contiguous with the RMS, contains a prolific source of neuronal progenitor cells. This suggests that the primate olfactory bulb also acquires newly generated neurons throughout life and that the mechanisms that regulate neurogenesis in the rodent may also apply to the primate.

Based on the evidence demonstrating similar organization and postnatal production of olfactory bulb neurons in rodents and nonhuman primates, it might be expected that the structural and functional features of olfactory bulb neuron production would also be similar in humans. Indeed, our preliminary data indicates that this is the case in neonatal humans (V. Pencea and M. B. Luskin, *unpublished data*). However, although there is evidence of ongoing neurogenesis in the SVZ in adult humans, a defined RMS has not been observed in adult human brain *(82)*. Taken together the primate studies described here demonstrate close parallels in the ongoing generation of rodent olfactory bulb neurons and primate olfactory bulb neurons (though there may be some structural differences in adult humans), just as there are parallels between neurogenesis in the rodent hippocampus *(83* and references therein) and human hippocampus *(4)*. Furthermore, the identification of an RMS in primates, including humans, advances the prospects for harvesting RMS cells and transplanting these harvested cells to treat human neurological disease.

INTRINSIC CONTROL OF SVZa-DERIVED NEURONAL PROGENITOR CELL PROLIFERATION BY THE CELL CYCLE INHIBITOR P19[INK4D]

The discovery of neuronal progenitor populations in the postnatal brain and the potential that such progenitors might be harnessed to replace neurons lost in neurological diseases has spurred interest in understanding the factors that regulate the proliferation, survival, and differentiation of these progenitors. For the remainder of this chapter we now consider what is known regarding the control of SVZa-derived neuronal progenitor cell proliferation. Whether a neuronal progenitor cell proceeds through the mitotic cycle and undergoes division or whether it becomes permanently postmitotic depends on its history and on pro- and antiproliferative signals it receives from its environment. We divide the control mechanisms involved into two categories: (1) intracellular regulators directly involved in cell cycle progression, which we refer to as "intrinsic controls" and (2) extracellular signals (including diffusible, membrane bound and ECM bound), which we refer to as "extrinsic signals." In the current section we discuss one family of intrinsic signals which are believed to regulate the cell cycle of SVZa-derived neuronal progenitors. In the two subsequent sections, we discuss cell-cell signaling proteins that regulate proliferation of SVZa-derived neuronal progenitors.

SVZa-derived neuronal progenitor cells express neuron-specific proteins and extend processes without becoming postmitotic (38,48), unlike the progenitor cells of the embryonic telencephalic ventricular zone, which give rise to the neurons of the cerebral cortex (22–24). This property of SVZa cells prompted us to examine whether they regulate their cell cycle in a fashion different from that of other CNS progenitor cells. Our strategy was to look at the expression pattern of proteins, the cyclin-dependent kinase inhibitors (CDKIs), whose expression usually commences when a cell is becoming postmitotic.

The CDKIs are regulators of the central cellular machinery controlling progression through the cell division cycle. In essentially all dividing cells the cell cycle is comprised of four phases: G_1, S, G_2, and M (where G = gap, S = synthesis, and M = mitosis). During S phase the cell duplicates its genomic DNA. On entering S phase, the cell is generally irreversibly committed to undergoing division. For all proliferating cells, extracellular and intracellular signals integrate at the G_1–S transition ("checkpoint") of the cell cycle to control whether a cell divides or becomes postmitotic (84). The cyclin-dependent kinases CDK4 and CDK6 are instrumental in the progression from G_1 to S phase (85). Conversely, CDK inhibitors (CDKIs) negatively regulate CDKs to block the cell cycle at the G_1 phase.

As a first step to investigating whether the expression pattern of CDKIs, and in particular one of the seven known CDKIs, p19[Ink4d], along the RMS can account for the unusual proliferative behavior of SVZa neuronal progenitor cells—that is, dividing after expressing the differentiation characteristics of immature neurons—Coskun and Luskin (49) analyzed the spatial–temporal expression pattern of p19[Ink4d] by the cells of the rat neonatal RMS and compared it to the expression pattern by cells of the developing cerebral cortex (for review *see* refs. 86 and 87). Their data confirmed and extended the study of Zindy et al. (88) demonstrating that as a cell in the developing telencephalon exits the cell cycle en route to the cortical plate, it expresses the CDKI p19[Ink4d]. This suggests that CDKIs, and specifically p19[Ink4d], are involved in the control of neuronal proliferation and maintaining cortical cells in the postmitotic state.

Analysis of p19[Ink4d] immunoreactivity in the RMS revealed that it is unlike the developing cerebral cortex. SVZa-derived cells exhibit a posterior[low]-anterior[high] gradient of p19[Ink4d] expression along the RMS: p19[Ink4d] expression is nearly absent in the SVZa and highest in the subependymal zone (sez), the most anterior portion of the RMS and the portion from which SVZa-derived cells migrate radially to become postmitotic, mature neurons of the olfactory bulb. Conversely, cell proliferation, measured by BrdU incorporation, is highest in the SVZa (most posterior portion of the RMS) and lowest in the sez. This pattern of p19[Ink4d] and BrdU expression leads to the predictions that (1) few cells withdraw from the cell cycle in the SVZa, (2) steadily more withdraw as their migration brings them closer to the olfactory bulb, and (3) p19[Ink4d] plays a role in cell cycle withdrawal.

To further investigate the role of the CDKI p19^{Ink4d}, Coskun and Luskin *(49)* determined the timing of p19^{Ink4d} expression by the SVZa-derived cells in the RMS relative to the S phase of the mitotic cycle. For these experiments, the proliferation marker BrdU was administered to neonatal rat pups at 3 and 9 h before perfusion and subsequently expression of p19^{Ink4d} by the BrdU(+) cells along the RMS was examined. The rationale for harvesting the rats 3 or 9 h after BrdU injection was based on the fact that the cell cycle time in the neonatal RMS is 14–17 h *(89)*. Thus, for rats perfused 3 h after BrdU administration, cells in S phase at the time of BrdU injection would likely be in G$_2$ phase; whereas, for animals perfused 9 h after BrdU administration, cells in S phase at the time of BrdU injection would likely have passed through mitosis and the daughters of that division would be in G$_1$.

A strikingly different result was exhibited by the cells along the posterior–anterior (caudal–rostral) axis of the RMS as a function of time post–BrdU administration. At 3 h following BrdU administration, very few SVZa-derived cells along the RMS co-localize BrdU and p19^{Ink4d}. However, 9 h post-BrdU administration a significant fraction of the BrdU(+) cells along the RMS, and most notably in the sez, are immunoreactive for both BrdU and p19^{Ink4d}. Based on these findings, Coskun and Luskin *(49)* hypothesized that SVZa-derived cells in the RMS successively down-regulate their p19^{Ink4d} expression prior to undergoing each division. They further conjectured that this cyclic up then down regulation of p19^{Ink4d} may enable these cells to repeatedly exit and re-enter the cell cycle. Once the SVZa-derived cells depart from the sez, destined for the granule cell and glomerular layers of the bulb, they no longer incorporate BrdU and they express p19^{Ink4d}, indicating that when SVZa-derived cells migrate to their final positions, they are terminally postmitotic. In summary, Coskun and Luskin *(49)* and others *(88,90)* have demonstrated that once the immature neurons of the prenatal telencephalic ventricular zone destined for the cerebral cortex begin to express p19^{Ink4d}, they differentiate and become permanently postmitotic. In contrast, Coskun and Luskin *(49)* propose that SVZa-derived cells in the RMS undergo repeated rounds of p19^{Ink4d} up-regulation and differentiation and then p19^{Ink4d} down-regulation and dedifferentiation followed by division.

p19^{Ink4d} is unlikely to be the only CDKI involved in regulating cell cycle progression and withdrawal of SVZa-derived neuronal progenitor cells. There are two families of CDKIs: the Ink4 proteins and the Cip/Kip proteins. Doetsch et al. *(91)* examined olfactory bulb neurogenesis in adult mice with a targeted mutation that prevented them from producing active p27^{Kip1}, a CDKI of the Cip/Kip family. In these mice there was both increased proliferation of olfactory bulb interneuron progenitors and increased apoptosis. Coskun and Luskin *(unpublished data)* have found that p27^{Kip1} is expressed along the posterior–anterior axis of the neonatal RMS, especially in the sez (anterior) portion of the RMS, suggesting that p27^{Kip1} may regulate olfactory bulb neurogenesis in the neonate as well. It should be noted, however, that Doetsch et al. *(91)* interpret their data as showing an effect on "C-type" cells of the adult, which are concentrated around the ventricles and are not found in the sez *(45)*, so the distribution of p27^{Kip1} observed by Coskun and Luskin in the neonate may reflect a different p27^{Kip1} function than that detected by Doetsch et al. *(91)*. Specifically, given its concentration in the sez, p27^{Kip1} may be involved in converting the cycling progenitors of the RMS to permanently postmitotic neurons of the olfactory bulb.

Taken together the data on CDKI expression patterns and the effects of targeted mutations indicate that both p19^{Ink4d} and p27^{Kip1} regulate cell cycle progression of SVZa-derived neuronal progenitor cells. The opposing gradients of p19^{Ink4d} and BrdU expression along the RMS may reflect a role of p19^{Ink4d} in controlling repeated differentiation/dedifferentiation of SVZa-derived neuronal progenitors as they divide while migrating along the RMS; whereas the concentration of p27^{Kip1} in the sez, the region of the RMS from which permanently postmitotic daughters of SVZa-derived neuronal progenitors migrate radially into the layers of the olfactory bulb, may reflect a role of p27^{Kip1} permanent in cell cycle exit.

EXTRINSIC CONTROL OF SVZa-DERIVED NEURONAL PROGENITOR CELL PROLIFERATION BY BMP SIGNALING PROTEINS

Coskun et al. *(92)* investigated whether the bone morphogenetic proteins (BMPs) expressed by the neonatal RMS control when and where SVZa-derived cells undergo cell cycle arrest. BMPs, a group of cytokines of the transforming growth factor-β superfamily, were selected for study because in some neural systems they play regulatory roles, in a cell type-specific manner, in the control of proliferation as well as in cell fate decisions *(25,93,94)*. For example, in cultures of neocortical ventricular zone cells, BMP4 increases the number of cells expressing the neuron-specific markers MAP-2 and neuron-specific type III β-tubulin (recognized by the antibody TuJ1) and expression of a dominant negative BMP receptor blocks migration and process formation of ventricular zone cells *(95)*. However, in cultured progenitor cells from the postnatal striatal SVZ, BMP2 or 7 treatment leads to the cessation of cell proliferation and induction of astrocyte differentiation *(96–98)*. In another study Yamato et al. *(99)* showed that in mouse hybridoma cells, BMPs act directly on the CDKI p21^{Cip1} to induce apoptosis or cell cycle exit. Therefore, BMPs can promote cell cycle exit, and in some contexts BMPs promote neuronal differentiation while in other contexts they promote glial differentiation.

To investigate whether BMPs regulate the proliferation and/or differentiation of SVZa-derived neuronal progenitor cells, Coskun et al. *(92)* altered the expression of the BMP receptor subtype Ia (BMPR-Ia) using retroviral-mediated gene expression. To augment BMP signaling, a replication-deficient retrovirus encoding the wild-type BMPR-Ia was injected into the neonatal SVZa. The virus was also engineered to express human alkaline phosphatase (AP), which allowed specific identification of the progeny of infected cells. The striking result was that the cells overexpressing the BMPR-Ia continued to exhibit a neuronal phenotype but essentially all became p19^{Ink4d}(+) even though p19^{Ink4d} is normally not detected in the SVZa. To block BMP signaling, a similar replication-deficient retroviral vector was constructed, but this vector caused expression of a dominant negative form of the BMPR-Ia. Eight days following infection with this virus, the progeny of infected cells had migrated to the sez, the terminal region of the RMS and an area where a large proportion of the cells normally express p19^{Ink4d}. However, expression of p19^{Ink4d} by infected (dominant negative BMPR-Ia expressing) cells within the sez was not observed. These findings suggest that BMP signaling is sufficient and necessary to induce p19^{Ink4d} expression in SVZa-derived neuronal progenitor cells in vivo.

In addition to regulating cell cycle progression, BMP signaling appears to have a second role in olfactory bulb neurogenesis: influencing the differentiation along the gliogenic vs neurogenic pathway in the adult. Lim et al. *(100)* found that BMPs acted on SVZ stem cells ("B-type" cells) to promote gliogenesis, whereas noggin, an inhibitor of BMPs, promoted neurogenesis by SVZ stem cells. If BMPs have a similar function in the neonate, they must act at an earlier stage in the lineage of olfactory bulb interneurons than the neuronal progenitors of the SVZa since, as described above, increasing BMP signaling did not alter the neuronal commitment of these cells. In summary, the consequence of altered BMP signaling may depend on the stage in the lineage of olfactory bulb neurons receiving the signal: when acting on stem cells (early stage in the lineage) the effect of BMPs may be to promote gliogenesis, but when acting on SVZa-derived neuronal progenitors (late stage in the lineage) the effect may be to inhibit cell cycle progression or promote cell cycle exit via action on p19[Ink4d]. In future studies we will directly test this second role by examining the effects of BMP signaling pathway activation and inhibition on the proliferation of neonatal SVZa-derived neuronal progenitor cells in vivo and in vitro.

EXTRINSIC CONTROL OF SVZa-DERIVED NEURONAL PROGENITOR CELL PROLIFERATION BY THE NEUROTROPHIN BDNF

Spurred by culture results demonstrating that the growth and differentiation factors bFGF and EGF have neurogenic properties, several investigators have attempted to induce neuronal proliferation in the postnatal brain by the intraventricular administration of these proteins. Infusion of bFGF or EGF into the lateral ventricles *(12,15,101–104)* or even peripherally *(15,102)* in rodents leads to proliferation in the striatal SVZ; however, astroglia seem to be preferentially generated by treatment with these trophic factors *(15,102)*. The finding that BDNF increased the number of neurons within neurospheres *(105)*, and evidence that p75, a low affinity receptor for neurotrophins, including BDNF, was highly expressed by cells of the RMS (S. Wiegand, T. Zigova and M. B. Luskin, *unpublished data*), and previous studies showing that in vitro BDNF promoted the neuronal differentiation or survival of SVZ progenitor cells *(37,105,106)* prompted Zigova et al. *(17)* to assess the effects of BDNF in vivo. As our focus in prior sections has been on studies of neurogenesis in the neonate, it is worthwhile emphasizing that these studies were conducted on adult rats. BDNF was infused into the right lateral ventricle of adult rat brains for twelve days in conjunction with either the intraventricular infusion or intraperitoneal injection of the cell proliferation marker BrdU, and BrdU immunohistochemistry was used to monitor the production of new cells. Significantly more BrdU-labeled cells in the RMS and olfactory bulb were observed on the BDNF-infused side than in the RMS and olfactory bulb of PBS-infused control animals. Using double-labeling with cell type-specific markers for neurons or glia, in conjunction with anti-BrdU, Zigova et al. *(17)* determined that the preponderance (>90%) of the newly generated cells in the RMS and postmitotic layers of the olfactory bulb on the BDNF-infused side of the treated rats were neurons and fewer than 5% were glia. Benraiss recently demonstrated that adenoviral delivery of BDNF also induces new neurons in the RMS *(107)*, a finding consistent with the results of the Zigova et al. *(17)* study. Moreover, Zigova et al. *(17)* demonstrated that trkB, the high-affinity tyrosine kinase receptor for BDNF, was heavily expressed by the RMS, including the SVZa. These results demonstrate that the generation and/or survival of new neurons in the adult brain can be increased substantially by the infusion of BDNF. Furthermore, the results support the idea that the SVZ, and in particular the SVZa, may constitute a reserve pool of progenitor cells available for neuronal replacement in the diseased or damaged brain.

SUMMARY AND FUTURE DIRECTIONS

Evidence has been presented supporting the ideas that SVZa-derived neuronal progenitor cells are true "neuronal restricted progenitors," that these cells have a different origin from the progenitors in the part of the SVZ posterior to the SVZa, that there are similar populations of SVZa-derived neuronal progenitors in rodents and primates, that SVZa-derived neuronal progenitors continue to proliferate and to produce neurons throughout life, and that the production of SVZa-derived neuronal progenitors can be enhanced by experimental manipulations. Three mechanisms implicated in controlling the proliferation of these cells have been discussed: intrinsic control via the cyclin-dependent kinase inhibitors (CDKIs), and extrinsic control by the cell–cell signaling proteins bone morphogenetic proteins (BMPs) and brain-derived neurotrophic factor (BDNF). The evidence described suggests that BMP inhibits proliferation by increasing the amount of the CDKI $p19^{Ink4d}$.

Future studies will directly test the hypothesis that BMPs acting through $p19^{Ink4d}$ inhibit the proliferation of SVZa-derived neuronal progenitors and will further examine the in vivo roles of BMPs and BDNF in regulating proliferation of these progenitors. Strong, but indirect, evidence suggests that SVZa-derived neuronal progenitors repeatedly divide after having differentiated, as evidenced by production of neuron-specific proteins and by the in vitro extension of neuronal processes *(38)*. Ongoing studies are directly testing the hypothesis that these cells dedifferentiate prior to each division and then redifferentiate following each division. If this hypothesis is supported, defining the mechanisms regulating this cyclic dedifferentiation will provide novel insights into the control of the neuronal cell cycle and of neuronal differentiation. Such understandings will contribute to development of strategies for neural repair.

ACKNOWLEDGMENTS

The authors thank Dr. Giri Venkatraman for work on the first edition of this manuscript. We also thank the members of the Luskin lab, past and present. This work was supported by grants to M. B. L. from the NIDCD.

REFERENCES

1. Gage, F. H. (2003) Brain, repair yourself. *Sci. Am.* **289,** 46–53.
2. Altman, J. and Das, G. D. (1966) Autoradiographic and histological studies of postnatal neurogenesis. I. A longitudinal investigation of the kinetics, migration and transformation of cells incorporating tritiated thymidine in neonate rats, with special reference to postnatal neurogenesis in some brain regions. *J. Comp. Neurol.* **126,** 337–389.
3. Rakic, P. (1985) Limits of neurogenesis in primates. *Science* **227,** 1054–1056.
4. Eriksson, P. S., Perfilieva, E., Bjork-Eriksson, T., et al. (1998) Neurogenesis in the adult human hippocampus. *Nat. Med.* **4,** 1313–1317.

5. Gould, E., Reeves, A. J., Fallah, M., Tanapat, P., Gross, C. G., and Fuchs, E. (1999) Hippocampal neurogenesis in adult Old World primates. *Proc. Natl. Acad. Sci. USA* **96,** 5263–5267.

6. Graziadei, P. P. and Graziadei, G. A. (1979) Neurogenesis and neuron regeneration in the olfactory system of mammals. I. Morphological aspects of differentiation and structural organization of the olfactory sensory neurons. *J. Neurocytol.* **8,** 1–18.

7. Graziadei, G. A. and Graziadei, P. P. (1979) Neurogenesis and neuron regeneration in the olfactory system of mammals. II. Degeneration and reconstitution of the olfactory sensory neurons after axotomy. *J. Neurocytol.* **8,** 197–213.

8. Graziadei, P. P. and Monti Graziadei, G. A. (1985) Neurogenesis and plasticity of the olfactory sensory neurons. *Ann. NY Acad. Sci.* **457,** 127–142.

9. Reynolds, B. A. and Weiss, S. (1992) Generation of neurons and astrocytes from isolated cells of the adult mammalian central nervous system. *Science* **255,** 1707–1710.

10. Luskin, M. B. (1993) Restricted proliferation and migration of postnatally generated neurons derived from the forebrain subventricular zone. *Neuron* **11,** 173–189.

11. Lois, C. and Alvarez-Buylla, A. (1993) Proliferating subventricular zone cells in the adult mammalian forebrain can differentiate into neurons and glia. *Proc. Natl. Acad. Sci. USA* **90,** 2074–2077.

12. Gage, F. H., Coates, P. W., Palmer, T. D., et al. (1995) Survival and differentiation of adult neuronal progenitor cells transplanted to the adult brain. *Proc. Natl. Acad. Sci. USA* **92,** 11879–11883.

13. Gage, F. H., Kempermann, G., Palmer, T. D., Peterson, D. A., and Ray, J. (1998) Multipotent progenitor cells in the adult dentate gyrus. *J. Neurobiol.* **36,** 249–266.

14. Huard, J. M., Youngentob, S. L., Goldstein, B. J., Luskin, M. B., and Schwob, J. E. (1998) Adult olfactory epithelium contains multipotent progenitors that give rise to neurons and non-neural cells. *J. Comp. Neurol.* **400,** 469–486.

15. Kuhn, H. G., Winkler, J., Kempermann, G., Thal, L. J., and Gage, F. H. (1997) Epidermal growth factor and fibroblast growth factor-2 have different effects on neural progenitors in the adult rat brain. *J. Neurosci.* **17,** 5820–5829.

16. Tao, Y., Black, I. B., and DiCicco-Bloom, E. (1997) In vivo neurogenesis is inhibited by neutralizing antibodies to basic fibroblast growth factor. *J. Neurobiol.* **33,** 289–296.

17. Zigova, T., Pencea, V., Wiegand, S. J., and Luskin, M. B. (1998) Intraventricular administration of BDNF increases the number of newly generated neurons in the adult olfactory bulb. *Mol. Cell. Neurosci.* **11,** 234–245.

18. Parent, J. M., Yu, T. W., Leibowitz, R. T., Geschwind, D. H., Sloviter, R. S., and Lowenstein, D. H. (1997) Dentate granule cell neurogenesis is increased by seizures and contributes to aberrant network reorganization in the adult rat hippocampus. *J. Neurosci.* **17,** 3727–3738.

19. Kokaia, Z., Arvidsson, A., Ekdahl, C., and Lindvall, O. (2004) Neurogenesis in stroke and epilepsy. In *Stem Cells in the Nervous System* (Gage, F. H., Bjorklund, A., Prochiantz, A., and Christen, Y., eds.), Springer-Verlag, New York.

20. Rao, M. S. (1999) Multipotent and restricted precursors in the central nervous system. *Anat. Rec.* **257,** 137–148.

21. Lendahl, U., Zimmerman, L. B., and McKay, R. D. (1990) CNS stem cells express a new class of intermediate filament protein. *Cell* **60,** 585–595.

22. McConnell, S. K. (1991) The generation of neuronal diversity in the central nervous system. *Annu. Rev. Neurosci.* **14,** 269–300.

23. McConnell, S. K. (1995) Constructing the cerebral cortex: neurogenesis and fate determination. *Neuron* **15,** 761–768.

24. Luskin, M. B. (1994) Neuronal cell lineage in the vertebrate central nervous system. *FASEB J.* **8,** 722–730.

25. Kalyani, A. J., Piper, D., Mujtaba, T., Lucero, M. T., and Rao, M. S. (1998) Spinal cord neuronal precursors generate multiple neuronal phenotypes in culture. *J. Neurosci.* **18,** 7856–7868.

26. Yang, H., Mujtaba, T., Venkatraman, G., Wu, Y. Y., Rao, M. S., and Luskin, M. B. (2000) Region-specific differentiation of neural tube-derived neuronal restricted progenitor cells after heterotopic transplantation. *Proc. Natl. Acad. Sci. USA* **97,** 13366–13371.

27. Zigova, T., Betarbet, R., Soteres, B. J., Brock, S., Bakay, R. A., and Luskin, M. B. (1996) A comparison of the patterns of migration and the destinations of homotopically trans-planted neonatal subventricular zone cells and heterotopically transplanted telencephalic ventricular zone cells. *Dev. Biol.* **173,** 459–474.

28. Bayer, S. A. (1983) ³H-thymidine-radiographic studies of neurogenesis in the rat olfac-tory bulb. *Exp. Brain Res.* **50,** 329–340.

29. Hinds, J. W. (1968) Autoradiographic study of histogenesis in the mouse olfactory bulb. II. Cell proliferation and migration. *J. Comp. Neurol.* **134,** 305–322.

30. Hinds, J. W. (1968) Autoradiographic study of histogenesis in the mouse olfactory bulb. I. Time of origin of neurons and neuroglia. *J. Comp. Neurol.* **134,** 287–304.

31. Kishi, K. (1987) Golgi studies on the development of granule cells of the rat olfactory bulb with reference to migration in the subependymal layer. *J. Comp. Neurol.* **258,** 112–124.

32. Luskin, M. B. and McDermott, K. (1994) Divergent lineages for oligodendrocytes and astrocytes originating in the neonatal forebrain subventricular zone. *Glia* **11,** 211–226.

33. Levison, S. W. and Goldman, J. E. (1993) Both oligodendrocytes and astrocytes develop from progenitors in the subventricular zone of postnatal rat forebrain. *Neuron* **10,** 201–212.

34. Levison, S. W., Chuang, C., Abramson, B. J., and Goldman, J. E. (1993) The migrational patterns and developmental fates of glial precursors in the rat subventricular zone are temporally regulated. *Development* **119,** 611–622.

35. Privat, A. (1975) Postnatal gliogenesis in the mammalian brain. *Int. Rev. Cytol.* **40,** 281–323.

36. Skoff, R. P. (1980) Neuroglia: a reevaluation of their origin and development. *Pathol. Res. Pract.* **168,** 279–300.

37. Kirschenbaum, B. and Goldman, S. A. (1995) Brain-derived neurotrophic factor promotes the survival of neurons arising from the adult rat forebrain subependymal zone. *Proc. Natl. Acad. Sci. USA* **92,** 210–214.

38. Luskin, M. B., Zigova, T., Soteres, B. J., and Stewart, R. R. (1997) Neuronal progenitor cells derived from the anterior subventricular zone of the neonatal rat forebrain con-tinue to proliferate in vitro and express a neuronal phenotype. *Mol. Cell. Neurosci.* **8,** 351–366.

39. Law, A. K., Pencea, V., Buck, C. R., and Luskin, M. B. (1999) Neurogenesis and neu-ronal migration in the neonatal rat forebrain anterior subventricular zone do not require GFAP-positive astrocytes. *Dev. Biol.* **216,** 622–634.

40. Lois, C. and Alvarez-Buylla, A. (1994) Long-distance neuronal migration in the adult mammalian brain. *Science* **264,** 1145–1148.

41. Levison, S. W. and Goldman, J. E. (1997) Multipotential and lineage restricted precur-sors coexist in the mammalian perinatal subventricular zone. *J. Neurosci. Res.* **48,** 83–94.

42. Suzuki, S. O. and Goldman, J. E. (2003) Multiple cell populations in the early postnatal subventricular zone take distinct migratory pathways: a dynamic study of glial and neu-ronal progenitor migration. *J. Neurosci.* **23,** 4240–4250.

43. Marshall, C. A., Suzuki, S. O., and Goldman, J. E. (2003) Gliogenic and neurogenic pro-genitors of the subventricular zone: Who are they, where did they come from, and where are they going? *Glia* **43,** 52–61.

44. Doetsch, F. and Alvarez-Buylla, A. (1996) Network of tangential pathways for neuronal migration in adult mammalian brain. *Proc. Natl. Acad. Sci. USA* **93,** 14895–14900.

45. Doetsch, F., Garcia-Verdugo, J. M., and Alvarez-Buylla, A. (1997) Cellular composition and three-dimensional organization of the subventricular germinal zone in the adult mammalian brain. *J. Neurosci.* **17**, 5046–5061.

46. Doetsch, F., Caille, I., Lim, D. A., Garcia-Verdugo, J. M., and Alvarez-Buylla, A. (1999) Subventricular zone astrocytes are neural stem cells in the adult mammalian brain. *Cell* **97**, 703–716.

47. Peretto, P., Merighi, A., Fasolo, A., and Bonfanti, L. (1997) Glial tubes in the rostral migratory stream of the adult rat. *Brain Res. Bull.* **42**, 9–21.

48. Menezes, J. R., Smith, C. M., Nelson, K. C., and Luskin, M. B. (1995) The division of neuronal progenitor cells during migration in the neonatal mammalian forebrain. *Mol. Cell. Neurosci.* **6**, 496–508.

49. Coskun, V. and Luskin, M. B. (2001) The expression pattern of the cell cycle inhibitor p19(INK4d) by progenitor cells of the rat embryonic telencephalon and neonatal anterior subventricular zone. *J. Neurosci.* **21**, 3092–3103.

50. Pencea, V., Bingaman, K. D., Freedman, L. J., and Luskin, M. B. (2001) Neurogenesis in the subventricular zone and rostral migratory stream of the neonatal and adult primate forebrain. *Exp. Neurol.* **172**, 1–16.

51. Lois, C., Garcia-Verdugo, J. M., and Alvarez-Buylla, A. (1996) Chain migration of neuronal precursors. *Science* **271**, 978–981.

52. Schubert, W., Coskun, V., Tahmina, M., Rao, M. S., Luskin, M. B., and Kaprielian, Z. (2000) Characterization and distribution of a new cell surface marker of neuronal precursors. *Dev. Neurosci.* **22**, 154–166.

53. Marin, O. and Rubenstein, J. L. (2003) Cell migration in the forebrain. *Annu. Rev. Neurosci.* **26**, 441–483.

54. Kishi, K., Peng, J. Y., Kakuta, S., et al. (1990) Migration of bipolar subependymal cells, precursors of the granule cells of the rat olfactory bulb, with reference to the arrangement of the radial glial fibers. *Arch. Histol. Cytol.* **53**, 219–226.

55. Rakic, P. (1971) Guidance of neurons migrating to the fetal monkey neocortex. *Brain Res.* **33**, 471–476.

56. Rousselot, P., Lois, C., and Alvarez-Buylla, A. (1995) Embryonic (PSA) N-CAM reveals chains of migrating neuroblasts between the lateral ventricle and the olfactory bulb of adult mice. *J. Comp. Neurol.* **351**, 51–61.

57. O'Rourke, N. A. (1996) Neuronal chain gangs: homotypic contacts support migration into the olfactory bulb. *Neuron* **16**, 1061–1064.

58. Thomas, L. B., Gates, M. A., and Steindler, D. A. (1996) Young neurons from the adult subependymal zone proliferate and migrate along an astrocyte, extracellular matrix-rich pathway. *Glia* **17**, 1–14.

59. Bonsall, J. M. and Luskin, M. B. (2003) Chondroitin sulfate proteoglycans (CSPGs) may restrict migrating SVZa - derived progenitor cells to the rostral migratory stream in the rat. *Soc. Neurosci. Abstr.* **33**, 138.135.

60. Bonsall, J. M. and Luskin, M. B. (2005) Extracellular matrix and/or cell surface associated molecules restrict neuronal progenitors to the rostral migratory stream. (in preparation)

61. Cremer, H., Lange, R., Christoph, A., et al. (1994) Inactivation of the N-CAM gene in mice results in size reduction of the olfactory bulb and deficits in spatial learning. *Nature* **367**, 455–459.

62. Hu, H., Tomasiewicz, H., Magnuson, T., and Rutishauser, U. (1996) The role of polysialic acid in migration of olfactory bulb interneuron precursors in the subventricular zone. *Neuron* **16**, 735–743.

63. Treloar, H., Tomasiewicz, H., Magnuson, T., and Key, B. (1997) The central pathway of primary olfactory axons is abnormal in mice lacking the N-CAM-180 isoform. *J. Neurobiol.* **32**, 643–658.

64. Wu, W., Wong, K., Chen, J., et al. (1999) Directional guidance of neuronal migration in the olfactory system by the protein Slit. *Nature* **400,** 331–336.

65. Nguyen-Ba-Charvet, K. T., Picard-Riera, N., Tessier-Lavigne, M., Baron-Van Evercooren, A., Sotelo, C., and Chedotal, A. (2004) Multiple roles for slits in the control of cell migration in the rostral migratory stream. *J. Neurosci.* **24,** 1497–1506.

66. Maricich, S. M., Gilmore, E. C., and Herrup, K. (2001) The role of tangential migration in the establishment of mammalian cortex. *Neuron* **31,** 175–178.

67. Marin, O. and Rubenstein, J. L. (2001) A long, remarkable journey: tangential migration in the telencephalon. *Nat. Rev. Neurosci.* **2,** 780–790.

68. Stewart, R. R., Zigova, T., and Luskin, M. B. (1999) Potassium currents in precursor cells isolated from the anterior subventricular zone of the neonatal rat forebrain. *J. Neurophysiol.* **81,** 95–102.

69. Stewart, R. R., Hoge, G. J., Zigova, T., and Luskin, M. B. (2002) Neural progenitor cells of the neonatal rat anterior subventricular zone express functional GABA(A) receptors. *J. Neurobiol.* **50,** 305–322.

70. Wang, D. D., Krueger, D. D., and Bordey, A. (2003) Biophysical properties and ionic signature of neuronal progenitors of the postnatal subventricular zone in situ. *J. Neurophysiol.* **90,** 2291–2302.

71. Zigova, T., Pencea, V., Betarbet, R., et al. (1998) Neuronal progenitor cells of the neonatal subventricular zone differentiate and disperse following transplantation into the adult rat striatum. *Cell Transplant.* **7,** 137–156.

72. Betarbet, R., Zigova, T., Bakay, R. A., and Luskin, M. B. (1996) Migration patterns of neonatal subventricular zone progenitor cells transplanted into the neonatal striatum. *Cell Transplant.* **5,** 165–178.

73. Betarbet, R., Zigova, T., Bakay, R. A., and Luskin, M. B. (1996) Dopaminergic and GABAergic interneurons of the olfactory bulb are derived from the neonatal subventricular zone. *Int. J. Dev. Neurosci.* **14,** 921–930.

74. Pencea, V. and Luskin, M. B. (2003) Prenatal development of the rodent rostral migratory stream. *J. Comp. Neurol.* **463,** 402–418.

75. Bonfanti, L. and Theodosis, D. T. (1994) Expression of polysialylated neural cell adhesion molecule by proliferating cells in the subependymal layer of the adult rat, in its rostral extension and in the olfactory bulb. *Neuroscience* **62,** 291–305.

76. Wichterle, H., Turnbull, D. H., Nery, S., Fishell, G., and Alvarez-Buylla, A. (2001) In utero fate mapping reveals distinct migratory pathways and fates of neurons born in the mammalian basal forebrain. *Development* **128,** 3759–3771.

77. Morshead, C. M., Garcia, A. D., Sofroniew, M. V., and van Der Kooy, D. (2003) The ablation of glial fibrillary acidic protein-positive cells from the adult central nervous system results in the loss of forebrain neural stem cells but not retinal stem cells. *Eur. J. Neurosci.* **18,** 76–84.

78. Anthony, T. E., Klein, C., Fishell, G., and Heintz, N. (2004) Radial glia serve as neuronal progenitors in all regions of the central nervous system. *Neuron* **41,** 881–890.

79. Kornack, D. R. and Rakic, P. (2001) The generation, migration, and differentiation of olfactory neurons in the adult primate brain. *Proc. Natl. Acad. Sci. USA* **98,** 4752–4757.

80. Bedard, A., Levesque, M., Bernier, P. J., and Parent, A. (2002) The rostral migratory stream in adult squirrel monkeys: contribution of new neurons to the olfactory tubercle and involvement of the antiapoptotic protein Bcl-2. *Eur. J. Neurosci.* **16,** 1917–1924.

81. Garcia-Verdugo, J., Doetsch, F., Wichterle, H., and Alvarez-Buylla, A. (1998) Architecture and cell types of the adult subventricular zone: in search of the stem cells. *J. Neurobiol.* **36,** 234–248.

82. Sanai, N., Tramontin, A. D., Quinones-Hinojosa, A., et al. (2004) Unique astrocyte ribbon in adult human brain contains neural stem cells but lacks chain migration. *Nature* **427,** 740–744.

83. Seaberg, R. M. and van der Kooy, D. (2002) Adult rodent neurogenic regions: the ventricular subependyma contains neural stem cells, but the dentate gyrus contains restricted progenitors. *J. Neurosci.* **22,** 1784–1793.

84. Cunningham, J. J. and Roussel, M. F. (2001) Cyclin-dependent kinase inhibitors in the development of the central nervous system. *Cell Growth Differ.* **12,** 387–396.

85. Sherr, C. J. (1994) G1 phase progression: cycling on cue. *Cell* **79,** 551–555.

86. Coskun, V. and Luskin, M. B. (2002) Intrinsic and extrinsic regulation of the proliferation and differentiation of cells in the rodent rostral migratory stream. *J. Neurosci. Res.* **69,** 795–802.

87. Luskin, M. B. and Coskun, V. (2002) The progenitor cells of the embryonic telencephalon and the neonatal anterior subventricular zone differentially regulate their cell cycle. *Chem. Senses* **27,** 577–580.

88. Zindy, F., Soares, H., Herzog, K. H., Morgan, J., Sherr, C. J., and Roussel, M. F. (1997) Expression of INK4 inhibitors of cyclin D-dependent kinases during mouse brain development. *Cell Growth Differ.* **8,** 1139–1150.

89. Smith, C. M. and Luskin, M. B. (1998) Cell cycle length of olfactory bulb neuronal progenitors in the rostral migratory stream. *Dev. Dyn.* **213,** 220–227.

90. Zindy, F., Cunningham, J. J., Sherr, C. J., Jogal, S., Smeyne, R. J., and Roussel, M. F. (1999) Postnatal neuronal proliferation in mice lacking Ink4d and Kip1 inhibitors of cyclin-dependent kinases. *Proc. Natl. Acad. Sci. USA* **96,** 13462–13467.

91. Doetsch, F., Verdugo, J. M., Caille, I., Alvarez-Buylla, A., Chao, M. V., and Casaccia-Bonnefil, P. (2002) Lack of the cell-cycle inhibitor p27Kip1 results in selective increase of transit-amplifying cells for adult neurogenesis. *J. Neurosci.* **22,** 2255–2264.

92. Coskun, V., Venkatraman, G., Yang, H., Rao, M. S., and Luskin, M. B. (2001) Retroviral manipulation of the expression of bone morphogenetic protein receptor Ia by SVZa progenitor cells leads to changes in their p19(INK4d) expression but not in their neuronal commitment. *Int. J. Dev. Neurosci.* **19,** 219–227.

93. Mabie, P. C., Mehler, M. F., Marmur, R., Papavasiliou, A., Song, Q., and Kessler, J. A. (1997) Bone morphogenetic proteins induce astroglial differentiation of oligodendroglial-astroglial progenitor cells. *J. Neurosci.* **17,** 4112–4120.

94. Mehler, M. F., Mabie, P. C., Zhu, G., Gokhan, S., and Kessler, J. A. (2000) Developmental changes in progenitor cell responsiveness to bone morphogenetic proteins differentially modulate progressive CNS lineage fate. *Dev. Neurosci.* **22,** 74–85.

95. Li, W., Cogswell, C. A., and LoTurco, J. J. (1998) Neuronal differentiation of precursors in the neocortical ventricular zone is triggered by BMP. *J. Neurosci.* **18,** 8853–8862.

96. Gross, R. E., Mehler, M. F., Mabie, P. C., Zang, Z., Santschi, L., and Kessler, J. A. (1996) Bone morphogenetic proteins promote astroglial lineage commitment by mammalian subventricular zone progenitor cells. *Neuron* **17,** 595–606.

97. Zhu, G., Mehler, M. F., Mabie, P. C., and Kessler, J. A. (1999) Developmental changes in progenitor cell responsiveness to cytokines. *J. Neurosci. Res.* **56,** 131–145.

98. Zhu, G., Mehler, M. F., Zhao, J., Yu Yung, S., and Kessler, J. A. (1999) Sonic hedgehog and BMP2 exert opposing actions on proliferation and differentiation of embryonic neural progenitor cells. *Dev. Biol.* **215,** 118–129.

99. Yamato, K., Hashimoto, S., Okahashi, N., et al. (2000) Dissociation of bone morphogenetic protein-mediated growth arrest and apoptosis of mouse B cells by HPV-16 E6/E7. *Exp. Cell Res.* **257,** 198–205.

100. Lim, D. A., Tramontin, A. D., Trevejo, J. M., Herrera, D. G., Garcia-Verdugo, J. M., and Alvarez-Buylla, A. (2000) Noggin antagonizes BMP signaling to create a niche for adult neurogenesis. *Neuron* **28,** 713–726.

101. Wagner, J. P., Black, I. B., and DiCicco-Bloom, E. (1999) Stimulation of neonatal and adult brain neurogenesis by subcutaneous injection of basic fibroblast growth factor. *J. Neurosci.* **19,** 6006–6016.

102. Craig, C. G., Tropepe, V., Morshead, C. M., Reynolds, B. A., Weiss, S., and van der Kooy, D. (1996) In vivo growth factor expansion of endogenous subependymal neural precursor cell populations in the adult mouse brain. *J. Neurosci.* **16,** 2649–2658.
103. Gritti, A., Parati, E. A., Cova, L., et al. (1996) Multipotential stem cells from the adult mouse brain proliferate and self-renew in response to basic fibroblast growth factor. *J. Neurosci.* **16,** 1091–1100.
104. Palmer, T. D., Ray, J., and Gage, F. H. (1995) FGF-2-responsive neuronal progenitors reside in proliferative and quiescent regions of the adult rodent brain. *Mol. Cell. Neurosci.* **6,** 474–486.
105. Shetty, A. K. and Turner, D. A. (1998) In vitro survival and differentiation of neurons derived from epidermal growth factor-responsive postnatal hippocampal stem cells: inducing effects of brain-derived neurotrophic factor. *J. Neurobiol.* **35,** 395–425.
106. Ahmed, S., Reynolds, B. A., and Weiss, S. (1995) BDNF enhances the differentiation but not the survival of CNS stem cell-derived neuronal precursors. *J. Neurosci.* **15,** 5765–5778.
107. Benraiss, A., Chmielnicki, E., Lerner, K., Roh, D., and Goldman, S. A. (2001) Adenoviral brain-derived neurotrophic factor induces both neostriatal and olfactory neuronal recruitment from endogenous progenitor cells in the adult forebrain. *J. Neurosci.* **21,** 6718–6731.

7

Glial Restricted Precursors

Mark Noble and Margot Mayer-Pröschel

The most numerous of the cells of the central nervous system (CNS) are the glia. These cells, which include the myelin-forming oligodendrocytes of the white matter and the ubiquitous astrocytes, play many roles in normal development and in disease. A subject of study since the time of del Rio de Hortega, a great deal of knowledge has been obtained regarding the development and function of these cells. Nonetheless, it must be recognized that we are still far from having a comprehensive understanding of the origins and biology of the glia. The extent to which our knowledge is still in its early stages is reflected in the often inadequate nomenclature with which to discuss the complexity already believed to exist.

In the context of developmental pathways, far the better understood of the glia is the oligodendrocyte, which is generally thought of as having the sole function of myelinating CNS axons. Such a view of this cell is certainly an oversimplification, for oligodendrocytes have multiple effects on neurons (discussed further in ref. *1*). For example, it has long been known that association of axons with oligodendrocytes has profound physical effects on the axon, and is associated with substantial increases in axons diameters. Animals in which oligodendrocytes are destroyed (e.g., by radiation) or defective (as in animals lacking proteolipid protein) show substantial axonal abnormalities *(2,3)*. In addition, axonal damage, leading eventually to axonal loss, may also occur in multiple sclerosis *(4)*.

One of the dramatic effects of oligodendrocytes on axons is to modulate axonal channel properties. During early development, both Na^+ and K^+ channels are distributed uniformly along axons, but become clustered into different axonal domains coincident with the process of myelination *(5,6)*. Na^+ channels specifically become clustered into the nodes of Ranvier, the regions of exposed axonal membrane that lie between consecutive myelin sheaths. K^+ channels, in contrast, become clustered in the juxtaparanodal region. It has become clear from multiple studies that Schwann cells in the peripheral nervous system, and oligodendrocytes in the CNS, play instructive roles in the clustering of axonal ion channels *(5–8)*.

While the study of trophic support derived from oligodendrocytes is still in its infancy, an increasing number of interesting proteins have been observed to be produced by these cells. For example, insulin-like growth factor I, nerve growth factor, brain-derived neurotrophic factor, and neurotrophin-3 and neurotrophin-4/mRNAs

From: *Neural Development and Stem Cells, Second Edition*
Edited by: M. S. Rao © Humana Press Inc., Totowa, NJ

and/or protein have been observed by *in situ* hybridization and via immunocytochemical studies in oliogdendrocytes *(9–11)*. Consistent with the idea that there might be
trophism-related differences in oligodendrocytes from different CNS regions, it does
appear that there is regional heterogeneity in the expression of these important proteins
(12). Still other proteins that have been suggested to be produced by oligodendrocytes include neuregulin-1 *(13–16)*, glia-derived neurotrophic factor *(17)*, fibroblast
growth factor-9 (FGF-9) *(18)*, and members of the transforming growth factor-β (TGF-
β) family *(19,20)*. Many of the factors that oligodendrocytes appear to produce have
been found to influence the development not only of neurons, but also of oligodendrocytes themselves. Thus, it may prove that one of the functions of oligodendrocytes is to
produce factors that modulate their own functions.

Oligodendrocytes and the precursor cells from which they are derived are also of
great interest due to their vulnerability to a wide range of insults, leading to neurological problems associated with failure of normal impulse conduction. Dysmyelination
(a failure of normal myelin production) occurs in such syndromes as hypothyroidism,
iron deficiency, and generalized nutritional deficiency. Demyelination (a destruction
of existing myelin) is seen in association with such traumatic injuries to the CNS as
hypoxic birth insults, in multiple leukodystrophies, in all instances of traumatic injury
to the CNS, and many chronic degenerative diseases. As enwrapment of projection
axons with myelin sheaths is essential for their normal impulse conduction, dysmyelination and demyelination are both associated with profound neurological consequences.
In addition, multiple physiological stressors appear to be associated with both
dysmyelination and demyelination.

Astrocytes are at least as important as oligodendrocytes, and play a wide range of
roles in the CNS, including providing trophic factor support, neurotransmitter uptake
and inactivation, induction of the blood–brain barrier, substrates for axonal outgrowth,
production of mitogens and inducers of differentiation, and even perhaps participating
in antigen presentation to cells of the immune system. In contrast with oligodendrocytes, however, very few studies have been carried out on precursor cells restricted to
the generation of astrocytes. Thus, this class of precursor cell is considered at the end
of this chapter, but the primary focus is on the much more extensively studied ancestry
of oligodendrocytes.

OLIGODENDROCYTE TYPE-2 ASTROCYTE PROGENITOR CELLS

The steps involved in the generation of oligodendrocytes have been analyzed in a
detailed manner that far exceeds that for neurons and astrocytes. Indeed, studies on
oligodendrocyte development are sophisticated enough to have allowed the asking of a
variety of questions in developmental biology that have not been possible with any
other cell type.

The key turning point in cellular biological analysis of the origin of oligodendrocytes came with the identification of a bipotential progenitor cell in cultures of optic
nerve *(21)* that can differentiate in vitro into an oligodendrocyte or into a particular
kind of astrocyte (called the type 2 astrocyte *[22]*). Numerous studies have confirmed
the ability of these precursor cells to generate oligodendrocytes following transplantation (e.g., refs. *23–25*), although it remains unknown whether there are circumstances
in which the potential of these cells to generate astrocytes is utilized in vivo *(26,27)*.

This uncertainty led to the use of two names for these cells, one being the oligodendrocyte type 2 astrocyte (O-2A) progenitor cell (to reflect the cells' developmental potential) and the other name being the oligodendrocyte precursor cell (OPC, to reflect the clear importance of this cell in oligodendrocyte generation). As both names are reflective of important properties of this cell, we use the combined abbreviation of *O-2A/OPC*. O-2A/OPCs have been isolated from many different regions of the CNS and from multiple species.

It is difficult to understate the extent to which the ability to study a defined precursor cell population revolutionized studies on oligodendrocyte development, as well as providing insights into problems of much broader relevance. In vitro studies on O-2A/OPCs have been essential in identifying signaling molecules that promote division, survival, migration and differentiation in this lineage (e.g., refs. *28–34*). They have led to the identification of vulnerabilities of these cells that may be of critical importance in understanding multiple pathological conditions, including such diverse situations as multiple sclerosis, spinal injury, leukomalacia in premature babies, lacunar infarcts, and multiple nutritional and hormonal deficiency disorder (as discussed later in this chapter). Studies on cells of the oligodendrocyte lineage have also provided insights into such general problems as the role of redox function in modulating precursor cell function *(35)*, the relationship between histone deacetylation and both biochemical and morphological differentiation *(36)* and the effects of toxicant exposure on precursor cell function *(37,38)*.

In vitro studies on O-2A/OPCs also provided some of the antigenic markers crucial to studying the early development of oligodendrocytes and their ancestors in vivo, thus enabling the discovery that ancestors of oligodendrocytes appear to arise at specific times in distinct regions of the ventral spinal cord or brain. Genes (or proteins) that have been studied as specific markers of progression along an oligodendrocyte pathway in the spinal cord include the platelet-derived growth factor receptor-α (PDGFR-α) *(39,40)*, the receptor for the major O-2A/OPC mitogen PDGF-AA *(28,34)*; the enzyme 2',3'-cyclic nucleotide 3'-phosphodiesterase; and DM20, an isoform of the major myelin proteolipid protein (PLP) gene *(41,42)*. In the avian spinal cord, antigens recognized by the monoclonal antibody O4 *(43)* also define a discrete ventral ventricular location of oligodendrocyte precursors *(44–46)*. The most extensively studied of these markers, PDGFRa, is first seen in the developing rat spinal cord at E14 -E14.5 *(40)*.

The discovery that putative ancestors of oligodendrocytes arise in discrete regions of the CNS has proven to be a central foundation stone of many further studies on the earliest stages of oligodendrocyte development in vivo. These observations—generally analyzed in conjunction with in vitro studies—have led to the identification of roles of particular signaling molecules, such as sonic hedgehog (Shh), in induction of oligodendrocyte generation. As discussed later, this localized generation of cells thought to give rise to oligodendrocytes has also been of critical importance in analysis of transcriptional regulation of differentiation along this pathway.

REGULATION OF OLIGODENDROCYTE GENERATION FROM DIVIDING O-2A/OPCS INVOLVES AT LEAST THREE DISTINCT PROCESSES

The process by which O-2A/OPCs generate oligodendrocytes has been the subject of extensive analysis. Of particular importance in such research has been the fact that

O-2A/OPCs can be readily grown in vitro as a purified cell population and in individual clones *(32,47,48)*. Studies on this lineage also benefit from the fact that the bipolar morphology of O-2A/OPCs and the multipolar morphology of oligodendrocytes is sufficiently distinct that it is possible to identify each of these cell types by visual inspection, thus allowing detailed clonal analysis of differentiation to be readily carried out.

Initial studies on the generation of oligodendrocytes from dividing O-2A/OPCs suggested that this differentiation process was controlled by a cell-intrinsic program that causes all clonally related cells to undergo differentiation in a synchronous and symmetric manner *(49)*. It now seems likely, however, that this symmetric clonal differentiation was the outcome of conducting experiments in the presence of both type 1 astrocytes and thyroid hormone (TH) *(47,48,50)*, and did not reflect the O-2A/OPCs most fundamental differentiation characteristics. We now know that these conditions are highly potent inducers of oligodendrocyte generation and cause what is basically an asymmetric system to read out as though the differentiation pattern were symmetric.

It currently appears that three distinct stages of oligodendrocyte generation can be recognized. The initial generation of oligodendrocytes seems to be controlled by a cell-intrinsic clock that, in a still unknown manner, causes dividing progenitor cells to begin to generate oligodendrocytes with a highly stereotyped timing. For example, in cultures derived from brain or optic nerve of embryonic rats of a variety of ages, the first oligodendrocytes appear at a time equivalent to the date of birth of the rat, the same time at which oligodendrocytes first appear in vivo in these tissues *(51,52)*. This appropriately timed initial generation of oligodendrocytes is a robust phenomenon that has been observed in a variety of conditions, including in high-density cultures from brain or optic nerve grown in medium supplemented with fetal calf serum (FCS) *(51)*, and in high- or low-density cultures supplemented with medium conditioned by type 1 astrocytes or with PDGF *(47,53,54)*.

One of the most remarkable features of the initial generation of oligodendrocytes is that it is a highly asymmetric process *(47)*. Clones of O-2A/OPCs derived from the brains of E15 rats induced to divide by exposure to PDGF will generate their first oligodendrocytes after 6 d of in vitro expansion. The percentage of oligodendrocytes generated per clone varies over a broad range, but in the great majority of clones represents <30% of the total cells and in many clones represents <10% of the total cells. There is little correlation between the size of the clone and the extent of oligodendrocyte generation that occurs, with some clones at this time containing fewer than 15 cells and others more than 300 cells. We interpret such an outcome to mean two things. First, the timer that controls initial oligodendrocyte generation does not count cell divisions but instead actually measures time in some manner. This interpretation is based on the fact that clones of 15 cells or less would have undergone four divisions and those with 300 cells or more would have undergone nine or more divisions, yet both types of clone, and all other sizes of clone, exhibit a high probability of generating their first oligodendrocytes with a highly stereotyped timing. For example, in our own experiments *(47)*, 60% of clones generated their first oligodendrocytes at a time equivalent to the date of birth of the rat, with virtually no clones generating any oligodendrocytes even 1 d earlier. The idea that the clock in these cells measure some aspect of elapsed time rather than the number of cell divisions is also supported by subsequent studies *(55)*. The second conclusion we draw is that the mechanism that causes oligodendrocyte generation is hard-wired to the extent that it can be "activated" nine divisions in advance (e.g., in those clones containing 300 or more cells) but is encoded in such a manner that the actual penetrance (i.e., the extent of differentiation) is asymmetric over a broad range. At present, no known molecular mechanism would account for a process that is temporally regulated with such precision yet allows for such a range of asymmetry and variability at the level of individual clones.

Detailed analysis of oligodendrocyte generation in individual clones of O-2A/OPCs isolated from embryonic rat brain or postnatal optic nerve indicates that once oligodendrocyte generation is initiated within a clone, a second process is initiated in which the balance between self-renewal and differentiation is modulated by environmental signals *(47)*. During this second period, O-2A/OPCs (isolated from optic nerves of postnatal rats and induced to divide by PDGF) exposed to certain signaling molecules (e.g., neurotrophin-3 [NT-3] or bFGF) tend to undergo self-renewing divisions in which progenitor cell expansion is dominant over differentiation. In contrast, exposure to other signaling molecules (e.g., TH or CNTF) promotes the generation of oligodendrocytes and reduces self-renewal *(47,48,50)*. The extent of plasticity that it is possible to achieve is impressive and can range from induction of differentiation of most cells within a clonal family within only a small number of divisions *(47–49)* to the almost complete suppression of differentiation and continuous promotion of self-renewal for many weeks *(56)*.

In the third stage of oligodendrocyte generation, cell-intrinsic mechanisms appear to cause dividing progenitor O-2A/OPCs to differentiate either into oligodendrocytes or into a second generation of O-2A/OPCs progenitor cells with properties more appropriate for the physiologic requirements of the adult CNS *(57)*, as discussed later in this chapter. The cell-intrinsic timing of differentiation in this third stage is not absolute, however, and can be environmentally overridden, for example, by continuous exposure to PDGF + bFGF *(56)*.

Studies on differentiation in the O-2A/OPC lineage provide a very different view of cellular aging than is derived from studies on cellular senescence. As the O-2A/OPC derived from optic nerves of perinatal rats goes through its continuing cell cycles, it does not appear to reach a stage where division is no longer possible. Instead, rapidly dividing cells from late embryos intrinsically mature into the less rapidly dividing cells of the postnatal animal *(58)*, which themselves give rise to the slowly dividing adult progenitor cells that will be discussed in detail later *(57,59)*. Thus, the transition that occurs with continued division of O-2A/OPCs in vitro is very different from that which occurs in, for example, dividing fibroblasts, which reach a point (termed senescence) at which they no longer divide at all. Aging in the O-2A/OPC lineage is associated instead with the emergence of a new population of precursor cells with fundamentally different properties, including a much slower cell cycle length. Such results give strong support to the view that maturational processes associated with aging of precursor cells include biologic alterations that may prove far more subtle than, for example, telomere shortening.

IDENTIFICATION OF THE TRIPOTENTIAL GRP CELL
AS AN EARLY GLIAL PRECURSOR CELL THAT ALSO GIVES RISE
TO OLIGODENDROCYTES

Cellular biological studies on the earliest events in spinal cord development have led to the identification of a second glial precursor cell that also appears to be a crucial ancestor of the oligodendrocyte. These studies originated with observations that neuroepithelial stem cells generate two antigenically distinct populations of lineage-restricted precursor cells in vitro, each restricted to the generation of either neurons or glia. Glial-restricted precursor (GRP) cells *(60)* were labeled with the A2B5 monoclonal antibody, and were shown to give rise to oligodendrocytes and two antigenically distinct populations of astrocytes (corresponding to previous descriptions of type 1 and type 2 astrocytes). Neuron-restricted precursor (NRP) cells, in contrast, expressed the polysialylated form of the neural cell adhesion molecule (PSA-NCAM) and were shown to give rise to multiple different kinds of neurons and not to glia *(61)*.

Both GRP cells and NRP cells can be directly isolated from the developing rat spinal cord and grown as purified populations *(61,62)*. Freshly isolated cells exhibit the same lineage restrictions as those cells derived from neuroepithelial stem cells in vitro. Clonal studies have demonstrated that GRP cells retain their tripotential nature even after weeks of in vitro expansion and several serial reclonings *(62)* and also exhibit these same restrictions following transplantation in vivo. GRP cells generate both oligodendrocytes and astrocytes following transplantation into brain or spinal cord, and do not generate neurons even when they migrate into such neurogenic zones as the rostral migratory stream and olfactory bulb *(63)*. NRP cells, in contrast, generate only neurons (including motor neurons), even upon transplantation into such CNS regions as the adult spinal cord *(64–66)*.

GRP cells differ from O-2A/OPCs in multiple ways *(62)*. Freshly isolated GRP cells from the E13.5 rat spinal cord are dependent on exposure to FGF-2 for both their survival and their division, while division and survival of O-2A/OPCs can be promoted by PDGF and other chemokines. Consistent with this difference in chemokine-response patterns, GRP cells freshly isolated from the E13.5 spinal cord do not express receptors for PDGF (although they do express such receptors with continued growth in vitro or in vivo, as discussed later). These populations also differ in their response to inducers of differentiation. For example, exposure of GRP cells to the combination of FGF-2 and ciliary neurotrophic factor (CNTF) induces these cells to differentiate into astrocytes (primarily expressing the antigenic phenotype of type 2 astrocytes *[62]*). In contrast, exposure of O-2A/OPCs to FGF-2 + CNTF promotes the generation of oligodendrocytes *(32,67,68)*. Moreover, the behavior of these two precursor cell populations following transplantation is strikingly different. The ability of GRP cells to readily generate astrocytes following transplantation into the adult CNS *(63)* stands in striking contrast to the behavior of primary O-2A/OPCs, which thus far only generate oligodendrocytes in such transplantations *(26)* (although it has been reported that O-2A/OPC cell lines will generate astrocytes if transplanted in similar circumstances *[69]*).

Antigenic and *in situ* analysis of development in vivo has confirmed that cells with the A2B5[+] antigenic phenotype of GRP cells arise in spinal development several days prior to the appearance of GFAP-expressing astrocytes, and also prior to the appearance of cells expressing markers of radial glia *(70)*. Thus, these cells can be isolated directly from the developing spinal cord, and cells with the appropriate antigenic phenotype have been found to exist in vivo at appropriate ages to play important roles in gliogenesis.

Thus far, analysis of A2B5$^+$ cells isolated from the early embryonic spinal cord reveals a great degree of homogeneity in their ability to generate oligodendrocytes, type 1 and type 2 astrocytes in vitro *(62,71)*. In addition, GRP cells have been isolated from multiple species and by multiple means. For example, such cells have been isolated from the rat spinal cord, the mouse spinal cord, and from murine embryonic stem cells *(72)*. In addition, A2B5$^+$ precursor cells restricted to the generation of astrocytes and oligodendrocytes have been derived from cultures of human embryonic brain cells *(73)*. Both mouse and human cells share the ability of rat GRP cells to generate oligodendrocytes and more than one antigenically defined population of astrocytes.

THE GRP CELL AS AN ANCESTOR OF THE O-2A/OPC

A number of questions arise from the fact that it is possible to isolate two distinct precursor cell populations (i.e., GRP cells and O2A/OPCs) from the developing animal, each of which can generate oligodendrocytes. Is the relationship between these two populations one of lineage restriction or lineage convergence? If GRP cells and O-2A/OPCs are related, what signals promote the generation of one from the other and how can the existence of both populations be integrated with existing studies on the generation of oligodendrocytes during spinal cord development?

In vitro studies have demonstrated that GRP cells can give rise to O-2A/OPCs if exposed to particular signaling molecules. In these experiments, cultures of GRP cells derived from E13.5 rats were grown in conditions known to induce the generation of oligodendrocytes *(71)*. At the initiation of these experiments no cells in the GRP cell cultures were labeled with the O4 antibody, which can be used to recognize O-2A/OPCs at a stage of development at which the generation of both oligodendrocytes and type 2 astrocytes in vitro is possible *(74–76)*. When GRP cells that originally had been grown in the presence of FGF-2 for several days were exposed to a combination of PDGF and thyroid hormone (TH), however, O4$^+$ cells were generated in the cultures. Purification of cells that were O4$^+$ but did not express galactocerebroside (GalC, a marker of oligodendrocytes), and subsequent examination of the differentiation potential of these cells at the clonal level, confirmed that they behaved like O-2A/OPCs rather than like GRP cells *(71)*. Moreover, we could find no GalC$^+$O4$^-$ oligodendrocytes in any conditions, which would have at least raised the possibility that oligodendrocytes might be generated directly from GRP cells. Such results are consistent with previous observations that passage through an O4$^+$/GalC$^-$ stage of development is required for oligodendrocyte generation from bipotential O2A/OPCs *(77–79)*.

Unlike PDGFR$^+$ cells, it does not appear that GRP cells are entirely restricted to the ventral spinal cord during early development. Even at E 13.5 (up to a full day before the appearance of PDGFR$^+$ cells in the rat ventral cord; *[40]*), both dorsal and ventral regions of spinal cord contain A2B5$^+$ cells that, when analyzed at the clonal level, were found to be tripotential GRP cells *(71)*. All clones contained both type 1 and type 2 astrocytes when exposed to fetal calf serum or BMP, and all clones were capable of generating both O4$^+$GalC$^-$ cells and GalC$^+$ oligodendrocytes. Antigenic analysis in vivo also confirms that the domain of A2B5$^+$ cells in the spinal cord at E14.5 includes the domain of PDGFR$^+$ cells but extends further laterally, dorsally and ventrally *(70)*.

Despite the presence of GRP cells in both dorsal and ventral spinal cord of E13.5 rats, there appear nonetheless to be potentially interesting differences in these two populations. The frequency of A2B5$^+$ cells was greater ventrally than dorsally at E13.5 (52 ± 7% vs 19 ± 8% of all cells, respectively), in agreement with immunohistochemical analysis of spinal cord development *(70)*. While both dorsal and ventral GRP cells responded similarly to exposure to PDGF$^+$ TH in their ability to generate O4$^+$GalC$^-$ cells, only ventral-derived cells generated a significant number of oligodendrocytes over a 5-d time period *(71)*. Ventral-derived cells may be generally more inclined to differentiate at this stage, as they also showed a greater tendency to generate astrocytes in response to low concentrations (1 ng/mL) of BMP-4. Strikingly, in the ventral-derived cultures, exposure to BMP-4 was also associated with differentiation of over half of the cells into O4$^+$GalC$^-$ cells (although not further into GalC$^+$ oligodendrocytes), whereas only 12% of the cells in the dorsal-derived cultures were O4$^+$GalC$^-$ in these conditions. Thus, it appears in general that although both dorsal and ventral-derived GRP cells can generate oligodendrocytes, the ventral-derived populations exhibit a greater tendency to readily progress along this pathway.

That the overall population of GRP cells may contain subsets of cells with different properties is also indicated by analysis of patterns of antigen and mRNA expression in the developing spinal cord *(70)*. For example, it appears that the domain of Nkx2.2-expressing cells in the E11.5–E.13.5 spinal cord forms a subdomain within the population of A2B5$^+$ cells. Whether such heterogeneity in patterns of transcription factor expression is associated with heterogeneity of biological properties may be revealed only by applying techniques of quantitative analysis of what might be subtle differences in clonal properties, as have been developed for analysis of O-2A/OPCs (e.g., refs. *80–83*).

It is intriguing to speculate whether the knowledge obtained thus far allows a description of the entire pathway of lineage restriction from the embryonic stem cell to the oligodendrocyte. Studies by Okabe et al. *(84)* and Fraichard et al. *(85)* have demonstrated that ES cells can give rise to totipotent neurospheres, which share the ability of the neural stem cells of the embryonic spinal cord to give rise to all the differentiated cell types of the CNS *(86)*. Although the oligodendrocyte precursor cells generated from neurospheres (e.g., as in ref. *87*) have not yet been characterized sufficiently to determine whether these cells are GRP cells, O-2A/OPCs, or still another population of glial precursor cells, it thus far appears that embryonic NSCs give rise directly to GRP cells *(60)*. As O-2A/OPCs give rise directly to oligodendrocytes *(21,54,60,88–90)*, the generation of O-2A/OPCs from GRP cells raises the possibility that the developmental lineage from embryonic stem cell to neuroepithelial stem cell to GRP cell to O-2A/OPC to oligodendrocyte might represent a complete description of one path to the creation of a differentiated oligodendrocyte. As more markers become available to allow the detailed study of other stages of gliogenesis, it will be possible to test this possibility more stringently.

THE ADULT-SPECIFIC O-2A/OPC

Complex as the picture of oligodendrocyte generation might seem thus far, it is already clear that this picture needs to be expanded to include consideration of multiple O-2A/OPC populations. At the time of this writing, we know of four distinct groups of O-2A/OPCs with different biologic properties.

The idea that a single precursor cell population, as defined by its lineage restriction, may actually contain multiple precursor cells with differing phenotypes was first indicated by findings that O-2A/OPCs isolated from the optic nerves of developing and adult rats expressed strikingly different properties *(91)*. We interpret the data discussed in the following in the context of observations that the physiologic demands made on precursor cell populations during different developmental epochs can be remarkably divergent, particularly in tissues that do not undergo constant turnover in the adult animal. In such tissues, with the CNS being a prime example, the rapid increase in numbers of precursor cells and their differentiated progeny becomes turned off over a relatively short period. Once this period of rapid cell generation ends, precursor cell populations may be maintained in the adult tissue, to participate in homeostatic cell replacement during normal function and to repair damaged tissue following injury. The regulation of the precursor cells resident in adult tissue must, however, be different in some manner from that which characterizes the explosive growth of early development.

STUDIES IN VITRO REVEAL NOVEL PROPERTIES OF ADULT O-2A/OPCS

There are a variety of substantial biological differences between O-2A/OPCs of the adult and perinatal CNS (originally termed O-2A^{perinatal} and O-2A^{adult} progenitor cells, respectively *(57,91–94)*. For example, in contrast with the rapid cell-cycle times (18 ± 4 h) and migration (21.4 ± 1.6 mm/h) of O-2A/OPC^{sperinatal}, O-2A/OPCs^{adult} exposed to identical concentrations of PDGF divide in vitro with cell cycle times of 65 ± 18 h and migrate at rates of 4.3 ± 0.7 mm/h. These cells are also morphologically and antigenically distinct. O-2A/OPCs^{adult} grown in vitro are unipolar cells, while O-2A/OPCs^{perinatal} express predominantly a bipolar morphology. Both progenitor cell populations are labeled by the A2B5 antibody, but *adult* O-2A/OPCs share the peculiar property of oligodendrocytes of expressing no intermediate filament proteins. In addition, it appears thus far that *adult* O-2A/OPCs are always labeled by the O4 antibody, while *perinatal* O-2A/OPCs may be either O4-negative or O4-positive (although the O4-positive cells *perinatal* cells do express different properties than their O4-negative ancestors [23,77]).

One of the particularly interesting features of *adult* O-2A/OPCs is that when these cells are grown in conditions that promote the differentiation into oligodendrocytes of all members of clonal families of O-2A/OPCs^{perinatal}, O-2A/OPCs^{adult} exhibit extensive asymmetric behavior, continuously generating both oligodendrocytes and more progenitor cells *(57)*. Thus, even though under basal division conditions both *perinatal* and *adult* O-2A/OPCs undergo asymmetric division and differentiation, this tendency is expressed much more strongly in the *adult* cells. Indeed, it is not yet known if there is a condition in which *adult* progenitor cells can be made to undergo the complete clonal differentiation that occurs in *perinatal* O-2A/OPC clones in certain conditions *(47)*.

Another feature of interest in regard to *adult* O-2A/OPCs is that these cells do have the ability to enter into limited periods of rapid division, which appear to be self-limiting in their extent. This behavior is manifested when cells are exposed to a combination of PDGF + FGF-2, in which conditions the *adult* O-2A/OPCs express a bipolar morphology and begin migrating rapidly (with an average speed of approx 15 mm/h. In addition, their cell cycle time shortens to an average of approx 30 h in these conditions *(94)*. These behaviors continue to be expressed for several days after which, even when maintained in the presence of PDGF + FGF-2, the cells reexpress the typical unipolar morphology, slow migration rate and long cell cycle times of freshly isolated *adult* O-2A/OPCs. Other growth conditions, such as exposure to glial growth factor (GGF) can elicit a similar response *(95)*.

As can be seen from the above, *adult* O-2A/OPCs in fact express many of the characteristics that normally are associated with stem cells in adult animals. They are relatively quiescent, yet have the ability to rapidly divide as transient amplifying populations of the sort generated by many stem cells in response to injury. They also appear to be present throughout the life of the animal, and can even be isolated from elderly rats (which, in the rat, equals about 2 yr of age). In this respect, the definition of a stem cell can be seen to be a complex one, for the *adult* O-2A/OPC would have to be classified as a narrowly lineage-restricted stem cell (in contrast with the pluripotent neuroepithelial stem cell).

The differing phenotypes of *adult* and *perinatal* O-2A/OPCs are strikingly reflective of the physiological requirements of the tissues from which they are isolated. O-2A/OPC*perinatal* progenitor cells express properties that might reasonably be expected to be required during early CNS development (e.g., rapid division and migration, and the ability to rapidly generate large numbers of oligodendrocytes). In contrast, O-2A/OPC*adult* progenitor cells express stem cell-like properties that appear to be more consistent with the requirements for maintenance of a largely stable oligodendrocyte population, and the ability to enter rapid division as might be required for repair of demyelinated lesions *(57,91,94)*.

It is of particular interest to consider the developmental relationship between *perinatal* and *adult* O-2A/OPCs in light of their fundamentally different properties. One might imagine, for example, that these two distinct populations are derived from different neuroepithelial stem cell populations, which produce lineage-restricted precursor cells with appropriate phenotypes as warranted by the developmental age of the animal. As it has emerged, the actual relationship between these two populations is even more surprising in its nature.

There are multiple indications that the ancestor of the O-2A/OPC*adult* is in fact the *perinatal* O-2A/OPC itself *(57)*. This has been shown both by repetitive passaging of *perinatal* O-2A/OPCs, which yields over the course of a few weeks cultures of cells with the characteristics of *adult* O-2A/OPCs. Moreover, time-lapse microscopic observation of clones of *perinatal* O-2A/OPCs provides a direct demonstration of the generation of unipolar, slowly dividing and slowly migrating *adult* cells from bipolar, rapidly dividing and rapidly migrating *perinatal* ones. The processes that modulate this transition remain unknown, but appear to involve a cell-autonomous transition that can be induced to happen more rapidly if *perinatal* cells are exposed to appropriate inducing factors. Intriguingly, one of the inducing factors for this transition appears to be thyroid hormone, which is also a potent inducer of oligodendrocyte generation *(59)*. How the choice of a *perinatal* O-2A/OPC to become an oligodendrocyte or an *adult* O-2A/OPC is regulated is wholly unknown.

The generation of *adult* O-2A/OPCs from *perinatal* O-2A/OPCs places the behavior of the *adult* cells exposed to PDGF + FGF-2 in an interesting context. It appears that the underlying genetic and metabolic changes that lead to expression of the *perinatal* phenotype are not irreversibly lost on generation of the *adult* phenotype. Instead, they are placed under a different control so that very specific combinations of signals are required to elicit them *(94)*.

Once the processes of development ends there is still a need for a pool of precursor cells for the purposes of tissue homeostasis and repair of injury. It is thus perhaps not surprising to find that the adult CNS also contains O-2A/OPCs. What is rather more remarkable is that current estimates are that these cells (or, at least cells with their antigenic characteristics) may be so abundant in both gray matter and white matter as to comprise 5–8% of all the cells in the adult CNS *(96)*. If such a frequency of these cells turns out to be accurate, then a strong argument can be made that they should be considered the fourth major component of the adult CNS, after astrocytes, neurons and oligodendrocytes themselves. Moreover, as discussed later, it appears that these cells may represent the major dividing cell population in the adult CNS.

STUDIES IN VIVO ON ADULT PROGENITORS

Based upon the expression of such antigens as NG2 and PDGFR-α, a great deal has been learned regarding the biology of cells *in situ* that are currently thought to be *adult* O-2A/OPCs. Using these antibodies, and the O4 antibody, to label cells, it has been seen that the behavior of putative *adult* O-2A/OPCs in vivo is highly consistent with observations made in vitro. Adult OPCs do divide *in situ* but, as in vitro, they are not rapidly dividing cells in most instances. For example, the labeling index for cells of the adult cerebellar cortex is only 0.2–0.3%. Nonetheless, as there are few other dividing cells in the brain outside of those found in highly specialized germinal zones (such as the subventricular zone and the dentate gyrus of the hippocampus), the adult OPC appears to represent the major dividing cell population in the parenchyma of the adult brain *(97,98)*. Indeed, of the dividing cells of the uninjured adult brain and spinal cord, it appears that 70% or more of these cells express NG2 (and thus, by current evaluations, would be considered to be adult OPCs) *(98)*. That these cells are engaged in active division is also confirmed by studies in which retroviruses are injected into the brain parenchyma. As the retroviral genome requires cell division in order to be incorporated into a host cell genome, only dividing cells express the marker gene encoded in the retroviral genome. In these experiments, 35% of all the CNS cells that label with retrovirus are NG-2-positive *(99)*. However, it must be stressed for all of these experiments that it is by no means clear that all of the NG2-expressing (or O4-expressing or PDGFR-α expressing) cells in the adult CNS are adult O-2A/OPCs.

One of the most likely functions of *adult* O-2A/OPCs is to provide a reservoir of cells that can respond to injury. As oligodendrocytes themselves do not appear to divide following demyelinating injury *(100–102)*, the O-2A/OPC*adult* is of particular interest as a potential source of new oligodendrocytes following demyelinating damage.

Observations made in vivo are also consistent with in vitro demonstrations that *adult* O-2A/OPCs can be triggered to enter transiently into a period of rapid division. When lesions are created in the adult CNS by injection of anti-oligodendrocyte antibodies *(101,103–105)* division of NG-2+ cells is observed in the area adjacent to lesion sites. Rapid increases in numbers of *adult* O-2A/OPCs are also seen following creation of demyelinated lesions by injection of ethidium bromide, viral infection or production of experimental allergic encephalomyelitis *(101,104,106–108)*. Most of the putative O-2A/OPCs*adult* in the region of a lesion have the bipolar appearance of immature perinatal glial progenitors rather than the unipolar morphology that appears to be more typical of the *adult* O-2A/OPC, just as in seen in vitro when O-2A/OPCs*adult* are induced to express a rapidly dividing phenotype by exposure to PDGF + FGF-2 *(94)*. It is also clear that cells that enter into division following injury are responsible for the later generation of oligodendrocytes *(108)*.

A variety of observations indicate that the *adult* O-2A/OPCs react differently depending on the nature of the CNS injury to which they are exposed. Adult OPCs seems to respond to almost any CNS injury *(101,103–109)*. Response is rapid, and reactive cells (as determined by morphology) can be seen within 24 h. Kainate lesions of the hippocampus produce the same kinds of changes in $NG2^+$ cells. It appears, however, that the occurrence of demyelination is required to induce *adult* O-2A/OPCs to undergo rapid division *in situ*, even though these cells do show evidence of reaction to other kinds of lesions. For example, *adult* O-2A/OPCs respond to inflammation by undergoing hypertrophy and upregulation of NG2 but, intriguingly, increases in cell division are only seen when inflammation is accompanied by demyelination or more substantial tissue damage *(101,104,109,110)*. It also appears that there is a greater increase in response to anti-GalC–mediated damage if there is concomitant inflammation *(103,104)*, indicating that the effects of demyelination on these cells are accentuated by the occurrence of concomitant injury. In this respect, the ability of GRO-α to enhance the response of spinal cord derived *perinatal* O-2A/OPCs to PDGF may be of particular interest *(111)*, although it is not yet known if *adult* O-2A/OPCs show any similar responses to Gro-α. Also in agreement with in vitro characterizations of *adult* O-2A/OPCs are observations that the progression of remyelination in the adult CNS, however, is considerably slower than is seen in the perinatal CNS *(112)*.

The wide distribution of O-2A/OPCs *in situ* also is consistent with the idea that these cells are stem cells with a primary role of participating in oligodendrocyte replacement in the normal CNS and in response to injury. It is not clear, however, whether these cells might also express other functions. For example, it is not clear whether *adult* O-2A/OPCs contribute to the astrocytosis that occurs in CNS injury. Glial scars made from astrocytes envelop axons after most types of demyelination *(113,114)*. It is known that O-2A/OPCs produce neurocan, phosphacan, NF2 and versican, all of which are present in sites of injury *(115–117)* and can inhibit axonal growth *(118–120)*. It is possible that much of the inhibitory chondroitin sulphate proteoglycans found at sites of brain injury is derived from *adult* O-2A/OPCS, or from adults made by *adult* O-2A/OPCs. Whether still other possible functions also need to be considered is a matter of some interest. For example, glutaminergic synapses have been described in the hippocampus on cells thought to be *adult* O-2A/OPCs *(121)*. What the cellular function of such synapses might be is not known.

If there are so many O-2A/OPCs in the adult CNS then why is remyelination not more generally successful? It seems clear that remyelination of initial lesions is well accomplished (at least if they are small enough), but that repeated episodes of myelin destruction eventually result in formation of chronically demyelinated axons. It seems that after the lesions are resolved, the O-2A/OPCs*adult* return to prelesion levels, consistent with their ability to undergo asymmetric division *(57,104,107)*. It also seems clear that there are *adult* O-2A/OPCs within chronically demyelinated lesions *(96,122–124)*. Thus, the stock of these does not appear to be completely exhausted. However, the O-2A/OPCs that are found in such sites as the lesions of individuals with multiple sclerosis are remarkably quiescent, showing no labeling with antibodies indicative of cells engaged in DNA synthesis *(124)*. The reasons for such quiescent behavior are unknown. There are claims that electrical activity in the axon is involved in regulating survival and differentiation of *perinatal* O-2A/OPCs in development *(125)*, and it is not known if similar principles apply in demyelinated lesions in which neuronal activity is perhaps compromised. It is also possible that lesion sites produce cytokines, such as TGF-β, that would actively inhibit O-2A/OPC division. At present, however, the reasons why the endogenous precursor pool is not more successful in remyelinating extensive, or repetitive, demyelinating lesions is not known.

It is also important to note that not all NG2$^+$ cells in the adult CNS are necessarily O-2A/OPCs. Recent studies have demonstrated that many of the NG2$^+$ progenitor cells isolated from the adult hippocampus are able to generate GABAergic neurons, astrocytes and oligodendrocytes in vitro *(126)*.

THE DEVELOPING CNS CONTAINS
MULTIPLE O-2A/OPC POPULATIONS WITH DIFFERENT PROPERTIES

The initial proposal that the differences between *perinatal* and *adult* O-2A/OPCs indicates that the specific physiologic requirements of a particular tissue are reflected in the intrinsic properties of the precursor cells resident in that tissue has recently been extended to consider different CNS regions of animals of the same age. In these studies, striking differences between the properties of O-2A/OPCs isolated from different regions of the CNS of 7-d-old rat pups have been found, differences that once again appear to be highly relevant to the understanding of development.

One of the striking aspects of CNS development is that different regions of this tissue develop according to different schedules, with great variations seen in the timing of both neurogenesis and gliogenesis. For example, neuron production in the rat spinal cord is largely complete by the time of birth, is still ongoing in the rat cerebellum for at least several days after birth, and continues in the olfactory system and in some regions of the hippocampus of multiple species throughout life. Similarly, myelination has long been known to progress in a rostral-caudal direction, beginning in the spinal cord significantly earlier than in the brain (e.g., refs. *127–129*). Even within a single CNS region, myelination is not synchronous. In the rat optic nerve, for example, myelinogenesis occurs with a retinal-to-chiasmal gradient, with regions of the nerve nearest the retina becoming myelinated first *(127,130)*. The cortex itself shows the widest range of timing for myelination, both initiating later than many other CNS regions (e.g., refs. *127–129*) and exhibiting an ongoing myelinogenesis that can extend over long periods of time. This latter characteristic is seen perhaps most dramatically in the human brain, for which it has been suggested that myelination may not be complete until after several decades of life *(131,132)*.

Variant time courses of development in different CNS regions could be due to two fundamentally different reasons. One possibility is precursor cells are sufficiently plastic in their developmental programs that local differences in exposure to modulators of division and differentiation may account for these variances. Alternatively, it may be that the precursor cells resident in particular tissues express differing biological properties related to the timing of development in the tissue to which they contribute.

As has been discussed earlier, there is ample evidence for extensive plasticity in the behavior of O-2A/OPCs, which appear to be the direct ancestor of oligodendrocytes. O-2A/OPCs obtained from the optic nerves of 7-d-old (P7) rat pups and grown in the presence of saturating levels of PDGF exhibit an approximately equal probability of undergoing a self-renewing division or exiting the cell cycle and differentiating into an oligodendrocyte *(81)*. The tendency of dividing O-2A/OPCs to generate oligodendrocytes is enhanced if cells are coexposed to such signaling molecules as thyroid hormone, ciliary neurotrophic factor or retinoic acid (e.g., refs. *32, 47*, and *48*). In contrast, coexposure to NT-3 or basic fibroblast growth factor inhibits differentiation and is associated with increased precursor cell division and self-renewal *(30,47,56)*. The balance between self-renewal and differentiation in dividing O-2A/OPCs can also be modified by the concentrations of the signaling molecules to which they are exposed, as well as by intracellular redox state *(35)*. Thus, the effects of the microenvironment could theoretically have considerable effects on the timing and extent of oligodendrocyte generation.

Recent experiments have raised the possibility that the differing timing of oligoendrocyte generation and myelination in different CNS regions is associated with the existence of regionally specialized O-2A/OPCs *(133)*. Characterization of O-2A/OPCs isolated from different regions indicates these developmental patterns are consistent with properties of the specific O-2A/OPCs resident in each region. In particular, cells isolated from optic nerve, optic chiasm and cortex of identically aged rats show marked differences in their tendency to undergo self-renewing division and in their sensitivity to known inducers of oligodendrocyte generation. Precursor cells isolated from the cortex, a CNS region where myelination is a more protracted process than in the optic nerve, appear to be intrinsically more likely to begin generating oligodendrocytes at a later stage and over a longer time period than cells isolated from the optic nerve. For example, in conditions where optic nerve-derived O-2A/OPCs generated oligodendrocytes within 2 d, oligodendrocytes arose from chiasm-derived cells after 5 d and from cortical O-2A/OPCs only after 7–10 d. These differences, which appear to be cell-intrinsic, were manifested both in reduced percentages of clones producing oligodendrocytes and in a lesser representation of oligodendrocytes in individual clones. In addition, responsiveness of optic nerve-, chiasm- and cortex-derived O-2A/OPCs to TH and CNTF, well-characterized inducers of oligodendrocyte generation, was inversely related to the extent of self-renewal observed in basal division conditions.

The preceding results indicate that the O-2A/OPC population may be more complex than initially envisaged, with the properties of the precursor cells resident in any particular region being reflective of differing physiological requirements of the tissues to which these cell contribute. For example, as discussed earlier, a variety of experiments have indicated that the O-2A/OPC population of the optic nerve arises from a germinal zone located in or near the optic chiasm and enters the nerve by migration *(44,134)*. Thus, it would not be surprising if the progenitor cells of the optic chiasm expressed properties expected of cells at a potentially earlier developmental stage than those cells that are isolated from optic nerve of the same physiological age. Such properties would be expected to include the capacity to undergo a greater extent of self-renewal, much as has been seen when the properties of O-2A/OPCs from optic nerves of embryonic rats and postnatal rats have been compared *(58)*. In respect to the properties of cortical progenitor cells, physiological considerations also appear to be consistent with our observations. The cortex is one of the last regions of the CNS in which myelination is initiated, and the process of myelination also can continue for extended periods in this region *(127–129)*. If the biology of a precursor cell population is reflective of the developmental characteristics of the tissue in which it resides, then one might expect that O-2A/OPCs isolated from this tissue would not initiate oligodendrocyte generation until a later time than occurs with O-2A/OPCs isolated from structures in which myelination occurs earlier. In addition, cortical O-2A/OPCs might be physiologically required to make oligodendrocytes for a longer time owing to the long period of continued development in this tissue, at least as this has been defined in the human CNS (e.g., refs. *131, 132*).

The observation that O-2A/OPCs from different CNS regions express different levels of responsiveness to inducers of differentiation adds a new level of complexity to attempts to understand how different signaling molecules contribute to the generation of oligodendrocytes. This observation also raises questions about whether cells from different regions also express differing responses to cytotoxic agents, and whether such differences can be biologically dissected so as to yield a better understanding of this currently mysterious form of biological variability.

If there are multiple biologically distinct populations of O-2A/OPCs, it is important to consider whether similar heterogeneity exists among oligodendrocytes themselves. Evidence for morphological heterogeneity among oligodendrocytes is well established. Early silver impregnation studies identified four distinct morphologies of myelinating oligodendrocytes and this was largely confirmed by ultrastructural analyses in a variety of species *(135–137)*. Oligodendrocyte morphology is closely correlated with diameter of the axons with which the cell associates *(138,139)*. Type I and II oligodendrocytes arise late in development, myelinate many internodes on predominantly small diameter axons while type III and IV oligodendrocyte arise later and myelinate mainly large diameter axons. Such morphological and functional differences between oligodendrocytes are associated with different biochemical characteristics. Oligodendrocytes that myelinate small diameter fibers (type 1 and 11) express higher levels of carbonic anhydrase II (CAII) *(138,140)*, while those myelinating larger axons (type III and IV) express a specific small isoform of the myelin-associated glycoprotein (MAG) *(138)*. Whether such differences represent the response of homogenous cells to different environments or distinct cell lineages is unclear. Transplant studies demonstrated that presumptive type I and II cells have the capacity to myelinate both small and large diameter axons suggesting that the morphological differences are environmentally induced *(141)*. By contrast, some developmental studies have been interpreted to suggest that the different classes of oligodendrocytes may be derived from biochemically distinct precursors *(142)* that differ in expression of PDGFR-α and PLP/Dm20, although more recent studies are not necessarily supportive of this hypothesis *(143)*.

OLIGODENDROCYTE DEVELOPMENT IN THE EMBRYONIC CORTEX: SIMILARITIES AND DIFFERENCES FROM THE SPINAL CORD

Just as there is heterogeneity among O-2A/OPCs, it also seems likely that heterogeneity exists among earlier glial precursor cell populations. Separate analysis of GRP cell populations derived from ventral and dorsal spinal cord demonstrates that ventral-derived GRPs may differ from dorsal cells in such a manner as to increase the probability that they will generate O2A/OPCs and/or oligodendrocytes, even in the presence of BMP *(71)*. Ventral-derived GRP cells yield several-fold larger numbers of oligodendrocytes over the course of several days of in vitro growth. When low doses of BMP-4 were applied to dorsal and ventral cultures, the dorsal cultures contained only a few cells with the antigenic characteristics of O-2A/OPCs. In contrast, over half of the cells in ventral-derived GRP cell cultures exposed to low doses of BMP differentiated into cells with the antigenic characteristics of O-2A/OPCs . Whether the O-2A/OPCs or oligodendrocytes derived from dorsal vs ventral GRP cells express different properties is not yet known.

Studies on oligodendrocyte development in the cortex are currently indicating that important similarities and differences are seen from the spinal cord even during the earliest stages of brain formation. As mentioned earlier, in both the brain and spinal cord, it currently appears that the ancestors of oligodendrocytes are generated in discrete locations. Analysis of expression of PDGR-α and plp/DM20 suggests the existence of a few localized ventral sites of origin *(142)*. In the early mouse forebrain, PDGFR-α expression is seen in the MGE and dorsal thalamus, and plp/DM20 is found in the basal (ventral) plate of the diencephalon, zona limitans intrathalamica, caudal hypothalamus, enteropeduncular area, amygdala, and olfactory bulb *(39,144,145)*, as is expression of the *Olig1* and *Olig2* genes *(145–147)*.

Two recent studies from the Temple *(148)* and Mehler *(149)* laboratories have analyzed several aspects of the cellular biology of early ancestors of oligodendrocytes. At least some of the stem cells that give rise to oligodendrocytes in the cortex appear to arise in the basal (ventral) forebrain and migrate into the overlying dorsal forebrain, including the ventricular zone, subventricular zone and intermediate zones *(150–153)*. These basal progeny, which express the members of the *dlx* family of homeodomain transcription factors, migrate dorsally and intermix with other cells to form the dorso-lateral SVZ *(153)*.

Prior to the tangential migration of stem/progenitor cells from ventral to dorsal forebrain regions it appears as if the early stages of specification are regionally biased. For example, when grown in medium supplemented with FGF-2 *(148)*, or FGF-2 + Shh *(149)*, MGE and LGE progenitors of the E13.0 ventral forebrain are biased toward the generation of GABAergic neurons compared to stem cells and progenitors derived from dorsal cortex. In addition, prior to E12.5 few of the progenitor cells from dorsal or basal regions produce glia-only clones: most glia arise from stem cells at this stage, suggesting that divergence of glial lineages with the appearance of glial restricted progenitors occurs predominantly at later stages. Indeed, it may be that the stem cells that are present in the dorsal forebrain prior to the period of tangential migration are not competent to make oligodendrocytes unless they are exposed to Shh *(149)*, although this was not found by others *(148,154)*.

The above results raise multiple questions. Are the stem cells or progenitor cells that make oligodendrocytes and/or GABAergic neurons truly migrating from the ventral to the dorsal cortex, or is instead the delayed appearance of such cells dorsally a reflection of a temporally regulated differentiation event that has a different timing in different regions of the CNS? To what extent is this specialization reflective of cell-intrinsic controlling mechanisms and to what extent do cell-extrinsic signaling molecules contribute to this specification? The association of oligodendrocytes with a particular class of neuron (the GABAergic neuron of the cortex, the motor neuron of the spinal cord) is also of particular interest, particularly in light of the ongoing discussions (to be considered in a following section) about whether or not oligodendrocytes and motor neurons are derived from a single lineage-restricted progenitor cell *(145,147,155–165)*. But does this generation of oligodendrocytes within a single clone of cells reflect a lineage restriction of a stem/progenitor cell to the generation of only a limited subset of cell types?

Current evidence suggests strongly that the appearance of cells in the dorsal cortex that are able to generate clones containing both GABAergic neurons and oligodendrocytes is truly reflective of a migration of cells from ventral to dorsal regions. Consistent with these observations, the analysis of *dlx2/tauLacZ* knock-in mouse *(166)* also indicates that cells derived from subpallial *dlx2*-expressing progenitors migrate dorsally and intermix with other cells to form the dorsolateral SVZ *(153)*. Moreover, in *dlx1/2-/-*mice, in which there is a generalized defect in tangential migration and a reduction in cortical GABAergic neurons *(152)*, there is a failure of such cells to populate the dorsal cortex *(148,149)*.

The consistent association of cell fate with position within a tissue raises the possibility that localized ventral and dorsal signals act on stem cells to make them generate particular, region appropriate, cell types. Hence, basal forebrain stem cells are biased early in development to generate GABAergic neurons that predominate in basal forebrain CNS areas *(148,149)*. It has been suggested that initial ventral forebrain specification and tangential cortical migration would expose these bipotent progenitors to sequential ventral and dorsal gradient morphogens that normally mediate opposing developmental programs *(149,167)*.

Two of the factors thought to play important roles in inducing ventral cortical stem cells to be biased toward the generation of GABAergic neurons and oligodendrocytes are Shh and BMPs. It appears to be a common principle along the neuraxis that Shh and BMPs are ventral and dorsal gradient morphogens, respectively *(168–170)*, and the role of these signaling molecules in development of the spinal cord has been discussed previously. The concentration of these molecules to which cells are exposed causes elaboration of specific sets of homeodomain and basic helix–loop–helix (bHLH) transcription factors that control the details of cell specification through their combinatorial interactions *(163,164,171)*. In dorsal domains of the spinal cord, BMP signaling is thought to promote the generation of astrocytes, while Shh promotes the localized generation of motor neurons and oligodendrocytes *(146,147,155–160,172–175)*.

Despite the apparent role of Shh and BMP in directing differentiation of cortical stem/progenitor cells, as well as spinal cord stem/progenitor cells, there are important differences between these two tissues. This difference is seen already at the level of genes induced in cortical stem cells by exposure to Shh. For example, it currently appears that while both cortical and spinal cord stem cells are induced to express *olig2* by exposure to Shh, the cortical cells are induced to express *mash1* while spinal cord stem cells are induced to express *neurogenin2 (149,171,176–178)*.

Data reported thus far indicates that the role of BMP may be more complex in the cortex than has thus far been revealed in the spinal cord. Shh promotes generation of GABAergic neurons and oligodendrocytes, but the sequential elaboration of these cells requires spatial and temporal modulation of cortical BMP signaling by BMP signaling and the BMP antagonist, noggin *(149)*. For example, coincident with the establishment of the cortical SVZ, BMPs from the BMP2/4 factor subgroup now enhance the specification of late-born cortical (GABAergic) neurons. It seems that Shh promotes lineage restriction of ventral forebrain stem cells, in part, by upregulation of *Olig2* and *Mash1*. BMP2 subsequently promotes GABAergic neuronal lineage elaboration by differential modulation of *Olig2* and *Mash1*. Thus, when applied together with Shh, BMP2 potentiates the elaboration of GABAergic neurons from cortical stem/progenitor cells and suppresses oligodendrocyte generation *(175,179)*, while the BMP antagonist noggin promotes the generation of oligodendrocytes *(175,180)*.

How can the above results indicating BMP-promoted generation of neurons be integrated with experiments in the spinal cord (and also on cells derived from the developing brain) indicating that BMPs promote the generation of astrocytes and suppress the generation of oligodendrocytes *(71,156,174,175,181–184)*? It is possible that BMP, a potent antimitotic agent, is generally able to stimulate differentiation of progenitor cells but that the pathway of differentiation that is promoted is dependent on as yet poorly understood changes in the target precursor cells themselves. One potentially interesting aspect of the studies of Yung et al. *(149)*, however, that may be relevant to BMP-mediated induction of neuron generation is that these studies address questions about what happens when cells are exposed to more than a single signaling molecule (i.e., Shh + BMP-2), a situation that seems likely to more closely resemble the realities of biology than exposure to a single agent. In this context, an attractive potential solution to this conundrum that needs to be explored is whether the combined exposure of cortical stem cells to BMP and Shh (the conditions applied in the studies of *[149]*) reveals an aspect of BMP signaling different from that which occurs when cells are exposed to BMP alone. Consistent with this possibility, continued Shh exposure also appears to suppress the generation of astrocytes in cortical stem/progenitor cells, which were only seen in cultures of these progenitor cells when expression of *Olig2* and *Mash1* was ablated by exposure to antisense oligonucleotide constructs *(149)*.

It will be of great interest to determine whether the correct paradigm for understanding the interactions between BMP-induced pathways and Shh-induced pathways might be that BMP always suppresses oligodendrocyte generation, but the directionality imposed by BMP is dependent upon the other signals to which the recipient cell is exposed, as well as on the differentiation potential of the target cell itself.

E13.5 RAT CORTEX CONTAINS A2B5+ CELLS
THAT CAN GENERATE OLIGODENDROCYTES,
TWO DIFFERENT ASTROCYTE POPULATIONS, AND NEURONS

As studies conducted by He et al. *(148)* and Yung et al. *(149)* indicate the existence of precursor cells that make neurons and glia, and other cells that are restricted to the generation of glia, it is of interest to know the identity of these precursor cells.

Analysis of the precursor cell populations in the cortex, although in its early stages, is suggesting a level of complexity not seen in the spinal cord at this age *(185)*. The E13.5 cortex contains abundant A2B5+ cells that do not express antigens associated with astrocytes or oligodendrocytes. In vitro characterization of the differentiation potential of these cells demonstrated that, in contrast with results in the spinal cord

(62), at least some of the cortex-derived A2B5⁺ cells appear to be able to generate neurons when grown in the presence of NT-3 and retinoic acid *(185)*.

A more detailed analysis of the A2B5⁺ cell population isolated from E13.5 cortex indicates the presence of antigenically distinct subpopulations, only one of which thus far has been found to generate neurons in vitro. The subpopulation of cells that is competent to generate neurons also expresses PSA-NCAM, an antigen that has been found in several instances to be expressed by precursor cells able to generate neurons *(61,186,187)*. Removal of the PSA-NCAM⁺ cells from the A2B5⁺ population was associated with the loss of generation of neurons from this population *(185)*.

Although the A2B5⁺/PSA-NCAM⁻ cells derived from E13.5 cortex appear to be restricted to the generation of glia in their differentiation potential, this population is more heterogeneous than antigenically identical cells isolated from the spinal cord. Unlike the spinal cord, only 44% of clones derived from A2B5⁺ cells contained both type 1 and type 2 astrocytes when exposed to BMP-4. Many of the cortex-derived clones contained only one astrocyte population, with 16% of clones containing only type 2 astrocytes, and 17% containing type 1 astrocytes only, with no progenitor-like cells found in any of these clones. Virtually all cells appeared to be competent to generate oligodendrocytes, however, as 86% of clones contained at least one oligodendrocyte after being exposed to PDGF + T3 for 5 d.

Thus, it appears that the E13.5 rat cortex contains cells with the same antigenic phenotype and differentiation potential of tripotential GRP cells isolated from the embryonic spinal cord. Further investigations are required to determine the degree of identity of these cells with GRP cells of the spinal cord, particularly due to the complexity of the A2B5⁺ populations isolated from the cortex. In addition, the embryonic cortex contains a further population of A2B5⁺ cells that coexpress PSA-NCAM, an antigen not expressed by GRP cells of the spinal cord. These cells, but not the PSA-NCAM⁻/A2B5⁺ cells, are able to generate neurons in vitro. Moreover, the observations that approx 16% of the clones derived from A2B5⁺/PSA-NCAM⁻ cells generated only type 2 astrocytes when exposed to BMP, and approx 17% generated clones containing only type 1 astrocytes in these conditions, demonstrates further differences between the A2B5⁺ population of the E13.5 cortex and the E13.5 spinal cord. In the cord, in contrast with the cortex, this population shows a striking homogeneity in respect to the cell types generated in different conditions *(62,71)*.

The full differentiation potential of the A2B5/PSA-NCAM double-positive cells that we have identified is still under study. Nonetheless, experiments thus far suggest that the embryonic rat cortex contains an A2B5⁺ precursor cell that is able to generate neurons and glia, in distinction from findings in other regions of the CNS, in which precursor cells labeled with this antibody generally appear to be glial-restricted in their lineage specification.

The heterogeneity of the A2B5⁺ populations derived from the E13.5 cortex underscores the need for clonal analysis and detailed cell purification protocols in order to analyze successfully the developmental potential of a putative precursor cell population. Any studies on cortical development that do not separate these populations of cells from each other will be impossible to interpret unambiguously. As almost none of the previous studies conducted have combined antigenic characterization of precursor cells with clonal analysis, it is not possible to interpret data contained therein in regard to the lineage potential of particular precursor cell populations. For example, the analysis of purified A2B5$^+$ cells from the E13.5 cortex would lead to the conclusion that cells with this antigenic phenotype can generate neurons. If one were to accept the conclusions of previous studies carried out in the developing rat CNS that A2B5$^+$ cells are glial-restricted progenitor cells (whether O-2A/OPCs, GRP cells, or astrocyte progenitor cells (e.g., refs. *21,62,133,188–190*), one might then draw the conclusion that growth in vitro is associated with generation of neurons from glial progenitor cells (as in, e.g., ref. *191*). It has been suggested, at least in the case of the studies of Kondo and Raff, that a potential complicating issue in such studies is the presence of a low frequency of true multipotent neuroepithelial stem cells in many regions of the perinatal CNS (D. Van der Kooy, *unpublished observations*). Another possibility is that the failure to distinguish between the PSA-NCAM-positive and negative subsets of A2B5$^+$ cells would lead to a misinterpretation of the behavior of what appears from our analysis thus far to represent two distinct populations of cells.

One of the other potentially intriguing differences between cortical and optic nerve-derived O-2A/OPCs that has been described is that only the cortical progenitor cells express members of the *dlx* family of transcriptional regulators *(148)*. While *dlx1/2* is not required for oligodendrocyte generation *(148)*, it is not known if such expression confers different properties on those precursor populations that are expression-positive. It is important to note, however, that just as generation of oligodendrocytes is an ongoing process in the cortex, so also is the generation of progenitor cells. For example, migration of cells from the LGE/MGE may continue after the earliest wave of tangential migration, as retroviral labeling of LGE/MGE cells in slice cultures harvested from E16 mice and grown in vitro for up to 72 h demonstrates migration of cells into the perintal SVZ of each slice *(153)*. Nothing is known at this time as to whether O-2A/OPCs express different properties if they are generated from ancestral populations that differ in the spatial *or* their temporal origin, or whether the differences between O-2A/OPCs isolated from cortex and optic nerve discussed in the following section of this chapter are the results of exposure to tissue-specific instructive signals after this stage of lineage restriction has been achieved.

OTHER OLIGODENDROCYTE PRECURSOR CELLS

One of the important aspects of oligodendrocyte development that has not yet been integrated into the information provided thus far is that there may be still other oligodendrocyte precursor cells whose biologic properties are currently less well understood. In particular, the precise relationship that the tripotential GRP cell or the O-2A/OPC has to other glial restricted progenitors, such as the polysialated neural cell adhesion molecule (PSA-NCAM)-expressing pre-progenitor cell *(192–196)*, or the cells generated by exposure of totipotent neuroepithelial stem cells to B104 conditioned medium *(197)*, is unclear at present. Moreover, it is clear that the totipotent NSCs isolated from a variety of regions of the CNS, and even from the adult CNS, are also able to generate oligodendrocytes in vitro and following transplantation *(198–204)*. It is not known whether the generation of oligodendrocytes from all these sources follows the same developmental sequence. It is certainly possible, for example, that the GRP cell is a specialized cell of the embryonic animal and that the NSCs of the adult animal generate glia without first progressing through a GRP cell stage. Unraveling these relationships remains an important challenge.

THE MOTOR NEURON/OLIGODENDROCYTE PRECURSOR (MNOP) CELL HYPOTHESIS

At the same time that studies have been ongoing on GRP cells and O-2A/OPCs, a wholly separate line of investigation has raised questions about whether oligodendrocytes are developmentally more closely related to motor neurons than they are to astrocytes. The MNOP hypothesis was based initially on observations that both motor neurons and oligodendrocytes arise in a similar (and possibly identical) discrete zone of the ventral spinal cord (reviewed in refs. *158* and *159*) Moreover, it was found that similar concentrations of Shh are required for the induction of both cell types *(157)* and in vitro the induction of oligodendrocytes (e.g., by ectopic Shh presentation) is frequently accompanied by the induction of motor neurons *(157,160)*.

The hypothesis that motor neurons and oligodendrocytes are developmentally related to each other has some intuitive attractiveness arising from the critical importance of this particular cell combination in evolution. The ensheathing of axons with myelin is associated with a large increase in conduction speed. In annelids and crustacea, pseudomyelin is preferentially associated with axons required for rapid escape responses *(205,206)*. It has been suggested that hagfish, which have no myelin, seem unable to accelerate to avoid capture *(158)*. One way to ensure that motor neurons and the cells that ensheath them arise at the same place would be to derive both cells from the same precursor (as suggested in refs. *158* and *159*).

The idea that motor neurons and oligodendrocytes might be developmentally related was given a further boost by the findings, from three separate laboratories, that compromising the function of members of the *Olig* gene family can prevent the generation of both motor neurons and oligodendrocytes *(161–163)*. (These studies have been discussed in detail in a number of detailed recent reviews *[158,164,165]*.)

Olig1 and *Olig2* genes are expressed in the developing mouse spinal cord within the specific region that appears to give rise to both oligodendrocytes and motor neurons *(147,207,208)*. Forced expression of *Olig1* or *Olig2* in neuroepithelial stem cells induces expression of early markers of the oligodendrocyte lineage *(147,171)*. Moreover, expression of *Olig2* in conjunction with *neurogenin2* appears to be critical for the generation of motor neurons *(176,177)*.

Perhaps most pertinent to discussions on the ancestors of oligodendrocytes are experiments showing that targeted disruption of *Olig2* prevents oligodendrocyte and motor neuron specification in the spinal cord *(161–163)*. (Disruption of *Olig1*, in contrast, disrupted normal maturation of oligodendrocytes *[161]*.) In these experiments, conducted independently by three different laboratories, mice strains were generated in which *Olig2* gene function was prevented by homologous recombination into the *Olig2* locus *(161,162)* (or, in one case, *Olig1* -/- *Olig2* -/- double mutant mice *[163]*). In all cases, generation of both oligodendrocytes and neurons was severely disrupted. Comparable results have also been obtained in studies in zebrafish, indicating the general applicability of these findings across species boundaries *(209)*. Thus, the evidence is quite clear that expression of *Olig2* is required for the generation of both oligodendrocytes and motor neurons.

The results of experiments on *Olig* gene disruption are consistent with several possible explanations. The strongest form, as taken from *(161)*, states that "our genetic analysis of *Olig* gene functions and our fate mapping of *Olig*-expressing progeny cells are incompatible with the view that oligodendrocytes arise from a glial-restricted precursor cell in the developing CNS." As represented in Fig. 8 of Lu et al. *(161)*, one possible hypothesis is that neuroepithelial stem cells give rise to an *Olig*$^+$ lineage-restricted precursor cell that is restricted to the generation of motor neurons and oligodendrocytes. The authors also state that "distinct unipotential *Olig*$^+$ progenitors for motor neurons or oligodendrocytes could be envisaged." Some authors *(165)* have interpreted the results of experiments on *Olig*-/- mice as "challenging the view that oligodendrocytes arise exclusively from a glial-restricted progenitor" and suggesting that the analysis of "fate mapping of *Olig*-expressing progeny cells are incompatible with the view that oligodendrocytes arise from a glial-restricted precursor cell in the developing CNS." Other authors have suggested that these data are consistent with a range of possible explanations, including the possibility of two separate precursor pools, such as NRP cells and GRP cells, in each of which *Olig* gene expression plays distinct roles in the promotion of particular cell fates *(158,162–164)*.

THE AMBIGUOUS CASE FOR A RESTRICTED OLIGODENDROCYTE: NEURON PRECURSOR CELL

Given the information discussed thus far, it is critical whether there exists any grounds—as some authors have suggested—for arguing that the GRP cell hypothesis should be abandoned in favor of an MNOP or MNP/OP hypothesis. Certainly, there is an intuitive attractiveness to the suggestion that if both oligodendrocytes and motor neurons are induced by Shh, both express *Olig* genes, require *Olig2* and both arise in the same location, they may be derived from an identical precursor cell. Nonetheless, whether the data is sufficient to support overthrowing the GRP cell hypothesis is far from clear. This topic has been reviewed in detail in *(210)*.

Data derived from studies on the expression and function of *Olig1* and *Olig2* genes contain substantial ambiguities. As these studies provide no evidence that has been presented of the derivation of both motor neurons and oligodendrocytes from a *single* lineage-restricted founder cell, the only conclusion that can be drawn from these experiments is that *Olig1* and *Olig2* genes are expressed in a population of ancestral cells of unknown heterogeneity. As has been pointed out in a notably careful recent review *(164)*, this population may well consist of separate *Olig1*$^+$/*Olig2*$^+$ precursors for neurons and for oligodendrocytes.

Critically, it is not yet possible to draw firm conclusions from existing studies on whether or not astrocytes are ever generated in vivo from cells that are at some point induced to express *Olig* genes. Suggestions that *Olig2*$^+$ cells do not generate astrocytes, and that disruption of *Olig* gene function does not alter astrocyte development *(161)*, are not without problems, as these suggestions may be difficult to test. It is the case, however, that in *Olig2* -/- mice in which the *Olig2* gene was disrupted by targeted replacement with tamoxifen-inducible Cre recombinase reveal at least some of the Cre expressing cells expressed the astrocyte marker S100β *(162)*. Similarly, in *Olig1*-/-*Olig2*-/- mice in which GFP was expressed in the *Olig2* locus, half of the GFP-expressing cells differentiated into astrocytes in vivo *(163)*. As these experiments are conducted in animals in which no functional *Olig* genes were expressed, no conclusions regarding *Olig* gene expression and lineage restriction can be drawn, but the conclusion can be drawn that the signals that induce *Olig* gene expression are not sufficient to cause restriction of the resultant precursor cells away from astrocytic pathways. If one believes, however, that disruption of the function of *Olig*1 and *Olig*2 genes in vivo is revealing of developmental plasticity (as contrasted with experimental plasticity), then the interpretation of the experiments of *(162)* and *(163)* would be that cells exposed to signals that induce expression of *Olig1/2* can readily generate astrocytes if *Olig* gene expression is disrupted. Recent experiments by Liu and Rao also have suggested that cells that express *Olig1* may even become astrocytes in vivo. Examination of sections of developing spinal cords of heterozygous *Olig1*-Cre/Rosa-LacZ mice *(161)* demonstrate the expression of β-galactosidase activity in cells that coexpressed astrocytic and radial glial markers *(211)*. The possibility that cells induced to express *Olig* gene products can still become astrocytes is consistent with observations that A2B5$^+$NG2$^+$ PDGFR$^+$ cells (which would be expected to express *Olig2*) derived from the ventral spinal cord of E16 rats readily generate oligodendrocytes and two populations of astrocytes in vitro when exposed to appropriate conditions, and thus appear to be GRP cells *(71)*.

It is also very important to ask whether the outcomes of developmental studies in vivo are at least consistent with an MNOP or MN/OPC hypothesis. This appears not to be the case. The view that *Olig1/2* expression represents restriction to the motor neuron/oligodendrocyte pathways makes a very specific prediction that labeling of a founder cell and its clonal derivatives at stages of spinal cord development after *Olig1/2* expression occurs will reveal that motor neuron-containing clones contain oligodendrocytes but not astrocytes. Highly relevant experiments appear to have been carried out over a decade ago, using the technique of injecting retroviral particles expressing bacterial β-galactosidase into the developing chick spinal cord, over a range of ages including up to one or two cell cycles before all motor neurons are born *(212)*. In these experiments, 82% of clones that contained motor neurons also had nonmotor neuron relatives. No evidence was found, however, for the occurrence of cell types in specific combinations. Forty-two percent of the multicellular clones that contained motor neurons also contained cells that were clearly glial in both gray and white matter, with many of these glial cells being clearly identifiable as astrocytes. Critically, in respect to the possible longevity of NSCs in the developing spinal cord, injection of retrovirus as late as one or two cell cycles before motor neurons are born revealed clones that contained motor neurons, interneurons and glia as relatives, with astrocytes prominently represented among the glia. Although the focus of this study was on motor neuron development, the authors also noted the existence of other clones that appeared to contain both oligodendrocytes and astrocytes (as would be predicted from the GRP cell hypothesis). The results of these studies are subject to multiple interpretations, but the reported frequency of motor neuron/astrocyte clones seems quite divergent from what one would expect were a restricted MNOP, or restricted MNP/OPCs, a critical contributor to spinal cord development.

At present, it appears that the most likely explanation of available data is that although *Olig* expression may indicate the likely fate(s) of an unperturbed cell in vivo, it does not define the developmental potential of the precursor cell population in which such expression was induced by local environmental signals. Such a hypothesis is consistent with the expression of *Olig2* at stages of spinal cord development *(178)* when current studies suggest that the whole cord appears to be composed of NSCs. Indeed, both *Olig1* and *Olig2* genes are expressed prior to the appearance of motor neurons or oligodendrocytes. Expression of *Olig1* and *Olig2* genes is seen in the ventral third of the spinal cord neuroepithelium of the embryonic mouse as early as E 8.5 *(147,208)*, long before the appearance of PDGFR-α-expressing cells in a more restricted region of the ventral cord of the embryonic mouse at E12.5 *(157,213)*. The suggestion that cells induced to express *Olig* genes are not committed is also consistent with the ability of cells that would have expressed *Olig* genes (or, in the heterozygotes discussed above, which do express *Olig* genes) to differentiate into astrocytes *(162,163)*. In addition, that precursor cells induced to express *Olig* genes in vivo might not generate astrocytes (if that is in fact the case) reveals nothing of the identity of the cellular populations in which expression of these genes is induced. It seems very clear that *Olig* gene expression is regulated by the microenvironment in which a precursor cell functions. Identical precursor cells (neural stem cells, for example) exposed to Shh or BMP clearly express *Olig* genes, or are repressed from expressing *Olig* genes, respectively *(145,147,155,156)*. In addition, A2B5$^+$PDGFR$^+$ cells (which would be expected to be *Olig2*$^+$ *[147,208]*) isolated from ventral spinal cord of E15 or E16 rats can readily generate type 1 astrocytes when exposed to BMP *(71)*. Thus, at these late post-motor-neuron stages of development it also appears likely that *Olig* gene expression is only indicative of how a precursor cell is likely to develop if it is not exposed to signals that induce other developmental pathways.

We suggest that current evidence most strongly favors the developmental model that neuroepithelial stem cell give rise to GRP cells, which then give rise to O-2A/OPCs and oligodendrocytes, if one makes the assumption that only one developmental pathway is involved in the generation of oligodendrocytes. This model is based on the integration of multiple avenues of analysis with what is known about those precursor cell populations that have been successfully isolated from the developing spinal cord. Within the developing spinal cord a restricted cohort of NSCs is induced to express *Olig1* and *Olig2* as a result of exposure to Shh. These cells are not committed to any particular fate, but if they are not exposed to conflicting signals will develop into motor neurons or oligodendrocytes. After the time that motor neurons are born, there exists both ventrally and dorsally a population of A2B5$^+$ GRP cells that all share the ability to generate oligodendrocytes and two populations of astrocytes in vitro. Many of the ventral GRP cells are PDGFR$^+$NG-2$^+$*Olig1/2*$^+$ and, under normal developmental circumstances, will go on to generate PDGFR$^+$NG-2$^+$*Olig1/2*$^+$ O-2A/OPCs. What happens during the period just before and during motor neuron generation is less fully defined. The strictest formulation of the GRP/NRP hypothesis makes the testable predictions, however, that intermediate between the *Olig1/2*$^+$ neural stem cell and the motor neuron is a PSA-N-CAM$^+$ NRP cell. Separate from this would be the A2B5$^+$ GRP cell. We stress, however, that there is no *a priori* reason to believe that there is only one developmental pathway that is utilized to generate any of the cell types of the CNS. Moreover, the failure to find a particular precursor cell population may represent the lack of appropriate isolation and growth conditions rather than the nonexistence of the population. Thus, it is important to remain open to the possibility that still new precursor cells will be identified as study of the developing spinal cord continues.

DEVELOPMENTAL TRANSITIONS AND DEVELOPMENTAL MALADIES

There are multiple reasons for attempting to understand the complexities of glial cell development. Deciphering the mysteries of differentiation is certainly a worthy challenge. Moreover, the use of precursor cells for CNS repair may allow treatment of medical disorders that at present have no treatment, and understanding the biology of these cells is important in such regard. Indeed, the possibility of using precursor cell transplantation to repair demyelinating damage has long been demonstrated and is the subject of active research in multiple locations. Still another reason for being vitally interested in precursor biology, however, and one that has perhaps not yet received the attention that it deserves is the opportunity to understand the cellular basis for defective development of the CNS.

Aberrant neurologic development is associated with a wide range of physiologic insults. The diverse causes of such problems include various nutritional deficiency disorders, hypothyroidism, fetal alcohol syndrome, treatment of CNS cancers of childhood by radiation, and treatment of even some non-CNS cancers of childhood by chemotherapy. Common to most—and perhaps even to all—of the physiologic challenges associated with neurologic impairment are problems related to formation or maintenance of myelin.

A number of the physiologic insults that result in neurologic impairment and defective myelination, such as deficiencies in TH or iron levels, as well as generalized nutritional deficiencies, are well known to have their most severe outcomes if they occur during critical developmental periods. In 1921 the suggestion was first made that perturbations to development have their maximal effect *(214)* if they occur during critical developmental periods, but it was not until 45 yr later that it was specifically hypothesized that the period of myelination represents a particularly important critical period in brain development *(215)*. This hypothesis is well-supported by a variety of observations (as discussed later). Still, relatively little is known about the actual biological processes involved in defining these critical periods, at either a biochemical or developmental level.

Several different kinds of developmental processes could be relevant to the existence of critical periods. These include cell survival, cell division, and expression of differentiated functions. Moreover, these processes could be altered in differentiated cells or in the precursor cells that give rise to the differentiated cells. For example, reductions in the number of a particular differentiated cell type could occur as a result of a failure of that cell to survive after it is generated. Reductions in cell number could equally result, however, from death or reduced division of ancestral precursor cells, from a failure of the precursor cells to undergo normal patterns of differentiation, or from other perturbations discussed in later portions of this application. Indeed, one of the critical realizations to emerge from developmental biology has been the recognition that reductions in the number of differentiated cells may occur for other reasons than cell death. Induction of premature differentiation of precursor cells (thus removing them from the mitotic cycle), or the absence of a substance required for their differentiation, both may lead to a relative paucity of differentiated cells. Such processes appear to be of profound importance in multiple developmental maladies.

Hypothyroidism

Fetal and early postnatal hypothyroidism, usually associated with iodine deficiency, is a major cause of mental retardation, myelination failure and other developmental disorders (e.g., refs. *216* and *217*). Children born to mothers with reduced TH levels during early stages of pregnancy perform poorly on later tests of neurological and cognitive function *(218–220)*. In addition, the thyroid status of neonates and children has a significant long-term impact on their behavior, locomotor ability, speech, hearing and cognition *(221)*. Hypothyroidism-associated deficiencies of myelination have been observed in the cerebral cortex, visual and auditory cortex, hippocampus and cerebellum *(222–224)*. In addition, TH can modulate such processes as dendritic and axonal growth, synaptogenesis and neuronal migration *(225–227)*. Hypothyroidism in developing rats causes a retarded elaboration of the neuropil in the cerebral cortex and adversely affects cerebellar Purkinje cells. Neuronal bodies are smaller and more densely packed, with diminished dendritic branching and elongation and altered distribution of dendritic spines *(228)*. Axonal density is decreased to such an extent as to reduce by as much as 80% the probability of appropriate axodendritic interaction *(229)*, a reduction that would greatly reduce the complexity of developing neural networks.

In both experimental animals and in human populations, hypothyroidism-associated neurological defects can be at least partially ameliorated if TH replacement therapy is initiated early enough in postnatal life (e.g., refs. *221,229–235*). Studies performed in iodine-deficient parts of the world have shown that iodine supplementation before pregnancy and in the first and second trimesters reduces the incidence of cretinism, but supplementation beginning later in pregnancy does not improve the neuro-developmental status of the offspring *(236,237)*. In the case of diagnosed neonatal TH deficiency, initiation of treatment within weeks after birth restores normal development, while treatment after this period is ineffective *(238,239)*.

Hypothyroidism provides an example of a syndrome in which the ability of precursor cells to differentiate normally is compromised. O-2A/OPCs cultured in the absence of TH generate only a fraction of the oligodendrocytes found when TH is present *(35,47,48,240)*. In vivo, the number of oligodendrocytes found in optic nerves of young postnatal hypothyroid rats is reduced by about 80%, the same level of reduction observed in vitro when cells are grown in the absence of TH *(47,241)*. Earlier points in the developmental sequence leading to oligodendrocytes may also be compromised, as TH also promotes the generation of O-2A/OPCs from GRP cells, at least in vitro *(71)*. Reductions in oligodendrocyte number associated with a failure of oligodendrocyte generation in hypothyroid animals may be further compounded by effects of TH on oligodendrocytes themselves, as TH promotes oligodendrocyte-specific gene expression *(233,242–244)* and possibly also survival *(245)*.

Studies on the effects of TH on neuronal precursor cells are less detailed than studies on glial precursors, but studies in the cerebellum indicate that TH deficiency is associated with abnormalities in migration and differentiation of granule neuron precursor cells *(246)*. In hypothyroid animals the external granular layer (the habitat of migrating and dividing granule neuron precursor cells) persists significantly longer than it does in normal animals, consistent with a failure to induce differentiation in an appropriately timely manner.

Iron Deficiency

Another example of a metabolic problem that impacts on CNS development is a lack of sufficient dietary iron, which has been estimated to afflict more than 2 billion people around the world *(247,248)*. Perinatal iron deficiency is associated with long-term cognitive abnormalities and neurological problems *(249–253)*. In children and in experimental animals, iron deficiency is associated with hypomyelination, changes in fatty acid composition, alterations in the blood-brain barrier and behavioral effects *(254–259)*. Internationally, an estimated 35–58% of healthy women show some degree of iron deficiency, with >90% of pregnant women estimated to be iron deficient in some populations *(260,261)*. In the United States, 9–11% of adolescent females and women of child-bearing age are iron deficient, with similar values reported for children 1–2 yr of age *(262)*. Other studies have suggested that the prevalence of iron deficiency for children under 2 yr of age may be 25% or more, as indicated by measurements of the latency of auditory brain responses (ABRs) to determine conduction speed. Changes in ABR latency have been related to the increased nerve conduction velocity that accompanies axonal myelination *(263–266)*, with differences in ABR latency between normal and iron-deficient children thought to be reflective of a myelination disorder. In addition, perturbation of normal hippocampal development may contribute to the cognitive abnormalities associated with perinatal iron deficiency. Electrophysiologic studies in infants at risk for perinatal iron deficiency suggest functional perturbations of the developing hippocampus, an area central to recognition memory *(249,250)*. Histochemical *(267)*, behavioral *(268)*, and biochemical studies *(269)* in rats also have demonstrated selective involvement of the developing hippocampus in perinatal iron deficiency. Preweaning or lactational exposure to low iron results in irreversible brain iron deficiency despite adequate therapy, in contrast with postweaning exposure, which is reversible *(270)*.

There is a relative lack of myelin lipids and proteins in iron-deficient animals, suggesting less myelin is produced *(257,259,271)*. Recent studies indicate that differentiation of both O-2A/OPCs and GRP cells, but not their survival, may be disrupted in iron deficiency *(272,273)*. O-2A/OPCs isolated from the optic nerves of P7 rats and exposed in vitro to the iron chelator desferrioxamine show a significant reduction in oligodendrocyte generation. Complementary to these data are observations that iron supplementation in vitro enhances the generation of oligodendrocytes in cultures of GRP cells. Although less studied, neuronal development may also be compromised by iron deficiency, through the regulation of enzymes controlling neurotransmitter synthesis *(274)*, cell division, and energy *(267,275)*. As mentioned above, there are some suggestions that the hippocampus may be particularly compromised by iron deficiency *(249,250,267–269)*.

Recent studies on iron-deficient rats have demonstrated the dramatic effects of maternal iron deprivation on fetal CNS iron stores and development. For a long time it was unclear whether maternal iron deprivation compromises fetal development. Studies indicating the fetus can accumulate sufficient iron in the face of mild or moderate maternal iron deficiency *(276–278)* contrasted with others indicating that maternal iron deficiency anemia during pregnancy compromises fetal iron reserves *(279–282)*. In our own studies, we found that raising pregnant rats on an iron-deficient diet was associated with 30–50% reduction in cortical and spinal cord iron levels by E17 *(273)*. Animals resulting from such pregnancies showed a 40% reduction in the numbers of oligodendrocytes in the postnatal (P7) spinal cord. It also bears note that in the corpus callosum, oligodendrocyte number was actually increased at this time point, although what happens at later time points (when myelination in the corpus callosum would be at its peak) is not yet known. As iron deficiency is particularly prevalent during pregnancy, findings that maternal iron deficiency is associated with reductions in brain iron levels and alterations in differentiation may have important implications for understanding developmental defects resulting from this widespread problem.

Nutritional Deficiency

Critical periods for the generation of defects in myelination also have been clearly established in the case of nutritional deficiency, with highly focused studies being carried out in rodent models. Lasting and significant myelin deficits are associated with undernourishment that is established at birth (or earlier, through maternal deprivation) and maintained through weaning *(283–285)*. Strikingly, the deficit in myelin can be quite specific, in that this parameter is affected even in cases of undernourishment in which brain weight remains normal. Moreover, nutritional rehabilitation post weaning may be associated with a restoration of brain weight to normal or near-normal levels, even in the absence of a restoration of myelin content to normal levels. That critical developmental periods are important in repair of this damage is indicated by observations that restoration of normal levels of myelin requires that normal nutrition be itself restored well before weaning. In addition, severe starvation imposed from 14 to 30 d after birth (i.e., after the critical period ends) produces no lasting deficit in myelin accumulation *(285)*, thus stressing the importance of critical periods in the establishment of this deficit.

We are not yet aware of any studies that have examined nutritional deficiency in a manner directly analogous to our studies on TH deficiency. Nonetheless, both in vitro and in vivo data raise the possibility that oligodendrocyte generation is impaired in at least some models of undernourishment. It has been reported that there is a relative reduction in the numbers of oligodendrocytes that are generated in glucose-deprived cultures *(286)*. In addition, severe malnutrition regimes are associated with a clear reduction in glial cell numbers in vivo *(287)*, although cell type-specific markers were not utilized to determine whether this reduction preferentially affected oligodendrocytes rather than astrocytes.

Regulation of myelin-specific genes by nutritional status has also been reported both in vivo and in vitro. In vivo, it is well established that the myelin deficits associated with undernutrition are even observed in animals in which oligodendrocyte number appears to be normal *(288)*. In such animals, however, it has been reported *(289)* that the mRNAs for three important myelin proteins (myelin-associated glycoprotein [MAG], proteolipid protein [PLP], and myelin basic protein [MBP]) do not undergo the normal increases seen in brains of well-nourished animals. Increases are delayed for several days beyond the normal time (i.e., d 7–9) at which they are observed, and the increases are lower in extent.

In vitro studies using glucose deprivation as a model for caloric undernutrition *(290)* have raised the surprising possibility that transient caloric restriction at critical periods may lead to long-term effects on differentiated function. In these experiments, mixed cultures were generated from newborn rat brain and exposed to different glucose concentrations, ranging from 0.55 to 10 mg/mL; the lower doses are within the range that occurs in clinical hypoglycemia. Low glucose concentrations were associated with markedly lower levels of increases in MAG, PLP, and MBP mRNA levels and with a subsequent and abnormal down-regulation in these mRNA levels. These effects were specific, in that total mRNA levels in the cultures were normal. Most importantly, these effects appeared to be irreversible if the glucose deprivation was applied over a time period that mirrored the critical period for nutritional deprivation in vivo. Deprivation coincident with the normal time of myelin gene activation and the period of rapid upregulation (6–14 d in vitro [DIV]) was irreversible. Deprivation at a later stage was instead associated with only transient depressing effects. These results are very important in raising the possibility that critical developmental periods may in part reflect the timing of nuclear events related to temporal and tissue-specific patterns of gene expression. It is also intriguing that recent studies have suggested that these effects are not seen if glucose deprivation is applied to cultures of purified oligodendrocytes, an observation the authors have suggested may indicate the involvement of an intermediary cell type to achieve suppression of myelin gene expression *(291)*. It is important to note, however, that the presence of other cells would promote division of O-2A/OPCs and generation of immature oligodendrocytes *(90)*, thus raising the possibility that the lack of any affect also may reflect effects at particular developmental stages.

ASTROCYTES AND THEIR PRECURSORS

We have focused the greatest attention in this review on precursor cells that meet the criteria of being able to be isolated directly from the animal and analyzed in clonal conditions to demonstrate their individual ability to generate diverse cell types. Moreover, both O-2A/OPCs and GRP cells have been transplanted in vivo, and shown to exhibit the same lineage restrictions in vitro and in vivo. It is of significant interest, however, to develop as comprehensive an understanding of the ancestry of astrocytes as we are beginning to have of oligodendrocytes.

The range of functions that have been attributed to astrocytes is broader than for any other cell type of which we know. Astrocytes provide substrates for axonal growth, secrete mitogens and survival factors for neurons and for O-2A/OPCs *(28,34,90,292–295)*, induce endothelial cells to differentiate to form the blood–brain barrier *(296,297)*, can function as antigen-presenting cells *(298–300)*, have been found to produce complement and inflammatory cytokines *(301,302)*, inactivate neurotransmitters and neuropeptides through both uptake and enzymatic inactivation *(303,304)*, modulate ion fluxes in the brain, may modulate neuronal activity through their own calcium fluxes *(305,306)*, can produce and secrete compounds with neurotransmitter activity *(307,308)*, play a central role in the generation of glial scar tissue *(309–311)*, and express a host of still other functions *(312–314)*.

The correlation between diversity of function in astrocytes and development of these cells, at this stage, represents wholly unknown territory. A number of astrocyte precursor cells have been described, including the A2B5$^+$ astrocyte precursor cell present in

E17 spinal cord and originally described by Miller and colleagues *(188,189)*, the putative astrocyte precursor cells from the embryonic mouse cerebellum described by Seidman et al. *(315)*, and the astrocyte precursor cell described by Mi and Barres *(190)*. Still another astrocyte precursor cell has been observed in cultures on human neural precursors *(316,317)*. In addition, Miller and colleagues *(318)* have described five distinct astrocyte populations in the spinal cord based on heritable morphologic differences. At this stage, little or nothing is known about how these various populations of astrocytes are developmentally related to each other, or what induces the appearance of specialized astrocyte functions. Moreover, little is known about the extent to which physiologic insults disrupt normal astrocytic development and function. Considering the multiple roles played by these cells, it would be very surprising if disruption of their function did not have profound neurologic consequences.

Still another potential astrocyte precursor is the GRP cell itself, which can give rise to two distinct antigenic classes of astrocytes. It has been suggested, however, that intermediate between GRP cells and astrocytes lies an astrocyte-restricted progenitor cell *(70)*, a suggestion analogous to our own suggestion that the O-2A/OPC is an intermediate stage between GRP cells and oligodendrocytes *(71)*.

One of the greatest problems hindering the study of astrocyte diversity is the lack of markers. The extensive characterization of O-2A/OPCs and the existence of markers (the O4 and anti-GalC antibodies) that enable purification of a specific subset of progeny cells derived from GRP cells allowed the demonstration of derivation of a bipotential O-2A/OPC-like cell from a tripotential GRP cell. We do not yet have sufficient markers and/or knowledge of growth conditions to determine whether GRP cells also can give rise to such other glial precursor cell populations as the astrocyte precursor cells that have been described by others *(188–190,315)* or perhaps even to the pre-O-2A/OPC described by Grinspan and colleagues *(193)*, although it has been suggested that it may be possible to study this problem with anti-CD44 antibodies *(70,316,317)*.

The extent of the need for new markers in the study of astrocytes is particularly well illustrated by the recent studies of Alvarez-Buylla and colleagues, who have described in the subventricular zone of the adult mammalian brain a precursor cell that expresses glial fibrillary acidic protein (GFAP), the supposedly "definitive" marker of an astrocyte *(319)*; yet is able to give rise to neuroblasts that migrate into the olfactory stream and differentiate into neurons when they reach the olfactory bulb *(320)*. That we currently have no suitable markers for differentiating even these GFAP$^+$ cells from astrocytes committed to the range of CNS functions mentioned in the beginning of this closing section is a stark indication of how far we must progress to analyze the development of what is the major cell type in the CNS. Considering the complexity of astrocytes, it seems most likely that their developmental history will be at least as filled with novel discoveries, as has been the case for their companion in the glial kingdom, the oligodendrocyte.

REFERENCES

1. Noble, M., Mayer-Proschel, M., and Miller, R. H. (2005) The oligodendrocyte. In *Developmental Neurobiology* (Rao, M. S., ed.).
2. Colello, R. J., Pott, U., and Schwab, M. E. (1994) The role of oligodendrocytes and myelin on axon maturation in the developing rat retinofugal pathway. *J. Neurosci.* **14,** 2594–2605.
3. Griffiths, I., Klugmann, M., Anderson, T., et al. (1998) Axonal swellings and degeneration in mice lacking the major proteolipid of myelin. *Science* **280,** 1610–1613.

4. Trapp, B., Peterson, J., Ransohoff, R., Rudick, R., Mork, S., and Bo, L. (1998) Axonal transection in the lesions of multiple sclerosis. *N. Engl. J. Med.* **338,** 278–285.

5. Peles, E. and Salzer, J. L. (2000) Molecular domains of myelinated fibers. *Curr. Opin. Neurobiol.* **10,** 558–565.

6. Rasband, M. N. and Shrager, P. (2000) Ion channel sequestration in central nervous system axons. *J. Physiol. (Lond.)* **525,** 63–73.

7. Kaplan, M. R., Meyer-Franke, A., Lambert, S., et al. (1997) Induction of sodium channel clustering by oligodendrocytes. *Nature* **386,** 724–728.

8. Kaplan, M. R., Cho, M.-H., Ullian, E. M., Isorn, L. L., Levinson, S. R., and Barres, B. A. (2001) Differential control of clustering of the sodium channels Na$_v$1. 2 and Na$_v$1. 6 at developing CNS nodes of Ranvier. *Neuron* **30,** 105–119.

9. Dai, X., Lercher, L. D., Yang, L., Shen, M., Black, I. B., and Dreyfus, C. F. (1997) Expression of neurotrophins by basal forebrain (BF) oligodendrocytes. *Soc. Neurosci. Abstr.* **23,** 331.

10. Dougherty, K. D., Dreyfus, C. F., and Black, I. B. (2000) Brain-derived neurotrophic factor in astrocytes, oligodendrocytes, and microglia/macrophages after spinal cord injury. *Neurobiol. Dis.* **7,** 574–585.

11. Dai, X., Lercher, L. D., Clinton, P. M., et al. (2003) The trophic role of oligodendrocytes in the basal forebrain. *J. Neurosci.* **23,** 5846–5853.

12. Krenz, N. R. and Weaver, L. C. (2000) Nerve growth factor in glia and inflammatory cells of the injured rat spinal cord. *J. Neurochem.* **74,** 730–739.

13. Vartanian, T., Corfas, G., Li, Y., Fischbach, G. D., and Stefansson, K. (1994) A role for the acetylcholine receptor-inducing protein ARIA in oligodendrocyte development. *Proc. Natl. Acad. Sci. USA* **91,** 11626–11630.

14. Raabe, T. D., Clive, D. R., Wen, D., and DeVries, G. H. (1997) Neonatal oligodendrocytes contain and secrete neuregulins in vitro. *J. Neurochem.* **69,** 1859–1863.

15. Cannella, B., Pitt, D., and Marchionni, M., Raine, C. S. (1999) Neuregulin and erbB receptor expression in normal and diseased human white matter. *J. Neuroimmunol.* **100,** 233–242.

16. Deadwyler, G. D., Pouly, S., Antel, J. P., and DeVries, G. H. (2000) Neuregulins and erbB receptor expression in adult human oligodendrocytes. *Glia* **32,** 304–312.

17. Strelau, J. and Unsicker, K. (1999) GDNF family members and their receptors: expression and functions in two oligodendroglial cell lines representing distinct stages of oligodendroglial development. *Glia* **26,** 291–301.

18. Nakamura, S., Todo, T., Motoi, Y., et al. (1999) Glial expression of fibroblast growth factor-9 in rat central nervous system. *Glia* **28,** 53–65.

19. McKinnon, R. D., Piras, G., Ida, J. A., Jr., and Dubois Dalcq, M. (1993) A role for TGF-beta in oligodendrocyte differentiation. *J. Cell Biol.* **121,** 1397–1407.

20. da Cunha, A., Jefferson, J. A., Jackson, R. W., and Vitkovic, L. (1993) Glial cell-specific mechanisms of TGF-beta 1 induction by IL-1 in cerebral cortex. *J. Neuroimmunol.* **42,** 71–85.

21. Raff, M. C., Miller, R. H., and Noble, M. (1983) A glial progenitor cell that develops in vitro into an astrocyte or an oligodendrocyte depending on the culture medium. *Nature* **303,** 390–396.

22. Raff, M. C., Abney, E. R., Cohen, J., Lindsay, R., and Noble, M. (1983) Two types of astrocytes in cultures of developing rat white matter: differences in morphology, surface gangliosides, and growth characteristics. *J. Neurosci.* **3,** 1289–1300.

23. Warrington, A. E., Barbarese, E., and Pfeiffer, S. E. (1993) Differential myelinogenic capacity of specific developmental stages of the oligodendrocyte lineage upon transplantation into hypomyelinating hosts. *J. Neurosci. Res.* **34,** 1–13.

24. Groves, A. K., Barnett, S. C., Franklin, R. J., et al. (1993) Repair of demyelinated lesions by transplantation of purified O-2A progenitor cells. *Nature* **362,** 453–455.

25. Utzschneider, D. A., Archer, D. R., Kocsis, J. D., Waxman, S. G., and Duncan, I. D. (1994) Transplantation of glial cells enhances action potential conduction of amyelinated spinal cord axons in the myelin-deficient rat. *Proc. Natl. Acad. Sci. USA* **91,** 53–57.

26. Espinosa de los Monteros, A., Zhang, M., and De Vellis, J. (1993) O2A progenitor cells transplanted into the neonatal rat brain develop into oligodendrocytes but not astrocytes. *Proc. Natl. Acad. Sci. USA* **90,** 50–54.

27. Knapp, P. E. (1991) Studies of glial lineage and proliferation in vitro using an early marker for committed oligodendrocytes. *J. Neurosci. Res.* **30,** 336–345.

28. Noble, M., Murray, K., Stroobant, P., Waterfield, M. D., and Riddle, P. (1988) Platelet-derived growth factor promotes division and motility and inhibits premature differentiation of the oligodendrocyte/type-2 astrocyte progenitor cell. *Nature* **333,** 560–562.

29. Bögler, O., Wren, D., Barnett, S. C., Land, H., and Noble, M. (1990) Cooperation between two growth factors promotes extended self-renewal and inhibits differentiation of oligodendrocyte-type-2 astrocytes (O-2A) progenitor cells. *Proc. Natl. Acad. Sci. USA* **87,** 6368–6372.

30. Barres, B. A., Raff, M. C., Gaese, F., Bartke, I., Dechant, G., and Barde, Y. A. (1994) A crucial role for neurotrophin-3 in oligodendrocyte development. *Nature* **367,** 371–375.

31. Barres, B. A., Schmidt, R., Sendtner, M., and Raff, M. C. (1993) Multiple extracellular signals are required for long-term oligodendrocyte survival. *Development* **118,** 283–295.

32. Mayer, M., Bhakoo, K., and Noble, M. (1994) Ciliary neurotrophic factor and leukemia inhibitory factor promote the generation, maturation and survival of oligodendrocytes in vitro. *Development* **120,** 142–153.

33. Pringle, N., Collarini, E. J., Mosley, M. J., Heldin, C. H., Westermark, B., and Richardson, W. D. (1989) PDGF A chain homodimers drive proliferation of bipotential (O-2A) glial progenitor cells in the developing rat optic nerve. *EMBO J.* **8,** 1049–1056.

34. Richardson, W. D., Pringle, N., Mosley, M. J., Westermark, B., and Dubois Dalcq, M. (1988) A role for platelet-derived growth factor in normal gliogenesis in the central nervous system. *Cell* **53,** 309–319.

35. Smith, J., Ladi, E., Mayer-Pröschel, M., and Noble, M. (2000) Redox state is a central modulator of the balance between self-renewal and differentiation in a dividing glial precursor cell. *Proc. Natl. Acad. Sci. USA* **97,** 10032–10037.

36. Marin-Husstege, M., Muggironi, M., Liu, A., and Casaccia-Bonnefil, P. (2002) Histone deacetylase activity is necessary for oligodendrocyte lineage progression. *J. Neurosci.* **22,** 10333–10345.

37. Deng, W., McKinnon, R. D., and Poretz, R. D. (2001) Lead exposure delays the differentiation of oligodendroglial progenitors in vitro, and at higher doses induces cell death. *Toxicol. Appl. Pharmacol.* **174,** 235–244.

38. Deng, W. and Poretz, R. D. (2002) Protein kinase C activation is required for the lead-induced inhibition of proliferation and differentiation of cultured oligodendroglial progenitor cells. *Brain Res.* **929,** 87–95.

39. Pringle, N. P. and Richardson, W. D. (1993) A singularity of PDGF alpha-receptor expression in the dorsoventral axis of the neural tube may define the origin of the oligodendrocyte lineage. *Development* **117,** 525–533.

40. Hall, A., Giese, N. A., and Richardson, W. D. (1996) Spinal cord oligodendrocytes develop from ventrally derived progenitor cells that express PDGF alpha receptors. *Development* **122,** 4085–4094.

41. Ikenaka, K., Kagawa, T., and Mikoshiba, K. (1992) Selective expression of DM-20, an alternatively spliced myelin proteolipid protein gene product, in developing nervous system and in nonglial cells. *J. Neurochem.* **58,** 2248–53.

42. Timsit, S., Martinez, S., Allinquant, B., Peyron, F., Puelles, L., and Zalc, B. (1995) Oligodendrocytes originate in a restricted zone of the embryonic ventral neural tube defined by DM-20 mRNA expression. *J. Neurosci.* **15,** 1012–1024.

43. Sommer, I. and Schachner, M. (1981) Monoclonal antibody (O1-O4) to oligodendrocyte cell surfaces: an immunocytological study in the central nervous system. *Dev. Biol.* **83,** 311–327.
44. Ono, K., Bansal, R., Payne, J., Rutishauser, U., and Miller, R. H. (1995) Early development and dispersal of oligodendrocyte precursors in the embryonic chick spinal cord. *Development* **121,** 1743–54.
45. Orentas, D. M. and Miller, R. H. (1996) The origin of spinal cord oligodendrocytes is dependent on local influences from the notochord. *Dev. Biol.* **177,** 43–53.
46. Orentas, D. and Miller, R. (1998) Regulation of oligodendrocyte development. *Mol. Neurobiol.* **18,** 247–259.
47. Ibarrola, N., Mayer-Proschel, M., Rodriguez-Pena, A., and Noble, M. (1996) Evidence for the existence of at least two timing mechanisms that contribute to oligodendrocyte generation in vitro. *Dev. Biol.* **180,** 1–21.
48. Barres, B. A., Lazar, M. A., and Raff, M. C. (1994) A novel role for thyroid hormone, glucocorticoids and retinoic acid in timing oligodendrocyte development. *Development* **120,** 1097–1108.
49. Temple, S. and Raff, M. C. (1986) Clonal analysis of oligodendrocyte development in culture: evidence for a developmental clock that counts cell division. *Cell* **44,** 773–779.
50. Mayer, M., Bogler, O., and Noble, M. (1993) The inhibition of oligodendrocytic differentiation of O-2A progenitors caused by basic fibroblast growth factor is overridden by astrocytes. *Glia* **8,** 12–19.
51. Abney, E., Bartlett, P., and Raff, M. (1981) Astrocytes, ependymal cells, and oligodendrocytes develop on schedule in dissociated cell cultures of embryonic rat brain. *Dev. Biol.* **83,** 301–310.
52. Miller, R. H., Ffrench Constant, C., and Raff, M. C. (1989) The macroglial cells of the rat optic nerve. *Annu. Rev. Neurosci.* **12,** 517–534.
53. Raff, M. C., Abney, E. R., and Fok-Seang, J. (1985) Reconstitution of a developmental clock in vitro: a critical role for astrocytes in the timing of oligodendrocyte differentiation. *Cell* **42,** 61–69.
54. Raff, M. C., Lillien, L. E., Richardson, W. D., Burne, J. F., and Noble, M. D. (1988) Platelet-derived growth factor from astrocytes drives the clock that times oligodendrocyte development in culture. *Nature* **333,** 562–565.
55. Gao, F., Durand, B., and Raff, M. (1997) Oligodendrocyte precursor cells count time but not cell divisions before differentiation. *Curr. Biol.* **7,** 152–155.
56. Bogler, O., Wren, D., Barnett, S. C., Land, H., and Noble, M. (1990) Cooperation between two growth factors promotes extended selfrenewal and inhibits differentiation of oligodendrocyte-type-2 astrocytes (O-2A) progenitor cells. *Proc. Natl. Acad. Sci. USA* **87,** 6368–6372.
57. Wren, D., Wolswijk, G., and Noble, M. (1992) In vitro analysis of the origin and maintenance of O-2A^adult progenitor cells. *J. Cell Biol.* **116,** 167–176.
58. Gao, F. and Raff, M. (1997) Cell size control and a cell-intrinsic maturation program in proliferating oligodendrocyte precursor cells. *J. Cell Biol.* **138,** 1367–1377.
59. Tang, D. G., Tokumoto, Y. M., and Raff, M. C. (2000) Long-term culture of purified oligodendrocyte precursor cells: evidence for an intrinsic maturation program that plays out over months. *J. Cell Biol.* **148,** 971–984.
60. Rao, M. and Mayer-Pröschel, M. (1997) Glial restricted precursors are derived from multipotent neuroepithelial stem cells. *Dev. Biol.* **188,** 48–63.
61. Mayer-Pröschel, M., Kalyani, A., Mujtaba, T., and Rao, M. S. (1997) Isolation of lineage-restricted neuronal precursors from multipotent neuroepithelial stem cells. *Neuron* **19,** 773–85.
62. Rao, M., Noble, M., and Mayer-Pröschel, M. (1998) A tripotential glial precursor cell is present in the developing spinal cord. *Proc. Natl. Acad. Sci. USA* **95,** 3996–4001.

63. Herrera, J., Yang, H., Zhang, S. C., et al. (2001) Embryonic-derived glial-restricted pre-
    cursor cells (GRP cells) can differentiate into astrocytes and oligodendrocytes in vivo.
    Exp. Neurol. **171,** 11–21.
64. Han, S. S., Kang, D. Y., Mujtaba, T., Rao, M. S., and Fischer, I. (2002) Grafted lineage-
    restricted precursors differentiate exclusively into neurons in the adult spinal cord.
    Exp. Neurol. **177,** 360–375.
65. Li, R., Thode, S., Zhou, J., et al. (2000) Motoneuron differentiation of immortalized
    human spinal cord cell lines. *J. Neurosci. Res.* **59,** 342–352.
66. Cao, Q. L., Howard, R. M., Dennison, J. B., and Whittemore, S. R. (2002) Differentiation
    of engrafted neuronal-restricted precursor cells is inhibited in the traumatically injured
    spinal cord. *Exp. Neurol.* **177,** 349–359.
67. Barres, B., Burne, J., Holtmann, B., Thoenen, H., Sendtner, M., and Raff, M. (1996)
    Ciliary neurotrophic factor enhances the rate of oligodendrocyte generation. *Mol. Cell.
    Neurosci.* **8,** 146–156.
68. Marmur, R., Kessler, J. A., Zhu, G., Gokhan, S., and Mehler, M. F. (1998) Differentiation
    of oligodendroglial progenitors derived from cortical multipotent cells requires extrinsic
    signals including activation of gp130/LIFbeta receptors. *J. Neurosci.* **18,** 9800–9811.
69. Franklin, R. J. and Blakemore, W. F. (1995) Glial-cell transplantation and plasticity in
    the O-2A lineage—implications for CNS repair. *Trends Neurosci.* **18,** 151–156.
70. Liu, Y., Wu, Y., Lee, J. C., et al. (2002) Oligodendrocyte and astrocyte development in
    rodents: an in situ and immunohistological analysis during embryonic development. *Glia* **40,**
    25–43.
71. Gregori, N., Proschel, C., Noble, M., and Mayer-Pröschel, M. (2002) The tripotential
    glial-restricted precursor (GRP) cell and glial development in the spinal cord: Generation
    of bipotential oligodendrocyte-type-2 astrocyte progenitor cells and dorsal-ventral differ-
    ences in GRP cell function. *J. Neurosci.* **22,** 248–256.
72. Mujtaba, J., Piper, D., Groves, A., Kalyani, A., Lucero, M., and Rao, M. S. (1999) Lin-
    eage restricted precursors can be isolated from both the mouse neural tube and cultures
    ES cells. *Dev. Biol.* **214,** 113–127.
73. Dietrich, J., Noble, M., and Mayer-Proschel, M. (2002) Characterization of A2B5+ glial
    precursor cells from cryopreserved human fetal brain progenitor cells. *Glia* **40,** 65–77.
74. Trotter, J. and Schachner, M. (1989) Cells positive for the O4 surface antigen isolated by
    cell sorting are able to differentiate into astrocytes or oligodendrocytes. *Brain Res. Dev.
    Brain Res.* **46,** 115–122.
75. Barnett, S. C., Hutchins, A. M., and Noble, M. (1993) Purification of olfactory nerve
    ensheathing cells from the olfactory bulb. *Dev. Biol.* **155,** 337–350.
76. Grzenkowski, M., Niehaus, A., and Trotter, J. (1999) Monoclonal antibody detects
    oligodendroglial cell surface protein exhibiting temporal regulation during development.
    Glia **28,** 128–137.
77. Gard, A. L. and Pfeiffer, S. E. (1993) Glial cell mitogens bFGF and PDGF differentially
    regulate development of O4+GalC- oligodendrocyte progenitors. *Dev. Biol.* **159,** 618–630.
78. Gard, A. L. and Pfeiffer, S. E. (1990) Two proliferative stages of the oligodendrocyte lin-
    eage (A2B5+O4- and O4+GalC-) under different mitogenic control. *Neuron* **5,** 615–625.
79. Gard, A. L., Williams, W. C., and Burrell, M. R. (1995) Oligodendroblasts distinguished
    from O-2A glial progenitors by surface phenotype (O4+GalC-) and response to cytokines
    using signal transducer LIFR beta. *Dev. Biol.* **167,** 596–608.
80. Boucher, K., Yakovlev, A., Mayer-Proschel, M., and Noble, M. (1999) A stochastic model
    of temporally regulated generation of oligodendrocytes in cell culture. *Math. Biosci.* **159,**
    47–78.
81. Yakovlev, A. Y., Boucher, K., Mayer-Pröschel, M., and Noble, M. (1998) Quantitative
    insight into proliferation and differentiation of O-2A progenitor cells in vitro: the clock
    model revisited. *Proc. Natl. Acad. Sci. USA* **95,** 14164–14167.

82. Yakovlev, A., Mayer-Proschel, M., and Noble, M. (1998) A stochastic model of brain cell differentiation in tissue culture. *J. Math. Biol.* **37,** 49–60.

83. Zorin, A., Mayer-Proschel, M., Noble, M., and Yakovlev, A. Y. (2000) Estimation problems associated with stochastic modeling of proliferation and differentiation of O-2A progenitor cells in vitro. *Math. Biosci.* **167,** 109–121.

84. Okabe, S., Forsberg-Nilsson, K., Spiro, A. C., Segal, M., and McKay, R. D. (1996) Development of neuronal precursor cells and functional postmitotic neurons from embryonic stem cells in vitro. *Mech. Dev.* **59,** 89–102.

85. Fraichard, A., Chassande, O., Bilbaut, G., Dehay, C., Savatier, P., and Samarut, J. (1995) In vitro differentiation of embryonic stem cells into glial cells and functional neurons. *J. Cell Sci.* **108,** 3181–3188.

86. Kalyani, A., Hobson, K., and Rao, M. S. (1997) Neuroepithelial stem cells: isolation, characterization and clonal analysis. *Dev. Biol.* **187,** 203–226.

87. Laywell, E. D., Kukekov, V. G., and Steindler, D. A. (1999) Multipotent neurospheres can be derived from forebrain subependymal zone and spinal cord of adult mice after protracted postmortem intervals. *Exp. Neurol.* **156,** 430–433.

88. Raff, M. C., Williams, B. P., and Miller, R. H. (1984) The in vitro differentiation of a bipotential glial progenitor cell. *EMBO J.* **3,** 1857–1864.

89. Noble, M., Barnett, S. C., Bogler, O., Land, H., Wolswijk, G., and Wren, D. (1990) Control of division and differentiation in oligodendrocyte-type-2 astrocyte progenitor cells. *Ciba Found. Symp.* **150,** 227–243.

90. Noble, M. and Murray, K. (1984) Purified astrocytes promote the in vitro division of a bipotential glial progenitor cell. *EMBO J.* **3,** 2243–2247.

91. Wolswijk, G. and Noble, M. (1989) Identification of an adult-specific glial progenitor cell. *Development* **105,** 387–400.

92. Wolswijk, G., Riddle, P. N., and Noble, M. (1990) Coexistence of perinatal and adult forms of a glial progenitor cell during development of the rat optic nerve. *Development* **109,** 691–698.

93. Wolswijk, G., Riddle, P. N., and Noble, M. (1991) Platelet-derived growth factor is mitogenic for O-2A*adult* progenitor cells. *Glia* **4,** 495–503.

94. Wolswijk, G. and Noble, M. (1992) Cooperation between PDGF and FGF converts slowly dividing O-2Aadult progenitor cells to rapidly dividing cells with characteristics of O-2Aperinatal progenitor cells. *J. Cell Biol.* **118,** 889–900.

95. Shi, J., Marinovich, A., and Barres, B. (1998) Purification and characterization of adult oligodendrocyte precursor cells from the rat optic nerve. *J. Neurosci.* **18,** 4627–4636.

96. Dawson, M. R., Levine, J. M., and Reynolds, R. (2000) NG2-expressing cells in the central nervous system: are they oligodendroglial progenitors? *J. Neurosci. Res.* **61,** 471–479.

97. Levine, J. M., Stincone, F., and Lee, Y. S. (1993) Development and differentiation of glial precursor cells in the rat cerebellum. *Glia* **7,** 307–321.

98. Horner, P. J., Power, A. E., Kempermann, G., et al. (2000) Proliferation and differentiation of progenitor cells throughout the intact adult rat spinal cord. *J. Neurosci.* **20,** 2218–2228.

99. Levison, S. W., Young, G. M., and Goldman, J. E. (1999) Cycling cells in the adult rat neocortex preferentially generate oligodendroglia. *J. Neurosci. Res.* **57,** 435–446.

100. Keirstead, H. S. and Blakemore, W. F. (1997) Identification of post-mitotic oligodendrocytes incapable of remyelination within the demyelinated adult spinal cord. *J. Neuropathol.* **56,** 1191–1201.

101. Redwine, J. M. and Armstrong, R. C. (1998) In vivo proliferation of oligodendrocyte progenitors expressing PDGFalphaR during early remyelination. *J. Neurobiol.* **37,** 413–428.

102. Carroll, W. M., Jennings, A. R., and Ironside, L. J. (1998) Identification of the adult resting progenitor cell by autoradiographic tracking of oligodendrocyte precursors in experimental CNS demyelination. *Brain* **121,** 293–302.

103. Keirstead, H., Hughes, H., and Blakemore, W. (1998) A quantifiable model of axonal regeneration in the demyelinated adult rat spinal cord. *Exp. Neurol.* **151,** 303–313.
104. Cenci di Bello, I., et al. (1999) Generation of oligodendroglial progenitors in acute inflammatory demyelinating lesions of the rat brain stem is associated with demyelination rather than inflammation. *J. Neurocytol.* **28,** 365–381.
105. Gensert, J. M. and Goldman, J. E. (1997) Endogenous progenitors remyelinate demyelinated axons in the adult CNS. *Neuron* **19,** 197–203.
106. Armstrong, R., Friedrich, V. L., Jr., Holmes, K. V., and Dubois Dalcq, M. (1990) In vitro analysis of the oligodendrocyte lineage in mice during demyelination and remyelination. *J. Cell Biol.* **111,** 1183–95.
107. Levine, J. M. and Reynolds, R. (1999) Activation and proliferation of endogenous oligodendrocyte precursor cells during ethidium bromide-induced demyelination. *Exp. Neurol.* **160,** 333–347.
108. Watanabe, M., Toyama, Y., and Nishiyama, A. (2002) Differentiation of proliferated NG2-positive glial progenitor cells in a remyelinating lesion. *J. Neurosci. Res.* **69,** 826–836.
109. Levine, J. M. (1994) Increased expression of the NG2 chondroitin-sulfate proteoglycan after brain injury. *J. Neurosci.* **14,** 4716–4730.
110. Nishiyama, A., et al. (1997) Normal and reactive NG2+ glial cells are distinct from resting and activated microglia. *J. Neurosci. Res.* **48,** 299–312.
111. Robinson, S., Tani, M., Strieter, R., Ransohoff, R., and Miller, R. H. (1998) The chemokine growth-regulated oncogene-alpha promotes spinal cord oligodendrocyte precursor proliferation. *J. Neurosci.* **18,** 10457–10463.
112. Shields, S., Gilson, J., Blakemore, W., and Franklin, R. (1999) Remyelination occurs as extensively but more slowly in old rats compared to young rats following gliotoxin-induced CNS demyelination. *Glia* **28,** 77–83.
113. Fok-Seang, J., et al. (1995) Migration of oligodendrocyte precursors on astrocytes and meningeal cells. *Dev. Biol.* **171,** 1–15.
114. Schnaedelbach, O., et al. (2000) N-Cadherin influences migration of oligodendrocytes on astrocyte monolayers. *Mol. Cell. Neurosci.* **15,** 288–302.
115. Asher, R. A., et al. (1999) Versican is up-regulated in CNS injury and is a product of O-2A lineage cells. *Soc. Neurosci. Abstr.* **25,** 750.
116. Asher, R. A., et al. (2000) Neurocan is upregulated in injured brain and in cytokine-treated astrocytes. *J. Neurosci.* **20,** 2427–2438.
117. Jaworski, D. M., et al. (1999) Intracranial injury acutely induces the expression of the secreted isoform of the CNS-specific hyaluronan-binding protein BEHAB brevican. *Exp. Neurol.* **157,** 327–337.
118. Dou, C. L. and Levine, J. M. (1994) Inhibition of neurite growth by the NG2 chondroitin sulfate proteoglycan. *J. Neurosci.* **14,** 7616–7628.
119. Fawcett, J. W. and Asher, R. A. (1999) The glial scar and CNS repair. *Brain Res. Bull.* **49,** 377–391.
120. Niederost, B. P., et al. (1999) Bovine CNS myelin contains neurite growth-inhibitory activity associated with chondroitin sulfate proteoglycans. *J. Neurosci.* **19,** 8979–8989.
121. Bergles, D. E., et al. (2000) Glutaminergic synapses on oligodendrocyte precursor cells in the hippocampus. *Nature* **405,** 187–191.
122. Nishiyama, A., Chang, A., and Trapp, B. D. (1999) NG2+ glial cells: a novel glial cell population in the adult brain. *J. Neuropathol. Exp. Neurol.* **58,** 1113–1124.
123. Chang, A., et al. (2000) NG2+ oligodendrocyte progenitor cells in adult human brain and multiple sclerosis lesions. *J. Neurosci.* **20,** 6404–6412.
124. Wolswijk, G. (2000) Oligodendrocyte survival, loss and birth in lesions of chronic-stage multiple sclerosis. *Brain* **123,** 105–115.
125. Barres, B. A. and Raff, M. C. (1993) Proliferation of oligodendrocyte precursor cells depends on electrical activity in axons. *Nature* **361,** 258–260.

126. Belachew, S., Chittajallu, R., Aguirre, A. A., et al. (2003) Postnatal NG2 proteoglycan–expressing progenitor cells are intrinsically multipotent and generate functional neurons. *J. Cell Biol.* **161,** 1–19.

127. Foran, D. R. and Peterson, A. C. (1992) Myelin acquisition in the central nervous system of the mouse revealed by an MBP-LacZ transgene. *J. Neurosci.* **12,** 4890–4897.

128. Kinney, H. C., Brody, B. A., Kloman, A. S., and Gilles, F. H. (1988) Sequence of central nervous system myelination in human infancy. II. Patterns of myelination in autopsied infants. *J. Neuropathol. Exp. Neurol.* **47,** 217–234.

129. Macklin, W. B. and Weill, C. L. (1985) Appearance of myelin proteins during development in the chick central nervous system. *Dev. Neurosci.* **7,** 170–178.

130. Skoff, R. P., Toland, D., and Nast, E. (1980) Pattern of myelination and distribution of neuroglial cells along the developing optic system of the rat and rabbit. *J. Comp. Neurol.* **191,** 237–253.

131. Benes, F. M., Turtle, M., Khan, Y., and Farol, P. (1994) Myelination of a key relay zone in the hippocampal formation occurs in the human brain during childhood, adolescence and adulthood. *Arch. Gen. Psychiatry* **51,** 477–484.

132. Yakovlev, P. L. and Lecours, A. R. (1967) The myelogenetic cycles of regional maturation of the brain. In *Regional Development of the Brain in Early Life* (Minkowski, A., et al., eds.), Blackwell, Oxford, pp. 3–70.

133. Power, J., Mayer-Proschel, M., Smith, J., and Noble, M. (2002) Oligodendrocyte precursor cells from different brain regions express divergent properties consistent with the differing time courses of myelination in these regions. *Dev. Biol.* **245,** 362–375.

134. Small, R. K., Riddle, P., and Noble, M. (1987) Evidence for migration of oligodendrocyte-type-2 astrocyte progenitor cells into the developing rat optic nerve. *Nature* **328,** 155–157.

135. Stensaas, L. J. and Stensaas, S. S. (1968) Astrocytic neuroglial cells, oligodendrocytes and microgliacytes in the spinal cord of the toad. 11. Electron microscopy. *Zeit. Zellforsch. Mikroskop. Anat.* **86,** 184–213.

136. Remahl, S. and Hildebrand, C. (1990) Relation between axons and oligodendroglial cells during myelination. 1. The glial unit. *J. Neurocytol.* **19,** 313–328.

137. Bjartmar, C., Hildebrand, C., and Loinder, K. (1968) Morphological heterogeneity of rat oligodendrocytes: electron microscopic studies on serial sections. *Glia* **11,** 235–244.

138. Butt, A. M., Ibrahim, M., Gregson, N., and Berry, M. (1998) Differential expression of the L and S isoforms of myelin associated glycoprotein (MAG) in oligodendrocyte unit phenotypes in the adult anterior medullary velum. *J. Neurocytol.* **27,** 271–280.

139. Butt, A. M., Ibrahim, M., and Berry, M. (1997) The relationship between developing oligodendrocyte units and maturing axons during myelinogenesis in the anterior velum of neonatal rats. *J. Neurocytol.* **26,** 327–338.

140. Butt, A. M., Ibrahim, M., Ruge, F. M., and Berry, M. (1995) Biochemical subtypes of oligodendrocytes in the anterior velum of the rat revealed by the monoclonal antibody Rip. *Glia* **14,** 185–197.

141. Fanarraga, M. L., Griffiths, I. R., Zhao, M., and Duncan, I. D. (1998) Oligodendrocytes are not inherently programmed to myelinate a specific size of axon. *J. Comp. Neurol.* **399,** 94–100.

142. Spassky, N., Olivier, C., Perez-Villegas, E., et al. (2000) Single or multiple oligodendroglial lineages: a controversy. *Glia* **29,** 143–148.

143. Mallon, B. S., Shick, H. E., Kidd, G. J., and Macklin, W. B. (2002) Proteolipid promoter activity distinguishes two populations of NG2-positive cells throughout neonatal cortical development. *J. Neurosci.* **22,** 876–885.

144. Spassky, N., Goujet-Zalc, C., Parmantier, E., et al. (1998) Multiple restricted origin of oligodendrocytes. *J. Neurosci.* **18,** 8331–8343.

145. Nery, S., Wichterle, H., and Fishell, G. (2001) Sonic hedgehog contributes to oligoden-drocyte specification in the mammalian forebrain. *Development* **128,** 527–540.
146. Zhou, Q., Wang, S., and Anderson, D. J. (2000) Identification of a novel family of oligoden-drocyte lineage-specific basis helix-loop-helix transcription factors. *Neuron* **25,** 331–343.
147. Lu, Q. R., Yuk, D., Alberta, J. A., et al. (2000) Sonic hedgehog–regulated oligodendro-cyte lineage genes encoding bHLH proteins in the mammalian central nervous system. *Neuron* **25,** 317–329.
148. He, W., Ingraham, C., Rising, L., Goderie, S., and Temple, S. (2001) Multipotent stem cells from the mouse basal forebrain contribute GABAergic neurons and oligodendro-cytes to the cerebral cortex during embryogenesis. *J. Neurosci.* **21,** 8854–8862.
149. Yung, S. Y., Gokhan, S., Jurcsak, J., Molero, A. E., Abrajano, J. J., and Mehler, M. F. (2002) Differential modulation of BMP signaling promotes the elaboration of cerebral cortical GABAergic neurons or oligodendrocytes from a common sonic hedgehog-responsive ventral forebrain progenitor species. *Proc. Natl. Acad. Sci. USA* **99,** 16273–16278.
150. Lavdas, A. A., Grigoriou, M., Pachnis, V., and Parnavelas, J. G. (1999) The medial gan-glionic eminence gives rise to a population of early neurons in the developing cerebral cortex. *J. Neurosci.* **19,** 7881–7888.
151. Wichterle, H., Garcia-Verdugo, J. M., Herrera, D. G., and Alvarez-Buylla, A. (1999) Young neurons from medial ganglionic eminence disperse in adult and embryonic brain. *Nat. Neurosci.* **2,** 461–466.
152. Anderson, S. A., Marin, O., Horn, C., Jennings, K., and Rubenstein, J. L. (2001) Distinct cortical migrations from the medial and lateral ganglionic eminences. *Development* **128,** 353–363.
153. Marshall, C. A. and Goldman, J. E. (2002) Subpallial dlx2-expressing cells give rise to astrocytes and oligodendrocytes in the cerebral cortex and white matter. *J. Neurosci.* **22,** 9821–9830.
154. Qian, X., Davis, A. A., Goderie, S. K., and Temple, S. (1997) FGF2 Concentration regu-lates the generation of neurons and glia from multipotent cortical stem cells. *Neuron* **18,** 81–93.
155. Tekki-Kessaris, N., Woodruff, R., Hall, A. C., et al. (2001) Hedgehog-dependent oligo-dendrocyte lineage specification in the telencephalon. *Development* **128,** 2545–2554.
156. Mekki-Dauriac, S., Agius, E., Kan, P., and Cochard, P. (2002) Bone morphogenetic pro-teins negatively control oligodendrocyte precursor specification in the chick spinal cord. *Development* **129,** 5117–5130.
157. Pringle, N. P., Wei-Ping, Y., Guthrie, S., et al. (1996) Determination of neuroepithelial cell fate: induction of the oligodendrocyte lineage by ventral midline cells and Sonic Hedgehog. *Dev. Biol.* **177,** 30–42.
158. Richardson, W. D., Smith, J. K., Sun, T., Pringle, N. P., Hall, A. C., and Woodruff, R. (2000) Oligodendrocyte lineage and the motor neuron connection. *Glia* **29,** 136–142.
159. Richardson, W. D., Pringle, N. P., Yu, W.-P., and Hall, A. C. (1997) Origins of spinal cord oligodendrocytes: possible developmental and evolutionary relationships with motor neurons. *Dev. Neurosci.* **19,** 54–64.
160. Orentas, D. M., Hayers, J. E., Dyer, K. L., and Miller, R. H. (1999) Sonic hedgehog signaling is required during the appearance of spinal cord oligodendrocyte precursors. *Development* **126,** 2419–2429.
161. Lu, Q. R., Sun, T., Zhu, Z., et al. (2002) Common developmental requirement for Olig function indicates a motor neuron/oligodendrocyte connection. *Cell* **109,** 75–86.
162. Takebayashi, H., Nabeshima, Y., Yoshida, S., et al. (2002) The basic helix–loop–helix factor olig2 is essential for the development of motoneuron and oligodendrocyte lineages. *Curr. Biol.* **12,** 1157–1163.
163. Zhou, Q. and Anderson, D. J. (2002) The bHLH transcription factors olig2 and olig1 couple neuronal and glial subtype specification. *Cell* **109,** 61–73.

164. Rowitch, D. H., Lu, R. Q., Kessaris, N., and Richardson, W. D. (2002) An 'oligarchy' rules neural development. *Trends Neurosci.* **25,** 417–422.
165. Sauvageot, C. M. and Stiles, C. D. (2002) Molecular mechanisms controlling cortical gliogenesis. *Curr. Opin. Neurobiol.* **12,** 244–249.
166. Corbin, J. G., Gaiano, N., Machold, R. P., Langston, A., and Fishell, G. (2000) The Gsh2 homeodomain gene controls multiple aspects of telencephalic development. *Development* **127,** 5007–5020.
167. Zhu, G., Mehler, M. F., Zhao, J., Yu Yung, S., and Kessler, J. A. (1999) Sonic hedgehog and BMP2 exert opposing actions on proliferation and differentiation of embryonic neural progenitor cells. *Dev. Biol.* **215,** 118–129.
168. Thomas, J. L., Spassky, N., Perez Villegas, E. M., et al. (2000) Spatiotemporal development of oligodendrocytes in the embryonic brain. *J. Neurosci. Res.* **59,** 471–476.
169. Briscoe, J. and Ericson, J. (1999) The specification of neuronal identity by graded Sonic Hedgehog signalling. *Semin. Cell Dev. Biol.* **10,** 353–362.
170. Miller, R. H., Hayes, J. E., Dyer, K. L., and Sussman, C. R. (1999) Mechanisms of oligodendrocyte commitment in the vertebrate CNS. *Int. J. Dev. Neurosci.* **17,** 753–763.
171. Zhou, Q., Choi, G., and Anderson, D. J. (2001) The bHLH transcription factor Olig2 promotes oligodendrocyte differentiation in collaboration with nkx2. 2. *Neuron* **31,** 791–807.
172. Davies, J. E. and Miller, R. H. (2001) Local sonic hedgehog signaling regulates oligodendrocyte precursor appearance in multiple ventricular domains in the chick metencephalon. *Dev. Biol.* **233,** 513–525.
173. Nery, S., Wichterle, H., and Fishell, G. (2001) Sonic hedghog contributes to oligodendrocyte specification in the mammalian forebrain. *Development* **128,** 527–540.
174. Mabie, P., Mehler, M., Marmur, R., Papavasiliou, A., Song, Q., and Kessler, J. (1997) Bone morphogenetic proteins induce astroglial differentiation of oligodendroglial–astroglial progenitor cells. *J. Neurosci.* **17,** 4112–4120.
175. Mehler, M. F., Mabie, P. C., Zhu, G., Gokhan, S., and Kessler, J. A. (2000) Developmental changes in progenitor cell responsiveness to bone morphogenetic proteins differentially modulate progressive CNS lineage fate. *Dev. Neurosci.* **22,** 74–85.
176. Mizuguchi, R., Sugimori, M., Takebayashi, H., et al. (2001) Combinatorial roles of olig2 and neurogenin2 in the coordinated induction of pan-neuronal and subtype-specific properties of motoneurons. *Neuron* **31,** 757–771.
177. Novitch, B. G., Chen, A. I., and Jessell, T. M. (2001) Coordinate regulation of motor neuron subtype identity and pan-neuronal properties by the bHLH repressor Olig2. *Neuron* **31,** 773–789.
178. Sun, T., Echelard, Y., Lu, R., et al. (2001) Olig bHLH proteins interact with homeodomain proteins to regulate cell fate acquisition in progenitors of the ventral neural tube. *Curr. Biol.* **11,** 1413–1420.
179. Mabie, P. C., Mehler, M. F., and Kessler, J. A. (1999) Multiple roles of bone morphogenetic protein signaling in the regulation of cortical cell number and phenotype. *J. Neurosci.* **19,** 7077–7088.
180. Li, W., Cogswell, C. A., and LoTurco, J. J. (1998) Neuronal differentiation of precursors in the neocortical ventricular zone is triggered by BMP. *J. Neurosci.* **18,** 8853–8862.
181. Gross, R. E., Mehler, M. F., Mabie, P. C., Zang, Z., Santschi, L., and Kessler, J. A. (1996) Bone morphogenetic proteins promote astroglial lineage commitment by mammalian subventricular zone progenitor cells. *Neuron* **17,** 595–606.
182. Grinspan, J. B., Edell, E., Carpio, D. F., et al. (2000) Stage-specific effects of bone morphogenetic proteins on the oligodendrocyte lineage. *J. Neurobiol.* **43,** 1–17.
183. Nakashima, K., Takizawa, T., Ochiai, W., et al. (2001) BMP2-mediated alteration in the developmental pathway of fetal mouse brain cells from neurogenesis to astrocytogenesis. *Proc. Natl. Acad. Sci. USA* **98,** 5868–5873.

184. Gomes, W. A., Mehler, M. F., and Kessler, J. A. (2003) Transgenic overexpression of BMP4 increases astroglial and decreases oligodendroglial lineage commitment. *Dev. Biol.* **255,** 164–177.

185. Noble, M., Arhin, A., Gass, D., and Mayer-Proschel, M. (2003) The cortical ancestry of oligodendrocytes: Common principles and novel features. *Dev. Neurosci.* **25,** 217–233.

186. Doetsch, F., Garcia-Verdugo, J. M., and Alvarez-Buylla, A. (1997) Cellular composition and three-dimensional organization of the subventricular germinal zone in the adult mammalian brain. *J. Neurosci.* **17,** 5046–5061.

187. Weickert, C. S., Webster, M. J., Colvin, S. M., et al. (2000) Localization of epidermal growth factor receptors and putative neuroblasts in human subependymal zone. *J. Comp. Neurol.* **423,** 359–372.

188. Fok-Seang, J. and Miller, R. H. (1994) Distribution and differentiation of A2B5+ glial precursors in the developing rat spinal cord. *J. Neurosci. Res.* **37,** 219–235.

189. Fok-Seang, J. and Miller, H. R. (1992) Astrocyte precursors in neonatal rat spinal cord cultures. *J. Neurosci.* **12,** 2751–2764.

190. Mi, H. and Barres, B. A. (1999) Purification and characterization of astrocyte precursor cells in the developing rat optic nerve. *J. Neurosci.* **19,** 1049–1061.

191. Kondo, T. and Raff, M. (2000) Oligodendrocyte precursor cells reprogrammed to become multipotential CNS stem cells. *Science* **289,** 1754–1757.

192. Ben-Hur, T., Rogister, B., Murray, K., Rougon, G., and Dubois-Dalcq, M. (1998) Growth and fate of PSA-NCAM+ precursors of the postnatal brain. *J. Neurosci.* **18,** 5777–5788.

193. Grinspan, J. B., Stern, J. L., Pustilnik, S. M., and Pleasure, D. (1990) Cerebral white matter contains PDGF-responsive precursors to O-2A cells. *J. Neurosci.* **10,** 1866–1873.

194. Keirstead, H., Ben-Hur, T., Rogister, B., O'Leary, M., Dubois-Dalcq, M., and Blakemore, W. (1999) Polysialylated neural cell adhesion molecule-positive CNS precursors generate both oligodendrocytes and Schwann cells to remyelinate the CNS after transplantation. *J. Neurosci.* **19,** 7529–7536.

195. Nait-Oumesmar, B., Decker, L., Lachapelle, F., Avellana-Adalid, V., Bachelin, C., and Van Evercooren, A. B. (1999) Progenitor cells of the adult mouse subventricular zone proliferate, migrate and differentiate into oligodendrocytes after demyelination. *Eur. J. Neurosci.* **11,** 4357–4366.

196. Vitry, S., Avellana-Adalid, V., Hardy, R., Lachapelle, F., and Baron-Van Evercooren, A. (1999) Mouse oligospheres: from pre-progenitors to functional oligodendrocytes. *J. Neurosci. Res.* **58,** 735–751.

197. Zhang, S. C., Lipsitz, D., and Duncan, I. D. (1998) Self-renewing canine oligodendroglial progenitor expanded as oligospheres. *J. Neurosci. Res.* **54,** 181–190.

198. Carpenter, M., Cui, X., Hu, Z., et al. (1999) In vitro expansion of a multipotent population of human neural progenitor cells. *Exp. Neurol.* **158,** 265–278.

199. Hammang, J., Archer, D., and Duncan, I. (1997) Myelination following transplantation of EGF-responsive neural stem cells into a myelin-deficient environment. *Exp. Neurol.* **147,** 84–95.

200. Milward, E., Lundberg, C., Ge, B., Lipsitz, D., Zhao, M., and Duncan, I. (1997) Isolation and transplantation of multipotential populations of epidermal growth factor-responsive, neural progenitor cells from the canine brain. *J. Neurosci. Res.* **50,** 862–871.

201. Svendsen, C., Caldwell, M., and Ostenfeld, T. (1999) Human neural stem cells: isolation, expansion and transplantation. *Brain Pathol.* **9,** 499–513.

202. Vescovi, A., Gritti, A., Galli, R., and Parati, E. (1999) Isolation and intracerebral grafting of nontransformed multipotential embryonic human CNS stem cells. *J. Neurotrauma* **16,** 689–693.

203. Vescovi, A., Parati, E., Gritti, A., et al. (1999) Isolation and cloning of multipotential stem cells from the embryonic human CNS and establishment of transplantable human neural stem cell lines by epigenetic stimulation. *Exp. Neurol.* **156,** 71–83.

204. Vescovi, A. and Snyder, E. (1999) Establishment and properties of neural stem cell clones: plasticity in vitro and in vivo. *Brain Pathol.* **9,** 569–598.
205. Roots, B. I. (1993) The evolution of myelin. *Adv. Neural Sci.* **1,** 187–213.
206. Davis, A. D., Weatherby, T. M., Hartline, D. K., and Lenz, P. H. (1999) Myelin-like sheaths in copepod axons. *Nature* **398,** 571.
207. Takebayashi, H., Yoshida, S., Sugimori, M., et al. (2000) Dynamic expression of basic helix-loop-helix Olig family members: implication of Olig2 in neuron and oligodendrocyte differentiation and identification of a new member, Olig3. *Mech. Dev.* **99,** 143–148.
208. Zhou, Q., Wang, S., and Anderson, D. J. (2000) Identification of a novel family of oligodendrocyte lineage-specific basic helix-loop-helix transcription factors. *Neuron* **25,** 331–343.
209. Park, H. C., Mehta, A., Richardson, J. S., and Appel, B. (2002) Olig2 is required for zebrafish primary motor neuron and oligodendrocyte development. *Dev. Biol.* **248,** 356–368.
210. Noble, M., Pröschel, C., and Mayer-Proschel, M. (2004) Getting a GR(i)P on oligodendrocyte development. *Dev. Biol.* **265,** 33–52.
211. Liu, Y. and Rao, M. S. (2003) Olig genes are expressed In a heterogeneous population of precursor cells in the developing spinal cord. *Glia* **45,** 67–74.
212. Leber, S. M., Breedlove, S. M., and Sanes, J. R. (1990) Lineage, arrangement, and death of clonally related motoneurons in chick spinal cord. *J. Neurosci.* **10,** 2451–2462.
213. Pringle, N. and Richardson, W. (1993) A singularity of PDGF alpha-receptor expression in the dorsoventral axis of the neural tube may define the origin of the oligodendrocyte lineage. *Development* **117,** 525–533.
214. Stockard, C. R. (1921) Developmental rate and structural expression in experimental study of twins, 'double monsters' and single deformities, and the interaction among embryonic organs during their origin and development. *Am. J. Anat.* **28,** 115–277.
215. Davison, A. N. and Dobbing, J. (1966) Myelination as a vulnerable period in brain development. *Br. Med. Bull.* **22,** 40–44.
216. Delange, F. (1994) The disorders induced by iodine deficiency. *Thyroid* **4,** 107–128.
217. Lazarus, J. H. (1999) Thyroid hormone and intellectual development: a clinician's view. *Thyroid* **9,** 659–660.
218. Pop, V. J., Kuijpens, J. L., van Baar, A. L., et al. (1999) Low maternal free thyroxine concentrations during early pregnancy are associated with impaired psychomotor development in infancy. *Clin. Endocrinol.* **50,** 149–155.
219. Man, E. B., Brown, J. F., and Scrunian, S. A. (1991) Maternal hypothyroxinemia: psychoneurological deficits of progeny. *Ann. Clin. Lab. Sci.* **21,** 227–239.
220. Haddow, J. E., Glenn, E., Palomaki, B. S., et al. (1999) Maternal thyroid deficiency during pregnancy and subsequent neuropsychological development of the child. *N. Engl. J. Med.* **341,** 549–555.
221. Legrand, J. (1986) Thyroid hormone effects on growth and development. In *Thyroid Hormone Metabolism* (Henneman, G., ed.), Marcel Dekker, New York, pp. 503–534.
222. Balazs, R., Kovacs, S., Cocks, W. A., Johnson, A. L., and Eayrs, J. T. (1971) Effect of thyroid hormone on the biochemical maturation of rat brain: postnatal cell formation. *Brain Res.* **25,** 555–570.
223. Balazs, R., Brooksbank, B. W., Davison, A. N., Eayrs, J. T., and Wilson, D. A. (1969) The effect of neonatal thyroidectomy on myelination in the rat brain. *Brain Res.* **15,** 219–232.
224. Rosman, N. P., Malone, M. J., Helfenstein, M., and Kraft, E. (1972) The effect of thyroid deficiency on myelination of brain. *Neurology* **22,** 99–106.
225. Eayrs, J. T. and Taylor, S. H. (1951) The effect of thyroid deficiency induced by methylthiouracil on the maturation of the central nervous system. *J. Anat.* **85,** 350–358.
226. Eayrs, J. T. (1955) The cerebral cortex of normal and hypothyroid rats. *Acta Anat.* **25,** 160–183.

227. Eayrs, J. T. and Horne, G. (1955) The development of cerebral cortex in hypothyroid and starved rats. *Anat. Rec.* **121,** 53–61.
228. Nicholson, J. L. and Altman, J. (1972) The effects of early hypo- and hyperthyroidism on the development of the rat cerebellar cortex. I. Cell proliferation and differentiation. *Brain Res.* **44,** 13–23.
229. Eayrs, J. T. (1971) Thyroid and developing brain: anatomical and behavioural effects. In *Hormones in Development* (Hamburgh, M. and Barrington, E., eds.), Appleton-Century-Crofts, New York.
230. Noguchi, T., Sugisaki, T., Satoh, I., and Kudo, M. (1985) Partial restoration of cerebral myelination of the congenitally hypothyroid mouse by parenteral or breast milk administration of thyroxine. *J. Neurochem.* **45,** 1419-1426.
231. Munoz, A., Rodriguez-Pena, A., Perez-Castillo, A., Ferreiro, B., Sutcliffe, J. G., and Bernal, J. (1991) Effects of neonatal hypothyroidism on rat brain gene expression. *Mol. Endocrinol.* **5,** 273–280.
232. Bernal, J. and Nunez, J. (1995) Thyroid hormones and brain development. *Eur. J. Endocrinol.* **133,** 390–398.
233. Ibarrola, N. and Rodriguez-Pena, A. (1997) Hypothyroidism coordinately and transiently affects myelin protein gene expression in most rat brain regions during postnatal development. *Brain Res.* **752,** 285–293.
234. Marta, C. B., Adamo, A. M., Soto, E. F., and Pasquini, J. M. (1998) Sustained neonatal hyperthyroidism in the rat affects myelination in the central nervous system. *J. Neurosci. Res.* **53,** 251–259.
235. Chan, S. and Kilby, M. D. (2000) Thyroid hormone and central nervous system development. *J. Endocrinol.* **165,** 1–8.
236. Pharoah, P., Buttfield, I. H., and Hotzel, B. S. (1971) Neurological damage to the fetus resulting from severe iodine deficiency during pregnancy. *Lancet* **i,** 308–310.
237. Cao, X. Y., X. M. J., Dou, Z. H., et al. (1994) Timing of vulnerability of the brain to iodine deficiency in endemic cretinism. *N. Engl. J. Med.* **331,** 1739–1744.
238. Klein, R. Z., Mitchell, M. L., and Foley, T. P. J. (1996) Hypothyroidism in infants and children. In *The Thyroid* (Braverman, L. E. and Utiger, R. D., eds.), Lippincott Williams & Wilkins, New York, pp. 984–989.
239. Klein, A. H., Meltzer, S., and Kenny, F. M. (1972) Improved prognosis in congenital hypothyroidism treated before age three months. *J. Pediatr.* **81,** 912–920.
240. Gao, F., Apperly, J., and Raff, M. (1998) Cell-intrinsic timers and thyroid hormone regulate the probability of cell-cycle withdrawal and differentiation of oligodendrocyte precursor cells. *Dev. Biol.* **197,** 54–66.
241. Ahlgren, S., Wallace, H., Bishop, J., Neophytou, C., and Raff, M. (1997) Effects of thyroid hormone on embryonic oligodendrocyte precursor cell development in vivo and in vitro. *Mol. Cell Neurosci.* **9,** 420–432.
242. Tosic, M., Torch, S., Comte, V., Dolivo, M., Honegger, P., and Matthieu, J. M. (1992) Triiodothyronine has diverse and multiple stimulating effects on expression of the major myelin protein genes. *J. Neurochem.* **59,** 1770–1777.
243. Pombo, P. M., Barettino, D., Ibarrola, N., Vega, S., and Rodriguez-Pena, A. (1999) Stimulation of the myelin basic protein gene expression by 9-cis-retinoic acid and thyroid hormone: activation in the context of its native promoter. *Mol. Brain. Res.* **64,** 92–100.
244. Pombo, P. M., Ibarrola, N., Alonso, M. A., and Rodriguez-Pena, A. (1998) Thyroid hormone regulates the expression of the MAL proteolipid, a component of glycolipid-enriched membranes, in neonatal rat brain. *J. Neurosci. Res.* **52,** 584–590.
245. Jones, S. A., Jolson, D. M., Cuta, K. K., Mariash, C. N., and Anderson, G. W. (2003) Triiodothyronine is a survival factor for developing oligodendrocytes. *Mol. Cell. Endocrinol.* **199,** 49–60.

246. Oppenheimer, J. H. and Schwartz, H. L. (1997) Molecular basis of thyroid hormone-dependent brain development. *Endocr. Rev.* **18,** 462–475.

247. Yip, R. (2002) Prevention and control of iron deficiency: policy and strategy issues. *J. Nutr.* **132,** 802S–805S.

248. Beard, J. L. (2001) Iron biology in immune function, muscle metabolism and neuronal functioning. *J. Nutr.* **131,** 568S–579S.

249. de Regnier, R. A., Nelson, C. A., Thomas, K., Wewerka, S., and Georgieff, M. K. (2000) Neurophysiologic evaluation of auditory recognition memory in healthy newborn infants and infants of diabetic mothers. *J. Pediatr.* **137,** 777–784.

250. Nelson, C. A., Wewerka, S., Thomas, K., Tribby-Walbridge, S., de Regnier, R. A., and Georgieff, M. K. (2000) Neurocognitive sequelae of infants of diabetic mothers. *Behav. Neurosci.* **114,** 950–956.

251. Tamura, T., Goldberg, R. L., Hou, J., et al. (2002) Cord serum ferritin concentrations and mental and psychomotor development of children at five years of age. *J. Pediatr.* **140,** 165–170.

252. Grantham-McGregor, S. and Ani, C. (2001) A review of studies on the effect of iron deficiency on cognitive development in children. *J. Nutr.* **131,** 649S–668S.

253. Yager, J. Y. and Hartfield, D. S. (2002) Neurological manifestations of iron deficiency in childhood. *Pediatr. Neurol.* **27,** 85–92.

254. Dobbing, J. (1990) *Brain, Behavior and Iron in the Infant Diet.* Springer-Verlag, London.

255. Honig, A. and Oski, F. (1978) Developmental scores of the iron deficient infants and the effect of therapy. *Infant Behav. Dev.* **1,** 168–176.

256. Pollitt, E. and Leibel, R. (1976) Iron deficiency and behavior. *J. Pediatr.* **88,** 732–781.

257. Yu, G., Steinkirchner, T., Rao, G., and Larkin, E. C. (1986) Effect of prenatal iron deficiency on myelination in rat pups. *Am. J. Pathol.* **125,** 620–624.

258. Lozoff, B. (2000) Perinatal iron deficiency and the developing brain. *Pediatr. Res.* **48,** 137–139.

259. Connor, J. R. and Menzies, S. L. (1996) Relationship of iron to oligodendrocytes and myelination. *Glia* **17,** 83–93.

260. Sacco, L. M., Caulfield, L. E., Zavaleta, N., and Retamozo, L. (1999) Usual mineral intakes of Peruvian women during pregnancy. *FASEB J.* **13,** A250 (Abstr).

261. O'Brien, K. O., Zavaleta, N., Abrams, S. A., and Caulfield, L. E. (2003) Maternal iron status influences iron transfer to the fetus during the third trimester of pregnancy. *Am. J. Clin. Nutr.* **77,** 924–930.

262. Looker, A. C., Dallman, P. R., Carroll, M. D., Gunter, M. T., and Johnson, C. L. (1997) Prevalence of iron deficiency in the United States. *JAMA* **277,** 973–976.

263. Hecox, K. and Burkard, R. (1982) Developmental dependencies of the human brainstem auditory evoked response. *Ann. NY Acad. Sci.* **388,** 538–556.

264. Jiang, Z. D. (1995) Maturation of the auditory brainstem in low risk-preterm infants: a comparison with age-matched full term infants up to 6 years. *Early Hum. Dev.* **42,** 49–65.

265. Salamy, A. and McKean, C. M. (1976) Postnatal development of human brainstem potentials during the first year of life. *Electroencephalogr. Clin. Neurophysiol.* **40,** 418–426.

266. Roncagliolo, M., Garrido, M., Walter, T., Peirano, P., and Lozoff, B. (1998) Evidence of altered central nervous system development in infants with iron deficiency anemia at 6 mo: delayed maturation of auditory brainstem responses. *Am. J. Clin. Nutr.* **68,** 683–690.

267. deUngria, M., Rao, R., Wobken, J. D., Luciana, M., Nelson, C. A., and Georgieff, M. K. (2000) Perinatal iron deficiency decreases cytochrome c oxidase (CytOx) activity in selected regions of neonatal rat brain. *Pediatr. Res.* **48,** 169–176.

268. Felt, B. T. and Lozoff, B. (1996) Brain iron and behavior of rats are not normalized by treatment of iron deficiency anemia during early development. *J. Nutr.* **126,** 693–701.

269. Rao, R., Tkac, I., Townsend, E. L., Gruetter, R., and Georgieff, M. K. (2003) Perinatal iron deficiency alters the neurochemical profile of the developing rat hippocampus. *J. Nutr.* **133,** 3215–3221.

270. Erikson, K. M., Pinero, D. J., Connor, J. R., and Beard, J. L. (1997) Regional brain iron, ferritin and transferrin concentrations during iron deficiency and iron repletion in developing rats. *J. Nutr.* **127,** 2030–2038.

271. Larkin, E. C. and Rao, G. A. (1990) Importance of fetal and neonatal iron: Adequacy for normal development of central nervous system. In *Brain, Behavior and Iron in the Infant Diet* (Dobbing, J., ed.), Springer-Verlag, London, pp. 43–63.

272. Morath, D. J. and Mayer-Proschel, M. (2001) Iron modulates the differentiation of a distinct population of glial precursor cells into oligodendrocytes. *Dev. Biol.* **237,** 232–243.

273. Morath, D. J. and Mayer-Proschel, M. (2002) Iron deficiency during embryogenesis and consequences for oligodendrocyte generation in vivo. *Dev. Neurosci.* **24,** 197–207.

274. Beard, J. L., Erikson, K. M., and Byron, C. J. (2003) Neonatal iron deficiency results in irreversible changes in dopamine function in rats. *J. Nutr.* **133,** 1174–1179.

275. Dallman, P. R. (1986) Biochemical basis for the manifestations of iron deficiency. *Annu. Rev. Nutr.* **6,** 13–40.

276. Harthoorn-Lasthuizen, E. J., Lindemans, J., and Langenhuijsen, M. M. (2001) Does iron-deficient erythropoiesis in pregnancy influence fetal iron supply? *Acta Obstet. Gynecol. Scand.* **80,** 392–396.

277. Wong, C. T. and Saha, N. (1990) Inter-relationships of storage iron in the mother, the placenta and the newborn. *Acta Obstet. Gynecol. Scand.* **69,** 613–616.

278. Lao, T. T., Loong, E. P., Chin, R. K., Lam, C. W., and Lam, Y. M. (1991) Relationship between newborn and maternal iron status and haematological indices. *Biol. Neonate* **60,** 303–307.

279. Allen, L. H. (1997) Pregnancy and iron deficiency: unresolved issues. *Nutr. Rev.* **55,** 91–101.

280. Halvorsen, S. (2000) Iron balance between mother and infant during pregnancy and breastfeeding. *Acta Paediatr.* **89,** 625–627.

281. Georgieff, M. K., Mills, M. M., Gordon, K., and Wobken, J. D. (1995) Reduced neonatal liver iron concentrations after uteroplacental insufficiency. *J. Pediatr.* **127,** 308–311.

282. Choi, J. W., Kim, C. S., and Pai, S. H. (2000) Erythropoietic activity and soluble transferrin receptor level in neonates and maternal blood. *Acta Paediatr.* **89,** 675–679.

283. Wiggins, R. C., Benjamins, J. A., Krigman, M. R., and Morell, P. (1974) Synthesis of myelin proteins during starvation. *Brain Res.* **80,** 345–349.

284. Wiggins, R. C., Miller, S. L., Benjamins, J. A., Krigman, M. R., and Morell, P. (1976) Myelin synthesis during postnatal nutritional deprivation and subsequent rehabilitation. *Brain Res.* **107,** 257–273.

285. Wiggins, R. C. and Fuller, G. N. (1978) Early postnatal starvation causes lasting brain hypomyelination. *J. Neurochem.* **30,** 1231–1237.

286. Zuppinger, K., Wiesmann, U., Siegrist, H. P., et al. (1981) Effect of glucose deprivation on sulfatide synthesis and oligodendrocytes in cultured brain cells of newborn mice. *Pediatr. Res.* **15,** 319–325.

287. Krigman, M. R. and Hogan, E. L. (1976) Undernutrition in the developing rat: effect upon myelination. *Brain Res.* **107,** 239–255.

288. Sikes, R. W., Fuller, G. N., Colbert, C., Chronister, R. B., DeFrance, J., and Wiggins, R. C. (1981) The relative numbers of oligodendroglia in different brain regions of normal and postnatally undernourished rats. *Brain Res. Bull.* **6,** 385–391.

289. Royland, J. E., Konat, G., and Wiggins, R. C. (1993) Abnormal upregulation of myelin genes underlies the critical period of myelination in undernourished developing rat brain. *Brain Res.* **607,** 113–116.

290. Royland, J. E., Konat, G. W., and Wiggins, R. C. (1993) Myelin gene activation: a glucose sensitive critical period in development. *J. Neurosci. Res.* **36**, 399–404.

291. Royland, J. E., Konat, G. W., and Wiggins, R. C. (1999) Differentiation dependent activation of the myelin genes in purified oligodendrocytes is highly resistant to hypoglycemia. *Metab. Brain Dis.* **14**, 189–195.

292. Carroll, P., Sendtner, M., Meyer, M., and Thoenen, H. (1993) Rat ciliary neurotrophic factor (CNTF): gene structure and regulation of mRNA levels in glial cell cultures. *Glia* **9**, 176–187.

293. Chernausek, S. D. (1993) Insulin-like growth factor-I (IGF-I) production by astroglial cells: regulation and importance for epidermal growth factor-induced cell replication. *J. Neurosci. Res.* **34**, 189–197.

294. Hammarberg, H., Risling, M., Hokfelt, T., Cullheim, S., and Piehl, F. (1998) Expression of insulin-like growth factors and corresponding binding proteins (IGFBP 1-6) in rat spinal cord and peripheral nerve after axonal injuries. *J. Comp. Neurol.* **400**, 57–72.

295. Moretto, G., Xu, R. Y., Walker, D. G., and Kim, S. U. (1994) Co-expression of mRNA for neurotrophic factors in human neurons and glial cells in culture. *J. Neuropathol. Exp. Neurol.* **53**, 78–85.

296. Janzer, R. C. and Raff, M. C. (1987) Astrocytes induce blood-brain barrier properties in endothelial cells. *Nature* **325**, 253–257.

297. Rubin, L. L., Hall, D. E., Porter, S., et al. (1991) A cell culture model of the blood–brain barrier. *J. Cell Biol.* **115**, 1725–1735.

298. Fierz, W., Endler, B., Reske, K., Wekerle, H., and Fontana, A. (1985) Astrocytes as antigen-presenting cells. I. Induction of Ia antigen expression on astrocytes by T cells via immune interferon and its effect on antigen presentation. *J. Immunol.* **134**, 3785–3793.

299. Fontana, A., Erb, P., Pircher, H., Zinkernagel, R., Weber, E., and Fierz, W. (1986) Astrocytes as antigen-presenting cells. Part II: Unlike H-2K-dependent cytotoxic T cells, H-2Ia-restricted T cells are only stimulated in the presence of interferon-gamma. *J. Neuroimmunol.* **12**, 15–28.

300. Frei, K. and Fontana, A. (1997) Antigen presentation in the CNS. *Mol. Psychiatry* **2**, 96–98.

301. Oh, J. W., Schwiebert, L. M., and Benveniste, E. N. (1999) Cytokine regulation of CC and CXC chemokine expression by human astrocytes. *J. Neurovirol.* **5**, 82–94.

302. Van Wagoner, N. J., Oh, J. W., Repovic, P., and Benveniste, E. N. (1999) Interleukin-6 (IL-6) production by astrocytes: autocrine regulation by IL-6 and the soluble IL-6 receptor. *J. Neurosci.* **19**, 5236–5244.

303. Hansson, E. and Ronnback, L. (1992) Adrenergic receptor regulation of amino acid neurotransmitter uptake in astrocytes. *Brain Res. Bull.* **29**, 297–301.

304. Mentlein, R. and Dahms, P. (1994) Endopeptidases 24. 16 and 24. 15 are responsible for the degradation of somatostatin, neurotensin, and other neuropeptides by cultivated rat cortical astrocytes. *J. Neurochem.* **62**, 27–36.

305. Araque, A., Sanzgiri, R. P., Parpura, V., and Haydon, P. G. (1999) Astrocyte-induced modulation of synaptic transmission. *Can. J. Physiol. Pharmacol.* **77**, 699–706.

306. Vesce, S., Bezzi, P., and Volterra, A. (1999) The highly integrated dialogue between neurons and astrocytes in brain function. *Sci. Prog.* **82**, 251–270.

307. Brand, A., Leibfritz, D., Hamprecht, B., and Dringen, R. (1998) Metabolism of cysteine in astroglial cells: synthesis of hypotaurine and taurine. *J. Neurochem.* **71**, 827–832.

308. Hertz, L., Dringen, R., Schousboe, A., and Robinson, S. R. (1999) Astrocytes: glutamate producers for neurons. *J. Neurosci. Res.* **57**, 417–428.

309. Bush, T. G., Puvanachandra, N., Horner, C. H., et al. (1999) Leukocyte infiltration, neuronal degeneration, and neurite outgrowth after ablation of scar-forming, reactive astrocytes in adult transgenic mice. *Neuron* **23**, 297–308.

310. Fitch, M. T., Doller, C., Combs, C. K., Landreth, G. E., and Silver, J. (1999) Cellular and molecular mechanisms of glial scarring and progressive cavitation: in vivo and in vitro

analysis of inflammation-induced secondary injury after CNS trauma. *J. Neurosci.* **19,** 8182–8198.

311. McKeon, R. J., Jurynec, M. J., and Buck, C. R. (1999) The chondroitin sulfate proteoglycans neurocan and phosphacan are expressed by reactive astrocytes in the chronic CNS glial scar. *J. Neurosci.* **19,** 10778–10788.

312. Drukarch, B., Schepens, E., Stoof, J. C., Langeveld, C. H., and Van Muiswinkel, F. L. (1998) Astrocyte-enhanced neuronal survival is mediated by scavenging of extracellular reactive oxygen species. *Free. Radic. Biol. Med.* **25,** 217–220.

313. Fillenz, M., Lowry, J. P., Boutelle, M. G., and Fray, A. E. (1999) The role of astrocytes and noradrenaline in neuronal glucose metabolism. *Acta Physiol. Scand.* **167,** 275–284.

314. Porter, J. T. and McCarthy, K. D. (1997) Astrocytic neurotransmitter receptors in situ and in vivo. *Prog. Neurobiol.* **51,** 439–455.

315. Seidman, K., Teng, A., Rosenkopf, R., Spilotro, P., and Weyhenmeyer, J. (1997) Isolation, cloning and characterization of a putative type-1 astrocyte cell line. *Brain Res.* **753,** 18–26.

316. Maragakis, N. J., Dietrich, J., Wong, V., et al. (2004) Glutamate transporter expression and function in human glial progenitors. *Glia* **45,** 133–143.

317. Mayer-Proschel, M., Liu, Y., Xue, H., Wu, Y., Carpenter, M. K., and Rao, M. S. (2002) Human neural precursor cells—an in vitro characterization. *Clin. Neurosci. Res.* **2,** 58–69.

318. Miller, R. H. and Szigeti, V. (1991) Clonal analysis of astrocyte diversity in neonatal rat spinal cord cultures. *Development* **113,** 353–362.

319. Bignami, A., Eng, L. F., Dahl, D., and Uyeda, C. T. (1972) Localization of the glial fibrillary acidic protein in astrocytes by immunofluorescence. *Brain Res.* **43,** 429–435.

320. Doetsch, F., Caille, I., Lim, D. A., Garcia-Verdugo, J. M., and Alvarez-Buylla, A. (1999) Subventricular zone astrocytes are neural stem cells in the adult mammalian brain. *Cell* **97,** 703–716.

8

PNS Precursor Cells in Development and Cancer

Houman D. Hemmati, Tanya A. Moreno, and Marianne Bronner-Fraser

INTRODUCTION

The peripheral nervous system (PNS) is comprised of groups of neurons and support cells whose cell bodies lie outside the spinal cord and brain. These peripheral ganglia relay sensory input back to the central nervous system (CNS), where the information is processed and physical responses are generated. The PNS is derived primarily from a population of precursor cells called neural crest cells that arise within the developing CNS but subsequently migrate to the periphery and are highly versatile with respect to the types of derivatives that they form.

The neural crest is one of the defining features of vertebrates. Neural crest cells originate in the ectoderm of the early embryo and develop as a ridge of cells flanking the rostrocaudal length of the open neural tube (Fig. 1), resembling a "crest." Initially, these cells appear to be multipotent and subsequently give rise to both neuronal and nonneuronal derivatives, including neurons and support cells of the PNS, pigment cells, smooth muscle cells, and cartilage and bone of the face and skull (1,2). Different populations of neural crest cells arise at different rostrocaudal levels of the neural axis. For example, at cranial levels, neural crest cells contribute to cranial sensory ganglia as well as skeletal elements of the face. In contrast, trunk neural crest cells never contribute to the bone or cartilage, but are the exclusive source of the peripheral ganglia and also contribute to the adrenal medulla (Fig. 2). Thus, neural crest cells at all axial levels appear to have multiple developmental potentials, but they differ from each other according to their level of origin. Recently, it has been shown that some neural crest cells are stem cells that self-renew in vivo and can contribute to at least some of the derivatives generated by the neural crest (3).

Interest in the mechanisms of induction, migration, and differentiation of neural crest cells has occupied developmental biologists for more than 130 yr (4–8), reprinted in ref. 9. Much is known about the later steps of neural crest development such as migration pathways and cell fate decisions (1,10–13). However, molecular aspects of these processes have only begun to be uncovered within the last two decades. This chapter summarizes recent findings regarding neural crest induction and the isolation and characterization of neural crest stem cells and discusses the involvement of neural

From: *Neural Development and Stem Cells, Second Edition*
Edited by: M. S. Rao © Humana Press Inc., Totowa, NJ

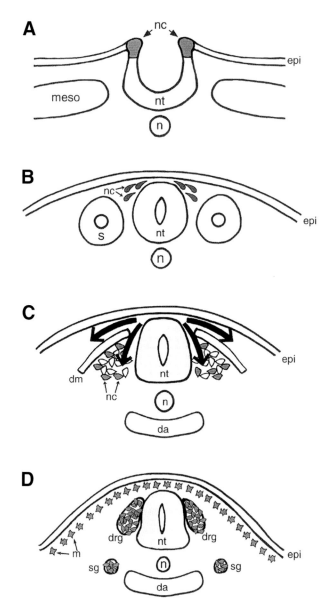

Fig. 1. Neural crest-forming regions and migration pathways in avians: cross-sectional view. **(A)** E1.5–2. Thickened epithelium at the midline begins to fold into a tube. The border of the neural and nonneural ectoderm is the site of neural crest formation. **(B)** E2–2.5. Neural crest cells delaminate from the dorsal neural tube and begin to migrate. **(C)** E3. Two migration pathways are shown in the trunk: the dorsolateral pathway passes between the dermomyotome and epidermis, and the ventral pathway passes through the sclerotome of the somites. **(D)** E4. Neural crest cells in the trunk populate the dorsal root ganglia and sympathetic ganglia and form melanocytes in the skin. da, Dorsal aorta; dm, dermomyotome; drg, dorsal root ganglion; epi, epidermis; m, melanocyte; meso, nonaxial mesoderm; nc, neural crest; nt, neural tube; s, somite; sg, sympathetic ganglion.

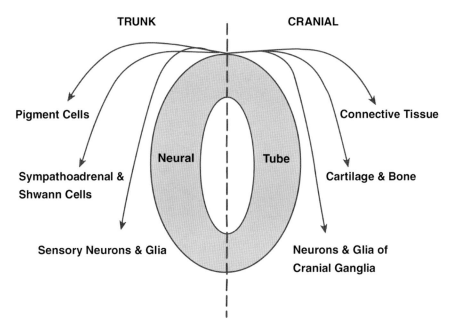

Fig. 2. Diagram illustrating the derivatives arising from trunk and cranial neural crest cells.

and neural crest stem cells in the development of tumors of the central and peripheral nervous systems.

ORIGIN AND INDUCTION OF THE NEURAL CREST

Neural Crest Origin

The ectoderm is the source of the tissues that eventually form the epidermis, CNS, and PNS of all vertebrates. It is initially patterned into neural and nonneural ectoderm by signals emanating from a mesodermal organizing center during gastrulation, that is, the dorsal lip of the blastopore (Spemann's organizer) in amphibians, Hensen's node in avians, the node in the mouse, and the embryonic shield in zebrafish. This process is called neural induction *(14–17)*. Later, the underlying mesoderm also plays a role in supplying rostrocaudal positional information to the neural ectoderm. At the start of neural induction, a broad domain of ectoderm adjacent to the midline thickens to form a columnar epithelium called the neural plate. The ectoderm outside of the neural plate will give rise to the epidermis and, in the head region, placodes. Placodes are regional thickenings of the ectoderm that will contribute to the cranial sensory ganglia and the sense organs of the head such as the eyes, ears, and nose *(18,19)*. They form the remainder of the PNS that is not generated by the neural crest.

Induction of the neural crest occurs at the border region between the future epidermis and the neural plate (reviewed in refs. *20* and *21*). As development proceeds, the neural plate begins to roll into a tube, causing its lateral edges to form folds that eventually approximate at the dorsal midline of the embryo. The neural folds typically contain the premigratory neural crest cells, although there are some exceptions. For example, in the frog, *Xenopus*, the cranial neural crest is not incorporated into the neural tube, but remains as a separate condensed mass of cells in the border region.

Thus, neural crest cells delaminate from the neuroepithelium and begin to migrate before neural tube closure in some species (e.g., mouse, *Xenopus*) *(9,22–26)*, whereas in other species (e.g., chicken), they migrate only after apposition of the neural folds *(27)*. Thus, the CNS is formed from the rolled-up neural plate, and the PNS is formed from the ectodermal placodes and the neural crest cells residing in and around the dorsal neural tube, which delaminate from the neural epithelium and migrate throughout the embryo (Fig. 1).

It was originally thought that the neural crest was a segregated population of cells, largely based on the fact that these cells appear morphologically distinct from neural tube cells in some species (e.g., axolotl and zebrafish). In other species, however, presumptive neural crest cells are not readily distinguishable from dorsal neural tube cells. Moreover, single-cell lineage analyses of the dorsal neural tube have shown that individual precursors in the neural tube can form both neural crest and neural tube derivatives in chick *(28,29)*, frog *(30)*, and mouse *(31,32)*. Even more strikingly, prior to neural tube closure, the neural folds can give rise to all three ectodermal derivatives: epidermis, neural tube, and neural crest *(13)*. Recently, genetic screens in zebrafish have identified a mutation called *narrowminded*, which supports a shared lineage between CNS and PNS cells. This mutant lacks both early neural crest cells (PNS) and sensory neurons in the neural tube (CNS) *(33)*. Further evidence for a common neural progenitor comes from isolation of stem cells from the spinal cord neuroepithelium (NEP) cells that can form both CNS and PNS derivatives *(34)*.

Not only has it been shown the neural tube/neural crest lineage is shared, but it has also been demonstrated that these cells are not irreversibly committed to either fate until relatively late in development. The ability of the neural tube to produce neural crest cells may persist for long periods. Sharma et al. *(35)* identified a late-emigrating population of neural tube cells that form neural crest-like derivatives. When transplanted into neural crest migratory pathways of younger embryos, these cells can migrate and differentiate into neural crest derivatives *(36)*. Conversely, it has been shown that early-migrating neural crest cells can reincorporate into the ventral neural tube and express markers characteristic of floor plate cells when challenged by transplantation *(37)*. In addition to neural crest cells that arise from the dorsal portion of the neural tube, there is evidence that multipotent precursors can arise from the ventral neural tube. These "VENT" cells appear to have the ability to form neural crest-like derivatives as well as other cell types *(38)*.

Neural Crest Induction

Cell–Cell Interaction at the Neural Plate Border

Several theories of neural crest induction exist (reviewed in ref. *19*). Both the mesoderm and the epidermal ectoderm have been shown to have the ability to induce neural crest. (This section discusses the evidence for ectodermal interactions; see later for a discussion of mesoderm.) The best supported model for neural crest induction is one in which cell–cell interaction at the border between neural and nonneural ectoderm is responsible for inducing the neural crest. In vivo grafting experiments suggest that interactions between presumptive epidermis and neural plate can form neural crest cells. In amphibians, epidermis grafted into the neural plate generates neural crest cells *(39,40)*. In avians and frogs, neural plate tissue grafted into the epidermal ectoderm results in the production of migratory cells expressing neural crest cell markers *(13,41,42)*. In vitro coculture experiments have similarly provided evidence for the sufficiency of the neural plate–epidermal ectoderm interaction to generate neural crest cells *(13,41,42)*. Interestingly, both the epidermis and the neural plate cells contributed to the neural crest cell population *(13,40)*.

The potential for more ventral neural tube cells to generate neural crest was examined in ablation experiments in which the dorsal region of the neural folds containing the presumptive neural crest cells was removed, thus bringing more ventral regions of the tube into contact with epidermal ectoderm. In this situation, neural crest cells were regenerated at the zone of contact *(43–47)*, for a limited period. These data show that a very important mechanism of neural crest induction is mediated through cell–cell interactions at the border between the epidermal ectoderm and the neural plate.

The Role of BMPs in Neural Crest Induction: Setting Up the Neural Plate Border Region

There is growing evidence, particularly from the *Xenopus* system, that members of the transforming growth factor-β (TGF-β) superfamily of signaling molecules play an integral role in setting up the border between neural and nonneural ectoderm. Given that neural crest cells arise at this border, it is likely that these cells are an important target of this signaling process.

Several lines of evidence support the idea that bone morphogenic protein (BMP) molecules play a role in neural induction (for review, see refs. *15* and *16*). *Xenopus* BMP-4 is expressed throughout the ectoderm prior to neural induction and then is lost from regions fated to become the neural plate *(48–50)*. The secreted BMP antagonists noggin *(51,52)*, chordin *(53,54)*, and follistatin *(55,56)* all are expressed in Spemann's organizer, the tissue responsible for patterning the ectoderm. Thus, the neural plate forms adjacent to the organizer, the source of BMP inhibition, whereas the nonneural ectoderm lies distal to the organizer (Fig. 3).

One possibility is that inhibition of BMP signaling is sufficient to generate both the neural plate and the neural crest, with high levels of inhibition yielding neural tissue and intermediate levels yielding neural crest. The idea that a diffusible morphogen could act to instruct the ectoderm to assume the various available fates was first proposed by Raven and Kloos *(57)*, who hypothesized that an "evocator" present in a graded fashion could generate neural crest at low levels and neural plate and neural crest at high levels (reviewed in ref. *19*). In *Xenopus* ectodermal explants (animal caps), varying the level of BMP activity leads to varying fates of ectoderm *(16,58)*. Overexpression of a dominant-negative BMP receptor *(59)* or the BMP antagonist chordin in *Xenopus* ectodermal explants causes neural crest marker expression and in whole embryos enhances the neural crest domain in a dose-dependent fashion *(60)*. In contrast, the reciprocal experiment of overexpressing BMP-4 itself in intact embryos does not influence the size of the neural crest domain. Instead, the size of the neural plate decreases in a dose-dependent fashion, thus moving the location, but not the extent, of the presumptive neural crest *(60)*. Furthermore, chordin by itself cannot induce robust expression of neural crest markers in *Xenopus* animal caps *(60)*. Taken together, these results indicate that inhibition of BMP signaling alone is not sufficient to induce neural crest formation.

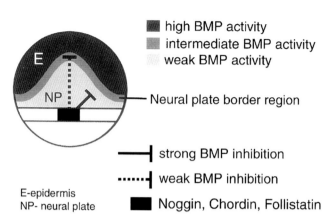

■ high BMP activity
■ intermediate BMP activity
  weak BMP activity

── Neural plate border region

──┤ strong BMP inhibition

┈┈┈┤ weak BMP inhibition

■ Noggin, Chordin, Follistatin

E-epidermis
NP- neural plate

Fig. 3. Schematic diagram of the *Xenopus* model of neural induction. The BMP antagonists *noggin*, *chordin*, and *follistatin* are secreted from Spemann's organizer (*black box*) to modulate BMP activity in the ectoderm. The activity of BMP molecules establishes three fates of ectoderm: lowest activity = neural plate; intermediate activity = neural crest; highest activity = epidermis. This simplistic model does not include the evidence for the involvement of other molecules in neural and neural crest induction, but is intended as a simplified model of neural induction. (Modified from ref. *60*.)

Genetic Evidence for the Involvement of TGF-β Family Members in Neural Crest Induction

Genetic evidence in the zebrafish supports a role for TGF-β family molecules influencing the fate of the ectoderm. Nguyen et al. *(61)* have investigated *swirl (62,63)*, a mutation in the zebrafish BMP-2 gene. *swirl* mutants display a loss of neural crest progenitors, whereas mutations in genes downstream of BMP-2b such as *somitabun* (mutation in Smad5, a BMP signal transducer) expand the neural crest domain *(61)*. The zebrafish mutant *radar*, which affects a dpp-Vg1-related molecule distinct from the BMP-2/4 and BMP-5/8 subgroups *(64;* and see ref. *65* for a review of TGF-β relationships), results in the loss of the neural crest marker msxC and selected neural crest derivatives. Conversely, overexpression of the *radar* gene causes up-regulation of msxC expression, but only in areas contiguous with the endogenous msxC domain *(64)*. In these mutants, however, the mesoderm underlying the neural crest is also affected, allowing for the possibility that the strength of the phenotype is not due solely to changes in BMP signaling in the ectoderm. This suggests that the activity of TGF-β family members contributes to the patterning of the ectoderm. However, only certain regions are competent to respond to these molecules, suggesting that other gene activities may be required for the establishment of the neural crest.

Transgenic mice bearing null mutations in BMP-4 *(66)*, follistatin *(67)*, or noggin *(68)* do not display the neural defects that would be expected by extrapolation from the experiments in *Xenopus* described earlier. It has been suggested that redundancy between different BMP family members, the antagonizing molecules, or other developmental defects may obscure the phenotype (reviewed in ref. *69*). Alternatively, there may be interesting species differences in the process of neural induction and neural crest formation. Indeed, many studies in the chick embryo have added to the interspecies discrepancies that are found on investigation of the role of TGF-β signaling as a mechanism for neural induction and neural crest formation.

BMPs Can Induce Neural Crest in Culture

In the chick embryo, BMP-4 and BMP-7 are expressed in the epidermal ectoderm that contacts the neural tube *(70,71)*. As development proceeds, however, expression is lost in the epidermal ectoderm but BMP-4 is expressed in the neural folds and dorsal neural tube *(72)*, along with another TGF-β family member, *dorsalin-1*, which is up-regulated after neural tube closure *(70,73)*. When added to isolated intermediate neural plates in tissue culture, both BMP-4 and -7 have been shown to induce neural crest markers and migratory cells *(70)*. This seemingly contrasts with the results in *Xenopus*, where inhibition of BMP signaling yields neural fates. However, the paradigm for neural induction by BMP repression in the neural plate does not appear to function in the chick embryo at the time of neural crest/neural plate border formation. *Chordin*, which inhibits BMP activity, is expressed in the avian organizer (Hensen's node) but alone cannot neuralize ectoderm *(73)*. In addition, neither BMP-4 nor -7 is sufficient to repress neural induction in the neural plate when ectopically expressed *(73)*.

Furthermore, by implanting noggin-producing cells into the neural tube or under the neural fold regions, it has been shown that BMP signaling is required in the chick neural tube for expression of neural crest markers, but not at the stage at which BMP is expressed in the ectoderm *(74)*. Pera et al. *(75)* found that ectopic expression of BMP-2 or -4 under the neural/nonneural border region distorts the neural plate and causes epidermal ectoderm marker expression in areas that would normally give rise to neural plate. Taken together, these results seem to indicate that BMP signaling plays several important roles in neural crest development, beginning with the positioning of the neural plate border and continuing with the maintenance of neural crest induction. Importantly, it is likely that other molecules are involved in the initiation of neural crest induction. Later, BMPs in the dorsal neural tube induce roof plate cells and sensory neurons *(76)*. Still later, BMPs are involved in the differentiation of sympathoadrenal precursors from neural crest cells *(77–79)*.

There is no direct evidence that either BMP-4 or -7 is the molecule that diffuses from the epidermal ectoderm to induce crest cells *(70)*. Indeed, it was shown that BMP-4 induces epidermis at the expense of neural tissue *(80)*. The ability of BMP-4 and -7 to induce neural crest from neural plate cultures *(70,76)* may be a reflection of the molecule having first induced epidermis, which in turn interacted with the neural plate to induce neural crest. Another possibility is that exogenous BMP bypasses an epidermal signaling event and mimics a later action of endogenous BMP signaling in the dorsal neural tube that is sufficient to generate neural crest cells. This possibility is supported by the later neural tube requirement for BMP signaling to produce neural crest cells, as demonstrated by Selleck et al. *(74)*. Thus, the action of BMPs may be required within the responding tissues to maintain crest production, rather than being a property of the initial induction (reviewed in ref. *21*).

It is important to bear in mind that although many experimental differences between species are reported in the literature, these are most likely to be a result of the rather striking differences among the organisms that are used for study. Differences in morphology and timing of development must require differences in gene expression to achieve the overall goal of properly forming the animal. For example, the frog embryo begins as a hollow ball of cells, whereas the chick embryo begins as a flat sheet of cells. In the frog embryo, development relies for a period on maternal stores of messenger

RNAs, which contrasts with the chick embryo. Moreover, the distances between signaling centers and their responding tissues may require different mechanisms in order to effect induction of neural tissue and other developmental events. Although there are many apparent species differences, these may reflect variations in the finer details that accommodate spatial and temporal variations among organisms; the general mechanisms are likely to be common for all vertebrates *(21)*.

Other Sources of Neural Crest-Inducing Signals

The Mesoderm

It would be overly simplistic to assume that a single signaling event within the ectoderm is sufficient to account for induction of the neural crest. Many lines of evidence suggest that the nonaxial mesoderm is also involved in inducing the neural crest. Although conjugating epidermis and neural plate in vitro is sufficient to induce neural crest markers in the absence of mesoderm *(13,40–42)*, mesoderm could represent an important modifier. Mesoderm–neural plate conjugates do not induce early neural crest markers *(13,81)*. However, it was demonstrated that paraxial mesoderm conjugated with neural plate could induce the formation of melanocytes, a neural crest derivative *(13)*. Similarly, nonaxial mesoderm from both chick and frog can induce neural crest markers in neural plate coculture experiments *(59,82,83)*, and removal of the nonaxial mesoderm before neural induction is complete results in a failure of the ectoderm to express neural crest markers *(59,83)*. The evidence that mesoderm can influence neural crest formation suggests that there may be other molecules involved in the early steps of neural crest induction.

Wnt Family Members

As discussed earlier, it seems likely that inhibition of BMP alone cannot account for neural crest induction, making it probable that other signaling systems are involved. Possible candidates for involvement in this process are secreted molecules expressed in both mesoderm and ectoderm, that have been implicated in patterning the neural tube. These include members of the wingless/int family known in vertebrates as Wnts *(84)* and the fibroblast growth factor (FGF) family *(85,86)*. In *Xenopus* ectodermal explants (animal caps), Wnt1 and Wnt3a *(87)*, Wnt7b *(17)*, and Wnt8 *(60)*, in conjunction with inhibition of BMP signaling (i.e., neural induction), can induce the expression of neural crest markers. Furthermore, overexpression of β-catenin (a downstream component of the Wnt signaling pathway) expands the neural crest domain; expression of a dominant-negative Wnt ligand eliminates the neural crest domain in *Xenopus* embryos *(60)*.

One of the earliest neural crest markers in *Xenopus* is the zinc finger transcription factor, Slug *(88)* (Fig. 4). When animal caps overexpressing Slug are juxtaposed to Wnt8-expressing explants, neural crest markers are induced, thus bypassing the requirement for inhibition of BMP signaling *(60)*. In contrast, Slug alone cannot induce neural crest *(60)*. Slug, in turn, can expand its own expression domain when overexpressed in the whole embryo *(60)*. These results suggest that a two-signal model may account for the events underlying neural crest formation, such that Wnt signaling together with inhibition of BMP signaling induces the neural crest marker, Slug, with Slug expression abrogating further need for BMP inhibition *(60)*. A recent study has

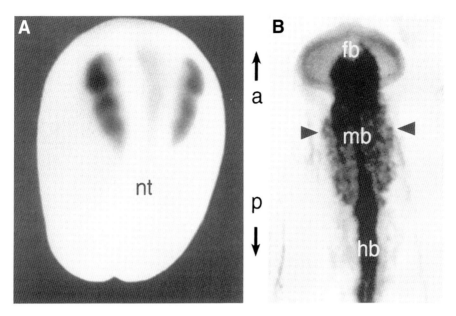

Fig. 4. *Slug* expression pattern in *Xenopus* and chick. The zinc-finger transcription factor *Slug* is an early marker for the neural crest in *Xenopus* and chick. (**A**) A late-neurula *Xenopus* embryo with *Slug* mRNA expression in the cranial neural crest on both sides of the closing neural tube. The groove down the central portion of the embryo is the forming neural tube. (**B**) An E1.5 (10-somite stage) chick embryo with *Slug* mRNA marking the early-migrating neural crest in the head (*arrowheads*) and premigratory neural crest at more posterior levels of the neural tube. a, Anterior; p, posterior; fb, forebrain; mb, midbrain; hb, hindbrain; nt, neural tube.

shown that in *Xenopus*, Wnt signals induce the expression of the proto-oncogene c-Myc in neural crest cells prior to the expression of Slug *(89)*. Knock-downs of c-Myc activity result in a loss of neural crest cells and their derivatives in vivo *(89)*.

Many Wnt molecules are expressed in spatiotemporal patterns appropriate for involvement in various aspects of neural crest development. *Xenopus* Wnt8 is expressed in the ventrolateral mesoderm *(90)*, a tissue that has been shown to be a neural crest inducer when conjugated with neural plate in vitro *(59,82,83)*, and avian Wnt-8C is similarly expressed in the nonaxial mesoderm *(91)*. In *Xenopus*, an early Wnt8 signal induces expression of Pax3 and Msx-1 in the lateral neural plate *(92)*. This establishes a posteriolateral domain from which neural crest cells will eventually arise *(92)*. *Xenopus* Wnt7b is expressed throughout the ectoderm at gastrulation *(17)*, and other Wnts may well be expressed in the ectoderm.

In chick *(41,93)*, frog *(94,95)*, and mouse embryos *(96,97)*, Wnt1 and Wnt3a are expressed in the dorsal neural tube well after the initial expression of neural crest markers, although *Xenopus* Wnt3a is also expressed before neural tube closure at the edges of the neural plate *(95)*. Furthermore, avian neural crest can be induced in conjugates of epidermis and neural plate without the concomitant expression of either Wnt1 or Wnt3a *(41)*. This suggests that Wnt1 and -3a are not involved in the initial induction of neural crest. However, Wnt1/3a double knockout mice have a reduction in neurogenic and gliogenic neural crest derivatives, suggesting that fewer neural crest cells emerge in embryos lacking both genes *(98)*. Not all neural crest derivatives are affected, with ventralmost derivatives such as sympathetic ganglia demonstrating normal morphology, whereas dorsal root ganglia are markedly reduced. This is consistent with the possibility that these Wnts play a later maintenance role in neural crest production by the neural tube. Wnts may be involved in the expansion of neural crest progenitors, most likely by regulating the proliferation of the cells after induction has occurred but prior to commencement of emigration *(98)*. Garcia-Castro et al. *(99)* have recently shown that a Wnt family member, Wnt6, is likely the early epidermal neural crest inducer in the chick. Wnt6 is expressed in the ectoderm adjacent to the neural folds, but not in the neural folds and neural plate, at a time when neural crest cells are being induced. *Drosophila* Wingless protein, which activates Wnt signaling in vertebrates, can induce neural crest from naïve neural plate in vitro in the absence of additives, whereas Wnt inhibition blocks neural crest formation in vivo. Taken together, these results demonstrating that Wnt signaling is both necessary and sufficient to induce neural crest in avian embryos *(99)*.

Wnt family members may also be able to control some aspects of neural crest cell fate. In zebrafish experiments, single neural crest cells overexpressing molecules of the Wnt signaling pathway form pigment cells at the expense of neurons or glia. Conversely, overexpressing inhibitors of the pathway biases the neural crest cells to form neurons at the expense of pigment cells *(100)*.

Recent work by Baker et al. *(101)* has put forward a novel model for Wnt function. These authors demonstrate that expression of *Xenopus* Wnt8, mouse Wnt8, and downstream Wnt targets in frog ectodermal explants can induce expression of the early panneural marker neural cell adhesion molecule (NCAM), without neural induction by BMP antagonists. In addition, they demonstrate that Wnt signaling components suppress BMP-4 expression in ectoderm explants as assayed by *in situ* hybridization. In fact, Wnt8, and not the BMP antagonist noggin, seems to be capable of blocking BMP-4 expression in the neural plate throughout gastrula stages, suggesting that an early Wnt signal and not a direct BMP antagonist is responsible for the early inhibition of BMP-4 expression in the neural plate. Finally, the authors suggest that there may be parallel pathways for the effects of Wnt signaling in neural induction because inhibition of Wnt8-mediated activation of the neural inducers Xnr3 and *siamois* did not abrogate Wnt8's ability to itself promote neural induction. These results suggest that Wnt signaling may be involved in multiple inductive events in early development. The ramifications of these data for the role of Wnt signaling in neural crest induction are unclear, as these investigators did not explore the effects of the perturbations on neural crest markers. Previous results showing that Wnts could not induce neural crest without a coexpressed neural inducer *(17,60,87)*, taken together with the results of Baker et al. *(101)*, may indicate that the precise levels of Wnt signaling are critical. Further investigation will be required to determine exactly what role Wnt plays during neural crest development.

Fibroblast Growth Factors

Other molecules expressed in the mesoderm have been shown to have neural crest inducing activities. FGF signaling can induce neural crest markers in frog ectodermal explants when in the presence of BMP antagonists *(60,102,103)*. Overexpression of a dominant-negative FGF receptor can inhibit expression of the early neural crest marker

XSlug in whole embryos *(102)*. Other investigators have demonstrated that FGF signaling has a posteriorizing effect on neural tissue *(52,103–106)*. Indeed, members of the FGF family are spatiotemporally expressed in a way that is consistent with their playing roles in the process of neural and/or neural crest induction *(107–113)*. Recent work by Streit et al. has shown that in the chick, an FGF signal from Hensen's node initiates neural induction prior to the onset of gastrulation, inducing the expression of early neural genes such as *ERNI*, *Sox2*, and *Sox3 (113)*. The results indicate that FGFs may be able to generate both posterior and lateral (i.e., neural crest) fates in the CNS and PNS. The role of FGFs becomes complicated in light of evidence from transgenic frog experiments, however, in which frog embryos expressing a dominant-negative FGF receptor have normally developing posterior neural tissue and border regions including the neural crest, although the investigators did not test a full range of neural crest markers *(114)*. Moreover, FGF-treated neural plate explants do not form neural crest tissue *(102)*. Another recent study suggests that FGF-8 may mediate the inductive effects of paraxial mesoderm on frog animal caps and may be sufficient to induce expression of several neural crest markers *(115)*. However, other assays suggest that neural crest induction by FGF may be a secondary result of its ability to induce a member of the Wnt family *(60)*.

Notch and Noelin

Recent work has implicated both Notch signaling and Noelin-1 in the generation of neural crest cells. Activation of the Notch receptor results in cleavage of its intracellular domain, which translocates to the nucleus and activates transcription *(116)*. Notch1 is expressed throughout the neural plate, with higher levels in the neural crest, whereas its ligand Delta1 is expressed in the epidermal ectoderm *(117–120)*. Notch signaling has been shown to be required for neural crest formation in avian, zebrafish, and *Xenopus* embryos *(118,121,122)*, perhaps by repressing Neurogenin-1 function *(121)*. In the chick and *Xenopus*, Notch promotes neural crest formation by modulating levels of BMP-4 expression: in the chick, Notch maintains BMP-4 expression *(118)*, whereas in *Xenopus* Notch represses BMP-4 transcription *(122)*. In zebrafish, Notch promotes formation of neural crest by repressing Neurogenin-1 function *(121)*.

Barembaum et al. have recently demonstrated that the secreted glycoprotein Noelin-1 plays a role in the competence of neural tissue to form neural crest formation *(123)*. Noelin-1 mRNA is restricted to the dorsal neural folds and migrating neural crest cells in avian embryos. Retroviral-mediated overexpression of Noelin-1 in the neural tube increases both the number of neural crest cells generated and the length of time neural crest cells continue to emigrate from the neural tube. These findings suggest that Noelin-1 may play a role in rendering the neural tube cells competent to form neural crest *(123)*.

Neural Crest Stem Cells

In the past decade, work by several investigators has led to the prospective identification and purification of neural crest stem cells—cells with the potential to self-renew and also to give rise to the diverse population of derivatives that are generated by the neural crest. The first neural crest stem cells were isolated in vitro by clonal analysis of cells that were fractionated from rat neural crest cultures by cell sorting based on expression of a cell surface epitope *(124)*. These cells can be replated to form new stem cells and also can give rise to "blast" cells that are partially restricted to form neurons or glia. These include the sympathoadrenal sublineage, which includes precursors to sympathetic neurons and adrenomedullary cells *(125,126)*, that, in the embryo, appear specified by the time that neural crest-derived cells reach their sites of localization around the dorsal aorta.

Specific molecules can instruct neural crest stem cells to adopt specific fates; for example, glial growth factor (neuregulin) causes the development of glia (Schwann cells) BMP-2 biases clones to develop into neurons (and a small number of smooth muscle cells), and TGF-β1 promotes development of smooth muscle cells *(127–129)*. It has recently been shown that transient Notch activation promotes glial production by neural crest stem cells at the expense of neurogenesis, even in the presence of BMP-2 *(130)*. Thus, it is interesting to note that members of the TGF-β superfamily are not only involved in induction of the neural crest but are also implicated in subsequent cell fate decisions.

Although the neural crest stem cells are very useful in testing the ability of factors to promote certain cell fate decisions, there are possible caveats; for example, the stem cell qualities of the purified cells may have been acquired in vitro and may not reflect an actual state that is present in the embryo. The findings of Frank and colleagues *(35,36)* that neural tubes can give rise to neural crest-like cells that emigrate long after the normal period of neural crest formation suggest that neural crest stem cells may persist within the spinal cord and other sites for long periods. Consistent with this possibility, Morrison et al. *(3)* have recently isolated neural crest stem cells from embryonic rat peripheral nerve at E14.5. The cells were isolated by fluorescence-activated cell sorting using cell surface epitopes p75 and P0. Under proper culture conditions, these cells self-renew and can differentiate into neurons, glia, and smooth muscle cells within single colonies. The cells are also instructively promoted to form neurons or glia by exposure to either BMP-2 or glial growth factor, respectively, in clonal cultures. An important test of the qualities of these neural crest stem cells is to determine whether newly isolated cells are multipotent when transplanted into an embryo. Indeed, freshly isolated cells that were p75$^+$/P0$^-$ have stem cell properties and can be back-transplanted into chick embryos, giving rise to both neurons and glia as assayed by differential marker expression *(3)*. However, neural crest stem cells sorted from embryonic day 14.5 (E14.5) rat spinal cords have been shown to have cell-intrinsic differences in developmental potential in vivo from their counterparts, cultured E10.5 neural tube explants *(131)*. The older, sorted neural crest cells produce fewer neurons and appear unable to give rise to noradrenergic neurons, owing to reduced sensitivity to the neurogenic signal BMP-2 *(131)*. This phenomenon suggests that neural crest stem cells can change as a function of time and perhaps in response to local environmental factors in the periphery. By labeling actively dividing cells in embryos with the thymidine analog bromodeoxyuridine, it was shown that endogenous neural crest stem cells persist in the embryo by self-renewing *(3)*.

Self-renewing neural crest stem cells have also recently been isolated by flow cytometry from both embryonic *(132)* and adult *(133)* gut. Gut neural crest stem cells can be sorted based on expression of both p75 and α4 integrin *(132)*. The prospective isolation of gut neural crest stem cells has proven particularly important toward the understanding of Hirschsprung disease, a common gut motility defect caused by the absence of enteric nervous system ganglia in the hindgut *(134)*. Gut neural crest stem cells from normal mice were found to express high levels of the glial cell line-derived neurotrophic factor (GDNF) receptor Ret, and GDNF promoted migration of neural crest stem cells *(134)*. Ret -/-null mice were found to have far fewer neural crest stem cells in the gut as compared to wild-type mice *(134)*. Yet there were no differences in proliferation, differentiation, or survival between neural crest stem cells from normal and mutant mice, suggesting that the absence of enteric ganglia in Ret null mice is caused by a failure of Ret null neural crest stem cells to migrate into the distal gut *(134)*.

LINEAGE AND CELL FATE DECISIONS IN THE NEURAL CREST

The existence of neural crest stem cells in the embryo supports the idea that the fate of neural crest cells in vivo is determined primarily by their environment *(135)*. Neural crest cell fate decisions and their relationships to cell lineage have been debated for many years. Although it has been accepted that at least some, if not most, neural crest cells are multipotent, some evidence indicates that other neural crest cells have restricted fates in vivo *(28,29,136)*. However, in these experiments, the potential of the cells has not actually been tested by challenging the cells with all possible factors that might influence cell fate choice. It is obviously difficult to quantify and compare the environment of one cell with another, beginning from their origins in the neural tube and following their migration trajectories through the periphery. In these lineage experiments, single dye-labeled or retrovirally tagged cells often gave rise to clones of progeny with multiple derivatives but sometimes gave rise to clones of only one cell type, suggesting an earlier specification for that progenitor cell. Thus, alternate methods of marking and challenging neural crest cells will be necessary to define the state of multipotency at the single cell level. This is an area in which the neural crest stem cells and their blast cells promise to provide new and important information.

Recent work has shown that the HMG-group transcriptional regulator Sox10 maintains the multipotency of neural crest stem cells *(137)*. In rodents, Sox10 is expressed in neural crest cells at the time of their emigration from the dorsal neural tube. Loss-of-function mutations in Sox10 result in defects in multiple neural crest derivatives *(138)*. Interestingly, overexpression of Sox10 in neural crest stem cells maintains their neurogenic and gliogenic potentials, despite challenges by opposing differentiation factors such as BMP2 or TGF-β *(137)*.

Mechanisms of Neural Crest Diversification

If neural crest cells are truly multipotent and receive instructions for differentiation only when migrating to or reaching their final destinations, then it is interesting to consider how cells are instructed to take on different fates. For example, neural crest cells in the dorsal root ganglia differentiate into both sensory neurons and glia. An asymmetric cell division could produce a blast cell of each type, which could in turn replicate. Alternatively, the progenitor may replicate itself and produce a more restricted daughter cell, which then goes on to form the final derivatives. The latter seems more likely given the ability of neural crest stem cells to self-renew.

Environmental Cues vs Timing of Emigration

Both the environment and the timing of emigration from the neural tube have been proposed to affect the cell fate decisions of the neural crest. A restriction in available cell fate accompanies the time of emigration from the neural tube: the latest migrating cells only populate the dorsal root ganglia as neurons and form melanocytes in the skin and feathers *(35,139)*. However, when transplanted into earlier embryos, neural crest-like cells derived from much older spinal cords were able to migrate more ventrally and make sympathetic and peripheral neurons *(36,140)*. Similarly, in the head, late-migrating cells formed dorsal derivatives only because of the presence, ventrally, of earlier migrating cells; however, they are not restricted in potential *(141)*. Furthermore, the latest migrating cells of the main wave of crest emigration make melanocytes in the skin, but skin culture experiments show that they have the potential to form neurons *(142)*. This suggests that the restriction in available fates in these cases is made by the environment that the cells occupy rather than the time that they emerge from the neural tube (Fig. 1).

Additional evidence for the influence of environment on neural crest cell fate comes from neural crest stem cells, in which single progenitor cells can generate smooth muscle cells when exposed to TGF-β molecules. However, a community effect takes place when denser cultures are exposed to TGF-β molecules, such that either neurons form or cell death occurs, rather than differentiation of smooth muscle cells *(143)*. These data suggest that cell fate in the embryo could also be determined by community effects in which cells respond differently to the same factors depending on the density of neighboring cells *(143)*. Other interesting studies on neural crest stem cells reveal that they can integrate multiple instructive cues and are biased to certain levels of responsiveness based on the growth factors to which they are exposed. If cultures of neural crest stem cells are exposed to saturating levels of both BMP-2 and glial growth factor (neuregulin), BMP-2 appears dominant and neurons differentiate. However, BMP-2 and TGF-β1 seem to be codominant *(129)*.

There is evidence, however, that some neural crest cell populations may undergo early fate restrictions. By culturing "early-migrating" and "late-migrating" trunk neural crest cells, Artinger and Bronner-Fraser *(144)* found that the latter are more restricted in their developmental potential than the former; although they can form pigment cells and sensory-like neurons, they fail to form sympathetic neurons. In addition, late-migrating cells transplanted into an earlier environment can colonize the sympathetic ganglia but failed to form adrenergic cells *(144)*. Thus, the time that a precursor leaves the neural tube may contribute to its potency. Perez et al. *(145)* have provided evidence for early specification of sensory neurons by the basic helix–loop–helix transcription factors Neurogenin-1 and -2. These molecules are expressed early in a subset of neural crest cells, and ectopic expression of the molecules biases migrating neural crest cells to localize in the sensory ganglia and express sensory neuron markers.

The mechanism for formation of sensory neurons from neural crest cells has remained a mystery until recently. In an elegant set of experiments, Lee et al. have demonstrated that activation of the canonical Wnt signaling pathway instructs neural crest cells to adopt a sensory neuronal fate *(146)*. Transgenic mice in which a constitutively active form of β-catenin, a key mediator in the canonical Wnt signaling pathway, was selectively expressed in neural crest cells produced only sensory neurons at the expense of other neural crest derivatives *(146)*. Moreover, exogenous Wnt added to clonal cultures of neural crest cells in vitro similarly biased the cells toward a sensory neuronal phenotype without altering their proliferation *(146)*.

Recent work implicates FGF and Wnt signaling in influencing the fate decisions of neural crest cells *(146,147)*. Hoxa2 expression in hindbrain neural crest appears to confer second branchial arch identity at, causing them to form second arch skeletal elements in the head *(148,149)*. Trainor et al. have shown that FGF-8 signals alone or from the isthmic organizer can inhibit Hoxa2, allowing second-arch cells to adopt a first-arch fate and duplicate first-arch skeletal structures *(147)*.

The study of neural crest stem cells has yielded new insight into the effects of environment and timing on the function of neural crest cells *(3,132,133)*. Bixby et al. have compared the properties of neural crest stem cells purified from the sciatic nerve and gut of rat embryos at E14, a time at when neurogenesis is predominant in the gut while gliogenesis is most prevalent in nerves *(132)*. In both cell culture and transplantation experiments, gut neural crest stem cells produced primarily neurons, a function of their increased sensitivity to BMP-4, whereas sciatic nerve neural crest stem cells formed mostly glia, owing to their enhanced sensitivity to neuregulin and the Notch ligand Delta *(132)*. These stem cells maintain their difference even after many days of culture and subcloning, suggesting that the differences are intrinsic to the cells *(132)*. In contrast, neural crest stem cells purified from postnatal rat gut formed primarily glia after they were transplanted into the peripheral nerves of chick embryos, demonstrating that gut neural crest stem cells undergo temporal changes that help determine their cell fates in vivo *(133)*. Some important questions arise from this work: What signals cause the spatial and temporal differences observed in different neural crest stem cells? What are the normal functions of neural crest stem cells that persist into adulthood?

Another way to account for the process of promoting two different cell fates from one precursor population within a single tissue is the proposal that temporal changes in the target environment bias the cell fate decision *(136)*. This is supported by the fact that first neurons and then glia are born in the dorsal root ganglia (e.g., ref. *150*). The target environment could be influenced to change by early differentiating neural crest cells themselves; for example, some neurons produce glial-promoting factors *(130,151–155)*. The strongest evidence of this phenomenon comes from the effects of Notch activation on cell fate of neural crest stem cells *(130)*. Notch activation by ligands such as Delta, which are expressed on differentiating neuroblasts, induces glial differentiation at the expense of neurogenesis, even in the presence of BMP-2 *(130)*. These findings suggest that differentiating neuroblasts might activate Notch in neighboring neural crest cells as a feedback signal to promote gliogenesis. Also, the loss of certain inhibitory glycoconjugates from the extracellular matrix in the dorsolateral migration pathway has been linked to the migration of late-emigrating neural crest cells along this pathway *(156)*, where they are exposed to melanogenic factors and hence adopt a melanocyte fate *(157)*. Thus, there is evidence for the influence of both the timing of emigration and environmental cues in determining neural crest fates.

Progressive Lineage Restriction

It has been proposed that neural crest cells adopt specific fates by progressive lineage restrictions *(12,77,158)*. One way to explain the intermingling of clonally related neurons and glia is that the choice is made stochastically, such that each cell has the capacity to adopt either fate, and environmental factors act by influencing the probability of a fate choice rather than imposing strict commitments *(136)*. Trentin et al. have recently taken individual avian neural crest cells through multiple rounds of serial recloning to demonstrate that both cranial and trunk neural crest cells give rise to progeny cells in a hierarchical manner, with progressively restricted developmental potentials, akin to the lineage hierarchy formed by hematopoietic stem cells *(159)*. Strikingly, they found that only two types of intermediate bipotent precursors, glial-melanocytic and glial-myofibroblast precursors had the ability to self-renew *(159)*. Support for the idea of progressive fate restriction comes also from the NEP, which can give rise to both CNS- and PNS-type stem cells. PNS stem cells (indistinguishable from neural crest stem cells, as described in ref. *11*) are formed on addition of BMP-2/-4 to the NEP cell cultures *(34)*. BMP-2, a molecule that is known to instruct neural crest stem cells toward an adrenergic neuronal fate, is expressed in the dorsal aorta, near where sympathetic ganglia form *(129,160,161)*. Thus, there is evidence that environmental cues may be able to promote progressive restriction of neural crest cell fates. Many factors act selectively by affecting the proliferation or survival of neural crest derivatives; others act instructively on multipotent progenitors to promote one fate over another. Further work will be required to answer the complex question of how individual cells within the same environment can adopt different fates. The evidence in support of both multipotentiality and lineage restriction may imply that neural crest cells take cues from both the timing of emigration from the neural tube and the environments to which they are exposed in cell lineage decisions. For more discussion on the topic of neural crest diversification, the reader is referred to several recent reviews *(162–164)*.

CANCER STEM CELLS IN THE CENTRAL AND PERIPHERAL NERVOUS SYSTEM

A great deal of recent interest has focused on the striking similarities between stem cells and cancer cells in the nervous and hematopoietic systems as well as in various epithelial cell types *(165,166)*. In particular, stem cells and some cancer cells share the fundamental properties of self-renewal and the ability to differentiate into multiple distinct cell types *(167–169)*. The mechanisms underlying self-renewal of normal stem cells are known to be tightly regulated *(170–173)*. In contrast, self-renewal of cancer cells is, by definition, aberrant.

The multipotency and self-renewal of some cancer cells raises the possibility that cancer might arise from the transformation of normal somatic stem or progenitor cells. In many cancers, it is known that only a small subset of cancer cells (called tumor or cancer stem cells) is able to drive the growth of the tumor and give rise to secondary tumors in vivo. However, the origins and phenotypes of those cells were unknown *(174)*. One interesting possibility is that these cancer stem cells may be lineally related to transformed stem or progenitor cells.

Recent work has identified and characterized cancer stem or stem-like cells in leukemia, breast cancer, and brain tumors, and shown that these cells can self-renew, are multipotent, and can recapitulate characteristics of the original tumor in vitro and/or in vivo *(169,175–179)*. The existence of cancer stem cells was first proven in acute myeloid leukemia *(169)*. Bonnet and Dick showed that a rare subset of cells from this cancer was able to proliferate extensively; in contrast, to the majority of leukemic cells have limited proliferative ability *(169)*. Moreover, these leukemia stem cells, but not nonstem cells from the same patients' population of leukemic cells, could transfer the disease after transplantation into immunodeficient mice *(169)*. This hyperproliferative subset of cells from these tumors was found to be phenotypically similar to normal hematopoietic stem cells based on expression of cell-surface antigens, suggesting that they might be related to the normal stem cells *(169)*. However, the possibility exists the leukemic stem cells arise from the transformed committed progenitor cells that have reacquired stem cell characteristics *(180)*. To address this question, Cozzio et al. recently transduced both hematopoietic stem cells and myeloid progenitor cells with a leukemogenic fusion protein, and found that transformation of both cell types produces an identical type of tumor in vivo *(181)*. Therefore, it is possible that cancer stem cells arise from cells other than multipotent stem cells *(181)*.

Similar experiments in breast cancer have demonstrated the existence of breast cancer stem cells *(175)*. Al-Hajj et al. used cell surface markers on uncultured breast cancer cells to fractionate them into different subsets, and transplanted the cells into immunodeficient mice *(175)*. Only cells that phenotypically resembled normally mammary epithelial progenitor cells were able to give rise to tumors in the mice *(175)*. Moreover, the tumors that formed in mice histologically resembled the tumors from which their stem cells were derived and themselves contained progenitor cells that formed tumors in other mice, suggesting that breast cancer stem cells can self-renew in vivo *(175)*.

The search for cancer stem-like cells in central nervous system malignancies has recently borne fruit *(176–179)*. It has been proposed for some time that brain tumors arise from the transformation of self-renewing neural stem or progenitor cells *(182–184)*. Aside from the fact that some brain tumors contain both neurons and glia, many brain tumors (particularly those occurring in children) arise from the ventricular zone, where neural stem cells reside postnatally *(185–188)*. Like neural stem cells, some brain tumors express the intermediate filament *nestin*, as well as other genes that regulate the proliferation of normal neural progenitor cells, such as epidermal growth factor receptor (EGFR) *(168,189–193)*. Moreover, expression of oncogenes in neural stem or progenitor cells in mice results in the formation of tumors that resemble primary human brain tumors *(184)*.

Ignatova et al. first showed that primary human cortical anaplastic astrocytoma and glioblastoma multiforme contain cells that, in clonal cultures, produce cells expressing neuronal and/or glial markers *(176)*. Two groups recently demonstrated that some cells from pediatric brain tumors (primarily medulloblastomas and astrocytomas), like normal neural stem cells, could be directly cultured in serum-free medium as floating aggregates known as neurospheres, which were multipotent and could self-renew for long periods of time to give rise to secondary neurospheres (Fig. 5) *(177,178)*. The neurosphere-forming subset was shown to reside in the fraction of cells expressing the cell-surface antigen CD133, a marker of human neural stem cells *(178,194)*. Hemmati et al. showed that tumor-derived progenitors from each patient had a stereotypic pattern of differentiation in vitro, yet those patterns were highly variable from one patient to another *(177)*. Strikingly, however, the proportions of neurons, glia, and *nestin*-expressing cells produced from differentiated brain tumor-derived progenitor

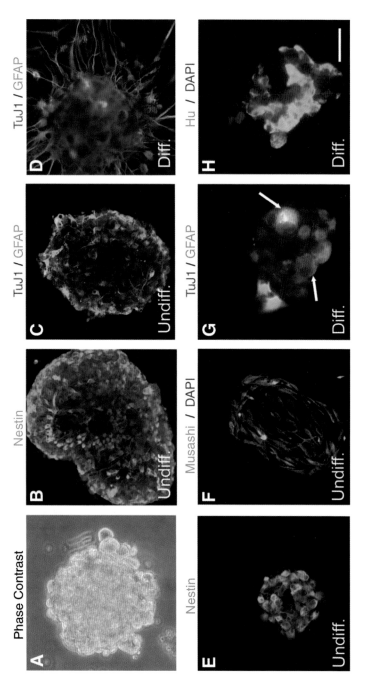

Fig. 5. Tumor-derived progenitors form neurospheres in culture that give rise to both neuronal and glial cells. Neurospheres from one tumor, BT1, were cultured at medium (**A–D**) and clonal (**E–H**) densities. (**A**) A typical primary neurosphere is round in morphology and contains numerous birefringent cells when viewed under phase-contrast optics. (**B,C**) Undifferentiated primary neurospheres expressed high levels of nestin protein (**B**, green) and low levels of (**C**) βIII-tubulin (red) and glial fibrillary acidic protein (GFAP) (green). (**D**) After 7 d of exposure to differentiation conditions, primary neurospheres significantly increased numbers of cells expressing βIII-tubulin and GFAP, and produced cells extending processes onto the substrate. (**E**) Undifferentiated clonal neurospheres expressed the neural stem cell marker musashi-1 (green) in nearly every cell. (**F**) Undifferentiated clonal neurospheres have high levels of *nestin* expression. (**G**) A neurosphere derived from a single cell that, under differentiation conditions, formed cells expressing βIII-tubulin (red) which is characteristic of neurons and GFAP (green), which is characteristic of astrocytes. Some cells expressed both markers. (**H**) Differentiated clonal neurospheres produced cells expressing the neuronal marker Hu (green) in similar proportions to βIII-tubulin. Some nuclei were counterstained with DAPI (**F,H**, blue). Scale bar = 30 μm in **A**, **G**, and **H**: 60 μm in **B–F**. (Reproduced with permission from *PNAS*.)

cells in vitro strongly correlated with their proportions in the primary tumor of origin *(177)*. Unlike neural stem cells, the tumor-derived progenitors proliferated aberrantly and differentiated into unusual cells that coexpressed both neuronal and glial markers (Fig. 5G) *(177)*. These results are consistent with the possibility that brain tumor-derived progenitors might be cancer stem cells *(177)*. Short-term studies have demonstrated that brain tumor-derived progenitors can migrate, proliferate, and differentiate after transplantation into rat brains, but tests of their ability to form tumors in immunodeficient mice are ongoing *(177)*.

In light of these data, might neural crest stem cells or their committed progenitor cells be the origins of peripheral nervous system tumors? This seems like a tractable possibility, as neural crest stem cells persist into adulthood and are therefore susceptible to acquiring transforming throughout life *(133)*. It has been posited that neuroblastomas, the most common solid extracranial tumor in children, arise from the transformation of neural crest stem cells or neural crest-derived sympathetic precursor cells *(195,196)*. The recent finding by Trentin et al. that multipotent neural crest cells form a hierarchy that contains lineage-restricted precursor cells that retain self-renewal ability suggests that those progenitor cells might be targets for transformation in the development of certain neural crest-derived malignancies *(159)*. Specifically, transformation of glial–melanocyte progenitor cells, which are able to self-renew in vivo, might lead to human tumors characterized by the overproduction of glia and melanocytes, such as neurofibromas and melanotic Schwannomas *(197,198)*. Likewise, glial–myofibroblast progenitor cells might give rise to tumors that involve both neural and mesectodermal cells, such as Ewing's sarcomas *(199,200)*. To address these possibilities, it will be necessary to prospectively isolate cancer stem cells from the aforementioned tumors using methods similar to those used for CNS tumors.

What molecular mechanisms might drive normal stem or progenitor cells to become malignant? One possibility is that failure of stem cells to regulate their endogenous self-renewal pathways causes their neoplastic transformation. One candidate molecule that has received much attention in this regard is bmi-1, a polycomb family transcriptional repressor that promotes proliferation partly by repressing the expression of two cyclin-dependent kinase inhibitors p16-ink4a and p19-Arf *(201,202)*. Bmi-1 was recently shown to be required for the self-renewal of both normal and leukemic hematopoietic stem cells *(171,172)*. In the nervous system, bmi-1 is required for the self-renewal of both neurosphere-forming CNS stem cells and neural crest stem cells *(173)*. Expression of bmi-1 has recently been shown to be elevated in cerebellar precursor cells, whole human medulloblastomas, and in tumor-derived progenitor cells from medulloblastomas and other pediatric brain tumors, even after differentiation *(177,203)*. Therefore it is possible that bmi-1 and other regulators of proliferation play a role in the pathogenesis of tumors of the CNS and PNS.

CONCLUSIONS

The demonstration that multiple molecules from different gene families have the capacity to induce neural crest implies that the mechanism of neural crest induction involves complex and perhaps parallel pathways. It is further interesting to note that the same molecules can have multiple inductive capabilities at different times in development. Although great strides have been made toward understanding the induction and cell fate decisions of the neural crest, many mysteries remain. The field of neural crest research is rich in unanswered questions whose solutions will not only offer deeper understanding of the mechanisms of neural crest development but will also give more general insight into phenomena such as cell migration and differentiation, as well as the development of cancers of the peripheral nervous system.

ACKNOWLEDGMENTS

We thank Clare Baker and Anne Knecht for invaluable comments on the manuscript and Carole LaBonne for helpful discussions. T. A. M. was a Fellow of the ARCS Foundation. H. D. H. was supported by the McCallum Fund at the California Institute of Technology, Medical Scientist Training Program Grant GM08042, and the Aesculapians Fund of the David Geffen School of Medicine at UCLA. This work was supported by U.S. Public Health Service Grants NS36585 and NS42287.

REFERENCES

1. Le Douarin, N. (1982) *The Neural Crest.* Cambridge University Press, Cambridge, UK.
2. Hall, A. (1998) Rho GTPases and the actin cytoskeleton. *Science* **279,** 509–514.
3. Morrison, S. J., White, P. M., Zock, C., and Anderson, D. J. (1999) Prospective identification, isolation by flow cytometry, and in vivo self-renewal of multipotent mammalian neural crest stem cells. *Cell* **96,** 737–749.
4. His, W. (1868) *Untersuchungen über die erste Anlage des Wirbeltierleibes. Die erste Entwicklung des Hühnchens im Ei.* F. C. W. Vogel, Leipzig.
5. Landacre, F. L. (1921) The fate of the neural crest in the head of the Urodeles. *J. Comp. Neurol.* **33,** 1–43.
6. Stone, L. S. (1922) Experiments on the development of the cranial ganglia and the lateral line sense organs in *Amblystoma punctatum. J. Exp. Zool.* **35,** 421–496.
7. Harrison, R. G. (1938) Die Neuralleiste Erganzheft. *Anat. Anz.* **85,** 3–30.
8. Hörstadius, S. (1950) *The Neural Crest.* Oxford University Press, Oxford.
9. Hall, B. K. and Hörstadius, S. (1988) *The Neural Crest.* Oxford University Press, Oxford.
10. Bronner-Fraser, M. (1993) Mechanisms of neural crest cell migration. *BioEssays* **15,** 221–230.
11. Erickson, C. A. and Perris, R. (1993) The role of cell–cell and cell-matrix interactions in the morphogenesis of the neural crest. *Dev. Biol.* **159,** 60–74.
12. Stemple, D. L. and Anderson, D. J. (1993) Lineage diversification of the neural crest: *in vitro* investigations. *Dev. Biol.* **159,** 12–23.
13. Selleck, M. A. J. and Bronner-Fraser, M. (1995) Origins of the avian neural crest: the role of neural plate-epidermal interactions. *Development* **121,** 525–538.
14. Sasai, Y. and De Robertis, E. M. (1997) Ectodermal patterning in vertebrate embryos. *Dev. Biol.* **182,** 5–20.
15. Weinstein, D. C. and Hemmati-Brivanlou, A. (1997) Neural induction in *Xenopus laevis:* evidence for the default model. *Curr. Opin. Neurobiol.* **7,** 7–12.
16. Wilson, P. A., Lagna, G., Suzuki, A., and Hemmati-Brivanlou, A. (1997) Concentration-dependent patterning of the *Xenopus* ectoderm by BMP4 and its signal transducer Smad1. *Development* **124,** 3177–3184.
17. Chang, C. and Hemmati-Brivanlou, A. (1998) Neural crest induction by Xwnt7B in *Xenopus. Dev. Biol.* **194,** 129–134.
18. Le Douarin, N. M., Fontaine-Perus, J., and Couly, G. (1986) Cephalic ectodermal placodes and neurogenesis. *Trends Neurosci.* **9,** 175–180.
19. Webb, J. F. and Noden, D. M. (1993) Ectodermal placodes: contributions to the development of the vertebrate head. *Am. Zool.* **33,** 434–447.

20. Baker, C. V. and Bronner-Fraser, M. (1997) The origins of the neural crest. Part I: embryonic induction. *Mech. Dev.* **69,** 3–11.

21. Labonne, C. and Bronner-Fraser, M. (1999) Molecular mechanisms of neural crest formation. *Annu. Rev. Cell Dev. Biol.* **15,** 81–112.

22. Olsson, L. and Hanken, J. (1996) Cranial neural-crest migration and chondrogenic fate in the Oriental fire-bellied toad *Bombina orientalis*: defining the ancestral pattern of head development in anuran amphibians. *J. Morphol.* **229,** 105–120.

23. Bartelmez, G. W. (1922) The origin of the otic and optic primordia. *J. Comp. Neurol.* **34,** 201–232.

24. Holmdahl, D. E. (1928) Die Enstehung und weitere Entwicklung der Neuralleiste (Ganglienleiste) bei Vogeln und Saugetieren. *Z. Mikrosk. Anat. Forsch.* **14,** 99–298.

25. Verwoerd, C. D. A. and van Oostrom, C. G. (1979) Cephalic neural crest and placodes. *Adv. Anat. Embryol. Cell Biol.* **58,** 1–75.

26. Nichols, D. H. (1981) Neural crest formation in the head of the mouse embryo as observed using a new histological technique. *J. Embryol. Exp. Morphol.* **64,** 105–120.

27. Bronner-Fraser, M. (1986) Analysis of the early stages of trunk neural crest migration in avian embryos using monoclonal antibody HNK-1. *Dev. Biol.* **115,** 44–55.

28. Bronner-Fraser, M. and Fraser, S. E. (1989) Developmental potential of avian neural crest cells in situ. *Neuron* **3,** 755–766.

29. Bronner-Fraser, M. and Fraser, S. E. (1988) Cell lineage analysis reveals multipotency of some avian neural crest cells. *Nature* **335,** 161–164.

30. Collazo, A., Bronner-Fraser, M., and Fraser, S. E. (1993) Vital dye labeling of *Xenopus-laevis* trunk neural crest reveals multipotency and novel pathways of migration. *Development* **118,** 363–376.

31. Serbedzija, G. N., Bronner-Fraser, M., and Fraser, S. E. (1992) Vital dye analysis of cranial neural crest cell migration in the mouse embryo. *Development* **116,** 297–307.

32. Serbedzija, G. N., Bronner-Fraser, M., and Fraser, S. E. (1994) Developmental potential of trunk neural crest cells in the mouse. *Development* **120,** 1709–1718.

33. Artinger, K. B., Chitnis, A. B., Mercola, M., and Driever, W. (1999) Zebrafish narrowminded suggests a genetic link between formation of neural crest and primary sensory neurons. *Development* **126,** 3969–3979.

34. Mujtaba, T., Mayer-Proschel, M., and Rao, M. S. (1998) A common neural progenitor for the CNS and PNS. *Dev. Biol.* **200,** 1–15.

35. Sharma, K., Korade, Z., and Frank, E. (1995) Late-migrating neuroepithelial cells from the spinal cord differentiate into sensory ganglion cells and melanocytes. *Neuron* **14,** 143–152.

36. Korade, Z. and Frank, E. (1996) Restriction in cell fates of developing spinal cord cells transplanted to neural crest pathways. *J. Neurosci.* **16,** 7638–7648.

37. Ruffins, S., Artinger, K., and Bronner-Fraser, M. (1998) Early migrating neural crest cells can form ventral neural tube derivatives when challenged by transplantation. *Dev. Biol.* **203,** 295–304.

38. Sohal, G. S., Bockman, D. E., Ali, M. M., and Tsai, N. T. (1996) DiI labeling and homeobox gene islet-1 expression reveal the contribution of ventral neural tube cells to the formation of the avian trigeminal ganglion. *Int. J. Dev. Neurosci.* **14,** 419–427.

39. Rollhäuser-ter Horst, J. (1980) Neural crest replaced by gastrula ectoderm in Amphibia. *Anat. Embryol.* **160,** 203–211.

40. Moury, J. D. and Jacobson, A. G. (1990) The origins of neural crest cells in the axolotl. *Dev. Biol.* **141,** 243–253.

41. Dickinson, M. E., Selleck, M. A. J., McMahon, A. P., and Bronner-Fraser, M. (1995) Dorsalization of the neural tube by the non-neural ectoderm. *Development* **121,** 2099–2106.

42. Mancilla, A. and Mayor, R. (1996) Neural crest formation in *Xenopus laevis*: mechanisms of *Xslug* induction. *Dev. Biol.* **177,** 580–589.

43. Scherson, T., Serbedzija, G., Fraser, S., and Bronner-Fraser, M. (1993) Regulative capacity of the cranial neural tube to form neural crest. *Development* **118,** 1049–1061.

44. Sechrist, J., Nieto, M. A., Zamanian, R. T., and Bronner-Fraser, M. (1995) Regulative response of the cranial neural tube after neural fold ablation: spatiotemporal nature of neural crest regeneration and upregulation of *Slug. Development* **121,** 4103–4115.

45. Hunt, P., Ferretti, P., Krumlauf, R., and Thorogood, P. (1995) Restoration of normal Hox code and branchial arch morphogenesis after extensive deletion of hindbrain neural crest. *Dev. Biol.* **168,** 584–597.

46. Suzuki, H. R. and Kirby, M. L. (1997) Absence of neural crest cell regeneration from the postotic neural tube. *Dev. Biol.* **184,** 222–233.

47. Couly, G., Grapin-Botton, A., Coltey, P., and Le Douarin, N. M. (1996) The regeneration of the cephalic neural crest, a problem revisited—the regenerating cells originate from the contralateral or from the anterior and posterior neural fold. *Development* **122,** 3393–3407.

48. Dale, L., Howes, G., Price, B. M. J., and Smith, J. C. (1992) Bone Morphogenetic Protein 4: a ventralizing factor in *Xenopus* development. *Development* **115,** 573–585.

49. Fainsod, A., Steinbeisser, H., and DeRobertis, E. (1994) On the function of BMP 4 in patterning the ventral marginal zone of the *Xenopus* embryo. *EMBO J.* **13,** 5015–5025.

50. Hemmati-Brivanlou, A. and Thomsen, G. H. (1995) Ventral mesodermal patterning in *Xenopus* embryos: expression patterns and activities of BMP-2 and BMP-4. *Dev. Genet.* **17,** 78–89.

51. Lamb, T. M., Knecht, A. K., Smith, W. C., et al. (1993) Neural induction by the secreted peptide noggin. *Science* **262,** 713–718.

52. Lamb, T. M. and Harland, R. M. (1995) Fibroblast growth factor is a direct neural inducer, which combined with noggin generates anterior-posterior neural pattern. *Development* **121,** 3627–3636.

53. Sasai, Y., Lu, B., Steinbesser, H., Geissert, D., Gont, L. K., and De Robertis, E. M. (1994) *Xenopus chordin*: a novel dorsalizing factor activated by organizer-specific homeobox genes. *Cell* **79,** 779–790.

54. Piccolo, S., Sasai, Y., Lu, B., and De Robertis, E. M. (1996) Dorsoventral patterning in *Xenopus*: inhibition of ventral signals by direct binding of chordin to BMP-4. *Cell* **86,** 589–598.

55. Hemmati-Brivanlou, A., Kelly, O. G., and Melton, D. A. (1994) Follistatin, an antagonist of activin is expressed in the Spemann organizer and displays direct neuralizing activity. *Cell* **77,** 283–295.

56. Fainsod A, Deissler, K., Yelin, R., et al. (1997) The dorsalizing and neural inducing gene follistatin is an antagonist of BMP4. *Mech. Dev.* **63,** 39–50.

57. Raven, C. P. and Kloos, J. (1945) Induction by medial and lateral pieces of the archenteron roof with special reference to the determination of the neural crest. *Acta Néerl. Morph.* **5,** 348–362.

58. Knecht, A. K., Good, P. G., Dawid, I. B., and Harland, R. M. (1995) Dorsal-ventral patterning and differentiation of noggin-induced neural tissue in the absence of mesoderm. *Development* **121,** 1927–1936.

59. Marchant, L., Linker, C., Ruiz, P., Guerrero, N., and Mayor, R. (1998) The inductive properties of mesoderm suggest that the neural crest cells are specified by a BMP gradient. *Dev. Biol.* **198,** 319–329.

60. LaBonne, C. and Bronner-Fraser, M. (1998) Neural crest induction in *Xenopus*: evidence for a two signal model. *Development* **125,** 2403–2414.

61. Nguyen, V. H., Schmid, B., Trout, J., Connors, S. A., Ekker, M., and Mullins, M. C. (1998) Ventral and lateral regions of the zebrafish gastrula, including the neural crest progenitors, are established by a bmp2b/swirl pathway of genes. *Dev. Biol.* **199,** 93–110.

62. Hammerschmidt, M., Serbedzija, G. N., and McMahon, A. P. (1996) Genetic analysis of dorsoventral pattern formation in the zebrafish: requirement of a BMP-like ventralizing activity and its dorsal repressor. *Genes Dev.* **10,** 2452–2461.

63. Kishimoto, Y., Lee, K. H., Zon, L., Hammerschmidt, M., and Schulte-Merker, S. (1997) The molecular nature of zebrafish *swirl*: BMP2 function is essential during early dorsoventral patterning. *Development* **124,** 4457–4466.

64. Delot, E., Kataoka, H., Goutel, C., et al. (1999) The BMP-related protein radar: a maintenance factor for dorsal neuroectoderm cells? *Mech. Dev.* **85,** 15–25.

65. Hogan, B. L. (1996) Bone morphogenetic proteins: multifunctional regulators of vertebrate development. *Genes Dev.* **10,** 1580–1594.

66. Winnier, G., Blessing, M., Labosky, P. A., and Hogan, B. L. (1995) Bone morphogenetic protein-4 is required for mesoderm formation and patterning in the mouse. *Genes Dev.* **9,** 2105–2116.

67. Matzuk, M. M., Lu, N., Vogel, H., Sellheyer, K., Roop, D. R., and Bradley, A. (1995) Multiple defects and perinatal death in mice deficient in follistatin. *Nature* **374,** 360–363.

68. McMahon, J. A., Takada, S., Zimmerman, L. B., Fan, C. M., Harland, R. M., and McMahon, A. P. (1998) Noggin-mediated antagonism of BMP signaling is required for growth and patterning of the neural tube and somite. *Genes Dev.* **12,** 1438–1452.

69. Lee, K. J. and Jessell, T. M. (1999) The specification of dorsal cell fates in the vertebrate central nervous system. *Annu. Rev. Neurosci.* **22,** 261–294.

70. Liem, K. F., Tremmi, G., Roelink, H., and Jessell, T. M. (1995) Dorsal differentiation of neural plate cells induced by BMP-mediated signals from epidermal ectoderm. *Cell* **82,** 969–979.

71. Schultheiss, T. M., Burch, J. B., and Lassar, A. B. (1997) A role for bone morphogenetic proteins in the induction of cardiac myogenesis. *Genes Dev.* **11,** 451–462.

72. Watanabe, Y. and Le Douarin, N. M. (1996) A role for BMP-4 in the development of subcutaneous cartilage. *Mech. Dev.* **57,** 69–78.

73. Streit, A., Lee, K. J., Woo, I., Roberts, C., Jessell, T. M., and Stern, C. D. (1998) Chordin regulates primitive streak development and the stability of induced neural cells, but is not sufficient forneural induction in the chick embryo. *Development* **125,** 507–519.

74. Selleck, M. A., Garcia-Castro, M. I., Artinger, K. B., and Bronner-Fraser, M. (1998) Effects of shh and noggin on neural crest formation demonstrate that BMP is required in the neural tube but not ectoderm. *Development* **125,** 4919–4930.

75. Pera, E., Stein, S., and Kessel, M. (1999) Ectodermal patterning in the avian embryo: epidermis versus neural plate. *Development* **26,** 63–73.

76. Liem, K. F., Tremml, G., and Jessell, T. M. (1997) A role for the roof plate and its resident TGFbeta-related proteins in neuronal patterning in the dorsal spinal cord. *Cell* **91,** 127–138.

77. Anderson, D. J. (1993) Cell fate determination in the peripheral nervous system: the sympathoadrenal progenitor. *J. Neurobiol.* **24,** 185–198.

78. Varley, J. E., McPherson, C. E., Zou, H., Niswander, L., and Maxwell, G. D. (1998) Expression of a constitutively active type I BMP receptor using a retroviral vector promotes the development of adrenergic cells in neural crest cultures. *Dev. Biol.* **196,** 107–118.

79. Schneider, C., Wicht, H., Enderich, J., Wegner, M., and Rohrer, H. (1999) Bone morphogenetic proteins are required in vivo for the generation of sympathetic neurons. *Neuron* **24,** 861–870.

80. Wilson, P. A. and Hemmati-Brivanlou, A. (1995) Induction of epidermis and inhibition of neural fate by Bmp-4. *Nature* **376,** 331–333.

81. Mitani, S. and Okamoto, H. (1991) Inductive differentiation of two neural lineages reconstituted in a microculture system from *Xenopus* early gastrula cells. *Development* **112,** 21–31.

82. Bang, A. G., Papalopulu, N., Kintne, R. C., and Goulding, M. D. (1997) Expression of Pax-3 is initiated in the early neural plate by posteriorizing signals produced by the orga- nizer and by posterior non-axial mesoderm. *Development* **124,** 2075–2085.

83. Bonstein, L., Elias, S., and Frank, D. (1998) Paraxial-fated mesoderm is required for neural crest induction in *Xenopus* embryos. *Dev. Biol.* **193,** 156–168.

84. Wodarz, A. and Nusse, R. (1998) Mechanisms of Wnt signaling in development. *Annu. Rev. Cell Dev. Biol.* **14,** 59–88.

85. Sieber-Blum, M. (1998) Growth factor synergism and antagonism in early neural crest development. *Biochem. Cell Biol.* **76,** 1039–1050.

86. Vaccarino, F. M., Schwartz, M. L., Raballo, R., Rhee, J., and Lyn-Cook, R. (1999) Fibro- blast growth factor signaling regulates growth and morphogenesis at multiple steps dur- ing brain development. *Curr. Top. Dev. Biol.* **46,** 179–200.

87. Saint-Jeannet, J., He, X., Varmus, H. E., and Dawid, I. B. (1997) Regulation of dorsal fate in the neuraxis by Wnt-1 and Wnt-3a. *Proc. Natl. Acad. Sci. USA* **94,** 13713–13718.

88. Mayor, R., Morgan, R., and Sargent, M. G. (1995) Induction of the prospective neural crest of *Xenopus. Development* **121,** 767–777.

89. Bellmeyer, A., Krase, J., Lindgren, J., and LaBonne, C. (2003) The protooncogene c-myc is an essential regulator of neural crest formation in *xenopus. Dev. Cell* **4,** 827–839.

90. Christian, J. L., McMahon, J. A., McMahon, A. P., and Moon, R. T. (1991) Xwnt-8, a *Xenopus* Wnt-1/int-1-related gene responsive to mesoderm-inducing growth factors, may play a role in ventral mesodermal patterning during embryogenesis. *Development* **111,** 1045–1055.

91. Hume, C. R. and Dodd, J. (1993) Cwnt-8C: a novel Wnt gene with a potential role in primitive streak formation and hindbrain organization. *Development* **119,** 1147–1160.

92. Bang, A. G., Papalopulu, N., Goulding, M. D., and Kintner, C. (1999) Expression of Pax-3 in the lateral neural plate is dependent on a Wnt-mediated signal from posterior nonaxial mesoderm. *Dev. Biol.* **212,** 366–380.

93. Hollyday, M., McMahon, J. A., and McMahon, A. P. (1995) Wnt expression patterns in chick embryo nervous system. *Mech. Dev.* **52,** 9–25.

94. Wolda, S. L., Moody, C. J., and Moon, R. T. (1993) Overlapping expression of *Xwnt-3a* and *Xwnt-1* in neural tissue of *Xenopus laevis* embryos. *Dev. Biol.* **155,** 46–57.

95. McGrew, L. L., Hoppler, S., and Moon, R. T. (1997) Wnt and FGF pathways coopera- tively pattern anteroposterior neural ectoderm in *Xenopus. Mech. Dev.* **69,** 105–114.

96. Roelink, H. and Nusse, R. (1991) Expression of two members of the Wnt family during mouse development—restricted temporal and spatial patterns in the developing neural tube. *Genes Dev.* **5,** 381–388.

97. Parr, B. A., Shea, M. J., Vassileva, G., and McMahon, A. P. (1993) Mouse Wnt genes exhibit discrete domains of expression in the early embryonic CNS and limb buds. *Devel- opment* **119,** 247–261.

98. Ikeya, M., Lee, S. M., Johnson, J. E., McMahon, A. P., and Takada, S. (1997) Wnt signal- ing required for expansion of neural crest and CNS progenitors. *Nature* **389,** 966–970.

99. Garcia-Castro, M. I., Marcelle, C., and Bronner-Fraser, M. (2002) Ectodermal Wnt func- tion as a neural crest inducer. *Science* **297,** 848–851.

100. Dorsky, R. I., Moon, R. T., and Raible, D. W. (1998) Control of neural crest cell fate by the Wnt signalling pathway. *Nature* **396,** 370–373.

101. Baker, J. C., Beddington, R. S., and Harland, R. M. (1999) Wnt signaling in *Xenopus* embryos inhibits bmp4 expression and activates neural development. *Genes Dev.* **13,** 3149–3159.

102. Mayor, R., Guerrero, N., and Martinez, C. (1997) Role of FGF and noggin in neural crest induction. *Dev. Biol.* **189,** 1–12.

103. Kengaku, M. and Okamoto, H. (1993) Basic fibroblast growth factor induces differentia- tion of neural tube and neural crest lineages of cultured ectoderm cells from *Xenopus* gastrula. *Development* **119,** 1067–1078.

104. Cox, W. G. and Hemmati-Brivanlou, A. (1995) Caudalization of neural fate by tissue recombination and bFGF. *Development* **121,** 4349–4358.

105. Launay, C., Fromentoux, V., Shi, D. L., and Boucaut, J. C. (1996) A truncated FGF receptor blocks neural induction by endogenous *Xenopus* inducers. *Development* **122,** 869–880.

106. Xu, R. H., Kim, J., Taira, M., Sredni, D., and Kung, H. (1997) Studies on the role of fibroblast growth factor signaling in neurogenesis using conjugated/aged animal caps and dorsal ectoderm-grafted embryos. *J. Neurosci.* **17,** 6892–6898.

107. Tannahill, D., Isaacs, H. V., Close, M. J., Peters, G., and Slack, J. M. W. (1992) Developmental expression of the *Xenopus int-2* (FGF-3) gene: activation by mesodermal and neural induction. *Development* **115,** 695–702.

108. Isaacs, H. V., Tannahill, D., and Slack, J. M. W. (1992) Expression of a novel FGF in the *Xenopus* embryo. A New candidate inducing factor for mesoderm formation and antero-posterior specification. *Development* **114,** 711–720.

109. Mahmood, R., Kiefer, P., Guthrie, S., Dickson, C., and Mason, I. (1995) Multiple roles for FGF-3 during cranial neural development in the chicken. *Development* **121,** 1399–1410.

110. Riese, J., Zeller, R., and Dono, R. (1995) Nucleo-cytoplasmic translocation and secretion of fibroblast growth factor-2 during avian gastrulation. *Mech. Dev.* **49,** 13–22.

111. Bueno, D., Skinner, J., Abud, H., and Heath, J. K. (1996) Spatial and temporal relationships between Shh, Fgf4, and Fgf8 gene expression at diverse signalling centers during mouse development. *Dev. Dyn.* **207,** 291–299.

112. Storey, K. G., Goriely, A., Sargent, C. M., et al. (1998) Early posterior neural tissue is induced by FGF in the chick embryo. *Development* **125,** 473–484.

113. Streit, A., Berliner, A. J., Papanayotou, C., Sirulnik, A., and Stern, C. D. (2000) Initiation of neural induction by FGF signalling before gastrulation. *Nature* **406,** 74–78.

114. Kroll, K. L. and Amaya, E. (1996) Transgenic *Xenopus* embryos from sperm nuclear transplantations reveal FGF signaling requirements during gastrulation. *Development* **122,** 3173–3183.

115. Monsoro-Burq, A. H., Fletcher, R. B., and Harland, R. M. (2003) Neural crest induction by paraxial mesoderm in *Xenopus* embryos requires FGF signals. *Development* **130,** 3111–3124.

116. Kopan, R. (2002) Notch: a membrane-bound transcription factor. *J. Cell Sci.* **115,** 1095–1097.

117. Williams, R., Lendahl, U., and Lardelli, M. (1995) Complementary and combinatorial patterns of Notch gene family expression during early mouse development. *Mech. Dev.* **53,** 357–368.

118. Endo, Y., Osumi, N., and Wakamatsu, Y. (2002) Bimodal functions of Notch-mediated signaling are involved in neural crest formation during avian ectoderm development. *Development* **129,** 863–873.

119. Coffman, C. R., Skoglund, P., Harris, W. A., and Kintner, C. R. (1993) Expression of an extracellular deletion of Xotch diverts cell fate in *Xenopus* embryos. *Cell* **73,** 659–671.

120. Bierkamp, C. and Campos-Ortega, J. A. (1993) A zebrafish homologue of the *Drosophila* neurogenic gene Notch and its pattern of transcription during early embryogenesis. *Mech. Dev.* **43,** 87–100.

121. Cornell, R. A. and Eisen, J. S. (2002) Delta/Notch signaling promotes formation of zebrafish neural crest by repressing Neurogenin 1 function. *Development* **129,** 2639–2648.

122. Glavic, A., Silva, F., Aybar, M. J., Bastidas, F., and Mayor, R. (2004) Interplay between Notch signaling and the homeoprotein Xiro1 is required for neural crest induction in *Xenopus* embryos. *Development* **131,** 347–359.

123. Barembaum, M., Moreno, T. A., LaBonne, C., Sechrist, J., and Bronner-Fraser, M. (2000) Noelin-1 is a secreted glycoprotein involved in generation of the neural crest. *Nat. Cell Biol.* **2,** 219–225.

124. Stemple, D. L. and Anderson, D. J. (1992) Isolation of a stem cell for neurons and glia derived from the mammalian neural crest. *Cell* **71,** 973–985.
125. Doupe, A. J., Patterson, P. H., and Landis, S. C. (1985) Small intensely fluorescent cells in culture: role of glucocorticoids and growth factors in their development and inter-conversions with other neural crest derivatives. *J. Neurosci.* **5,** 2143–2160.
126. Doupe, A. J., Landis, S. C., and Patterson, P. H. (1985) Environmental influences in the development of neural crest derivatives: glucocorticoids, growth factors, and chromaffin cell plasticity. *J. Neurosci.* **5,** 2119–2142.
127. Shah, N. M., Marchionni, M. A., Isaacs, I., Stroobant, P. W., and Anderson, D. J. (1994) Glial growth factor restricts mammalian neural crest stem cells to a glial fate. *Cell* **77,** 349–360.
128. Shah, N. M., Groves, A. K., and Anderson, D. J. (1996) Alternative neural crest cell fates are instructively promoted by TGFb superfamily members. *Cell* **85,** 331–343.
129. Shah, N. M. and Anderson, D. A. (1997) Integration of multiple instructive cues by neural crest stem cells reveals cell-intrinsic biases in relative growth factor responsiveness. *Proc. Natl. Acad. Sci. USA* **94,** 11369–11374.
130. Morrison, S. J., Perez, S. E., Qiao, Z., et al. (2000) Transient Notch activation initiates an irreversible switch from neurogenesis to gliogenesis by neural crest stem cells. *Cell* **101,** 499–510.
131. White, P. M., Morrison, S. J., Orimoto, K., Kubu, C. J., Verdi, J. M., and Anderson, D. J. (2001) Neural crest stem cells undergo cell-intrinsic developmental changes in sensitivity to instructive differentiation signals. *Neuron* **29,** 57–71.
132. Bixby, S., Kruger, G. M., Mosher, J. T., Joseph, N. M., and Morrison, S. J. (2002) Cell-intrinsic differences between stem cells from different regions of the peripheral nervous system regulate the generation of neural diversity. *Neuron* **35,** 643–656.
133. Kruger, G. M., Mosher, J. T., Bixby, S., Joseph, N., Iwashita, T., and Morrison, S. J. (2002) Neural crest stem cells persist in the adult gut but undergo changes in self-renewal, neuronal subtype potential, and factor responsiveness. *Neuron* **35,** 657–669.
134. Iwashita, T., Kruger, G. M., Pardal, R., Kiel, M. J., and Morrison, S. J. (2003) Hirschsprung disease is linked to defects in neural crest stem cell function. *Science* **301,** 972–976.
135. Le Douarin, N. M. (1986) Cell lineage segregation during peripheral nervous system ontogeny. *Science* **231,** 1515–1522.
136. Frank, E. and Sanes, J. R. (1991) Lineage of neurons and glia in chick dorsal root ganglia: analysis in vivo with a recombinant retrovirus. *Development* **111,** 895–908.
137. Kim, J., Lo, L., Dormand, E., and Anderson, D. J. (2003) SOX10 maintains multipotency and inhibits neuronal differentiation of neural crest stem cells. *Neuron* **38,** 17–31.
138. Southard-Smith, E. M., Kos, L., and Pavan, W. J. (1998) Sox10 mutation disrupts neural crest development in Dom Hirschsprung mouse model. *Nat. Genet.* **18,** 60–64.
139. Serbedzija, G., Bronner-Fraser, M., and Fraser, S. E. (1989) Vital dye analysis of the timing and pathways of avian trunk neural crest cell migration. *Development* **106,** 806–816.
140. Weston, J. A. and Butler, S. L. (1966) Temporal factors affecting the localization of neural crest cells in chick embryos. *Dev. Biol.* **14,** 246–266.
141. Baker, C. V. H., Bronner-Fraser, M., Le Douarin, N. M., and Teillet, M. (1997) Early- and late-migrating cranial neural crest cell populations have equivalent developmental potential in vivo. *Development* **124,** 3077–3087.
142. Richardson, M. K. and Sieber-Blum, M. (1993) Pluripotent neural crest cells in the developing skin of the quail embryo. *Dev. Biol.* **157,** 348–358.
143. Hagedorn, L., Suter, U., and Sommer, L. (1999) P0 and PMP22 mark a multipotent neural crest-derived cell type that displays community effects in response to TGF-beta family factors. *Development* **126,** 3781–3794.

144. Artinger, K. B. and Bronner-Fraser, M. (1992) Partial restriction in the developmental potential of late emigrating avian neural crest cells. *Dev. Biol.* **149,** 149–157.

145. Perez, S. E., Rebelo, S., and Anderson, D. J. (1999) Early specification of sensory neuron fate revealed by expression and function of neurogenins in the chick embryo. *Development* **126,** 1715–1728.

146. Lee, H. Y., Kleber, M., Hari, L., et al. (2004) Instructive role of Wnt/beta-catenin in sensory fate specification in neural crest stem cells. *Science* **303,** 1020–1023.

147. Trainor, P. A., Ariza-McNaughton, L., and Krumlauf, R. (2002) Role of the isthmus and FGFs in resolving the paradox of neural crest plasticity and prepatterning. *Science* **295,** 1288–1291.

148. Pasqualetti, M., Ori, M., Nardi, I., and Rijli, F. M. (2000) Ectopic Hoxa2 induction after neural crest migration results in homeosis of jaw elements in *Xenopus*. *Development* **127,** 5367–5378.

149. Grammatopoulos, G. A., Bell, E., Toole, L., Lumsden, A., and Tucker, A. S. (2000) Homeotic transformation of branchial arch identity after Hoxa2 overexpression. *Development* **127,** 5355–5365.

150. Carr, V. M. and Simpson, S. B., Jr. (1978) Proliferative and degenerative events in the early development of chick dorsal root ganglia. II. Responses to altered peripheral fields. *J. Comp. Neurol.* **182,** 741–755.

151. Marchionni, M. A., Goodearl, A., Chen, M. S., et al. (1993) Glial growth factors are alternatively spliced erbB2 ligand expressed in the nervous system. *Nature* **362,** 312–318.

152. Orr-Utreger, A., Trakhtenbrot, L., Ben-Levy, R., et al. (1993) Neural expression and chromosomal mapping of Neu differentiation factor to 8p12-p21. *Proc. Natl. Acad. Sci. USA* **90,** 1867–1871.

153. Meyer, D. and Birchmeier, C. (1995) Multiple essential functions of neuregulin in development. *Nature* **378,** 386–390.

154. Lemke, G. (1996) Neuregulins in development. *Mol. Cell Neurosci.* **7,** 247–262.

155. Meyer, D., Yamaai, T., Garratt, A., et al. (1997) Isoform-specific expression and function of neuregulin. *Development* **124,** 3575–3586.

156. Oakley, R. A., Lasky, C. J., Erickson, C. A., and Tosney, K. W. (1994) Glycoconjugates mark a transient barrier to neural crest migration in the chicken embryo. *Development* **120,** 103–114.

157. Perris, R. (1997) The extracellular matrix in neural crest-cell migration. *Trends Neurosci.* **20,** 23–31.

158. Anderson, D. J. (1999) Lineages and transcription factors in the specification of vertebrate primary sensory neurons. *Curr. Opin. Neurobiol.* **9,** 517–524.

159. Trentin, A., Glavieux-Pardanaud, C., Le Douarin, N. M., and Dupin, E. (2004) Self-renewal capacity is a widespread property of various types of neural crest precursor cells. *Proc. Natl. Acad. Sci. USA* **101,** 4495–4500.

160. Bitgood, M. J. and McMahon, A. P. (1995) Hedgehog and BMP genes are coexpressed at many diverse sites of cell-cell interaction in the mouse embryo. *Dev. Biol.* **172,** 126–138.

161. Lyons, K. M., Hogan, B. L. M., and Robertson, E. J. (1995) Colocalization of BMP2 and BMP7 RNAs suggests that these factors cooperatively mediate tissue interaction during murine development. *Mech. Dev.* **50,** 71–83.

162. Ito, K. and Sieber-Blum, M. (1993) Pluripotent and developmentally restricted neural-crest-derived cells in posterior visceral arches. *Dev. Biol.* **156,** 191–200.

163. LaBonne, C. and Bronner-Fraser, M. (1998) Induction and patterning of the neural crest, a stem cell-like precursor population. *J. Neurobiol.* **36,** 175–189.

164. Groves, A. and Bronner-Fraser, M. (1999) Neural crest diversification. *Curr. Top. Dev. Biol.* **43,** 221–258.

165. Reya, T., Morrison, S. J., Clarke, M. F., and Weissman, I. L. (2001) Stem cells, cancer, and cancer stem cells. *Nature* **414,** 105–111.

166. Pardal, R., Clarke, M. F., and Morrison, S. J. (2003) Applying the principles of stem-cell biology to cancer. *Nat. Rev. Cancer* **3,** 895–902.
167. Sell, S. and Pierce, G. B. (1994) Maturation arrest of stem cell differentiation is a common pathway for the cellular origin of teratocarcinomas and epithelial cancers. *Lab. Invest.* **70,** 6–22.
168. Wechsler-Reya, R. and Scott, M. P. (2001) The developmental biology of brain tumors. *Annu. Rev. Neurosci.* **24,** 385–428.
169. Bonnet, D. and Dick, J. E. (1997) Human acute myeloid leukemia is organized as a hierarchy that originates from a primitive hematopoietic cell. *Nat. Med.* **3,** 730–737.
170. Reya, T., Duncan, A. W., Ailles, L., et al. (2003) A role for Wnt signalling in self-renewal of haematopoietic stem cells. *Nature* **423,** 409–414.
171. Lessard, J. and Sauvageau, G. (2003) Bmi-1 determines the proliferative capacity of normal and leukaemic stem cells. *Nature* **423,** 255–260.
172. Park, I. K., Qian, D., Kiel, M., et al. (2003) Bmi-1 is required for maintenance of adult self-renewing haematopoietic stem cells. *Nature* **423,** 302–305.
173. Molofsky, A. V., Pardal, R., Iwashita, T., Park, I. K., Clarke, M. F., and Morrison, S. J. (2003) Bmi-1 dependence distinguishes neural stem cell self-renewal from progenitor proliferation. *Nature* **425,** 962–967.
174. Hamburger, A. W. and Salmon, S. E. (1977) Primary bioassay of human tumor stem cells. *Science* **197,** 461–463.
175. Al-Hajj, M., Wicha, M. S., Benito-Hernandez, A., Morrison, S. J., and Clarke, M. F. (2003) Prospective identification of tumorigenic breast cancer cells. *Proc. Natl. Acad. Sci. USA* **100,** 3983–3988.
176. Ignatova, T. N., Kukekov, V. G., Laywell, E. D., Suslov, O. N., Vrionis, F. D., and Steindler, D. A. (2002) Human cortical glial tumors contain neural stem-like cells expressing astroglial and neuronal markers in vitro. *Glia* **39,** 193–206.
177. Hemmati, H. D., Nakano, I., Lazareff, J. A., et al. (2003) Cancerous stem cells can arise from pediatric brain tumors. *Proc. Natl. Acad. Sci. USA* **100,** 15178–15183.
178. Singh, S. K., Clarke, I. D., Terasaki, M., et al. (2003) Identification of a cancer stem cell in human brain tumors. *Cancer Res.* **63,** 5821–5828.
179. Kondo, T., Setoguchi, T., and Taga, T. (2004) Persistence of a small subpopulation of cancer stem-like cells in the C6 glioma cell line. *Proc. Natl. Acad. Sci. USA* **101,** 781–786.
180. Passegue, E., Jamieson, C. H., Ailles, L. E., and Weissman, I. L. (2003) Normal and leukemic hematopoiesis: are leukemias a stem cell disorder or a reacquisition of stem cell characteristics? *Proc. Natl. Acad. Sci. USA* **100(Suppl 1),** 11842–11849.
181. Cozzio, A., Passegue, E., Ayton, P. M., Karsunky, H., Cleary, M. L., and Weissman, I. L. (2003) Similar MLL-associated leukemias arising from self-renewing stem cells and short-lived myeloid progenitors. *Genes Dev.* **17,** 3029–3035.
182. Brustle, O. and McKay, R. D. (1995) The neuroepithelial stem cell concept: implications for neuro-oncology. *J. Neurooncol.* **24,** 57–59.
183. Holland, E. C. (2000) A mouse model for glioma: biology, pathology, and therapeutic opportunities. *Toxicol. Pathol.* **28,** 171–177.
184. Holland, E. C., Celestino, J., Dai, C., Schaefer, L., Sawaya, R. E., and Fuller, G. N. (2000) Combined activation of Ras and Akt in neural progenitors induces glioblastoma formation in mice. *Nat. Genet.* **25,** 55–57.
185. Mischel, P. S., Shai, R., Shi, T., et al. (2003) Identification of molecular subtypes of glioblastoma by gene expression profiling. *Oncogene* **22,** 2361–2373.
186. Sutton, L. N., Phillips, P., and Lange, B. (1992) Midline supratentorial tumors. *Neurosurg. Clin. N. Am.* **3,** 821–837.
187. Koos, W. T. and Horaczek, A. (1985) Statistics of intracranial midline tumors in children. *Acta Neurochir. Suppl. (Wien)* **35,** 1–5.

188. Sanai, N., Tramontin, A. D., Quinones-Hinojosa, A., et al. (2004) Unique astrocyte ribbon in adult human brain contains neural stem cells but lacks chain migration. *Nature* **427,** 740–744.

189. Tohyama, T., Lee, V. M., Rorke, L. B., Marvin, M., McKay, R. D., and Trojanowski, J. Q. (1992) Nestin expression in embryonic human neuroepithelium and in human neuroepithelial tumor cells. *Lab. Invest.* **66,** 303–313.

190. Rorke, L. B., Trojanowski, J. Q., Lee, V. M., et al. (1997) Primitive neuroectodermal tumors of the central nervous system. *Brain Pathol.* **7,** 765–784.

191. Almqvist, P. M., Mah, R., Lendahl, U., Jacobsson, B., and Hendson, G. (2002) Immunohistochemical detection of nestin in pediatric brain tumors. *J. Histochem. Cytochem.* **50,** 147–158.

192. Taipale, J. and Beachy, P. A. (2001) The Hedgehog and Wnt signalling pathways in cancer. *Nature* **411,** 349–354.

193. Gilbertson, R., Hernan, R., Pietsch, T., et al. (2001) Novel ERBB4 juxtamembrane splice variants are frequently expressed in childhood medulloblastoma. *Genes Chromosomes Cancer* **31,** 288–294.

194. Uchida, N., Buck, D. W., He, D., et al. (2000) Direct isolation of human central nervous system stem cells. *Proc. Natl. Acad. Sci. USA* **97,** 14720–14725.

195. Brodeur, G. M. (2003) Neuroblastoma: biological insights into a clinical enigma. *Nat. Rev. Cancer* **3,** 203–216.

196. Nakagawara, A. and Ohira, M. (2004) Comprehensive genomics linking between neural development and cancer: neuroblastoma as a model. *Cancer Lett.* **204,** 213–224.

197. Riccardi, V. M. (1991) Neurofibromatosis: past, present, and future. *N. Engl. J. Med.* **324,** 1283–1285.

198. Ferner, R. E. and O'Doherty, M. J. (2002) Neurofibroma and schwannoma. *Curr. Opin. Neurol.* **15,** 679–684.

199. Thiele, C. J. (1991) Biology of pediatric peripheral neuroectodermal tumors. *Cancer Metastas. Rev.* **10,** 311–319.

200. Cavazzana, A. O., Miser, J. S., Jefferson, J., and Triche, T. J. (1987) Experimental evidence for a neural origin of Ewing's sarcoma of bone. *Am. J. Pathol.* **127,** 507–518.

201. Jacobs, J. J., Kieboom, K., Marino, S., DePinho, R. A., and van Lohuizen, M. (1999) The oncogene and Polycomb-group gene bmi-1 regulates cell proliferation and senescence through the ink4a locus. *Nature* **397,** 164–168.

202. Jacobs, J. J., Scheijen, B., Voncken, J. W., Kieboom, K., Berns, A., and van Lohuizen, M. (1999) Bmi-1 collaborates with c-Myc in tumorigenesis by inhibiting c-Myc-induced apoptosis via INK4a/ARF. *Genes Dev.* **13,** 2678–2690.

203. Leung, C., Lingbeek, M., Shakhova, O., et al. (2004) Bmi1 is essential for cerebellar development and is overexpressed in human medulloblastomas. *Nature* **428,** 337–341.

9

Stem Cells of the Adult Olfactory Epithelium

James E. Schwob and Woochan Jang

INTRODUCTION

The peripheral olfactory system consists of the olfactory (neuro)epithelium lining the posterodorsal nasal cavity, and the olfactory nerve connecting the sensory neurons in the periphery with their central nervous system (CNS) target, the olfactory bulb (1,2). The epithelium is composed of a handful of easily distinguishable cell types, including basal cells, olfactory sensory neurons (OSNs), nonneuronal supporting or sustentacular (Sus) cells, and Bowman duct/gland assemblies (3). The peripheral olfactory system is readily accessible and can be safely biopsied with minimal discomfort or risk, thereby offering a unique glimpse of a part of the nervous system (4–6). In addition, the capacity of the peripheral olfactory system to accomplish anatomical reconstitution and functional restoration from injury has suggested that the epithelium retains a population of neurocompetent stem cells (i.e., capable of producing neurons) which, given their accessibility, may be a valuable addition to our therapeutic and analytical armamentarium. Moreover, the ensheathing cells of the olfactory nerve have been effective in promoting behavioral and neuroanatomical recovery after spinal cord injury in experimental animals (7).

During embryological development, all components of the peripheral olfactory system as well as the other, nonolfactory parts of the nasal lining, derive from the olfactory placode (8,9). The placode emerges at the rostrolateral aspect of the head shortly after closure of the neural tube and may ultimately derive from the anterior neural ridge (10). Subsequently, the placode invaginates to form an olfactory pit—the anlage of the nasal lining—out of which some cells also migrate toward and into the forebrain (11). Some of the epithelial emigrants differentiate into the ensheathing glia of the olfactory nerve and come to surround the olfactory bulb, while others become the gonadotropin-releasing hormone (GnRH)-secreting cells of the nervus terminalis and of the hypothalamus after invading the CNS along axons of the olfactory nerve (12,13).

The purpose of this chapter is to demonstrate that the adult olfactory epithelium retains a cell that is as broadly potent (or nearly so) as the placodal cells of the early embryo and to describe what is known of the regulation of the progenitor populations of the olfactory epithelium. In addition, this review is intended to inform the controlled manipulation of these cells in vitro and in vivo.

From: *Neural Development and Stem Cells, Second Edition*
Edited by: M. S. Rao © Humana Press Inc., Totowa, NJ

AN HISTORICAL PERSPECTIVE

The peripheral olfactory system's capacity to regenerate a population of neurons after injury has been known since the 1930s and 40s from both observations in humans (the recovery of olfactory function in children irrigated intranasally with zinc sulfate as prophylaxis against poliomyelitis) and experimental studies in animals *(14,15)*. Research into the nature of "the" purported olfactory neural stem cell was invigorated by demonstrations that actively proliferating cells were present at relatively high density in the basal region of the olfactory epithelium *(16,17)*. Pulse-chase experiments using [3H]thymidine demonstrated the promotion of the labeled progenitors into the neural zone in the middle of the epithelium *(18–21)*. Moreover, a component of the neuronal population in the normal adult epithelium was shown to be immature, that is, expressing the protein GAP-43 and lacking cilia, in contrast with the larger set of mature neurons, that is, expressing olfactory marker protein (OMP) and having elaborated cilia *(21–24)*. As a consequence, the notion arose that the neural population of the epithelium undergoes constitutive turnover *(18–20)*. Originally, it was thought that the generation of new OSNs was required for the replacement of preexisting mature neurons that died after a fixed lifespan on the order of 30 or perhaps as many as 90 d *(25)*. There is surprisingly little direct evidence that mature, synaptically connected, functionally active sensory neurons have a finite lifespan in the manner of skin or intestinal epithelial cells. Rather, it has become evident that OSNs require contact with, and trophic support from, the olfactory bulb to survive beyond the immature-to-mature transition *(24)*. Thus, a more conservative hypothesis for the production of new neurons throughout life posits that neurogenesis persists in order to form a population of "ready reserve" neurons, which differentiate and survive when preexisting OSNs die as a consequence of environmental toxin or injury.

Whatever their purpose in the protected laboratory environment, it quickly became clear that the neurocompetent progenitors of the olfactory epithelium were needed for and capable of reconstituting the neuronal population rapidly following experimental lesions that kill neurons either directly (irrigation with zinc sulfate or detergents or exposure by inhalation or injection of olfactotoxins) or indirectly (damage to the olfactory axons by transecting the olfactory nerve or ablating the olfactory bulb) *(26–32)*. In these settings, the reconstitution of the neuronal population proceeds rapidly and completely when the olfactory bulb and nerve have not been damaged by the lesion.

THE IDENTIFICATION OF NEUROCOMPETENT PROGENITORS IN THE ADULT OE

Two phenotypically distinct categories of basal cells and a third, intermediate type are evident in the basal region. The first, termed horizontal or dark basal cells (HBCs), resembles basal cells of the epithelium lining other parts of the respiratory tree; they form desmosomal attachments to the basal lamina and express markers in common with them, including cytokeratins 5 and 14, intercellular adhesion molecule-1 (ICAM-1), epidermal growth factor receptor (EGF-R), and the sugar moiety recognized by the lectin from *Bandaierea (Griffonia) simplicifolia (21,33)*. The second, termed globose or light basal cells (GBCs) are remarkable in their morphological simplicity, being round with scant cytoplasm, and are situated between the HBCs and the population of

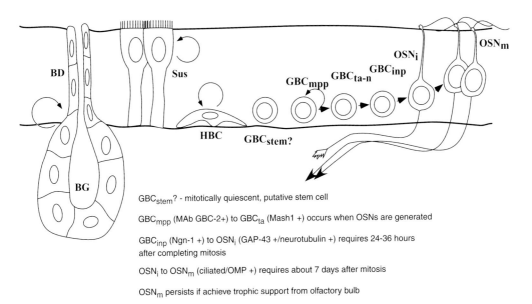

Fig. 1. Cellular consitutuents and progenitor–progeny relationships in the "neuropoietic" olfactory epithelium (where only the neuronal population is undergoing substantial turnover). Each cell type occupies its own lineage *in this context*. Expression of bHLH factors can distinguish transit amplifying and immediate precursor classes of neuronally fated GBCs. However, the multipotent variant is mitotically active in the normal or bulbectomized epithelium. In addition, a set of quiescent, that is, BrdU label-retaining, GBCs is evident in the normal epithelium.

immature OSNs *(21)*. The vast majority of proliferating cells in the olfactory epithelium are classified as GBCs, which operationally fall into a category defined by being "not"—cells near the base of the epithelium that are *not* HBCs, *not* OSNS, and *not* ducts by phenotypic criteria *(34,35)*. Less well appreciated is the existence of a third morphological type that is neither GBC-like, as it is polygonal and touches the basal lamina, nor HBC-like as it lacks the morphological specializations of the HBC, that is, keratin filaments and desmosomes *(21,33)*. This third type has been described as a "transitional" form, implying intermediacy between HBCs and GBCs; however, no data are available to suggest any such relationship.

A wealth of evidence indicates that the population of GBCs includes the progenitor cells that are fated to make neurons in normal epithelium or in epithelium undergoing accelerated turnover limited to the neuronal population (i.e., following bulb ablation) (Fig. 1). Among these findings are the pulse-chase data indicated earlier, selective enhancement of GBC proliferation—and not HBC proliferation—when neuronal turnover is enhanced, and lineage tracing experiments using fluorescent markers or infection of dividing GBCs with replication-incompetent, retrovirally derived vectors (RVV) *(18–21,34,36–38)*. In the latter instance, the expression of the RVV-encoded enzyme is limited to GBCs and OSNs, indicating that the actively proliferating (hence RVV-infectable) GBCs are fated to make neurons in the olfactory epithelium. Finally, the gene encoding *Mash1*, a member of the family of basic helix–loop–helix (bHLH) transcription factors, is selectively expressed in GBCs, and elimination of functional Mash1 protein aborts neuron production in the OE *(39–41)*. One important caveat attaches to the usual conclusion drawn from the foregoing observations. On the basis of these data, one can conclude that GBCs are fated to make neurons and nothing else in epithelium in which only the neuronal population is being replaced in large numbers, that is, undergoing substantial turnover. The data do NOT elucidate the full differentiative capacity of GBCs in other settings.

Nonetheless, the capacity to generate neurons over the long term indicates that the OE retains cells that are competent to serve as neural stem cells throughout life. Indeed, a rare population in the OE is capable of producing large colonies of neurons in vitro, and may be a stem cell in the same sense as used to characterize the CNS cells that give rise to neurospheres in culture *(42,43)*. In keeping with the terminology used to describe other self-renewing tissues (e.g., skin and gut), GBCs in the OE that have some capacity for proliferative expansion *and* are committed to a particular lineage have been termed transit amplifying cells; *Mash1*⁺ GBCs have been identified as transit amplifying cells committed to the neuronal lineage on correlative and genetic grounds *(40,41,44)*. Those GBCs that are downstream of the *Mash1*⁺ transit amplifying cells are considered to be immediate neuronal precursors (INPs) and are presumed to have a very limited capacity for division before terminal differentiation into OSNs *(44,45)*.

MULTIPOTENCY AND THE SINGLE GBC

Much has been learned by exploration of the neuropoietic OE. However, an in-depth understanding of cellular renewal requires a broader perspective. By analogy to the formation of blood, the differentiative capacity of hematopoetic stem cells is much broader than their apparent fate when only one population, say platelets, has been depleted and requires selective replenishment. Accordingly, for the past 10-plus years, we have been exploiting a model for direct epithelial injury that is initiated by passive inhalation of the gas methyl bromide (MeBr) *(32)*. Quite remarkably, rats and several strains of mice (including C57 and DBA2, although not CD-1) when exposed for a single period of 6–10 h develop a profound lesion limited to the OE. In the affected area (> 95% of the epithelium's tangential extent) all Sus cells and all OSNs are destroyed and the populations of basal, duct, and gland cells are partially depleted *(32)*. Despite the severity of the original lesion, the vast majority of the affected OE recovers to a condition that is indistinguishable from normal by 6–8 wk after lesion, including the restoration of the spatial patterns of expression of individual members of the odorant receptor gene family. It is worth noting that direct epithelial injury is more typical of the life of animals in the wild than any form of lesion that causes selective destruction of olfactory neurons *(32,46)*.

As a consequence of the cell loss in the OE occasioned by MeBr exposure, the residual progenitors are challenged with the need to replace a myriad of cell types: both kinds of basal cells, duct cells, sustentacular cells (including the microvillar subset), and, of course, neurons. Under these conditions, to a first approximation, epithelial stem cells should be activated.

Stem cells of the OE are expected to express the characteristics of other tissue stem cells. These include quiescence except in time of need, totipotency, and a capacity for infinite (or nearly infinite) self-renewal *(47–52)*. Although we do no yet have an epithelial stem cell in hand, we have glimpsed them almost within reach. At this point, the data indicate that a multipotent progenitor (MPP) cell is present in the adult OE, which approaches the potency of the cells of the olfactory placode. Furthermore, the MPP appears to be a kind of GBC.

The data indicating multipotency include marker studies, in which cells are caught in phenotypic transition between GBCs and Sus cells on the one hand and GBCs and HBCs on the other *(53)*. In addition, RVV-lineage tracing studies reveal the shift in progenitor cell capacity in response to the lesioned state of the OE *(38,54)*. In contrast to the results in normal epithelium, clones derived from a single infected progenitor in the MeBr-lesioned rat epithelium were composed of neurons, Sus cells (including microvillar cells), HBCs and GBCs, or some combination of the foregoing types. In addition, clones composed of Sus cells only *or* duct/gland and Sus cells were also observed. Given the disappearance of HBCs from the ventral OE in rats, the data suggest that GBCs are the most likely cell type for the MPP, and that duct cells are an alternate source for regenerating Sus cells *(32,54)*.

Other indirect evidence suggesting that some GBCs are multipotent comes from the analysis of expression of the truncated *Mash1* mRNA in mice in with the *Mash1* gene has been disrupted by homologous recombination *(55)*. Although the OE is aneuronal, truncated *Mash1* mRNA remains expressed in Sus cells as well as basal cells of the mutant mice. The most parsimonious explanation for the expanded expression of *Mash1* message is the derivation of Sus cells and neurons from a common progenitor.

The foregoing data are certainly suggestive, although indirect, evidence in favor of the existence of a multipotent GBC. However, direct demonstration of GBC capacity required the development of antibodies suitable for fluorescence-activated cell sorting (FACS) of the various epithelial cell types and of the technologies for promoting progenitor engraftment and for monitoring descendants of transplant-derived progenitors following transplantation.

Unlike most parts of the nervous system, progenitors transplant into the OE easily and engraft productively under conditions where the donor cells are differentiating in parallel with host cells, that is, recovery after a lesion analogous to ones that occur in nature. Thus, dissociated sorted or unsorted cells can be injected into the nasal cavity of either rats or mice lesioned by exposure to MeBr 1 d prior to infusion. The transplanted cells engraft as single cells, and differentiate to produce a panoply of clonally related descendants. Thus, our transplantation paradigm is the equivalent of the colony forming unit-spleen assay that revolutionized the understanding of hematopoiesis.

In mice, GBCs that were FACS-isolated based on surface labeling with the monoclonal antibody GBC-2, and marked by constitutive expression of a marker (e.g., the enhanced form of the green fluorescent protein [eGFP] or β-galactosidase) or by *ex vivo* labeling with RVV, were infused into the nasal cavity of a wild-type host previously lesioned by exposure to MeBr *(56)*. The engrafted GBCs give rise, in aggregate, to GBCs, neurons, sustentacular cells, duct/gland cells, and even columnar respiratory epithelial cells (Fig. 2). Individual clones were composed of OSNs *or* Sus cells *or* OSNs, GBCs and Sus cells, *or* OSNs and duct/gland cells *or* OSNs and respiratory epithelial cells. The neurons that derive from the transplanted GBCs mature to the point of OMP and odorant receptor expression, and extend axons to the OB. Interestingly, the axons grow to that portion of the bulb to which the surrounding, host-derived neurons project their axons normally and after regeneration. However, the question remains open as to whether the donor-derived descendant neurons retain a memory of

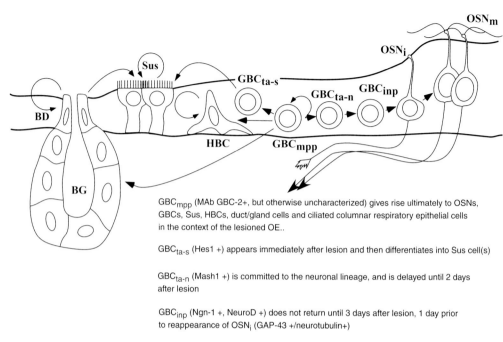

GBC$_{mpp}$ (MAb GBC-2+, but otherwise uncharacterized) gives rise ultimately to OSNs, GBCs, Sus, HBCs, duct/gland cells and ciliated columnar respiratory epithelial cells in the context of the lesioned OE..

GBC$_{ta-s}$ (Hes1 +) appears immediately after lesion and then differentiates into Sus cell(s)

GBC$_{ta-n}$ (Mash1 +) is committed to the neuronal lineage, and is delayed until 2 days after lesion

GBC$_{inp}$ (Ngn-1 +, NeuroD +) does not return until 3 days after lesion, 1 day prior to reappearance of OSN$_i$ (GAP-43 +/neurotubulin+)

Fig. 2. Cellular consitutuents and progenitor–progeny relationships in MeBr-lesioned olfactory epithelium where wholesale replacement of several different cell types, both neurons and nonneuronal cells, must take place to restore the epithelium to its normal state. In this context, multipotent GBCs give rise to all of the cell types that have been depleted in full or in part. A set of GBCs express *Hes1* acutely after lesion and differentiate subsequently into Sus cells. The expression of *Hes1* precedes and may prevent the expression of proneural bHLH transcription factors (first *Mash1* and then *Ngn1* and *NeuroD*).

the original location of their clones' founding progenitor, or whether the precursors and/or differentiating neurons acquire cues from the region in which they engraft that drive such spatially regulated phenotypes as odorant receptor expression.

In rats, the evidence is less direct, but suggests that transplanted GBCs can give rise to HBCs as well as GBCs, OSNs, and Sus cells *(57)*.

In contrast, sorted duct/gland/Sus cells give rise only to themselves. HBCs fail to engraft in mice. In this species the HBC population does *not* disappear from the OE after MeBr lesion, but instead remains as a continuous layer. In rats, bead-labeled HBCs engraft and remain evident as HBCs several days later. However, a more complete examination of the differentiation capacity of HBCs in the latter setting awaits the use of rats that express markers constitutively *(56)*.

Thus, GBCs and no other cell types in the adult OE give evidence of a multipotency that approaches the capacity of the original placodal cells of the embryo. In addition, it is notable that the generation of duct/gland cells from GBCs in the lesioned OE closes the lineage loop between GBCs and Sus cells; that is, Sus cells can arise directly from GBCs (as shown by transplantation and lineage studies) as well as via duct cell intermediate (as shown by the RVV lineage studies).

The multipotency of GBCs and the HBCs' lack thereof stand in some contrast to previous formulations of cellular renewal in the OE. In the past, HBCs have been assigned stem cell status on grounds of relative quiescence, the existence of the ostensibly transitional forms (although evidence for conversion in either direction is lacking), and culture results in which putative HBCs and HBC-derived cell lines can express proteins characteristic of neurons *(21,58,59)*. It is worth noting that the extent of neuronal differentiation in these settings is limited. Against these are the lack of multipotency following engraftment and the absence of lineage relationships with neurons in vivo *(37,38,54)*. Moreover, HBCs are a relatively late-appearing cell type during the differentiation of the embryonic OE, as they appear just prior to birth and may actually invade olfactory epithelium from the neighboring respiratory epithelium *(33)*. In addition, they are very similar in most respects to respiratory epithelial basal cells, all of which makes them less attractive as a stem cell candidate *(33)*.

The lineage and transplantation data assaying the differentiative capacity of GBCs come close to satisfying the totipotency requirement for "stemness." Of the other criteria, mitotic quiescence (or conservation of proliferative potential) has been cited as a characteristic of stem cells in other tissues. A small subset of GBCs is also quiescent, that is, they retain BrdU for an extended period (on the order of weeks), are activated by MeBr lesion, and then are restored within a few days after recovery from the lesion begins *(60)*.

In sum, GBCs show evidence of near-totipotency (by reference to their olfactory placodal ancestors), self-renewal (at least to the limited extent shown by the persistence of donor-derived GBCs after transplantation), and mitotic quiescence. Thus, the best candidate at present for an epithelial stem cell in the adult OE is a kind of GBC.

MOLECULAR AND FUNCTIONAL CLASSES OF GBCS

The progression of GBC progenitors from less to more terminally differentiated has been tied to the expression of members of the bHLH family of transcription factors, which are known to drive cellular differentiation in other settings. A combination of embryological analyses, the identification of epistatic relationships following gene mutation by homologous recombination, and studies of gene expression following lesion have associated particular transcription factors with defined differentiative capacity.

As mentioned earlier, the expression of *Mash1* is required for maintained (although not initial) production of neurons *(39)*. The timing of its expression in the developing epithelium, after bulbectomy, and during recovery from MeBr lesion strongly supports the assignment of *Mash1* expression to transit amplifying cells that are committed to the neuronal lineage *(40,41,44,61)*. The epistatic relationships between bHLH family members and the relative timing of their expression suggest that *Ngn1* and *NeuroD* are downstream of *Mash1* and characteristic of INPs *(41,44)*. On timing grounds, *NeuroD* quickly follows on *Ngn1* expression *(41)*.

What of the multipotent GBCs? Other markers of the bHLH family are known to act as transcriptional repressors, are expressed by multipotent progenitors, and act, in part, by suppressing the proneuronal bHLH factors *(62)*. For example, *Hes1*, the mammalian homolog of the neurogenic gene *hairy* in *Drosophila*, is often expressed in counterpoint to *Mash1 (63,64)*. *Hes1* mRNA is expressed by mature Sus cells in the normal adult OE or after bulbectomy *(61)*. In contrast, *Hes1* is expressed by a subset of GBCs at 1 d post-MeBr lesion, which is perhaps not surprising given the rapid generation of

Sus cells by GBCs acutely after MeBr lesion. Over the next few days during recovery, the *Hes1⁺* basal cells lose their close association with the basal lamina, are displaced apicalward as the neuronal population is reconstituted, and differentiate into Sus cells. Thus, *Hes1* expression seems to mark commitment to the execution of a sustentacular cell differentiation program and not the multipotent GBCs *per se*. Interestingly, the resumption of *Mash1* expression by GBCs lags that of *Hes1* by a day during the recovery from MeBr lesion (reappearing in large numbers on d 2 postlesion), and *Ngn1* and *NeuroD* are delayed yet another day beyond *Mash1* (d 3 postlesion). Finally, neurons reappear a day after *Ngn1* and *NeuroD* (d 4 postlesion). Given the prevalence of active multipotent cells at 1 d after MeBr lesion, none of the proneural factors are candidates for expression by the multipotent cells. Thus, it appears that the generation of Sus cells is the first task undertaken by the reconstituting epithelium.

The expression of *Hes1* vs *Mash1* is apparently reciprocal. In the absence of functional *Mash1* gene product, *Hes1* expression is eliminated while expression of the truncated *Mash1* mRNA is maintained even into Sus cells *(41,64)*. Conversely, elimination of *Hes1* is known to expand the *Mash1* expression domain and the production of neurons in the developing placode *(64)*. In contrast, *Hes6*, also a transcriptional repressor, seems to act as a promoter of neuronal differentiation in OE, perhaps by suppressing Hes1 *(65)*.

Two conclusions derive from the foregoing. First, *Hes1* expression is tied to, and probably required for, the suppression of *Mash1* in OE progenitors. Second, *Hes1* is not required, *per se*, for the differentiation of Sus cells, because they form in the *Mash1*-knockout animals despite their failure to express *Hes1*. However, it is striking that *Hes1* expression continues as the cells differentiate and is maintained as they mature, raising the issue of whether a neuronal differentiation program might reactivate if *Hes1* expression is suppressed in the Sus cells.

Furthermore, the central role of *Hes1* during the early recovery of the epithelium after MeBr lesion hints at the identity of the regulatory pathway that sits upstream of the gene. In several other settings in vertebrates, signaling via the Notch cascade is known to activate *Hes1* and thereby suppress its downstream targets including *Mash1* *(62,66)*. Here, too, in the OE, *Notch1* is expressed by a subset of GBCs and may be marking those that have the capacity to serve as MPPs *(61)*.

REGULATION OF PROGENITOR CELL CAPACITY

Implicit in the foregoing discussion is the idea that progenitor cell behavior is regulated by the status of the epithelial environment. The lineage data indicate that GBCs are fated to make neurons in one setting (where only OSNs need replacing) but shift actively to making nonneuronal cells if nonneuronal populations are depleted. That statement holds true even for GBCs that are in the mitotic cycle at the time of transplantation from neuropoietic (normal OE or after bulbectomy) to MeBr-lesioned epithelium. Thus, it appears that some MPPs are actively proliferating in the normal OE and primed to respond to external cues by shifting to a multipotent fate *(56,57)*. In addition, the rate at which neurons are made is responsive to conditions of increased need for replacement neurons. For example, the rate of GBC proliferation and of neuronal production is accelerated following injury to the ON or bulb, which elicit the retrograde degeneration of OSNs, or as a consequence of the accelerated turnover

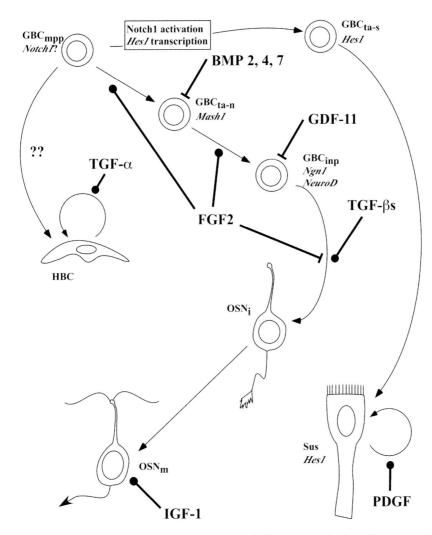

Fig. 3. Growth factor regulate the processes of cellular renewal in the olfactory epithelium by means of negative feedback on cellular production (BMPs and GDF-11), positive feedback on cellular production (TGF-α and platelet-derived growth factor [PDGF]), and effects on the differentiation state of the target cells (TGF-β and FGF-2). Lines ending in *circles* indicate a stimulatory effect; lines ending in a *perpendicular line* indicate inhibition.

occasioned by the failure of OSNs born in the absence of the bulb to achieve trophic support *(24,27,34,67)*. Conversely, the mitotic rate falls following naris occlusion, possibly owing to a protective effect of reducing environmental exposure to the OE on the occluded side *(68,69)*.

Given evidence of regulation, what kinds of cues are acting on the progenitors and how are the shifts in proliferation and differentiation accomplished within the cell? Both aspects of the regulatory process are relatively poorly understood, but several key mediators and regulatory process have been identified (Fig. 3).

Work from Calof's and Mackay-Sim's laboratories has focused on signals that have clearly played a role in other differentiating settings. Thus, fibroblast growth factors

(FGFs) are present in the OE and cause modest stimulation of GBC proliferation in vitro, which also express FGF receptors *(70–74)*. In addition, activation of the FGF signaling cascade apparently suppressed differentiation of GBC-derived cell lines toward neurons and thus is a candidate factor for playing a role in the regulation of multipotency *(75)*. Ligands that activate members of the ErbB family of tyrosine kinase receptors also seem to play a role *(76)*. EGF and transforming growth factor-α (TGF-α) stimulate the proliferation of HBCs both in vivo and in vitro *(77–79)*. Likewise, neu differentiation factor is found in the OE and activates its receptor in the OE after infusion in vivo *(80)*.

The enhancement of proliferation that follows retrograde degeneration of OSNs looks to be due at least in part to the release of an inhibitory feedback loop of the OSN-derived factors onto the GBCs. Calof's laboratory has identified two such loops. In the first, members of the bone morphogenetic protein (BMP) family can reduce olfactory neurogenesis in vitro *(81)*. In keeping with their role as feedback factors, OSNs express the genes for BMP-4 and possibly 7 (if in neurons, only in immature ones) *(82)*. BMPs suppress neurogenesis in vitro by causing the proteosome-mediated proteolysis of the proneural transcription factor *Mash1* and the death of the transit amplifying GBCs that make it *(81)*.

In the second, a strong case can be made for the participation of GDF-11 (glial differentiation factor 11, a member of the TGF-β-activin wing of the TGF-β superfamily) as a negative feedback regulator *(45)*. GDF-11 is expressed by a least a subset of OSNs, possibly concentrated in the deeper and probably more immature neurons. Elimination of GDF-11 by gene "knockout" causes an increase in the size of the neuronal population in the embryonic OE. Conversely, application of GDF-11 in vitro or elimination of follistatin, a GDF inhibitor by gene knockout, in vivo decreases neurogenesis. In contrast to the effect of BMPs, manipulation of the GDF-11 pathway apparently acts downstream of the transit amplifying cells by reducing either the production or expansion of the immediate neuronal precursor (INP) population judging by the reduction in the number of cells that express a *Ngn1* transgene. In contrast to the effects of BMPs, no increase in apoptosis is observed, and removal of GDF-11 releases the inhibition partially.

Other members of the TGF-β superfamily seem to promote neuronal differentiation. Thus, TGF-β1 or 2 can push the differentiation of primary cultures or cell lines toward more pronounced differentiation *(76)*.

Other factors, no doubt, exist that promote or repress neurogenesis, and accelerate or retard neuronal differentiation following terminal mitosis, but remain obscure.

SUMMARY, CONCLUSIONS, AND UNANSWERED QUESTIONS

Analysis of the OE has shown that GBCs exhibit an unexpected breadth and power as progenitors. Beyond their commonly accepted role as neuronal precursors, it has become apparent that GBCs in the adult OE retain a differentiative capacity that is as broad—or nearly so—as that of the original placodal cells that give rise to the peripheral olfactory system during embryonic development. In functional terms, the GBCs more closely resemble their embryonic forerunners than do the progenitors of the adult CNS, which are apparently fairly limited in their differentiative capacity normally. In addition, GBCs may not resemble the progenitors of the adult CNS very closely with respect to biochemical phenotype. GBCs do not express many of the markers that are typical of the CNS neural stem cells, such as *nestin*.

Unfortunately, we cannot say precisely what genetic profile DOES characterize the stem cells of the olfactory epithelium, nor can we isolate the stem cells specifically. The GBC population is clearly heterogeneous with respect to differentiative capacity, and the identity of the bHLH family member whose expression apparently correlates with those differences. It may be feasible to take advantage of selective expression of bHLH family members, for example, by using BAC transgenic mice that express eGFP from a bHLH transgene, to isolate and then define the functional capacity of defined GBC subsets in more detail using our transplantation assay, and to assess whether their patterns of gene expression are equivalent to neural and other kinds of stem cells.

Progress in understanding the regulation of epitheliopoiesis in the olfactory system requires a better characterization of these cells and the development of more facile and potent assays for their functional characterization. The time is ripe to take advantage of the facility for manipulating the system in vivo using, for example, retro- or lentiviral vectors to boost or block gene expression without having to resort to the time-consuming and expensive generation of transgenic or gene-knockout lines, which will lack targeted expression in most cases. In addition, the field desperately needs a cell culture system that supports full cellular differentiation in order to investigate the regulation of cellular renewal by soluble factors.

The potential payoff for pursuing these lines of investigation is substantial. For better or worse, studies are already underway attempting to exploit essentially uncharacterized olfactory tissue, isolated by autologous harvest, to generate cell lines for therapeutic interventions in spinal cord injury and demyelinating diseases. True progress in the understanding of the biology of olfactory stem cells, and their responsible use as a form of cellular therapy will necessarily go hand-in-hand.

ACKNOWLEDGMENTS

The authors thank present and past members of the Schwob laboratory for their myriad contributions to the success of the work. The laboratory's work and the preparation of the review were supported by grants from the NIH R01 DC00467, R01 DC02167, and R21 DC006517.

REFERENCES

1. Graziadei, P. P. C. (1990) Olfactory development. In *Development of Sensory Systems in Mammals* (Coleman, J. R., ed.), John Wiley, New York.
2. Graziadei, P. P. C. (1974) The olfactory organ of vertebrates: a survey. In *Essays on Structure and Function in the Nervous System* (Bellairs, R. and Gray, E. G., eds.), Clarendon, London, pp. 191–222.
3. Schwob, J. E. (2002) Neural regeneration and the peripheral olfactory system. *Anat. Rec.* **269,** 33–49.
4. Rawson, N. E., Gomez, G., Cowart, B., and Restrepo, D. (1998) The use of olfactory receptor neurons (ORNs) from biopsies to study changes in aging and neurodegenerative diseases. *Ann. NY Acad. Sci.* **855,** 701–707.
5. Lane, A. P., Gomez, G., Dankulich, T., Wang, H., Bolger, W. E., and Rawson, N. E. (2002) The superior turbinate as a source of functional human olfactory receptor neurons. *Laryngoscope* **112,** 1183–1189.

6. Rawson, N. E. and Gomez, G. (2002) Cell and molecular biology of human olfaction. *Microsc. Res. Tech.* **58,** 142–151.

7. Raisman, G. (2001) Olfactory ensheathing cells—another miracle cure for spinal cord injury? *Nat. Rev. Neurosci.* **2,** 369–375.

8. Cuschieri, A. and Bannister, L. H. (1975) The development of the olfactory mucosa in the mouse: light microscopy. *J. Anat.* **119,** 277–286.

9. Cuschieri, A. and Bannister, L. H. (1975) The development of the olfactory mucosa in the mouse: electron microscopy. *J. Anat.* **119,** 471–498.

10. Couly, G. F. and Le Douarin, N. M. (1985) Mapping of the early neural primordium in quail-chick chimeras. I. Developmental relationships between placodes, facial ectoderm, and prosencephalon. *Dev. Biol.* **110,** 422–439.

11. Farbman, A. I. and Squinto, L. M. (1985) Early development of olfactory receptor cell axons. *J. Neurochem.* **44,** 1459–1464.

12. Schwanzel-Fukuda, M. and Pfaff, D. W. (1990) The migration of luteinizing hormone-releasing hormone (LHRH) neurons from the medial olfactory placode into the medial basal forebrain. *Experientia* **46,** 956–962.

13. Schwanzel-Fukuda, M. (1999) Origin and migration of luteinizing hormone-releasing hormone neurons in mammals. *Microsc. Res. Tech.* **44,** 2–10.

14. Nagahara, Y. (1940) Experimentelle Studien uber die histologiischen Veranderungen des Geruchsorgan nach der Olfactoriusdurschneidung. Beitrage zur Kenntnis des feineren Baus des Geruchsorgans. *Jpn. J. Med. Sci. V. Pathol.* **5,** 165–169.

15. Bodian, D. A. and Howe, H. A. (1941) Experimental studies on intraneural spread of poliomyelitis virus. *Bull. Johns Hopkins Hosp.* **68,** 248–267.

16. Moulton, D. G., Celebi, G., and Fink, R. P. (1970) Olfaction in mammals—two aspects: proliferation of cells in the olfactory epithelium and sensitivity to odours. In *Ciba Foundation Symposium on Taste and Smell in Vertebrates* (Wolstenholme, G. E. W. and Knight, J., eds.), Churchill, London, pp. 227–250.

17. Graziadei, P. P. C. and Metcalf, J. F. (1971) Autoradiographic and ultrastructural observations on the frog's olfactory mucosa. *Z. Zellforsch. Mikrosk. Anat.* **116,** 305–318.

18. Moulton, D. G. (1975) Cell renewal in the olfactory epithelium. In *Olfaction and Taste,* V (Denton, D. A. and Coghlan, J. P., eds.), Academic Press, New York, pp. 111–114.

19. Graziadei, P. P. C. (1973) Cell dynamics in the olfactory mucosa. *Tissue Cell* **5,** 113–131.

20. Graziadei, P. P. C. and Monti Graziadei, G. A. (1978) Continuous nerve cell renewal in the olfactory system. In *Handbook of Sensory Physiology,* Vol. IX (Jacobson, M., ed.), Springer-Verlag, Berlin, pp. 55–82.

21. Graziadei, P. P. C. and Monti Graziadei, G. A. (1979) Neurogenesis and neuron regeneration in the olfactory system of mammals. I. Morphological aspects of differentiation and structural organization of the olfactory sensory neurons. *J. Neurocytol.* **8,** 1–18.

22. Verhaagen, J., Oestreicher, A. B., Gispen, W. H., and Margolis, F. L. (1989) The expression of the growth associated protein B50/GAP43 in the olfactory system of neonatal and adult rats. *J. Neurosci.* **9,** 683–691.

23. Meiri, K. F., Bickerstaff, L. E., and Schwob, J. E. (1991) Monoclonal antibodies show that kinase C phosphorylation of GAP-43 during axonogenesis is both spatially and temporally restricted in vivo. *J. Cell Biol.* **112,** 991–1005.

24. Schwob, J. E., Szumowski, K. E., and Stasky, A. A. (1992) Olfactory sensory neurons are trophically dependent on the olfactory bulb for their prolonged survival. *J. Neurosci.* **12,** 3896–3919.

25. Mackay-Sim, A. and Kittel, P. W. (1991) On the life span of olfactory receptor neurons. *Eur. J. Neurosci.* **3,** 209–215.

26. Harding, J., Graziadei, P. P. C., Monti Graziadei, G. A., and Margolis, F. L. (1977) Denervation in the primary olfactory pathway of mice. IV. Biochemical and morphological evidence for neuronal replacement following nerve section. *Brain Res.* **132,** 11–28.

27. Monti Graziadei, G. A. and Graziadei, P. P. C. (1979) Neurogenesis and neuron regeneration in the olfactory system of mammals. II. Degeneration and reconstitution of the olfactory sensory neurons after axotomy. *J. Neurocytol.* **8,** 197–213.
28. Costanzo, R. M. and Graziadei, P. P. C. (1983) A quantitative analysis of changes in the olfactory epithelium following bulbectomy in hamster. *J. Comp. Neurol.* **215,** 370–381.
29. Costanzo, R. M. (1984) Comparison of neurogenesis and cell replacement in the hamster olfactory system with and without a target (olfactory bulb). *Brain Res.* **307,** 295–301.
30. Costanzo, R. M. (1985) Neural regeneration and functional reconnection following olfactory nerve transection in hamster. *Brain Res.* **361,** 258–266.
31. Costanzo, R. M. (2000) Rewiring the olfactory bulb: changes in odor maps following recovery from nerve transection. *Chem. Senses* **25,** 199–205.
32. Schwob, J. E., Youngentob, S. L., and Mezza, R. C. (1995) Reconstitution of the rat olfactory epithelium after methyl bromide-induced lesion. *J. Comp. Neurol.* **359,** 15–37.
33. Holbrook, E. H., Szumowski, K. E. and Schwob, J. E. (1995) An immunochemical, ultrastructural, and developmental characterization of the horizontal basal cells of rat olfactory epithelium. *J. Comp. Neurol.* **363,** 129–146.
34. Schwartz Levey, M., Chikaraishi, D. M., and Kauer, J. S. (1991) Characterization of potential precursor populations in the mouse olfactory epithelium using immunocytochemistry and autoradiography. *J. Neurosci.* **11,** 3556–3664.
35. Huard, J. M. and Schwob, J. E. (1995) Cell cycle of globose basal cells in rat olfactory epithelium. *Dev. Dyn.* **203,** 17–26.
36. Schwartz Levey, M., Cinelli, A. R., and Kauer, J. S. (1992) Intracellular injection of vital dyes into single cells in the salamander olfactory epithelium. *Neurosci. Lett.* **140,** 265–269.
37. Caggiano, M., Kauer, J. S., and Hunter, D. D. (1994) Globose basal cells are neuronal progenitors in the olfactory epithelium: a lineage analysis using a replication-incompetent retrovirus. *Neuron* **13,** 339–352.
38. Schwob, J. E., Huard, J. M., Luskin, M. B., and Youngentob, S. L. (1994) Retroviral lineage studies of the rat olfactory epithelium. *Chem. Senses* **19,** 671–682.
39. Guillemot, F., Lo, L. C., Johnson, J. E., Auerbach, A., Anderson, D. J., and Joyner, A. L. (1993) Mammalian achaete-scute homolog 1 is required for the early development of olfactory and autonomic neurons. *Cell* **75,** 463–476.
40. Gordon, M. K., Mumm, J. S., Davis, R. A., Holcomb, J. D., and Calof, A. L. (1995) Dynamics of MASH1 expression in vitro and in vivo suggest a non-stem cell site of MASH1 action in the olfactory receptor neuron lineage. *Mol. Cell. Neurosci.* **6,** 363–379.
41. Cau, E., Gradwohl, G., Fode, C., and Guillemot, F. (1997) Mash1 activates a cascade of bHLH regulators in olfactory neuron progenitors. *Development* **124,** 1611–1621.
42. Mumm, J. S., Shou, J., and Calof, A. L. (1996) Colony-forming progenitors from mouse olfactory epithelium: evidence for feedback regulation of neuron production. *Proc. Natl. Acad. Sci. USA* **93,** 11167–11172.
43. Calof, A. L., Mumm, J. S., Rim, P. C., and Shou, J. (1998) The neuronal stem cell of the olfactory epithelium. *J. Neurobiol.* **36,** 190–205.
44. Cau, E., Casarosa, S., and Guillemot, F. (2002) Mash1 and Ngn1 control distinct steps of determination and differentiation in the olfactory sensory neuron lineage. *Development* **129,** 1871–1880.
45. Wu, H. H., Ivkovic, S., Murray, R. C., et al. (2003) Autoregulation of neurogenesis by GDF11. *Neuron* **37,** 197–207.
46. Iwema, C. L., Fang, H., Kurtz, D. B., Youngentob, S. L., and Schwob, J. E. (2004) Odorant receptor expression patterns are restored in lesion-recovered rat olfactory epithelium. *J. Neurosci.* **24,** 356–369.
47. Cotsarelis, G., Cheng, S. Z., Dong, G., Sun, T. T., and Lavker, R. M. (1989) Existence of slow-cycling limbal epithelial basal cells that can be preferentially stimulated to proliferate: implications on epithelial stem cells. *Cell* **57,** 201–209.

48. Potten, C. S. and Loeffler, M. (1990) Stem cells: attributes, cycles, spirals, pitfalls and uncertainties. Lessons for and from the crypt. *Development* **110**, 1001–1020.
49. Morris, R. J. and Potten, C. S. (1994) Slowly cycling (label-retaining) epidermal cells behave like clonogenic stem cells in vitro. *Cell Prolif.* **27**, 279–289.
50. Potten, C. S. (1998) Stem cells in gastrointestinal epithelium: numbers, characteristics and death. *Philos. Trans. R. Soc. Lond. B Biol. Sci.* **353**, 821–830.
51. Watt, F. M. and Hogan, B. L. (2000) Out of Eden: stem cells and their niches. *Science* **287**, 1427–1430.
52. Lavker, R. M. and Sun, T. T. (2003) Epithelial stem cells: the eye provides a vision. *Eye* **17**, 937–942.
53. Goldstein, B. J. and Schwob, J. E. (1996) Analysis of the globose basal cell compartment in rat olfactory epithelium using GBC-1, a new monoclonal antibody against globose basal cells. *J. Neurosci.* **16**, 4005–4016.
54. Huard, J. M., Youngentob, S. L., Goldstein, B. J., Luskin, M. B., and Schwob, J. E. (1998) Adult olfactory epithelium contains multipotent progenitors that give rise to neurons and non-neural cells. *J. Comp. Neurol.* **400**, 469–486.
55. Murray, R. C., Navi, D., Fesenko, J., Lander, A. D., and Calof, A. L. (2003) Widespread defects in the primary olfactory pathway caused by loss of *Mash1* function. *J. Neurosci.* **23**, 1769–1780.
56. Chen, X., Fang, H., and Schwob, J. E. (2004) Multipotency of purified, transplanted globose basal cells in olfactory epithelium. *J. Comp. Neurol.* **469**, 457–474.
57. Goldstein, B. J., Fang, H., Youngentob, S. L., and Schwob, J. E. (1998) Transplantation of multipotent progenitors from the adult olfactory epithelium. *NeuroReport* **9**, 1611–1617.
58. Satoh, M. and Yoshida, T. (2000) Expression of neural properties in olfactory cytokeratin-positive basal cell line. *Brain Res. Dev. Brain Res.* **121**, 219–222.
59. Satoh, M. and Takeuchi, M. (1995) Induction of NCAM expression in mouse olfactory keratin-positive basal cells in vitro. *Brain Res. Dev. Brain Res.* **87**, 111–119.
60. Chen, X. C. (2003) *Functional Capacity of Progenitor Cells in the Olfactory Epithelium.* Ph. D. thesis in Cell, Molecular, and Developmental Biology, Tufts University, Boston, MA.
61. Manglapus, G. L. (2003) *Molecular Mechanisms for Progenitor Cell Regulation in the Mammalian Peripheral Olfactory System.* Ph. D. thesis in Neuroscience and Physiology, SUNY-Syracuse.
62. Davis, R. L. and Turner, D. L. (2001) Vertebrate *hairy* and *Enhancer of split* related proteins: transcriptional repressors regulating cellular differentiation and embryonic patterning. *Oncogene* **20**, 8342–8357.
63. Fisher, A. and Caudy, M. (1998) The function of *hairy*-related bHLH repressor proteins in cell fate decisions. *BioEssays* **20**, 298–306.
64. Cau, E., Gradwohl, G., Casarosa, S., Kageyama, R., and Guillemot, F. (2000) *Hes* genes regulate sequential stages of neurogenesis in the olfactory epithelium. *Development* **127**, 2323–2332.
65. Suzuki, Y., Mizoguchi, I., Nishiyama, H., Takeda, M., and Obara, N. (2003) Expression of *Hes6* and *NeuroD* in the olfactory epithelium, vomeronasal organ and nonsensory patches. *Chem Senses* **28**, 197–205.
66. Iso, T., Kedes, L., and Hamamori, Y. (2003) HES and HERP families: multiple effectors of the Notch signaling pathway. *J. Cell. Physiol.* **194**, 237–255.
67. Carr, V. M. and Farbman, A. I. (1992) Ablation of the olfactory bulb up-regulates the rate of neurogenesis and induces precocious cell death in olfactory epithelium. *Exp. Neurol.* **115**, 55–59.
68. Farbman, A. I., Brunjes, P. C., Rentfro, L., Michas, J., and Ritz, S. (1988) The effect of unilateral naris occlusion on cell dynamics in the developing rat olfactory epithelium. *J. Neurobiol.* **19**, 681–693.

69. Farbman, A. I. (1990) Olfactory neurogenesis: genetic or environmental controls? *Trends Neurosci.* **13,** 362–365.
70. Calof, A. L. and Chikaraishi, D. M. (1989) Analysis of neurogenesis in a mammalian neuroepithelium: proliferation and differentiation of an olfactory neuron precursor in vitro. *Neuron* **3,** 115–127.
71. DeHamer, M. K., Guevara, J. L., Hannon, K., Olwin, B. B., and Calof, A. L. (1994) Genesis of olfactory receptor neurons in vitro: regulation of progenitor cell divisions by fibroblast growth factors. *Neuron* **13,** 1083–1097.
72. Calof, A. L. (1995) Intrinsic and extrinsic factors regulating vertebrate neurogenesis. *Curr. Opin. Neurobiol.* **5,** 19–27.
73. Newman, M. P., Feron, F., and Mackay-Sim, A. (2000) Growth factor regulation of neurogenesis in adult olfactory epithelium. *Neuroscience* **99,** 343–350.
74. Hsu, P., Yu, F., Feron, F., Pickles, J. O., Sneesby, K., and Mackay-Sim, A. (2001) Basic fibroblast growth factor and fibroblast growth factor receptors in adult olfactory epithelium. *Brain Res.* **896,** 188–197.
75. Goldstein, B. J., Wolozin, B. L., and Schwob, J. E. (1997) FGF2 suppresses neuronogenesis of a cell line derived from rat olfactory epithelium. *J. Neurobiol.* **33,** 411–428.
76. Mahanthappa, N. K. and Schwarting, G. A. (1993) Peptide growth factor control of olfactory neurogenesis and neuron survival in vitro: roles of EGF and TGF-betas. *Neuron* **10,** 293–305.
77. Farbman, A. I. and Buchholz, J. A. (1996) Transforming growth factor-alpha and other growth factors stimulate cell division in olfactory epithelium in vitro. *J. Neurobiol.* **30,** 267–280.
78. Ezeh, P. I. and Farbman, A. I. (1998) Differential activation of ErbB receptors in the rat olfactory mucosa by transforming growth factor-alpha and epidermal growth factor in vivo. *J. Neurobiol.* **37,** 199–210.
79. Getchell, T. V., Narla, R. K., Little, S., Hyde, J. F., and Getchell, M. L. (2000) Horizontal basal cell proliferation in the olfactory epithelium of transforming growth factor-alpha transgenic mice. *Cell Tissue Res.* **299,** 185–192.
80. Salehi-Ashtiani, K. and Farbman, A. I. (1996) Expression of neu and Neu differentiation factor in the olfactory mucosa of rat. *Int. J. Dev. Neurosci.* **14,** 801–811.
81. Shou, J., Rim, P. C., and Calof, A. L. (1999) BMPs inhibit neurogenesis by a mechanism involving degradation of a transcription factor. *Nat. Neurosci.* **2,** 339–345.
82. Shou, J., Murray, R. C., Rim, P. C., and Calof, A. L. (2000) Opposing effects of bone morphogenetic proteins on neuron production and survival in the olfactory receptor neuron lineage. *Development* **127,** 5403–5413.

10

Retinal Stem Cells

Ani V. Das, Jackson James,
Sreekumaran Edakkot, and Iqbal Ahmad

INTRODUCTION

The vertebrate retina is a well-characterized central nervous system (CNS) structure, consisting of seven major cell types, which in adult are arranged in a stereotypical laminar organization. These cell types are born in an evolutionarily conserved temporal sequence: the majority of retinal ganglion cells (RGCs), horizontal cells, amacrine cells, and cone photoreceptors are born during early histogenesis, whereas the majority of rod photoreceptors, bipolar cells, and the Müller glia are generated during late histogenesis *(1)*. Thus, as elsewhere in the CNS *(2)*, neurogenesis in the retina precedes gliogenesis. Underlying cellular diversity in the retina is population of neural progenitors that generate stage-specific neurons and glia *(3)*. Evidence from a variety of experimental approaches including cell ablation studies and in vivo lineage analyses demonstrated that neural progenitors in the developing retina were multipotential, possessing capacity to generate all seven retinal cell types, including the Müller glia *(4–8)*. Although retinal progenitors have not been demonstrated to possess the potential of self-renewal *(9,10)*, a hallmark of stem cells, they are included within the broad description of stem cells, with the assumption that they possess the potential of self-renewal. Potentially this is not demonstrable in vitro because of a lack of a conducive environment *(3)*. In mammals and other warm-blooded vertebrates, neural stem cells are found only in the embryonic retina *(11–13)*. Recently a quiescent population of neural stem cells with retinal potential has been identified in the ciliary epithelium of warm-blooded vertebrates *(13–15)*. These cells are regarded as analogous to those found in the ciliary marginal zone (CMZ) of adult fish and frog retina *(11,16,17)*. In adult fish, neural stem cells are not confined to CMZ but are also located in the inner retina and are regarded to generate rod photoreceptors during regeneration and in response to injury *(16)*.

ISOLATION AND ENRICHMENT OF RETINAL STEM CELLS

Neural stem cells from the embryonic retina and adult ciliary epithelium can be isolated and enriched as neurospheres in response to exposure to mitogens *(10,14,15,18)*. Cells in the neurospheres express universal molecular characteristics of neural stem

From: *Neural Development and Stem Cells, Second Edition*
Edited by: M. S. Rao © Humana Press Inc., Totowa, NJ

cells *(3,19)*. For example, they express cell surface carbohydrate Lex/SSEA1/CD15 *(20)*; transcription factor Sox2 *(21–23)*; telomerase reverse transcriptase (TERT) *(22,24)*; RNA binding protein, Musashi *(25,26)*; nestin, an intermediate filament marker *(25,27,28)*; and neuralstemnin, a nucleolar protein *(29)*. In addition, they express multiple genes encoding transcription factors that play important roles during patterning and development of optic neuroepithelium. These include Pax6 *(30,31)*, Chx10 *(32,33)*, Lhx2 *(34,35)*, and Six6 *(36,37)*. The expression of a combination of transcription factors and universal neural stem cell markers may help identify neural stem cells in the developing retina and adult ciliary epithelium. For example, the relatively low expression of Musashi, Lhx2, Sox2, and Chx10 (Musashi^{low}, Lhx2^{low}, Sox2^{low}, Chx10^{low}) distinguishes ciliary epithelial stem cells from their retinal counterparts.

Like neural stem cells in the CNS, retinal and ciliary epithelial stem cells have been isolated retrospectively, based on their responsiveness to mitogens *(10,14,15)*. In the past few years, several strategies have been adopted for the direct identification of neural stem cells from fresh tissues (prospective identification). For example, a positive selection strategy using cell surface markers and fluorescence-activated cell sorting (FACS) has been used successfully to isolate stem cells from the peripheral nervous system (PNS) *(38)* and CNS *(20,39)*. More recently, a negative selection strategy to exclude cells expressing differentiation epitopes has been used for the direct isolation of embryonic neural stem cells *(40)*. Another approach to identify stem cells is based on the ability of stem cells/progenitors to selectively exclude Hoechst Dye 33342. These cells can be enriched as a minor population, called side population (SP) cells *(41)*. The Hoechst dye exclusion assay has been used for the direct identification of retinal and ciliary epithelial stem cells *(3,42)*. The emergence of retinal and ciliary epithelial stem cells, using the Hoechst dye exclusion assay, is sensitive to verapamil and correlates with the expression of ATP-binding cassette transporter, ABCG2 *(43)*. A comparison of retinal SP cells, isolated from fresh embryonic retina and mitogen-exposed neurospheres, has shown that these two populations of cells are similar in characteristics and potential *(42)*.

PROLIFERATIVE POTENTIAL OF RETINAL STEM CELLS

The generation of distinct cell types in two stages of retinal histogenesis is underpinned by two temporally segregated subpopulations of retinal stem cells: early and late. Their competence for stage-dependent cell fate specification is accompanied by differential responsiveness to growth factors and potential to generate neurons and glia. Like their counterparts in other regions of the CNS during neurogenesis *(2,44)*, the early and late retinal stem cells show preference for fibroblast growth factor-2 (FGF-2) and epidermal growth factor (EGF), respectively, for proliferation (Fig. 1). The responsiveness of early retinal stem cells to FGF-2 is likely due to relatively high expression of FGFR-1, the receptor that is thought primarily to mediate the effects of FGF-2 *(45)* (Fig. 1). The role of FGFR-1 in sustaining the proliferation of stem cells/progenitors in early stages of neurogenesis is supported by observations that FGFR-1 is expressed during early neurogenesis *(46,47)* (James and Ahmad, *unpublished observation*) and that the loss of functional FGFR-1 compromises the proliferation of early neural progenitors *(44)*. There is a significant decrease in levels of both FGFR-1 transcripts in late retinal stem cells that may explain their lack of responsiveness to FGF-2 for prolif-

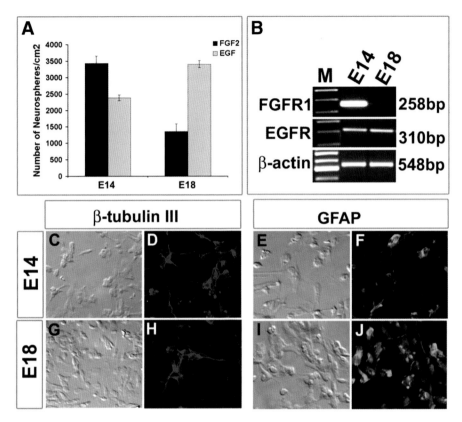

Fig. 1. Early and late retinal stem cells display distinct proliferative and differentiation potential. Retinal stem cells representing early and late stages of histogenesis display differential ability to generate neurospheres in the presence of FGF-2 and EGF (**A**). Reverse transcriptase-polymerase chain reaction (RT-PCR) analysis reveals that transcripts corresponding to FGFR-1 and EGFR are expressed differentially in early and late retinal stem cells (**B**). Neurospheres generated by early and late retinal stem cells were cultured in differentiating condition and potential of cells in neurospheres to express β-tubulin and GFAP was examined by immunocytochemical analysis. E14 neurospheres contained more β-tubulin-positive cells, whereas E18 neurospheres contained more GFAP-positive cells (**C–J**).

eration. Their proliferative responsiveness to EGF is correlated with high levels of EGFR expression in neurospheres. Such responsiveness to EGF, which has been observed to be a characteristic of the late neural progenitors, is severely affected when activity of EGFR is blocked *(44,48)*. The mechanism underlying the temporal changes in the proliferative behavior of early and late retinal stem cells is not well understood. Because early and late retinal stem cells represent two temporally segregated subpopulations of retinal stem cells, it is tempting to speculate that the former may influence the proliferative properties of the latter. This notion is supported by several lines of evidence, emerging from studies carried out in the CNS progenitors *(44,49)*. First, lineage analysis carried out in the developing cortex, using retrovirus coexpressing EGFR and a lineage marker, has shown that the late neural progenitors expressing high levels of EGFR are descendants of early neural progenitors *(50)*. Second, analysis of early neural progenitors in explant culture demonstrated that their responsiveness to EGF is accelerated by exposure to FGF-2 *(49)*. Also, loss of functional FGFR-1 has been shown to compromise the emergence of EGF-responsive late neural progenitors *(44)*.

The ciliary epithelial stem cells appear similar to early retinal stem cells in terms of their proliferative responsiveness *(3)*, in the sense that they are more responsive to FGF2 than EGF. However, they are distinct from retinal stem cells in one respect: unlike retinal stem cells they can self-renew in vitro *(3)*. Limiting dilution analysis of neurosphere generation suggests that the ability of retinal stem cells to generate a clone is a noncell autonomous process, that is, requires cell–cell interactions, whereas ciliary epithelial stem cells can generate neurospheres at clonal density *(3,14,15)*. Such distinctions may represent tissue-specific differences in competence, which is reflected in different transcriptional profiles of retinal and ciliary epithelial stem cells. Analysis has shown that these two stem cell populations share 80% of 2968 expressed genes *(3)*. The transcriptional profile also sheds valuable light on the possible relationships between retinal and ciliary epithelial stem cells; the ciliary epithelial stem cells have more expressed genes in common with early (6.68%) than with late (0.61%) retinal stem cells, therefore, lineally closer to the former than to the latter. Based on the fact that they share more expressed genes with early retinal stem cells and have express self-renewal properties, the ciliary epithelial stem cells can be regarded as the antecedent of retinal stem cells.

The importance of the maintenance of a pool of retinal stem cells/progenitors for sustaining both early and late histogenesis suggests that multiple signaling mechanisms, besides those mediated by FGF-2 and EGF, may regulate their proliferation and the state of commitment. In addition to EGF/FGF-2–mediated receptor tyrosine kinase (RTK) signaling, intracellular signaling mediated by Notch and Wnt may play important role in the maintenance of retinal and ciliary epithelial stem cells. The Notch signaling pathway defines an evolutionarily conserved cell–cell interaction mechanism that has been shown to regulate stem cells in a broad spectrum of tissues of both invertebrates and vertebrates *(51)*. Recent studies have demonstrated an essential role of Notch signaling in the maintenance of neural stem cells. For example, a dramatic reduction in the generation of neurospheres was observed by cells lacking functional *Notch1* genes or those that encode intracellular components of the canonical Notch pathway, such as *Hes1*, *Hes5*, *presenilin*, or *CSL* as compared to wild-type controls *(52,53)*. Similarly, perturbations of Notch signaling significantly affect the generation of neurospheres by retinal and ciliary epithelial stem cells. Therefore, Notch signaling, whose role in retinal development is well established *(54–58)*, is likely to play an important role in the maintenance of retinal stem cells. Signaling mediated by Wnt through Frizzled receptors is known to modulate multiple developmental events, such as patterning, proliferation, and cell-fate determination *(59,60)*. Wnt signaling is implicated in the regulation of self-renewal of hematopoietic stem cells *(61)*. Emerging evidence suggests that Wnt signaling may similarly regulate neural stem cells in vertebrate eyes. For example, various components of the canonical Wnt signaling pathway are expressed both in chick and rat retina and ciliary epithelium. Perturbations of this pathway influence the proliferation and differentiation of retinal and CE stem cells *(3,62–64)*. Transcription profiling of early and late retinal stem cells under proliferating conditions identified two additional signaling pathways for the regulation of stem cell proliferation *(3)* (Das and Ahmad, *unpublished observations*). Signaling mediated by insulin-like growth factors (IGFs) is known to promote cell proliferation *(65,66)*. The relatively high expression levels of IGF-II and IGF binding proteins and positive influence of IGF-II on the generation of neurospheres by early and late retinal stem cells/progenitors, suggests that IGF-II–mediated signaling may play an important role in proliferation and may represent an evolutionarily conserved mechanism for the maintenance of retinal stem cells/progenitors (Das and Ahmad, *unpublished observation*). This notion is further supported by evidence of insulin and IGFs-mediated signaling in the developing fish and chick retina and the recent observation that IGFs-mediated signaling sustains the proliferative phase of persistent retinal neurogenesis in the adult fish *(67–69)*. Signaling mediated by stem cell factor (SCF) through the c-Kit receptor is known to regulate proliferation of stem cells during hematopoiesis, gametogenesis, and melanogenesis *(70)*. The expression of SCF and its receptor c-Kit in retinal and ciliary epithelial stem cells and the observation that SCF promotes their proliferation and keeps them undifferentiated, suggests that SCF signaling also represents a part of signaling hierarchy employed to maintain retinal and ciliary epithelial stem cells *(71)*.

DIFFERENTIATION POTENTIAL OF RETINAL STEM CELLS

The early and late retinal stem cells not only differ in their capacity to give rise to neurons and glia, that is, the former preferentially generating neurons as compared to the latter that show proclivity toward glial differentiation, but they also have distinct potentials to generate specific retinal cell types. Evidence from the developing cerebral cortex and retina suggest that the competence of neural progenitors is progressively altered, such that they become fated to give rise to specific neurons of a particular developmental stage *(72–74)*. An alternative hypothesis is that the change in competence is not irreversible, but rather, progenitors are constrained by overwhelming epigenetic influences from giving rise to any other neuronal types than those born during that particular stage. This notion was tested by examining the ability of enriched late retinal stem cells to give rise to early born neurons, specifically RGCs *(58)*. It was observed that mitogen-enriched late retinal stem cells, when shifted to differentiating conditions, expressed RGC-specific markers, suggesting a potential to give rise to early born neurons. Exposure of early stem cells to conditioned medium, obtained from culture of retinal cells from chick embryonic stage 3 that is known to promote RGC differentiation, doubled the number of cells expressing RGC-specific markers as compared to controls. In addition, the differentiating late retinal stem cells established contacts with cells in superior colliculus explants, an RGC target, and displayed electrophysiological properties suggestive of RGCs. For example, the majority of cells displayed voltage-dependent currents characteristics of RGCs the have been observed across species in that they displayed a fast inward current, attributed to I_{Na} ($n = 10/12$), followed by a rapidly inactivating outward current, attributed to I_a ($n = 9/12$) and a sustained outward current (Fig. 2). These observations suggested that late retinal stem cells are competent to respond to cues that promote RGC differentiation. In addition, it was demonstrated that the acquisition of the RGC phenotype by late retinal stem cells, involved the recruitment of normal mechanism of RGC differentiation, that is, Notch signaling and was preceded by, or accompanied with, the expression of regulators of RGC differentiation, for example, Ath5 *(75)* and Brn3b *(76)*. These observations revealed plasticity within the subpopulation of retinal stem cells and suggested that

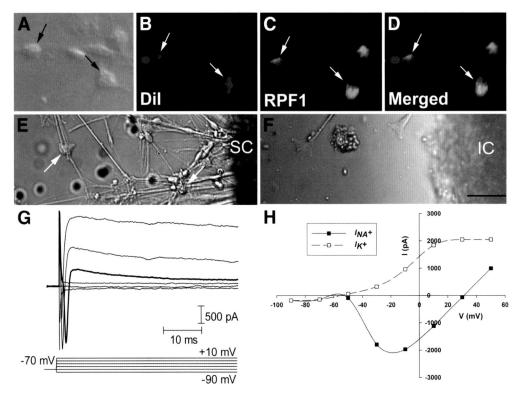

Fig. 2. Late retinal stem cell–derived RGCs display target selectivity and electrophysiological properties characteristic of RGCs. Late retinal stem cells were labeled with DiI and cultured in the presence of E3 chick retinal conditioned medium for 5–7 d. DiI-positive cells can be observed expressing RPF-1 (**A–D**). DiI-labeled late retinal stem cells were cultured in the presence of explants from superior (SC) and inferior colliculi (IC). DiI-positive cells were observed sending processes to their natural target, the SC (**E**, *arrows*) and not to IC explants (**F**). DiI-positive cells, similarly cultured, were chosen for patch-clamp recording. Patched cell was stimulated with a series of 20-mV voltage steps (150 ms) from –110 mV to +50mV. The first 50 ms of current is displayed in (**G**). Current-voltage relationship (**H**) shows that the depolarization above –50 mV evoked transient inward current attributed to voltage-dependent Na^+ currents. The outward currents consisted of both transient and sustained components. The transient outward current, which appears rather slow because of the rapid time scale, is attributed to the A-type K^+ current (I_a).

retinal stem cells may not be irreversibly fated but, appeared as such, under the constraints dictated by specific epigenetic cues.

The specification of retinal stem cells requires the acquisition of competence to respond to temporally and spatially arrayed epigenetic cues. Emerging evidence suggests that the competence of neural stem cells is generally regulated by the basic helix–loop–helix (bHLH) class of transcription factors such as Neurogenin, Achaete-scute, Atonal, and NeuroD *(77)*. The regulation of bHLH transcription factors in response to Notch signaling offers a link between the maintenance of stem cells and their acquisition of competence to differentiate. Several studies have suggested that one of the mechanisms by which Notch signaling maintains these cells in an uncommitted state is by suppressing the expression of bHLH transcription factors. For example, the absence of Notch pathway genes such as *Notch1*, *CSL*, or *Hes1* leads to up-regulation of bHLH transcription factors and premature neuronal differentiation *(78,79)*. The up-regulated bHLH transcription factors move the cells farther away from the stem cell state by unleashing a cascading expression of downstream bHLH factors that facilitate cell-cycle exit *(80–82)* and sub specification of progenitors/precursors into RGCs *(75,83)*; amacrine cells *(84,85)*, bipolar cells *(86)*, and rod photoreceptors *(87,88)*. Such processes are also facilitated by transcription factors belonging to homeo-domain gene families including *Brn3b* (RGCs) *(76)*, *Chx10* (bipolar cells) *(86)*, *Pax6* and *Six3* (amacrine cells) *(85)*, *Prox1* (bipolar cells) *(89)*, and *Otx2* (photoreceptors) *(90)*. In addition to facilitation of neuronal differentiation, the bHLH factors are likely to prevent premature gliogenesis *(86,91)*, most likely by sequestering the transcriptional coactivator CBP/p300 needed for STAT-mediated activation of glial-specific genes *(92)*. Notch signaling, which plays a primary role in the maintenance of retinal stem cells/progenitors, may be recruited during late retinal histogenesis to promote differentiation of Müller glia *(93)*. The role of Notch signaling in specifying Müller glia is consistent with Notch-mediated instructive gliogenesis in the central and peripheral nervous systems *(94)*. However, the mechanisms underlying the stage-dependent switch in Notch functions are not well known. It is likely that Notch signaling may directly activate glial-specific genes as demonstrated for neural progenitors where Notch signaling activated a GFAP promoter in a CBP/p300-STAT independent manner *(95)*. The question remains as to why the Notch signaling is not gliogenic during early stages of neurogenesis. One likely explanation could be the inaccessibility of transcription factors to promoters of glial-specific genes during early stages of neurogenesis. The sequential acquisition of competence may be accompanied by chromatin remodeling that may provide accessibility of DNA to transcription factors that was not previously available. Recently, involvement of epigenetic factor dependent chromatin remodeling has been shown to regulate the expression of glial fibrillary acidic protein (GFAP) and astrocyte differentiation *(96)*.

MÜLLER GLIA AS RETINAL STEM CELLS

A series of studies have suggested that glia or cells expressing glial features possess neural potentials *(97)*. Radial glia have long been suspected of being neural precursors, capable of generating neurons, based on observations from developing neuroepithelium of rats where radial glia were found expressing the neural stem cell marker, nestin *(98)*, on the basis of lineage analysis in chick optic tectum *(99)* and thymidine labeling of adult avian brain *(100)*. Later, Doetsch et al. *(101)* and Sanai et al. *(108)*, using a variety of experimental approaches, demonstrated that astrocytes in the subventricular zone of rodents and human, respectively, possess the potential of neural stem cells. Using a Cre-Lox approach, it was shown that the majority of neurons in the CNS are generated by progenitors that expressed GFAP, thus confirming the glial nature of neural progenitors *(102)*. Can Müller glia in the retina serve as neural precursors? This possibility was first raised in a regeneration study involving laser lesion that selectively ablated photoreceptors in the goldfish retina *(103)*. It was observed that the Müller glia proliferated in response to this injury and migrated into space vacated by degenerated photoreceptors, raising the possibility that a dedifferentiated Müller cells

Purified Muller glia   **Neurospheres**

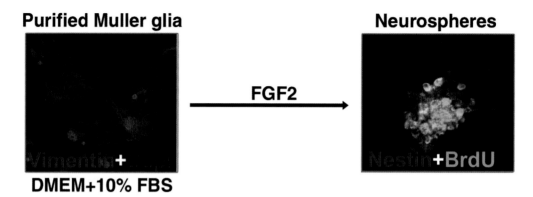

DMEM+10% FBS

Fig. 3. Purified Müller glia generate neurospheres. Müller glia, enriched as previously described *(107)*, were cultured in the presence of FGF-2 for 3–4 d. Clonal neurospheres were generated that contained BrdU-positive cells expressing Nestin.

might have participated in the replacement the lost photoreceptors. More recently, studies involving neurotoxin damage to postnatal chick *(13)* and mouse *(104)* retina have suggested that Müller glia proliferate in response to injury, and in the case of the former might serve as a source of regenerative neurogenesis. For example, following the injury, Müller glia proliferate, transiently express neural bHLH transcription factors, and a small proportion of these cells expressed neuronal markers *(13)*. In addition, it has been suggested that the injury-activated Müller cells possess the capacity to replace specific cell types, selectively activated by neurotoxins *(105)*. We have begun investigating factors that regulate the neurogenic potential of Müller glia *(106)*. We have observed that purified adult Müller cells when exposed to mitogens proliferate and generate neurospheres apparently indistinguishable from those derived from neural progenitors (Fig. 3). Cells in neurospheres are proliferating and express nestin and glial markers, such as vimentin. Preliminary study from our laboratory shows that they possess self-renewal capability and are multipotent, generating both neurons and glia. These and previous observations suggest that Müller glia, under certain conditions, can acquire the properties and potential of neural stem cells and therefore, may serve as a target for therapeutic regeneration in retinal diseases.

ACKNOWLEDGMENTS

The authors thank Graham Sharp for critical reading of the manuscript, and Kavita Mallya and Frank Soto for excellent technical assistance. This work was supported by NIH, Nebraska Research Foundation and Research to Prevent Blindness.

REFERENCES

1. Robinson, S. R. (1991) Neuroanatomy of the Visual Pathways and their development. In *Vision and Visual Dysfunction* Vol. 3 (Dreher, B. and Robinson, S. R., eds.), Macmillan, London, pp. 59–128.
2. Temple, S. (2001) The development of neural stem cells. *Nature* **414,** 112–117.
3. Ahmad, I., Das, A. V., James, J., Bhattacharya, S., and Zhao, X. (2004) Neural stem cells in the mammalian eye:types and regulation. *Semin. Cell Dev. Biol.* **15,** 53–62.

4. Negishi, K., Teranishi, T., and Kato, S. (1982) New dopaminergic and indoleamine-accumulating cells in the growth zone of goldfish retinas after neurotoxic destruction. *Science* **216,** 747–749.

5. Reh, T. A. and Tully, T. (1986) Regulation of tyrosine hydroxylase-containing amacrine cell number in larval frog retina. *Dev. Biol.* **114,** 463–469.

6. Turner, D. L. and Cepko, C. L. (1987) Common progenitor for neurons and glia persists in rat retina late in development. *Nature* **328,** 131–136.

7. Wetts, R. and Fraser, S. E. (1988) Multipotent precursors can give rise to all major cell types of the frog retina. *Science* **239,** 1142–1145.

8. Turner, D. L., Snyder, E. Y., and Cepko, C. L. (1990) Lineage-independent determination of cell type in the embryonic mouse retina. *Neuron* **4,** 833–845.

9. Jensen, A. M. and Raff, M. C. (1997) Continuous observation of multipotential retinal progenitor cells in clonal density culture. *Dev. Biol.* **188,** 267–279.

10. Ahmad, I., Dooley, C. M., Thoreson, W. B., Rogers, J. A., and Afiat, S. (1999) In vitro analysis of a mammalian retinal progenitor that gives rise to neurons and glia. *Brain Res.* **831,** 1–10.

11. Perron, M. and Harris, W. A. (2000) Retinal stem cells in vertebrates. *Bioessays* **22,** 685–688.

12. Ahmad, I. (2001) Stem cells: new opportunities to treat eye disease. *Invest. Ophthalmol. Vis. Sci.* **42,** 2743–2748.

13. Reh, T. A. and Fischer, A. J. (2001) Stem cells in the vertebrate retina. *Brain Behav. Evol.* **58,** 296–305.

14. Ahmad, I., Tang, L., and Pham, H. (2000) Identification of neural progenitors in the adult mammalian eye. *Biochem. Biophys. Res. Commun.* **270,** 517–521.

15. Tropepe, V., Coles, B. L., Chiasson, B. J., et al. (2000) Retinal stem cells in the adult mammalian eye. *Science* **287,** 2032–2036.

16. Raymond, P. A. and Hitchcock, P. F. (1997) Retinal regeneration: common principles but a diversity of mechanisms. *Adv. Neurol.* **72,** 171–184.

17. Otteson, D. C. and Hitchcock, P. F. (2003) Stem cells in the teleost retina: persistent neurogenesis and injury-induced regeneration. *Vision Res.* **43,** 927–936.

18. Yang, P., Seiler, M. J., Aramant, R. B., and Whittemore, S. R. (2002) Differential lineage restriction of rat retinal progenitor cells in vitro and in vivo. *J. Neurosci. Res.* **69,** 466–476.

19. Pevny, L. and Rao, M. S. (2003) The stem-cell menagerie. *Trends Neurosci.* **26,** 351–359.

20. Capela, A. and Temple, S. (2002) LeX/ssea-1 is expressed by adult mouse CNS stem cells, identifying them as nonependymal. *Neuron* **35,** 865–875.

21. Zappone, M. V., Galli, R., Catena, R., et al. (2000) Sox2 regulatory sequences direct expression of a (beta)-geo transgene to telencephalic neural stem cells and precursors of the mouse embryo, revealing regionalization of gene expression in CNS stem cells. *Development* **127,** 2367–2382.

22. Cai, J., Wu, Y., Mirua, T., et al. (2002) Properties of a fetal multipotent neural stem cell (NEP cell). *Dev. Biol.* **251,** 221–240.

23. Graham, V., Khudyakov, J., Ellis, P., and Pevny, L. (2003) SOX2 functions to maintain neural progenitor identity. *Neuron* **39,** 749–765.

24. Klapper, W., Shin, T., and Mattson, M. P. (2001) Differential regulation of telomerase activity and TERT expression during brain development in mice. *J. Neurosci. Res.* **64,** 252–260.

25. Kayahara, T., Sawada, M., Takaishi, S., et al. (2003) Candidate markers for stem and early progenitor cells, Musashi-1 and Hes1, are expressed in crypt base columnar cells of mouse small intestine. *FEBS Lett.* **535,** 131–135.

26. Maslov, A. Y., Barone, T. A., Plunkett, R. J., and Pruitt, S. C. (2004) Neural stem cell detection, characterization, and age-related changes in the subventricular zone of mice. *J. Neurosci.* **24,** 1726–1733.

27. Lendahl, U., Zimmerman, L. B., and McKay, R. D. (1990) CNS stem cells express a new class of intermediate filament protein. *Cell* **60,** 585–595.
28. Frederiksen, K. and McKay, R. D. (1988) Proliferation and differentiation of rat neuroepithelial precursor cells in vivo. *J. Neurosci.* **8,** 1144–1151.
29. Tsai, R. Y. and McKay, R. D. (2002) A nucleolar mechanism controlling cell proliferation in stem cells and cancer cells. *Genes Dev.* **16,** 2991–3003.
30. Cook, T. (2003) Cell diversity in the retina: more than meets the eye. *Bioessays* **25,** 921–925.
31. Wargelius, A., Seo, H. C., Austbo, L., and Fjose, A. (2003) Retinal expression of zebrafish six3.1 and its regulation by Pax6. *Biochem. Biophys. Res. Commun.* **309,** 475–481.
32. Liu, I. S., Chen, J. D., Ploder, L., et al. (1994) Developmental expression of a novel murine homeobox gene (Chx10): evidence for roles in determination of the neuroretina and inner nuclear layer. *Neuron* **13,** 377–393.
33. Chen, C. M. and Cepko, C. L. (2000) Expression of Chx10 and Chx10-1 in the developing chicken retina. *Mech. Dev.* **90,** 293–297.
34. Porter, F. D., Drago, J., Xu, Y., et al. (1997) *Lhx2,* a LIM homeobox gene, is required for eye, forebrain, and definitive erythrocyte development. *Development* **124,** 2935–2944.
35. Zuber, M. E., Gestri, G., Viczian, A. S., Barsacchi, G., and Harris, W. A. (2003) Specification of the vertebrate eye by a network of eye field transcription factors. *Development* **130,** 5155–5167.
36. Jean, D., Bernier, G., and Gruss, P. (1999) Six6 (Optx2) is a novel murine *Six3*-related homeobox gene that demarcates the presumptive pituitary/hypothalamic axis and the ventral optic stalk. *Mech. Dev.* **84,** 31–40.
37. Bernier, G., Panitz, F., Zhou, X., Hollemann, T., Gruss, P., and Pieler, T. (2000) Expanded retina territory by midbrain transformation upon overexpression of Six6 (Optx2) in *Xenopus* embryos. *Mech. Dev.* **93,** 59–69.
38. Morrison, S. J., White, P. M., Zock, C., and Anderson, D. J. (1999) Prospective identification, isolation by flow cytometry, and in vivo self-renewal of multipotent mammalian neural crest stem cells. *Cell* **96,** 737–749.
39. Rietze, R. L., Valcanis, H., Brooker, G. F., Thomas, T., Voss, A. K., and Bartlett, P. F. (2001) Purification of a pluripotent neural stem cell from the adult mouse brain. *Nature* **412,** 736–739.
40. Maric, D., Maric, I., Chang, Y. H., and Barker, J. L. (2003) Prospective cell sorting of embryonic rat neural stem cells and neuronal and glial progenitors reveals selective effects of basic fibroblast growth factor and epidermal growth factor on self-renewal and differentiation. *J. Neurosci.* **23,** 240–251.
41. Goodell, M. A., Brose, K., Paradis, G., Conner, A. S., and Mulligan, R. C. (1996) Isolation and functional properties of murine hematopoietic stem cells that are replicating in vivo. *J. Exp. Med.* **183,** 1797–1806.
42. Bhattacharya, S., Jackson, J. D., Das, A. V., et al. (2003) Direct identification and enrichment of retinal stem cells/progenitors using hoechst dye efflux assay. *Invest. Ophthalmol. Vis. Sci.* **44,** 2764–2773.
43. Bhattacharya, S., Das, A., Cowan, K. H., and Ahmad, I. (2003) Role of ABCG2 transporter in Notch and c-Kit mediated maintenance of retinal stem cells. *Invest. Ophthalmol. Vis. Sci.,* ARVO 2003, 1668/B564.
44. Tropepe, V., Sibilia, M., Ciruna, B. G., Rossant, J., Wagner, E. F., and van der Kooy, D. (1999) Distinct neural stem cells proliferate in response to EGF and FGF in the developing mouse telencephalon. *Dev. Biol.* **208,** 166–188.
45. Johnson, D. E. and Williams, L. T. (1993) Structural and functional diversity in the FGF receptor multigene family. *Adv. Cancer Res.* **60,** 1–41.
46. Orr-Urtreger, A., Givol, D., Yayon, A., Yarden, Y., and Lonai, P. (1991) Developmental expression of two murine fibroblast growth factor receptors, flg and bek. *Development* **113,** 1419–1434.

47. Wanaka, A., Milbrandt, J., and Johnson, E. M., Jr. (1991) Expression of FGF receptor gene in rat development. *Development* **111,** 455–468.
48. Kilpatrick, T. J. and Bartlett, P. F. (1995) Cloned multipotential precursors from the mouse cerebrum require FGF-2, whereas glial restricted precursors are stimulated with either FGF-2 or EGF. *J. Neurosci.* **15,** 3653–3661
49. Lillien, L. and Raphael, H. (2000) BMP and FGF regulate the development of EGF-responsive neural progenitor cells. *Development* **127,** 4993–5005.
50. Burrows, R. C., Wancio, D., Levitt, P., and Lillien, L. (1997) Response diversity and the timing of progenitor cell maturation are regulated by developmental changes in EGFR expression in the cortex. *Neuron* **19,** 251–267.
51. Artavanis-Tsakonas, S., Rand, M. D., and Lake, R. J. (1999) Notch signaling: cell fate control and signal integration in development. *Science* **284,** 770–776.
52. Ohtsuka, T., Sakamoto, M., Guillemot, F., and Kageyama, R. (2001) Roles of the basic helix–loop–helix genes *Hes1* and *Hes5* in expansion of neural stem cells of the developing brain. *J. Biol. Chem.* **276,** 30467–30474.
53. Hitoshi, S., Alexson, T., Tropepe, V., et al. (2002) Notch pathway molecules are essential for the maintenance, but not the generation, of mammalian neural stem cells. *Genes Dev.* **16,** 846–858.
54. Dorsky, R. I., Rapaport, D. H., and Harris, W. A. (1995) Xotch inhibits cell differentiation in the *Xenopus* retina. *Neuron* **14,** 487–496.
55. Ahmad, I., Zaqouras, P., and Artavanis-Tsakonas, S. (1995) Involvement of Notch-1 in mammalian retinal neurogenesis: association of Notch-1 activity with both immature and terminally differentiated cells. *Mech. Dev.* **53,** 73–85.
56. Austin, C. P., Feldman, D. E., Ida, J. A., Jr., and Cepko, C. L. (1995) Vertebrate retinal ganglion cells are selected from competent progenitors by the action of Notch. *Development* **121,** 3637–3650.
57. Ahmad, I., Dooley, C. M., and Polk, D. L. (1997) Delta-1 is a regulator of neurogenesis in the vertebrate retina. *Dev. Biol.* **185,** 92–103.
58. James, J., Das, A. V., Bhattacharya, S., Chacko, D. M., Zhao, X., and Ahmad, I. (2003) In vitro generation of early-born neurons from late retinal progenitors. *J. Neurosci.* **23,** 8193–8203.
59. Wodarz, A. and Nusse, R. (1998) Mechanisms of Wnt signaling in development. *Annu. Rev. Cell Dev. Biol.* **14,** 59–88.
60. Patapoutian, A. and Reichardt, L. F. (2000) Roles of Wnt proteins in neural development and maintenance. *Curr. Opin. Neurobiol.* **10,** 392–399.
61. Reya, T., Duncan, A. W., Ailles, L., et al. (2003) A role for Wnt signalling in self-renewal of haematopoietic stem cells. *Nature* **423,** 409–414.
62. Jasoni, C., Hendrickson, A., and Roelink, H. (1999) Analysis of chicken Wnt-13 expression demonstrates coincidence with cell division in the developing eye and is consistent with a role in induction. *Dev. Dyn.* **215,** 215–224.
63. Kubo, F., Takeichi, M., and Nakagawa, S. (2003) Wnt2b controls retinal cell differentiation at the ciliary marginal zone. *Development* **130,** 587–598.
64. Liu, H., Mohamed, O., Dufort, D., and Wallace, V. A. (2003) Characterization of Wnt signaling components and activation of the Wnt canonical pathway in the murine retina. *Dev. Dyn.* **227,** 323–334.
65. Heyner, S., Smith, R. M., and Schultz, G. A. (1989) Temporally regulated expression of insulin and insulin-like growth factors and their receptors in early mammalian development. *Bioessays* **11,** 171–176.
66. Ferry, R. J., Jr., Katz, L. E., Grimberg, A., Cohen, P., and Weinzimer, S. A. (1999) Cellular actions of insulin-like growth factor binding proteins. *Horm. Metab. Res.* **31,** 192–202.
67. Mack, A. F. and Fernald, R. D. (1993) Regulation of cell division and rod differentiation in the teleost retina. *Brain Res. Dev. Brain Res.* **76,** 183–187.

68. Garcia-de Lacoba, M., Alarcon, C., de la Rosa, E. J., and de Pablo, F. (1999) Insulin/ insulin-like growth factor-I hybrid receptors with high affinity for insulin are developmentally regulated during neurogenesis. *Endocrinology* **140,** 233–243.

69. Otteson, D. C., Cirenza, P. F., and Hitchcock, P. F. (2002) Persistent neurogenesis in the teleost retina: evidence for regulation by the growth-hormone/insulin-like growth factor-I axis. *Mech. Dev.* **117,** 137–149.

70. Ashman, L. K. (1999) The biology of stem cell factor and its receptor c-kit. *Int. J. Biochem. Cell Biol.* **31,** 1037–1051.

71. Das, A., James, J., Zhao, X., Bhattacharya, S., and Ahmad, I. (2004) Involvement of c-Kit receptor tyrosine kinase in the maintenance of ciliary epithelial neural stem cells; interaction with Notch signaling. *Dev. Biol.* **273,** 87–105.

72. Frantz, G. D. and McConnell, S. K. (1996) Restriction of late cerebral cortical progenitors to an upper-layer fate. *Neuron* **17,** 55–61.

73. Morrow, E. M., Belliveau, M. J., and Cepko, C. L. (1998) Two phases of rod photoreceptor differentiation during rat retinal development. *J. Neurosci.* **18,** 3738–3748.

74. Belliveau, M. J. and Cepko, C. L. (1999) Extrinsic and intrinsic factors control the genesis of amacrine and cone cells in the rat retina. *Development* **126,** 555–566.

75. Vetter, M. L. and Brown, N. L. (2001) The role of basic helix–loop–helix genes in vertebrate retinogenesis. *Semin. Cell Dev. Biol.* **12,** 491–498.

76. Liu, W., Mo, Z., and Xiang, M. (2001) The Ath5 proneural genes function upstream of Brn3 POU domain transcription factor genes to promote retinal ganglion cell development. *Proc. Natl. Acad. Sci. USA* **98,** 1649–1654.

77. Bertrand, N., Castro, D. S., and Guillemot, F. (2002) Proneural genes and the specification of neural cell types. *Nat. Rev. Neurosci.* **3,** 517–530.

78. Ishibashi, M., Moriyoshi, K., Sasai, Y., Shiota, K., Nakanishi, S., and Kageyama, R. (1994) Persistent expression of helix–loop–helix factor HES-1 prevents mammalian neural differentiation in the central nervous system. *EMBO J.* **13,** 1799–1805.

79. de la Pompa, J. L., Wakeham, A., Correia, K. M., et al. (1997) Conservation of the Notch signalling pathway in mammalian neurogenesis. *Development* **124,** 1139–1148.

80. Farah, M. H., Olson, J. M., Sucic, H. B., Hume, R. I., Tapscott, S. J., and Turner, D. L. (2000) Generation of neurons by transient expression of neural bHLH proteins in mammalian cells. *Development* **127,** 693–702.

81. Kay, J. N., Finger-Baier, K. C., Roeser, T., Staub, W., and Baier, H. (2001) Retinal ganglion cell genesis requires lakritz, a Zebrafish atonal homolog. *Neuron* **30,** 725–736.

82. Ohnuma, S., Hopper, S., Wang, K. C., Philpott, A., and Harris, W. A. (2002) Coordinating retinal histogenesis: early cell cycle exit enhances early cell fate determination in the *Xenopus* retina. *Development* **129,** 2435–2446.

83. Wang, S. W., Kim, B. S., Ding, K., et al. (2001) Requirement for math5 in the development of retinal ganglion cells. *Genes Dev.* **15,** 24–29.

84. Marquardt, T., Ashery-Padan, R., Andrejewski, N., Scardigli, R., Guillemot, F., and Gruss, P. (2001) Pax6 is required for the multipotent state of retinal progenitor cells. *Cell* **105,** 43–55.

85. Inoue, T., Hojo, M., Bessho, Y., Tano, Y., Lee, J. E., and Kageyama, R. (2002) Math3 and NeuroD regulate amacrine cell fate specification in the retina. *Development* **129,** 831–842.

86. Hatakeyama, J., Tomita, K., Inoue, T., and Kageyama, R. (2001) Roles of homeobox and bHLH genes in specification of a retinal cell type. *Development* **128,** 1313–1322.

87. Ahmad, I., Acharya, H. R., Rogers, J. A., Shibata, A., Smithgall, T. E., and Dooley, C. M. (1998) The role of NeuroD as a differentiation factor in the mammalian retina. *J. Mol. Neurosci.* **11,** 165–178.

88. Morrow, E. M., Furukawa, T., Lee, J. E., and Cepko, C. L. (1999) NeuroD regulates multiple functions in the developing neural retina in rodent. *Development* **126,** 23–36.

89. Dyer, M. A., Livesey, F. J., Cepko, C. L., and Oliver, G. (2003) Prox1 function controls progenitor cell proliferation and horizontal cell genesis in the mammalian retina. *Nat. Genet.* **34,** 53–58.

90. Nishida, A., Furukawa, A., Koike, C., et al. (2003) Otx2 homeobox gene controls retinal photoreceptor cell fate and pineal gland development. *Nat. Neurosci.* **6,** 1255–1263.

91. Cai, L., Morrow, E. M., and Cepko, C. L. (2000) Misexpression of basic helix–loop–helix genes in the murine cerebral cortex affects cell fate choices and neuronal survival. *Development* **127,** 3021–3030.

92. Vetter, M. L. and Moore, K. B. (2001) Becoming glial in the neural retina. *Dev. Dyn.* **221,** 146–153.

93. Furukawa, T., Mukherjee, S., Bao, Z. Z., Morrow, E. M., and Cepko, C. L. (2000) rax, Hes1, and notch1 promote the formation of Muller glia by postnatal retinal progenitor cells. *Neuron* **26,** 383–394.

94. Wang, S. and Barres, B. A. (2000) Up a notch: instructing gliogenesis. *Neuron* **27,** 197–200.

95. Tanigaki, K., Nogaki, F., Takahashi, J., Tashiro, K., Kurooka, H., and Honjo, T. (2001) Notch1 and Notch3 instructively restrict bFGF-responsive multipotent neural progenitor cells to an astroglial fate. *Neuron* **29,** 45–55.

96. Song, M. R. and Ghosh, A. (2004) FGF2-induced chromatin remodeling regulates CNTF-mediated gene expression and astrocyte differentiation. *Nat. Neurosci.* **7,** 229–235.

97. Goldman, S. (2003) Glia as neural progenitor cells. *Trends Neurosci.* **26,** 590–596.

98. Frederiksen, K., Jat, P. S., Valtz, N., Levy, D., and McKay, R. (1988) Immortalization of precursor cells from the mammalian CNS. *Neuron* **1,** 439–448.

99. Gray, G. E. and Sanes, J. R. (1992) Lineage of radial glia in the chicken optic tectum. *Development* **114,** 271–283.

100. Alvarez-Buylla, A. (1990) Mechanism of neurogenesis in adult avian brain. *Experientia* **46,** 948–955.

101. Doetsch, F., Caille, I., Lim, D. A., Garcia-Verdugo, J. M., and Alvarez-Buylla, A. (1999) Subventricular zone astrocytes are neural stem cells in the adult mammalian brain. *Cell* **97,** 703–716.

102. Zhuo, L., Theis, M., Alvarez-Maya, I., Brenner, M., Willecke, K., and Messing, A. (2001) hGFAP-cre transgenic mice for manipulation of glial and neuronal function in vivo. *Genesis* **31,** 85–94.

103. Braisted, J. E., Essman, T. F., and Raymond, P. A. (1994) Selective regeneration of photoreceptors in goldfish retina. *Development* **120,** 2409–2419.

104. Dyer, M. A. and Cepko, C. L. (2000) Control of Muller glial cell proliferation and activation following retinal injury. *Nat. Neurosci.* **3,** 873–880.

105. Fischer, A. J. and Reh, T. A. (2001) Muller glia are a potential source of neural regeneration in the postnatal chicken retina. *Nat. Neurosci.* **4,** 247–252.

106. Ahmad, I., Das, A. V., and Mallya, K. B. (2004) Are Muller glia stem cells? *Invest. Ophthalmol. Vis. Sci. (ARVO, 2004)* 5401/B725.

107. Hicks, D. and Courtois, Y. (1990) The growth and behaviour of rat retinal Muller cells in vitro. 1. An improved method for isolation and culture. *Exp. Eye Res.* **51,** 119–129.

108. Sanai, N., Tramontin, A. D., Quinones-Hinojose, A., et al. (2004) Unique astrocyte ribbon in adult human brain contains neural stem cells but lacks chain migration. *Nature* **427,** 740–744.

11

Transdifferentiation in the Nervous System

Ying Liu and Mahendra S. Rao

NORMAL CENTRAL NERVOUS SYSTEM (CNS) DEVELOPMENT

In the nervous system, neural stem cells follow a sequential process of development. More differentiated cells have a more limited repertoire of fate choices while fully differentiated cells do not have any alternative fates and may not be able to reenter the cell cycle at all (reviewed in refs. *1* and *2*). This progressive restriction of developmental potential is a normal aspect of development, and phenotypic plasticity appears uncommon. To a large part, analysis with gene specific promoters, culture of isolated populations of cells, clonal analysis, and challenge perturbation experiments *(3)* have confirmed this lack of plasticity and suggested that cells acquire an identity prior to terminal mitosis and this positional and phenotypic identity is difficult to alter *(4,5)*. Overall the idea that there is a cell intrinsic change that restricts the potential of initially pluripotent cells is appealing, as it helps explain how the same regulatory molecules can be reiteratively used at multiple stages and in different tissues to direct differentiation and different fates in multiple distinct lineages *(2,6)*.

However, even during development there are several examples of divergence from this process of progressive lineage restriction. For example, radial glia do not in general form non-neural tissue or mature to form astrocytes in rodents and human in normal development *(7)*. However, in the axlotl tail, where this has been examined in detail, radial glia, in response to amputation of the tail, regenerate all tail structures including mesodermal and endodermal derivatives *(8)*. Rodent and avian tail bud formation has not been examined in much detail, but even in these species, it has been suggested that a similar transdifferentiation occurs *(9)*. In zebrafish, as well, contributions from the notochord to the floor plate and vice versa have been recognized *(10,11)*.

Similar ectoderm to mesoderm cross-lineage differentiation is normally seen in cranial neural crest. Neural crest cells derived from the craniofacial ectoderm, or generated from neural epithelial stem cells *(12)*, can generate muscle, bone, cartilage, melanocytes, fibroblasts, and smooth muscle as well as neural components of the peripheral nervous system (PNS) and other mesenchymal derivatives *(13*, reviewed in ref. *1)*. This is an example of a cross-lineage development ability that appears to be restricted to cranial crest. It is possible, however, to induce caudal crest to generate muscle, cartilage, and bone either in culture (M.S. Rao, *unpublished result*) or after

From: *Neural Development and Stem Cells, Second Edition*
Edited by: M. S. Rao © Humana Press Inc., Totowa, NJ

transplantation. Thus, ectoderm to mesoderm transdifferentiation is a normal aspect of development for cranial crest and may be an ability shared by caudal crest.

Likewise, placode derived stem cells (which also undergo an epithelial to mesenchymal transition) have been shown to give rise to both neural and nonneural tissue. In the otic placode, for example, single cells have been shown to be multipotential and generate fibroblasts, cartilage cells, hair cells, as well as neurons *(14)*. A late epithelial to mesenchymal differentiation has been described for the neural tube as well *(15–17)*, with the generation of a novel cell type. This cell type was first described by Sohal and colleagues and termed ventrally emigrating neural tube (VENT) cells *(15–17)*. These cells migrate from the CNS to the periphery and appear to be capable of participating in the tissue organization of multiple distinct nonneural organs *(16,17)*.

Similar epithelial to mesenchymal transitions have been described in other tissues and organ as well *(18–21)*. These include ureteric development in the kidney, lung alveolar development, and placodal delamination to generate cranial ganglia (reviewed in ref. *22*). Other examples of transdifferentiation or dedifferentiation include primordial germ cells that under appropriate conditions become totipotent, as evidenced by differentiating into all types of somatic cells after transplantation *(23,24)*. These and other uncited examples all suggest that while progressive restriction in cell fate may be the form for most normal development, there clearly appears some flexibility in fate determination and indeed this flexibility has been exploited during normal development.

Thus, fetal maturation provides numerous examples of exceptions to the normal sequential process of progressive restriction in developmental fate and suggests that cells may retain a broader differentiation potential than that reflected in vivo, and that this broad potential could be harnessed if the mechanisms that regulate this process were better understood. We do not believe that these examples discussed should be defined as transdifferentiation. Rather, these examples suggest that linear progressive restriction in cell fate, although common, is not the only way an organism develops. Cells are plastic, daughter cells may have a wider differentiation potential and in many cases cells may be more plastic than previously realized. This plasticity has been exploited during aspects of development and may be important in repair and regeneration.

PLASTICITY AND TRANSDIFFERENTIATION— REVEALED COMPETENCE AND DEDIFFERENTIATION

Recent evidence from multiple investigators has provided additional proof that the nervous system may be more plastic than previously thought and that tissue-specific stem cells, intermediate precursors, and even fully differentiated postmitotic cells can be induced to alter their phenotypic profile in dramatic ways that are not predicted by their normal development and differentiation *(25)*. This process has been termed transdifferentiation in the case of stem and precursor cells, or dedifferentiation, in the case of fully differentiated cells changing their phenotype. Both dedifferentiation and transdifferentiation should be distinguished from competence and the normal fate of cells (reviewed in refs. *22* and *26*). Cells may be competent to differentiate into a particular phenotype but this competence may not have been recognized, or not be expressed during normal development (absence of cues), or be actively repressed. Such competence, although not observed in normal development fate, may be readily revealed by altering the environment or providing the appropriate cue. Such demonstration of competence is not evidence for transdifferentiation or dedifferentiation; rather, it illustrates plasticity of cells. Neural crest differentiating into cartilage or bone is an example of revealed competence but not of transdifferentiation. Acquisition of neural markers by mesenchymal cells on exposure to dimethyl sulfoxide (DMSO, ref. *27*) may be a transdifferentiation event while the presence of neural and connective tissue elements in Ewing's sarcoma *(28)* may be an example of dedifferentiation. Oligodendrocyte precursors giving rise to neurons is a transdifferentiation event *(29)*, while radial glia or mature astrocytes or postmitotic neurons generating neurons or precursor cells of other lineages can be classified as a dedifferentiation phenomenon *(30–33)*.

It is important to note that classifying a process as dedifferentiation or transdifferentiation depends on information available about the system and in many cases it will be impossible to distinguish between the two and in some instances may be academic. The differentiation of skin cells into neurons (e.g., ref. *34*) may be a dedifferentiation event if the skin cells used have been demonstrated to have mature markers and to have the functions of terminally differentiated cells. If solely hair cell precursors were present then this may be an example of transdifferentiation. On the other hand, if harvested skin cells include placodal or crest precursors then this may be an example of revealed competence.

It is also important to distinguish transdifferentiation/dedifferentiation from atypical differentiation seen as a result of the presence of contaminating populations of cells. This is particularly true when considering neuronal transdifferentiation, given our knowledge of the ability of neural precursors to differentiate normally into mesodermal and other nonneural derivatives. Neural crest and VENT cells are widely distributed during development, and recent reports suggest that neural crest cells may persist in peripheral organs *(15–17,35,36)*. Nerve endings with associated Schwann cells are present in virtually all tissue, and many of the conditions in which cells are cultured allow for survival of these populations. It is therefore possible that some results reported as transdifferentiation may be due to such contamination. Indeed, skin differentiation into neurons has been explained in some part to the presence of neural crest *(34)*. Likewise in lens epithelial differentiation into neuronal cells, it appears as if separate populations of ectodermal and neural progenitors are present *(37)*.

The converse is also true when neural stem cells are harvested. In most cases neurospheres are used for transplantation and the selection methodology uses selective growth in fibroblast growth factor (FGF) and epidermal growth factor (EGF, refs. *38* and *39*). It is useful to remember that connective tissue and blood vessels are an integral component of all tissue and may be present in neurospheres. To our knowledge markers to demonstrate their absence are not used routinely. Hematopoietic stem cells (HSCs) transit through blood vessels and can be harvested with tissues. Such examples of contaminating stem cell populations have been provided by Magrassi et al. *(40)*. In particular, HSCs have been shown to contaminate neural cells and muscle cells *(41,42)*. The existence of multipotent adult progenitor cells (MAPCs, refs. *43* and *44*) and other embryonic stem (ES)-like cells, including pluripotent epiblastic-like stem cells (PPELSCs), ectodermal germ-layer lineage stem cells (EctoGLLSCs), mesodermal germ-layer lineage stem cells (MGLLSCs), endodermal germ-layer lineage stem cells (EndoGLLSCs) and pancreatic progenitor cells (PanPCs), in the adult, also raises the possibility of contamination of tissue specific populations with a more global undifferentiated population *(45)*.

In general, the presence of rare populations of cells can often be safely ignored in assessing the differentiation potential of harvested tissue. However, in cases in which the frequency of dedifferentiation or transdifferentiation observed is low, it becomes imperative that this be ruled out. For example, the number of neuronal cells seen after mesenchymal cell injections was disturbingly small and could be accounted for by less than 0.1% contamination. Indeed, several reports have shown that some of the previously recognized transdifferentiation phenomena are due to contamination of stem cells of different lineages *(42,46–50)*. Based on these results, it has been suggested that either purified populations of cells be used, the transdifferentiation process be robust and/or clonal analysis be performed before labeling an observation as evidence of transdifferentiation *(2,51)*. Thus, before determining an event is a transdifferentiation phenomenon, one must rule out alternate explanations, such as contaminating populations of cells, revealed competence, and the normal developmental potential of cells. Even when apparently authentic dedifferentiation or transdifferentiation is observed, one needs to be careful about assessing cell fusion. It has been shown that cells, rather than altering their fate, can fuse with other cells such that the resultant cells have a mixture of these properties. Such cells are usually polyploid. Cell fusion may be more common in some tissues or cell types than others *(47,48,52–54)*. Smith and colleagues, for example, cocultured neurospheres derived from green fluorescent protein (GFP)-labeled, puromycin resistant transgenic mice (with expression of GFP and puromycin controlled under Oct4 promoter), together with HT2 ES cells which had both hygromycin resistance and ganciclovir sensitivity. After selection by puromycin, the resulting cultured cells had characteristics of ES cells, expressed GFP, were resistant to hygromycin and sensitive to ganciclovir, and could differentiation into nonneural cells. The initial assumption was that neural stem cells (in this case the neurospheres) have transdifferentiated into pluripotent ES cells. More detailed analysis showed that the cells displayed multiple nucleoli and their karyotype was mostly tetraploid, indicating that fusion with ES cells rather than transdifferentiation gave rise to nonneural derivatives in this experiment *(53)*. In other cases where diploid cells were seen, opponents of the concept of transdifferentiation have suggested fusion followed by resolution to maintain a diploid phenotype *(54)*. Detailed analysis has suggested that many of the reports of transdifferentiation were actually attributable to unrecognized cell fusion *(47,48,52–54)*.

We believe however that the possibility that transdifferentiation can occur under suitable environmental stimuli has been compellingly addressed by somatic nuclear transplantation experiments *(55–57)*. Nuclei from postmitotic committed cells that are fated to make only particular types of cells can be reprogrammed under appropriate environment to reorder their fate choices. Thus a nucleus of a skin cell can generate authentic CNS and kidney cells, and importantly does it in sufficient numbers and fidelity to generate a functional animal with functional organs. Nuclear transfer experiments have also suggested that it is not just reprogramming in the oocyte or blastocyst is required, but that some degree of reprogramming can occur when nuclei are transferred from one cell type to another *(25,51)*. For example, more mature erythroblasts can be reprogrammed to express fetal hemoglobin by transferring the nucleus to an earlier state.

Transdifferentiation is also a common phenomenon in many cancers (reviewed in refs. *58* and *59*). For example, prostate cancer cells have been reported to trans-differentiate into neuroendocrine-like cells *(60)*, and Ewing's sarcoma often shows the presence of neural or nonneural elements *(28)*. Teratocarcinomas derived from germ cells show differentiation foci of ectoderm, endoderm, and mesoderm *(61)*. Over-expression of master regulatory proteins can also alter/transdifferentiate cells (discussed later). Misexpression of neurogenic genes can induce skin cells transdifferentiate into neural cells *(62,63)* or overexpression of myogenic genes can cause ectodermal tissue to generate skeletal muscle *(64)*. Such misexpression clearly shows that cells are more plastic than previously supposed and can respond to signals to alter their fate.

These examples of transdifferentiation cannot be explained by involving cell fusion, presence of contamination population, or unexpected or revealed competence. Overall we believe that transdifferentiation is a rare event. It requires a critical review of the evidence, test for contaminating populations of cells, experiments of clonality and fluo-rescence *in situ* hybridization (FISH) analysis and careful assessment of the robustness of the phenomenon. We believe that many of the reports documenting transdif-ferentiation can be explained by overenthusiasm in interpretation, presence of con-taminating crest/vent or circulating HSCs, or by cell fusion. However, these alternate mechanisms cannot explain the transdifferentiation seen during development *(22)*, the transdifferentiation seen in somatic nuclear transfer experiments *(56)*, and the transdifferentiation and metaplasia seen in carcinogenesis *(25,64,65)*. We would sug-gest that although any report on transdifferentiation must be examined carefully to rule out alternate explanations, evidence supports the idea that transdifferentiation occurs as a normal aspect of development and mechanisms to direct the process likely exist.

TRANSDIFFERENTIATION AND DEDIFFERENTIATION IN THE NERVOUS SYSTEM

In the CNS, oligodendrocyte precursors, astrocytes, and radial glia have all been shown to be capable of dedifferentiating/transdifferentiating into mature neurons (Fig. 1 and Table 1; refs. *29–31*). Even postmitotic neurons can be induced to reenter the cell cycle and generate dividing progenitor cells *(32,33)*.

The well-characterized A2B5[+] glial progenitors have been shown to differentiate into astrocytes, and subsequently transdifferentiate/dedifferentiate into stem cell that can generate neurons, astrocytes and oligodendrocytes *(29)*. The authors applied a sequential exposure of A2B5[+] glial precursors to fetal calf serum (FCS) or bone mor-phogenetic proteins (BMPs), and then after the addition of basic FGF (bFGF), the cells were induced to revert to a state that resembles that of multipotential CNS stem cells. These experiments included clonal culture as well, making it difficult to be explained by any mechanism other than transdifferentiation. Anderson and colleagues further showed glial precursors dedifferentiated into multipotent stem cells when they were cultured in FGF-2 *(66)*. The dorsoventral patterning of these glial cells was modulated and the positional identity altered.

Radial glia and astrocytes have been shown to be capable of differentiating into neurons under the appropriate conditions *(30,67–70)*. Given the careful analysis and

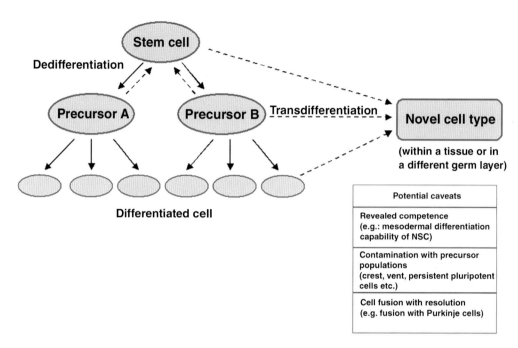

Fig. 1. Transdifferentiation and dedifferentiation. Multipotent stem cells give rise to lineage restricted precursors that then differentiate into mature terminal cells. Under certain conditions, more differentiated cells can acquire properties of stem cells (dedifferentiation) or generate new cell types (transdifferentiation).

Table 1
Transdifferentiation and Dedifferentiation in the Nervous System

Original cell type	Transdifferentiation	Reference
Oligodendrocyte precursor	Neural stem cell	*(29)*
Astrocyte	Neural stem cell	*(30,70)*
Radial glia	Neuron and glia	*(31)*
Neuron	Neural stem cell	*(32,33)*

temporal profile and the labeling experiments performed with radial glia, it appears unlikely that these results could all be attributed to artifact, overinterpretation of data, or cell fusion. Not all astrocytes appear to share this property, and this property appears to decay with time *(71)*. The multipotential nature of some astrocytes has been shown in quite convincing fashion by several laboratories demonstrating some reliability and reproducibility. However, given the observation that some stem cell populations express glial fibrillary acidic protein (GFAP), it is difficult to rule out a contaminating population of GFAP⁺ stem cells. Such cells have been described (reviewed in ref. *72*) and remain a possible explanation.

Macklis and colleagues *(73)*, in an elegant neuronal loss experiment, showed that these neurons were replaced by cells present in the vicinity rather than by stem cells migrating to the appropriate location form the ventricular zone (VZ) or the subventricular zone (SVZ). The identity of the replacing cells remains unclear and these could represent transdifferentiating glia or a quiescent population of stem cells. Neurons isolated from adult rat brain have also been shown to be able to proliferate and dedifferentiate into neural stem cells under certain culture conditions such as B27/ Neurobasal and FGF-2 *(32,33)*. Alexanian and Nornes retrogradely labeled adult rat corticospinal tract neurons by dextran dyes in vivo and showed that these adult neurons on dissociation and culture were able to incorporate BrdU and appeared to divide and regenerate daughter cells *(32)*. It is difficult to explain these results by cell fusion, contamination with precursors, or any other alternate possibility.

Overall the data provide intriguing evidence that plasticity is more common than previously supposed and that under appropriate conditions cells can be induced to alter their phenotype. This process is not limited to stem cells or early fetal cells but can occur in postmitotic neurons, adult astrocytes, as well as in more restricted precursor cell populations. Indeed, one may well argue that calling a cell a restricted precursor (our terminology and one used in this book) is a misnomer given abundant evidence of plasticity; the term biased precursor cell rather than restricted precursor cell should be used.

Intriguingly some cells do not readily transdifferentiate even when they appear closely related, present in the same environment or share lineal (albeit distant) relationship. Schwann cells, for example, will dedifferentiate into melanocytes but do not appear to transdifferentiate into astrocytes even though they will invade a damaged spinal cord and functionally are related. Likewise even when myelinating central axons Schwann cells will lay down myelin that has the characteristics of peripheral myelin rather than central myelin. Neural crest cells when transplanted in vivo even early in development do not populate the CNS or differentiate into CNS derivatives. In contrast, ablation of the neural tube *(74,75)* or overexpression of Fox-D3 *(76)* appears to be sufficient to direct the fate of CNS cells to neural crest and PNS early in development. Trunk crest does not appear to acquire the properties of cranial crest even when back-transplanted early in development. The ability of skin to convert to placodal derivatives appears to be restricted to a narrow temporal window *(77)* and is lost early in development.

Thus, although transdifferentiation may exist, it is not completely random and there appear to be biases in transdifferentiated fate. These biases are environment and cell dependent and may not be easily generalized to all cell types, that is, the same environmental cocktail may not transdifferentiate all cells along the same lineage and different environments may not necessarily expand the repertoire of a particular cell type. These results, however, raise the possibility that understanding the mechanisms that regulate the process of transdifferentiation may allow one to manipulate it with some fidelity and predictive ability.

TRANSDIFFERENTIATION AND DEDIFFERENTIATION OF NONNEURAL CELLS INTO NEURONS

The relative abundance of dedifferentiation or transdifferentiation within the nervous system raises the possibility that not only will this be possible within a tissue but all across other tissues as well. Indeed several lines of evidence suggest that this can occur. This review does not cover these examples in detail, but it is sufficient to say that mesodermal and endodermal differentiation in neural tissue has been reported by

Table 2
Transdifferentiation into Neural Cells

Original cell type	Transdifferentiation	Reference
Skin cell	Neuron	*(34)*
Bone marrow derived stem cell	Neuron	*(98,99)*
Marrow derived stromal cells	Neuron	*(100)*
Mesenchymal tissue	Neuron	*(27)*
Hematopoietic stem cells	Astrocyte	*(101)*
Melanoma cell line	Myelin expressing oligodendrocyte	*(102)*

multiple investigators, and in particular stem cells from bone marrow and mesenchyme have been shown to generate neurons, astrocytes, and oligodendrocytes in vitro and in vivo. A brief list of some reports is summarized in Table 2.

Although no doubt many of these examples can be explained by alternative mechanisms including cell fusion, presence of contaminating cells, and perhaps some overinterpretation, it is important to emphasize that these criticisms do not suggest that transdifferentiation itself does not occur. Rather, they raise questions on the frequency and utility of the process and the mechanism employed to induce transdifferentiation.

IF TRANSDIFFERENTIATION EXISTS, CAN WE UNDERSTAND AND REGULATE THE PROCESS?

As discussed in previous sections, although much of development involved progressive restriction in developmental fate, although examples of plasticity and transdifferentiation exist that cannot be explained by fusion, contamination, revealed competence, or fusion followed by resolution. Examples where clonal analysis was performed, or where nuclei were transferred in certain cancers, suggest that transdifferentiation can occur as well. Reconciling those apparently diametrically opposing ideas is not difficult. One can examine the cases of transdifferentiation as examples in which cells have bypassed the normal process of fate restriction or reversed such a restriction. We expect that useful insights will be obtained by examining the process of cell fate restriction and assessing the importance of these factors in transdifferentiating cells.

Cell specification broadly requires expression of cell type specific genes that are present in regions of open chromatin, while genes that will not be expressed are in regions of condensed chromatin with associated changes in the epigenome to maintain a heritable euchromatin and heterochromatin structure typical of a particular cell type. Many results suggest that lineage-specific genes are operative in a totipotent/pluripotent stem cell, such as an ES cell prior to lineage commitment, and suggest that stem cells express a multilineage transcriptosome. Most genes (including tissue specific genes) appear to be maintained in an open state with low but detectable levels of transcription with higher levels of specific transcription seen in appropriate cell types. Maintenance of an open transcriptosome in multipotent cells likely requires both the presence of positive factors as well as the absence of negative regulators. Factors that maintain an open transcriptosome include demethylases, reprogramming molecules present in blastocyst cytoplasm, regulators of heterochromatin modeling, and perhaps additional unidentified pathways. These positive factors are segregated as early progenitor cells undergo asymmetric cell division. The cell that receives these factors remains undifferentiated while the other daughter either degrades these factors, or does not receive them to activate cell type specific programs *(78)*. Global activators, global repressors, and master regulatory genes play important regulatory roles in switching on or off cassettes of genes while methylation *(79)*; reviewed in *(80)*, heterochromatin remodeling *(81)*, and perhaps small interfering RNA (siRNA, ref. *82*) maintain a stable phenotype by specifically regulating the overall transcriptional status of a cell. This epigenetic modulation also includes regulation of cell cycle. Most adult cells are postmitotic and are held in either transient or permanent (irreversible G_0) stage *(83)*. Reentry into mitosis is actively regulated and activation of cell cycle genes leads to apoptosis in cells held in irreversible G_0 stage *(83)*. Overall, the establishment and maintenance of the differentiated cell type appears to be tightly regulated by multiple mechanisms that operate at different stages during development. It is important to emphasize that not every mechanism is equally active in all cells and complex interactions occur between the various regulatory molecules.

It is thus reasonable to assume that if these epigenetic regulators of cell type specific gene expression could be altered or if cell type specific patterns of gene regulation could be activated (perhaps by activation of master regulators), then the pattern of gene expression would be changed to reflect acquisition of a different phenotype, much as what happens in development. As long as the epigenetic change could be modulated by external stimuli, cells should be capable of transdifferentiation and such transdifferentiation by extrinsic signal is exemplified by somatic nuclear transfer. Further, if this change occurred sufficiently precisely, the altered cell would be transdifferentiated into an unexpected phenotype that is indistinguishable from a normally developing cell. Multiple studies have indeed suggested that this can occur in specific instances, perhaps best exemplified by somatic nuclear transfer. In somatic nuclear transfer experiments, a somatic cell nucleus is inserted into an enucleated egg. This results in a major reprogramming of gene expression and switch in cell fate, and blastocysts derived from such experiments can generate normal fertile animals (e.g., ref. *84* and *85*) or apparently normal ES cell lines *(86)*. These results suggest that extrinsic stimuli exist that can alter the state/differentiation potential of a fully differentiated cells.

Forced expression of a global regulator can activate a cassette of cell type specific genes. Loss of single regulatory genes can alter the fate of the cells or cause them to acquire a new unexpected fate. Examples from *Drosophila* and *C. elegans* abound and suggest that if gene expression is altered at appropriate times, cells are sufficiently plastic that they can acquire a new fate *(87,88)*. In *Xenopus*, for example, misexpression of neurogenic genes in early development can induce neurogenic differentiation in skin cells *(62,63)*. In mice expression of muscle specific HLH genes can induce differentiation of myoblasts from ectodermal derivatives *(64)*.

Altering methylation patterns can induce reexpression of important regulatory molecules. For example it has been shown that expression of Oct3/4 is regulated by methylation and that alteration of methylation can reinduce expression of Oct3/4 and activate downstream target genes. Loss of a global repressor such as repressor element-1 silencing transcription factor/neuron restrictive silencer factor (REST/NRSF) can activate the expression of neuronal genes in mesenchymal cells *(89)*.

Table 3
Reagents that May Affect Transdifferentiation

Reagent	Example	Result	Reference
Demethylating reagent	5-Aza 2'deoxycytidine (5azaD)	Altered dedifferentiation	(92,93)
HDAC inhibitor	Trichostatin-A (TSA)	Increased dedifferentiation and altered differentiation	(93,97,103)
	Dimethyl sulfoxide (DMSO)	Transdifferentiate from mesenchymal tissue to neurons	(27)
	Butyrates	Transdifferentiate exocrine acini to pancreatic islet and duct-like complexes	(104)
	Suberolyanilide hydroxamic acid (SAHA)	Altered differentiation of erythroleukemia cell line	(105)
	Phorbol esters	Altered transdifferentiation of striatal neurons	(106)

Schwann cells will transdifferentiate into melanocytes when the neurofibromatosis gene is mutated *(90)*, and tumors often show evidence of metaplasia or trans-differentiation *(91)*. Forced expression of global regulators or treatment with 5-aza-cytidine or drugs that modulate heterochromatin remodeling will result in altered dedifferentiation *(92)*. Trichostatin A (TSA) has been shown to alter the differentiation of HSCs and to dedifferentiate progenitor cells *(93)*. TSA also has been shown to inhibit ES cell differentiation *(94)*.

Perhaps the most intriguing examples have come from data on heterochromatin remodeling and histone deacetylases (HDACs) and cancer *(95)*. Although these data are too voluminous to review here, it is intriguing in our opinion that many of the reagents that are known to affect chromatin remodeling have been used to alter transdifferentiation in culture (Table 3).

What becomes clear from these examples is that the maintenance of the appropriate epigenetic state requires active processes that are in dynamic flux with methylation of CpG islands, activation of master regulatory genes, inhibition by global repressors, and histone methylation/phosphorylation/acetylation acting in concert to define the state of a cell. For transdifferentiation to occur, some or all of these pathways that regulate the differentiation process must be susceptible to extrinsic manipulation. Available evidence from a variety of sources suggests that it is indeed possible. Thus, most of the mechanisms that regulate phenotypic specification are reversible and altering these regulatory mechanisms will permit expression of genes normally never expressed by particular cell types or alter their phenotypic differentiation. However, clearly our understanding of these pathways is limited and we lack precise control of the process. For example, generating DNMT1 (a methylase) null mice has effects only on subsets of neurons in the nervous system rather than a global effect, as one would predict based on its postulated function and expression pattern. Further, the resultant outcome is not transdifferentiation of the cells but cell death, although there is clear up-regulation of genes that are regulated by methylation *(96)*. More importantly, however, these studies identify a variety of small molecules, some of which are already used in the clinics (see, e.g., suberolyanilide hydroxamic acid [SAHA]), that can be used to assess the ability of a cell to transdifferentiate and provide a mechanism for the process of transdifferentiation *(95)*.

We would urge readers, however, to assess the cautionary moral of these results as well. These results clearly indicate that although modulating certain markers is well within our means, ectopic expression of these markers does not imply a change in phenotype. For example, β-III tubulin expression in fibroblasts in NRSF/REST knock-outs does not make these cells neurons. TSA treatment also has been shown to inhibit HSC transdifferentiation *(97)*. These results strongly suggest that multiple markers and functional integration will be required to demonstrate adequate and effective trans-differentiation.

These results suggest that a robust, reliable system of transdifferentiation is needed, in which each of these pathways can be systematically manipulated to assess the relative importance of each of these regulatory process. Understanding how critical each component is will allow one to realistically assess the fidelity of the process and its persistence and heritability. Unfortunately such robust systems appear unavailable and the few mammalian systems described have been controversial or difficult to reproduce.

Overall we would suggest that pathways to dedifferentiating or transdifferentiating cells exist and virtually every mechanism that regulates a stable differentiated phenotype can be subverted or modulated in one system or the other. This modulation is sufficient to produce relatively dramatic changes in phenotype, although we lack a detailed understanding or a precise control of the process. Framing transdifferentiation as an alteration of the normal regulators of progressive differentiation may allow us to plan more defined experiments and make predictions as to the outcome.

IS TRANSDIFFERENTIATION OF CLINICAL RELEVANCE?

In the previous section we have argued that transdifferentiation is possible, and that we know something about the process, and even have some indications of small molecules that could regulate this process. However, this does not to us suggest that transdifferentiated cells are of clinical relevance as yet. Unless we have precise control of transdifferentiation, we cannot translate this research to clinical treatment.

For clinical utility, the process has to be reliable, reproducible, heritable, and robust. In none of the systems examined so far are these criteria fulfilled. Indeed, because this process may involve a cell conversion not typically found in normal development, for the most part it is unclear how reliable and reproducible it will be in vivo. Although transdifferentiation itself may not be of clinical utility, we believe that studying transdifferentiation is important, as one needs to carefully address its potential. The current evidence on cell fusion, contamination, and lack of reproducibility *(47,48,52–54)* raises important legitimate questions about the efficiency of the process, its practical utility, and the rationale for using an attempt to transdifferentiate and the assumptions associated with a successful experiment validating the process of transdifferentiation.

Examining the process of transdifferentiation as aberrant fate restriction suggests some therapeutic strategies to achieve controlled transdifferentiation. Identifying the cytoplasmic factors that regulate nuclear reprogramming may identify important global regulators of fate restriction. Molecules regulating methylation and heterochromatin remodeling are likely to be useful candidates to regulate transdifferentiation. Equally useful we predict will be siRNAs to enable us to coopt a natural regulatory process to selectively derepress or activate specific subsets of genes. Finally, we would suggest that if forced senescence is a commonly used mechanism to prevent reentry into the cell cycle and to inhibit dedifferentiation or transdifferentiation, then apoptosis inhibitors may be useful both for understanding and for manipulating the process of transdifferentiation.

We would further suggest that resolving the controversies in the literature is worthwhile, because if transdifferentiation can be manipulated, one fell swoop can solve two major problems that bedevil cell therapy advocates. It provides a potential for obtaining sufficient numbers of cells that are otherwise in short supply. For example, we know that transplanting dopaminergic neurons of the appropriate type or β islet cells can treat Parkinson's disease or diabetes. However, we do not have enough cells to treat all possible patients who would benefit from this therapy. Transdifferentiation also offers the potential of using autologous cells for therapy thus solving the problem of immune rejection, side effects of suppressive therapy, and the mortality associated with these regimens.

It is useful to remember that many attempts have been made to solve these twin issues of number and immunologically matched cell type that range from using transgenic pigs to somatic nuclear transfer. In each of these attempts, initially the assumption by the proponents was that this problem has been solved and by its opponents was that these particular technologies were unlikely to succeed. In the case of transdifferentiation, we would suggest that the only way to find out is to perform the experiments as rigorously as possible with a clear hypothesis based on our understanding of the process of development in a robust and reliable system. Such experiments are in progress and it will be interesting to evaluate their outcome.

REFERENCES

1. Rao, M. S. (1999) Multipotent and restricted precursors in the central nervous system. *Anat. Rec.* **257**, 137–148.
2. Weissman, I. L., Anderson, D. J., and Gage, F. (2001) Stem and progenitor cells: origins, phenotypes, lineage commitments, and transdifferentiations. *Annu. Rev. Cell Dev. Biol.* **17**, 387–403.
3. Gilbert, S. F. (2003) Developmental Biology. 7th edition. Sinauer Associates, Inc., p. 838.
4. Morshead, C. M. and van der Kooy, D. (2004) Disguising adult neural stem cells. *Curr. Opin. Neurobiol.* **14**, 125–131.
5. Murayama, A., Matsuzaki, Y., Kawaguchi, A., Shimazaki, T., and Okano, H. (2002) Flow cytometric analysis of neural stem cells in the developing and adult mouse brain. *J. Neurosci. Res.* **69**, 837–847.
6. Gage, F. H. (2000) Mammalian neural stem cells. *Science* **287**, 1433–1438.
7. Rakic, P. (2003) Elusive radial glial cells: historical and evolutionary perspective. *Glia* **43**, 19–32.
8. Echeverri, K. and Tanaka, E. M. (2002) Ectoderm to mesoderm lineage switching during axolotl tail regeneration. *Science* **298**, 1993–1996.

9. Schoenwolf, G. C. (2000) Molecular genetic control of axis patterning during early embryogenesis of vertebrates. *Ann. NY Acad. Sci.* **919,** 246–260.

10. Rastegar, S., Albert, S., Le Roux, I., et al. (2002) A floor plate enhancer of the zebrafish netrin1 gene requires Cyclops (Nodal) signalling and the winged helix transcription factor FoxA2. *Dev. Biol.* **252,** 1–14.

11. Placzek, M., Dodd, J., and Jessell, T. M. (2000) Discussion point. The case for floor plate induction by the notochord. *Curr. Opin. Neurobiol.* **10,** 15–22.

12. Mujtaba, T., Mayer-Proschel, M., and Rao, M. S. (1998) A common neural progenitor for the CNS and PNS. *Dev. Biol.* **200,** 1–15.

13. Ziller, C., Dupin, E., Brazeau, P., Paulin, D., and Le Douarin, N. M. (1983) Early segregation of a neuronal precursor cell line in the neural crest as revealed by culture in a chemically defined medium. *Cell* **32,** 627–638.

14. Lang, H. and Fekete, D. M. (2001) Lineage analysis in the chicken inner ear shows differences in clonal dispersion for epithelial, neuronal, and mesenchymal cells. *Dev. Biol.* **234,** 120–137.

15. Sohal, G. S., Ali, M. M., Ali, A. A., and Bockman, D. E. (1999) Ventral neural tube cells differentiate into hepatocytes in the chick embryo. *Cell. Mol. Life Sci.* **55,** 128–130.

16. Sohal, G. S., Ali, M. M., Ali, A. A., and Dai, D. (1999) Ventrally emigrating neural tube cells contribute to the formation of Meckel's and quadrate cartilage. *Dev. Dyn.* **216,** 37–44.

17. Sohal, G. S., Ali, M. M., Ali, A. A., and Dai, D. (1999) Ventrally emigrating neural tube cells differentiate into heart muscle. *Biochem. Biophys. Res. Commun.* **254,** 601–604.

18. Bariety, J., Hill, G. S., Mandet, C., et al. (2003) Glomerular epithelial-mesenchymal transdifferentiation in pauci-immune crescentic glomerulonephritis. *Nephrol. Dial. Transplant.* **18,** 1777–1784.

19. Yanez-Mo, M., Lara-Pezzi, E., Selgas, R., et al. (2003) Peritoneal dialysis and epithelial-to-mesenchymal transition of mesothelial cells. *N. Engl. J. Med.* **348,** 403–413.

20. Torday, J. S., Torres, E., and Rehan, V. K. (2003) The role of fibroblast transdifferentiation in lung epithelial cell proliferation, differentiation, and repair in vitro. *Pediatr. Pathol. Mol. Med.* **22,** 189–207.

21. Lim, Y. S., Kim, K. A., Jung, J. O., et al. (2002) Modulation of cytokeratin expression during in vitro cultivation of human hepatic stellate cells: evidence of transdifferentiation from epithelial to mesenchymal phenotype. *Histochem. Cell Biol.* **118,** 127–136.

22. Liu, Y. and Rao, M. S. (2003) Transdifferentiation—fact or artifact. *J. Cell. Biochem.* **88,** 29–40.

23. Donovan, P. J. (1994) Growth factor regulation of mouse primordial germ cell development. *Curr. Top. Dev. Biol.* **29,** 189–225.

24. Matsui, Y., Zsebo, K., and Hogan, B. L. (1992) Derivation of pluripotential embryonic stem cells from murine primordial germ cells in culture. *Cell* **70,** 841–847.

25. Tosh, D. and Slack, J. M. (2002) How cells change their phenotype. *Nat. Rev. Mol. Cell. Biol.* **3,** 187–194.

26. Tsonis, P. A. (2000) Regeneration in vertebrates. *Dev. Biol.* **221,** 273–284.

27. Woodbury, D., Schwarz, E. J., Prockop, D. J., and Black, I. B. (2000) Adult rat and human bone marrow stromal cells differentiate into neurons. *J. Neurosci. Res.* **61,** 364–370.

28. Franchi, A., Pasquinelli, G., Cenacchi, G., et al. (2001) Immunohistochemical and ultrastructural investigation of neural differentiation in Ewing sarcoma/PNET of bone and soft tissues. *Ultrastruct. Pathol.* **25,** 219–225.

29. Kondo, T. and Raff, M. (2000) Oligodendrocyte precursor cells reprogrammed to become multipotential CNS stem cells. *Science* **289,** 1754–1757.

30. Laywell, E. D., Rakic, P., Kukekov, V. G., Holland, E. C., and Steindler, D. A. (2000) Identification of a multipotent astrocytic stem cell in the immature and adult mouse brain. *Proc. Natl. Acad. Sci. USA* **97,** 13883–13888.

31. Malatesta, P., Hartfuss, E., and Gotz, M. (2000) Isolation of radial glial cells by fluorescent-activated cell sorting reveals a neuronal lineage. *Development* **127,** 5253–5263.
32. Alexanian, A. R. and Nornes, H. O. (2001) Proliferation and regeneration of retrogradely labeled adult rat corticospinal neurons in culture. *Exp. Neurol.* **170,** 277–282.
33. Brewer, G. J. (1999) Regeneration and proliferation of embryonic and adult rat hippocampal neurons in culture. *Exp. Neurol.* **159,** 237–247.
34. Toma, J. G., Akhavan, M., Fernandes, K. J., et al. (2001) Isolation of multipotent adult stem cells from the dermis of mammalian skin. *Nat. Cell Biol.* **3,** 778–784.
35. Sieber-Blum, M. (2004) Cardiac neural crest stem cells. *Anat. Rec.* **276A,** 34–42.
36. Kruger, G. M., Mosher, J. T., Bixby, S., Joseph, N., Iwashita, T., and Morrison, S. J. (2002) Neural crest stem cells persist in the adult gut but undergo changes in self-renewal, neuronal subtype potential, and factor responsiveness. *Neuron* **35,** 657–669.
37. Tsonis, P. A. and Del Rio-Tsonis, K. (2004) Lens and retina regeneration: transdifferentiation, stem cells and clinical applications. *Exp. Eye Res.* **78,** 161–172.
38. Reynolds, B. A. and Weiss, S. (1996) Clonal and population analyses demonstrate that an EGF-responsive mammalian embryonic CNS precursor is a stem cell. *Dev. Biol.* **175,** 1–13.
39. Vescovi, A. L., Reynolds, B. A., Fraser, D. D., and Weiss, S. (1993) bFGF regulates the proliferative fate of unipotent (neuronal) and bipotent (neuronal/astroglial) EGF-generated CNS progenitor cells. *Neuron* **11,** 951–966.
40. Magrassi, L., Castello, S., Ciardelli, L., et al. (2003) Freshly dissociated fetal neural stem/progenitor cells do not turn into blood. *Mol. Cell. Neurosci.* **22,** 179–187.
41. Benca, R. M., Wemhoff, G., and Quintans, J. (1986) Functional studies of pluripotential hemopoietic stem cells in mouse brain. *J. Neuroimmunol.* **10,** 341–352.
42. McKinney-Freeman, S. L., Jackson, K. A., Camargo, F. D., Ferrari, G., Mavilio, F., and Goodell, M. A. (2002) Muscle-derived hematopoietic stem cells are hematopoietic in origin. *Proc. Natl. Acad. Sci. USA* **99,** 1341–1346.
43. Jiang, Y., Jahagirdar, B. N., Reinhardt, R. L., et al. (2002) Pluripotency of mesenchymal stem cells derived from adult marrow. *Nature* **418,** 41–49.
44. Song, L. and Tuan, R. S. (2004) Transdifferentiation potential of human mesenchymal stem cells derived from bone marrow. *FASEB J.*
45. Young, H. E., Duplaa, C., Romero-Ramos, M., et al. (2004) Adult reserve stem cells and their potential for tissue engineering. *Cell Biochem. Biophys.* **40,** 1–80.
46. Morshead, C. M., Benveniste, P., Iscove, N. N., and van der Kooy, D. (2002) Hematopoietic competence is a rare property of neural stem cells that may depend on genetic and epigenetic alterations. *Nat. Med.* **8,** 268–273.
47. Terada, N., Hamazaki, T., Oka, M., et al. (2002) Bone marrow cells adopt the phenotype of other cells by spontaneous cell fusion. *Nature* **416,** 542–545.
48. Vassilopoulos, G., Wang, P. R., and Russell, D. W. (2003) Transplanted bone marrow regenerates liver by cell fusion. *Nature* **422,** 901–904.
49. Geiger, H., True, J. M., Grimes, B., Carroll, E. J., Fleischman, R. A., and Van Zant, G. (2002) Analysis of the hematopoietic potential of muscle-derived cells in mice. *Blood* **100,** 721–723.
50. McKinney-Freeman, S. L., Majka, S. M., Jackson, K. A., Norwood, K., Hirschi, K. K., and Goodell, M. A. (2003) Altered phenotype and reduced function of muscle-derived hematopoietic stem cells. *Exp. Hematol.* **31,** 806–814.
51. Camargo, F. D., Chambers, S. M., and Goodell, M. A. (2004) Stem cell plasticity: from transdifferentiation to macrophage fusion. *Cell Prolif.* **37,** 55–65.
52. Eto, K., Murphy, R., Kerrigan, S. W., et al. (2002) Megakaryocytes derived from embryonic stem cells implicate CalDAG-GEFI in integrin signaling. *Proc. Natl. Acad. Sci. USA* **99,** 12819–12824.
53. Ying, Q. L., Nichols, J., Evans, E. P., and Smith, A. G. (2002) Changing potency by spontaneous fusion. *Nature* **416,** 545–548.

54. Wang, X., Willenbring, H., Akkari, Y., et al. (2003) Cell fusion is the principal source of bone-marrow-derived hepatocytes. *Nature* **422,** 897–901.

55. Broyles, R. H. (1999) Use of somatic cell fusion to reprogram globin genes. *Semin. Cell Dev. Biol.* **10,** 259–265.

56. Wilmut, I., Beaujean, N., de Sousa, P. A., et al. (2002) Somatic cell nuclear transfer. *Nature* **419,** 583–586.

57. Wilmut, I. and Paterson, L. (2003) Somatic cell nuclear transfer. *Oncol. Res.* **13,** 303–307.

58. Reya, T., Morrison, S. J., Clarke, M. F., and Weissman, I. L. (2001) Stem cells, cancer, and cancer stem cells. *Nature* **414,** 105–111.

59. Joshi, C. V. and Enver, T. (2002) Plasticity revisited. *Curr. Opin. Cell Biol.* **14,** 749–755.

60. Bang, Y. J., Pirnia, F., Fang, W. G., et al. (1994) Terminal neuroendocrine differentiation of human prostate carcinoma cells in response to increased intracellular cyclic AMP. *Proc. Natl. Acad. Sci. USA* **91,** 5330–5334.

61. Martin, G. R. (1980) Teratocarcinomas and mammalian embryogenesis. *Science* **209,** 768–776.

62. Moreno, T. A. and Bronner-Fraser, M. (2001) The secreted glycoprotein Noelin-1 promotes neurogenesis in *Xenopus. Dev. Biol.* **240,** 340–360.

63. Anderson, D. J. (1995) Neural development. Spinning skin into neurons. *Curr. Biol.* **5,** 1235–1238.

64. Boukamp, P. (1995) Transdifferentiation induced by gene transfer. *Semin. Cell Biol.* **6,** 157–163.

65. Sparks, R. L., Seibel-Ross, E. I., Wier, M. L., and Scott, R. E. (1986) Differentiation, dedifferentiation, and transdifferentiation of BALB/c 3T3 T mesenchymal stem cells: potential significance in metaplasia and neoplasia. *Cancer Res.* **46,** 5312–5319.

66. Gabay, L., Lowell, S., Rubin, L. L., and Anderson, D. J. (2003) Deregulation of dorsoventral patterning by FGF confers trilineage differentiation capacity on CNS stem cells in vitro. *Neuron* **40,** 485–499.

67. Gotz, M. and Steindler, D. (2003) To be glial or not-how glial are the precursors of neurons in development and adulthood? *Glia* **43,** 1–3.

68. Hartfuss, E., Galli, R., Heins, N., and Gotz, M. (2001) Characterization of CNS precursor subtypes and radial glia. *Dev. Biol.* **229,** 15–30.

69. Seri, B., Garcia-Verdugo, J. M., McEwen, B. S., and Alvarez-Buylla, A. (2001) Astrocytes give rise to new neurons in the adult mammalian hippocampus. *J. Neurosci.* **21,** 7153–7160.

70. Doetsch, F., Caille, I., Lim, D. A., Garcia-Verdugo, J. M., and Alvarez-Buylla, A. (1999) Subventricular zone astrocytes are neural stem cells in the adult mammalian brain. *Cell* **97,** 703–716.

71. Steindler, D. A. and Laywell, E. D. (2003) Astrocytes as stem cells: nomenclature, phenotype, and translation. *Glia* **43,** 62–69.

72. Pevny, L. and Rao, M. S. (2003) The stem-cell menagerie. *Trends Neurosci.* **26,** 351–359.

73. Eyding, D., Macklis, J. D., Neubacher, U., Funke, K., and Worgotter, F. (2003) Selective elimination of corticogeniculate feedback abolishes the electroencephalogram dependence of primary visual cortical receptive fields and reduces their spatial specificity. *J. Neurosci.* **23,** 7021–7033.

74. Kulesa, P., Bronner-Fraser, M., and Fraser, S. (2000) In ovo time-lapse analysis after dorsal neural tube ablation shows rerouting of chick hindbrain neural crest. *Development* **127,** 2843–2852.

75. Sechrist, J., Nieto, M. A., Zamanian, R. T., and Bronner-Fraser, M. (1995) Regulative response of the cranial neural tube after neural fold ablation: spatiotemporal nature of neural crest regeneration and up-regulation of Slug. *Development* **121,** 4103–4115.

76. Hanna, L. A., Foreman, R. K., Tarasenko, I. A., Kessler, D. S., and Labosky, P. A. (2002) Requirement for Foxd3 in maintaining pluripotent cells of the early mouse embryo. *Genes Dev.* **16,** 2650–2661.
77. Stark, M. R., Sechrist, J., Bronner-Fraser, M., and Marcelle, C. (1997) Neural tube-ectoderm interactions are required for trigeminal placode formation. *Development* **124,** 4287–4295.
78. Knoblich, J. A. (1997) Mechanisms of asymmetric cell division during animal development. *Curr. Opin. Cell Biol.* **9,** 833–841.
79. Bird, A. P. and Wolffe, A. P. (1999) Methylation-induced repression—belts, braces, and chromatin. *Cell* **99,** 451–454.
80. Surani, M. A. (2001) Reprogramming of genome function through epigenetic inheritance. *Nature* **414,** 122–128.
81. Wu, J. and Grunstein, M. (2000) 25 Years after the nucleosome model: chromatin modifications. *Trends Biochem. Sci.* **25,** 619–623.
82. Ahlquist, P. (2002) RNA-dependent RNA polymerases, viruses, and RNA silencing. *Science* **296,** 1270–1273.
83. Sommer, L. and Rao, M. (2002) Neural stem cells and regulation of cell number. *Prog. Neurobiol.* **66,** 1–18.
84. Wakayama, T., Perry, A. C., Zuccotti, M., Johnson, K. R., and Yanagimachi, R. (1998) Full-term development of mice from enucleated oocytes injected with cumulus cell nuclei. *Nature* **394,** 369–374.
85. Hwang, W. S., Ryu, Y. J., Park, J. H., et al. (2004) Evidence of a pluripotent human embryonic stem cell line derived from a cloned blastocyst. *Science* **303,** 1669–1674.
86. Wakayama, T., Tabar, V., Rodriguez, I., Perry, A. C., Studer, L., and Mombaerts, P. (2001) Differentiation of embryonic stem cell lines generated from adult somatic cells by nuclear transfer. *Science* **292,** 740–743.
87. Baker, N. E. (2001) Master regulatory genes; telling them what to do. *Bioessays* **23,** 763–766.
88. Baker, N. E. (2001) Cell proliferation, survival, and death in the *Drosophila* eye. *Semin. Cell Dev. Biol.* **12,** 499–507.
89. Kallunki, P., Edelman, G. M., and Jones, F. S. (1997) Tissue-specific expression of the L1 cell adhesion molecule is modulated by the neural restrictive silencer element. *J. Cell Biol.* **138,** 1343–1354.
90. Stocker, K. M., Baizer, L., Coston, T., Sherman, L., and Ciment, G. (1995) Regulated expression of neurofibromin in migrating neural crest cells of avian embryos. *J. Neurobiol.* **27,** 535–552.
91. Kameyama, M., Ishikawa, Y., Shibahara, T., and Kadota, K. (2000) Melanotic neurofibroma in a steer. *J. Vet. Med. Sci.* **62,** 125–128.
92. Robertson, K. D. and Jones, P. A. (2000) DNA methylation: past, present and future directions. *Carcinogenesis* **21,** 461–467.
93. Milhem, M., Mahmud, N., Lavelle, D., et al. (2004) Modification of hematopoietic stem cell fate by 5aza 2'deoxycytidine and trichostatin A. *Blood* **103,** 4102–4110.
94. Lee, J. H., Hart, S. R., and Skalnik, D. G. (2004) Histone deacetylase activity is required for embryonic stem cell differentiation. *Genesis* **38,** 32–38.
95. Marks, P., Rifkind, R. A., Richon, V. M., Breslow, R., Miller, T., and Kelly, W. K. (2001) Histone deacetylases and cancer: causes and therapies. *Nat. Rev. Cancer* **1,** 194–202.
96. Fan, G., Beard, C., Chen, R. Z., et al. (2001) DNA hypomethylation perturbs the function and survival of CNS neurons in postnatal animals. *J. Neurosci.* **21,** 788–797.
97. Rombouts, K., Niki, T., Wielant, A., Hellemans, K., and Geerts, A. (2001) Trichostatin A, lead compound for development of antifibrogenic drugs. *Acta Gastroenterol. Belg.* **64,** 239–246.
98. Brazelton, T. R., Rossi, F. M., Keshet, G. I., and Blau, H. M. (2000) From marrow to brain: expression of neuronal phenotypes in adult mice. *Science* **290,** 1775–1779.

99. Mezey, E., Chandross, K. J., Harta, G., Maki, R. A., and McKercher, S. R. (2000) Turning blood into brain: cells bearing neuronal antigens generated in vivo from bone marrow. *Science* **290,** 1779–1782.

100. Kohyama, J., Abe, H., Shimazaki, T., et al. (2001) Brain from bone: efficient "meta-differentiation" of marrow stroma-derived mature osteoblasts to neurons with Noggin or a demethylating agent. *Differentiation* **68,** 235–244.

101. Hao, H. N., Zhao, J., Thomas, R. L., Parker, G. C., and Lyman, W. D. (2003) Fetal human hematopoietic stem cells can differentiate sequentially into neural stem cells and then astrocytes in vitro. *J. Hematother. Stem Cell Res.* **12,** 23–32.

102. Slutsky, S. G., Kamaraju, A. K., Levy, A. M., Chebath, J., and Revel, M. (2003) Activation of myelin genes during transdifferentiation from melanoma to glial cell phenotype. *J. Biol. Chem.* **278,** 8960–8968.

103. Niki, T., Rombouts, K., De Bleser, P., et al. (1999) A histone deacetylase inhibitor, trichostatin A, suppresses myofibroblastic differentiation of rat hepatic stellate cells in primary culture. *Hepatology* **29,** 858–867.

104. Rooman, I., Heremans, Y., Heimberg, H., and Bouwens, L. (2000) Modulation of rat pancreatic acinoductal transdifferentiation and expression of PDX-1 in vitro. *Diabetologia* **43,** 907–914.

105. Richon, V. M., Emiliani, S., Verdin, E., et al. (1998) A class of hybrid polar inducers of transformed cell differentiation inhibits histone deacetylases. *Proc. Natl. Acad. Sci. USA* **95,** 3003–3007.

106. Guo, Z., Du, X., and Iacovitti, L. (1998) Regulation of tyrosine hydroxylase gene expression during transdifferentiation of striatal neurons: changes in transcription factors binding the AP-1 site. *J. Neurosci.* **18,** 8163–8174.

12

Neural Progenitor Cells of the Adult Human Brain

Steven A. Goldman

Over the past two decades, studies of cell genesis in the adult vertebrate brain have revealed the persistence of neural progenitor cells in both the neuroepithelial lining of the cerebral ventricles and the developmentally contiguous hippocampal dentate gyrus. Competent neural progenitor cells have been identified in adult fish, reptiles, birds, rodents, monkeys, and humans *(1,2)*. Across phylogeny, both multipotential and phenotypically restricted progenitors populate the ventricular lining *(3–7)*, within which they appear to be largely subependymal in origin *(8,9)*. These subependymal neural progenitor cells extend throughout the adult ventricular system *(10–12)*, persist throughout adult life *(13,14)*, and may include or derive from multipotential founders *(15–17)*. Although ependymal cells have also been reported to include multipotential progenitors *(18)*, this observation remains controversial and as yet unverified. Rather, most studies have pointed to the existence in adults of a subependymal progenitor cell population, which remains neurogenic in selected regions, such as the avian neostriatum and rodent olfactory bulb, but that more typically is quiescent unless activated *(17,19)*, then yielding either glia or short-lived neuronal progeny *(18,20)*.

Humans, like their lower species counterparts, retain competent neural progenitor cells in adulthood *(6,21–23)*. We review here the identification, initial isolation, relative distributions, and lineage competence of the three major progenitor cell phenotypes that have been isolated from the adult human forebrain: the ventricular zone neural progenitor cell, the hippocampal neuronal progenitor, and the white matter glial progenitor *(23–28)*. Each of these cell types has been prospectively identified and selected from adult human brain tissue, and isolated to near purity (reviewed in ref. *29*). The isolation of adult progenitor cells has advanced our understanding not only of their lineage potential and growth factor dependence, but also of their potential utility as both transplantable cellular vectors *(30–32)*, and as targets for endogenous induction *(33–40)*. In this chapter, we limit our discussion to the identification, isolation, lineage competence, and interrelationships among the major progenitor cell types thus far characterized in the adult human brain.

From: *Neural Development and Stem Cells, Second Edition*
Edited by: M. S. Rao © Humana Press Inc., Totowa, NJ

NEURONAL PRECURSOR CELLS RESIDE
IN THE ADULT HUMAN FOREBRAIN VENTRICULAR ZONE

In adult primates, the forebrain ventricular zone (VZ), composed of the apposing ependymal and subependymal cell layers, continues to harbor dividing cells, predominantly if not exclusively within the subependymal cell population *(41,42)*. In adult rodents, subependymal cell division is followed by the migration of neuronal daughter cells rostrally to the olfactory bulb *(5,43)*, and at least developmentally, to the subgranular zone of the hippocampus. On this basis, we postulated that the adult human brain might retain a reservoir of such subependymal progenitor cells, which cease generating neurons in vivo yet retain the capacity for neurogenesis in vitro. To test this possibility, we sought evidence of neurogenesis in cultures of adult human temporal lobe *(6)*. In our initial studies, both explants and dissociates were prepared from temporal lobe tissue obtained during surgical resection; these samples were dissected into cortical, subcortical, and periventricular zone (VZ), and cultured under conditions permissive for neuronal differentiation. The VZ cultures, and only these, gave rise to neurons, as identified both antigenically and physiologically. In addition, antigenically verified neurons that incorporated [^{3}H]thymidine were found in VZ cultures, indicating that these cells arose from precursor division in vitro (Fig. 1).

The new VZ-derived neurons were functionally competent: When depolarized during confocal imaging, they showed rapid, 4- to 10-fold elevations in Ca^{2+}_i in response to 60 mM K^+, responses typical of neuronal voltage-gated calcium channels. These were the first indications that progenitor cells derived from the adult human VZ might continue to exhibit mitotic neurogenesis, and that daughter cells generated from adult human VZ progenitor cells could indeed develop mature neuronal function *(6,22,44,45)*.

PROGENITOR CELLS MAY BE IDENTIFIED HISTOLOGICALLY
IN THE ADULT HUMAN SUBEPENDYMA

The study of the neural and committed neuronal progenitor cell populations of the adult central nervous system (CNS) had been hampered for decades by the lack of any available antigenic markers by which these cells might be specifically identified. The identification of nestin protein as an intermediate filament expressed at high levels by neuroepithelial cells aided and accelerated the study of these cells *(46)*, despite nestin's lack of absolute phenotypic specificity *(47)*. In addition, recent discoveries of RNA-binding proteins specific for neural phenotype have led to the identification and development of several new probes for neurons and their progenitors. Musashi protein is one such RNA-binding protein, which is expressed only by mitotic, uncommitted progenitors in development, and by VZ cells and parenchymal astrocytes in adulthood *(48)*. Musashi was first identified in *Drosophila* and *Xenopus (49,50)*, in which it is expressed by CNS stem cells and their mitotic daughters. Musashi binds numb protein, and as such acts as a positive regulator of notch signaling, as such promoting progenitor cell self-maintenance. In mammalian development, musashi expression is limited to cycling cells in the ventricular and subventricular zones, and diminishes rapidly with cell migration. It is not expressed by neurons or oligodendrocytes, but is sustained at a relatively low level by parenchymal astrocytes *(51)*. In adults, musashi expression is limited largely to the ventricular and olfactory subependyma, a distribution pattern

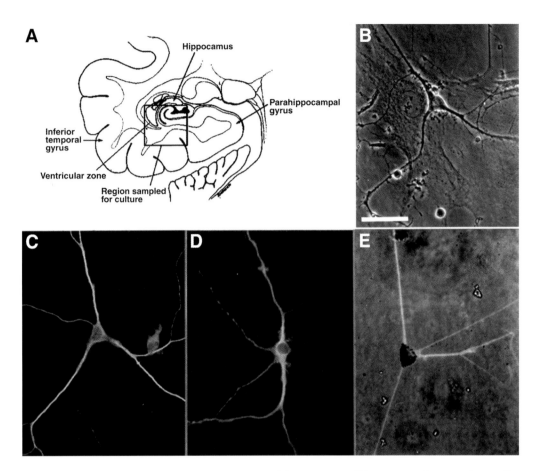

Fig. 1. The adult human temporal lobe provides an accessible source of progenitor cells. Samples were taken during temporal lobectomy, typically either for decompressive resection or refractory epilepsy. (**A**) Schematic of a typical temporal lobe resection; each sample was dissected into cortical, subcortical, and periventricular portions, the latter including the ependyma and adjacent subventricular tissue. When the hippocampus was included in the resection, it was dissected from the temporal lobe, and the dentate gyrus then dissected clean of its overlying ventricular wall. (**B**) The outgrowth from an adult SZ explant, in which a presumptive neuron is seen on a layer of flat substrate cells at 19 DIV. (**C**) A MAP-2⁺ neuron, found in a subcortical culture at 18 DIV. (**D**) An NCAM⁺ neuron in an SZ dissociate at 12 DIV. (**E**) A MAP-5⁺ cell that incorporated [³H]thymidine in vitro, suggesting its origin from precursor cell mitosis. Scale = 50 µm. (Adapted from ref. *6*.)

similar to that of nestin *(46)*; its sequence is highly conserved, allowing antibodies against mouse musashi to identify precursor cells in the adult human VZ *(22)*.

The Hu proteins constitute another such family of neuronal RNA-binding proteins *(52)*; three of its four known members appear to be expressed only by neurons, perhaps at different phases of neuronal ontogeny. As a result, the anti-Hu MAb 16A11, which recognizes a conserved epitope on the Hu proteins HuC, HuD, and Hel-N1, recognizes only neurons and their committed progenitors *(53–55)*. As in musashi, the sequences of the Hu proteins are highly conserved, allowing antibodies against avian Hu to recognize neuronally committed progenitor cells in the adult human VZ *(22,55)*.

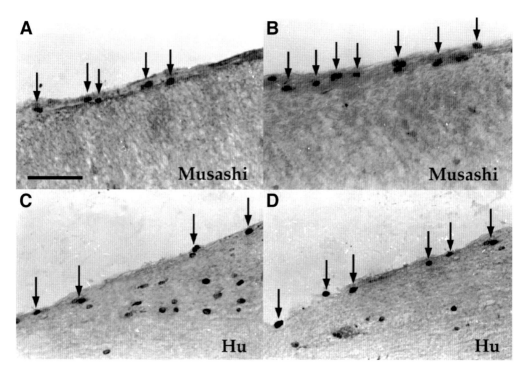

Fig. 2. Musashi and Hu proteins recognize uncommitted progenitor cells and their neuronal daughters in the adult temporal VZ. These sections were taken from the ependyma/sub-ependyma lining of the lateral ventricle, deep to the inferior temporal gyrus, in a 27-yr-old man with mesial temporal sclerosis. **(A,B)** Scattered islands of ventricular cells, generally subependymal, immunoperoxidase stained for musashi protein, an RNA-binding protein of neural progenitors. Musashi expression was limited to the VZ of these adult human temporal resections. **(C,D)** Loose aggregates of adult SZ cells also expressed Hu, a triad of early, neuron-specific RNA-binding proteins recognized by MAb 16A11. Scale = 50 μm. (From ref. *22*.)

On the basis of these studies, the distribution of neural and neuronal progenitor cells has been estimated in the adult human temporal VZ, respectively using musashi and Hu proteins as immunomarkers *(22)* (Fig. 2). Overall, 7.8 ± 2.2% of subependymal cells expressed Hu, and 6.2 ± 2.6% were musashi[+]; together, >10% of temporal VZ cells expressed one or the other of these markers. However, this estimate of the frequency of progenitor cells and their derivatives in the adult subependyma must be viewed in the context of the patchy distribution and evanescent thinness of the adult VZ, which is but a noncontiguous cellular monolayer along the adult human temporal horn. As a result, the incidence of potentially neurogenic progenitor cells in the adult temporal VZ would appear to be quite low. However, a more recent study of the human VZ, which used labeling for glial fibrillary acidic protein (GFAP) to identify subependymal astrocytes, demonstrated not only the neurogenic competence of at least some of these astrocytes *(23)*, but also that the reservoir of potentially neurogenic VZ progenitor cells might be higher than previously recognized. This point remains unsettled, and will require further investigation of the homogeneity, or lack thereof, of subependymal progenitor cell populations and their derived lineages.

ADULT VZ CELLS RESPOND TO FIBROBLAST GROWTH FACTOR-2 (FGF-2)/ BRAIN-DERIVED NEUROTROPHIC FACTOR (BDNF) WITH EXPANSION AND NEURONAL DIFFERENTIATION

In rodents, the proliferation of adult VZ precursor cells is promoted by FGF-2 *(16,56,57)*, whereas the differentiation, maturation, and survival of their neuronal daughters is supported by BDNF *(10,58)*. On this basis, we sequentially treated explants of the adult human temporal VZ with FGF-2 followed by BDNF, and found that neurogenesis could indeed be induced and supported with this combination of agents *(22)*. Neuronal number and survival in explants raised for 1 wk in 20 ng/mL of FGF-2, followed by 8 wk in 40 ng/mL of BDNF, were both substantially greater than in unsupplemented plates or those given *either* FGF-2 *or* BDNF. After 9 wk in vitro, many explants raised in FGF-2/BDNF exhibited elaborate networks of scores of healthy neurons (Fig. 3). These cells expressed MAP-2, and displayed sharp calcium increments to K^+-depolarization, suggesting their functional maturation. Many had incorporated [^{3}H]thymidine during their first week in vitro, indicating their genesis during that week in FGF-2, 8 wk earlier. No surviving neurons were noted beyond 2 wk in plates not treated with FGF-2 and BDNF. These data indicated that serial application of FGF-2 and BDNF allowed the generation of complex networks of new neurons from subependymal progenitors of the adult human brain *(22,59)*.

THE INACCESSIBILITY OF HUMAN NEURAL PRECURSORS HAS ENCOURAGED EXPANSION STRATEGIES

The harvest of primary neuronal precursor cells from the adult human forebrain has been limited by the low yields attending its enzymatic dissociation, and the difficulty in recognizing and purifying surviving precursor cells as such. To improve the yield of adult-derived neural progenitors, several groups have taken the approach of raising neural cell lines derived from single precursors, exposed continuously to mitogens in serum-deficient culture. Although first established for use in the adult rodent brain *(15,17,60)*, the propagation of clonally derived neurospheres was extended to the propagation of fetal human neural progenitor cells as well *(61–63)*. Steindler and colleagues then propagated adult human VZ progenitor cells in suspension cultures, and reported the multilineage potential of the nominally clonal neurospheres thereby generated *(64)*. The generation of both neurons and glia by these adult VZ-derived neurospheres suggested that the neuronal progenitor cells identified in adult human VZ explant cultures *(6,22)*, might be derivatives of periventricular neural stem cells.

It is important to note that despite the abundance of cells obtained through the sustained propagation of VZ cells in vitro, this strategy for preparing engraftable neural progenitors has a number of limitations: First, the directed differentiation of tissue-derived neural stem cells into desired phenotypes remains a largely unrealized goal, despite some progress in modifying or biasing the phenotypic choice and fate of these cells by defined neurotrophic and gliotrophic agents *(10,58,65–69)*. Second, the lineage potential, transformation state, and karyotype of propagated neural stem cells remain uncertain; after prolonged passage at high split ratios, the antigenic expression patterns of repetitively passaged precursors often manifest mixed lineages *(56)*. Indeed, under the stress of prolonged mitogenic stimulation in serum-free culture, neither the

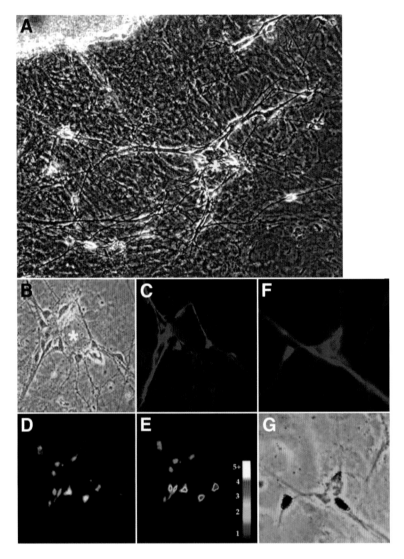

Fig. 3. Adult human VZ progenitor cells can be stimulated to expand in vitro, and generate functional neurons. Cultures from this patient were grown in added FGF-2 for 1 wk and BDNF thereafter. **(A)** A field of neurons that have arisen from a neocortical explant after 9 wk in vitro; highly neuritic neurons lie on ependymal cells and glia. **(B)** Higher magnification (*asterisk*). **(C)** MAP-2 staining confirms the neuronal identity of these cells. **(D)** Laser-scanning confocal microscopy at 488-nm images the basal calcium signal of the neuronal outgrowth, after loading with fluo-3. **(E)** A sharp increase in fluo-3 fluorescence, typical of neuronal calcium responses, to K$^+$ depolarization. **(F,G)** Of 11 MAP-2$^+$ cells in **B**, 4 incorporated [^{3}H]thymidine$^+$ during their first week in vitro. (From ref. *22*.)

clonality nor karyotypic integrity of these cells can be assumed. Although the reversion to a mixed-antigenic phenotype may represent the emergence or reversion to a stem-cell phenotype *(70)*, it might also manifest the degradation of committed lineages into lines that are at best unrepresentative of their founders, and at worst, into transformed neuroectodermal blasts. Third, it remains unclear whether neurons generated from repetitively passaged precursors retain the normal characteristics of neuronal electro-physiological function, although recent observations of action potential generation from extensively expanded human fetal progenitor cell lines have been reassuring in this regard *(71,72)*.

HUMAN NEURAL PROGENITOR CELLS
MAY ACT AS SUCH UPON XENOGRAFT

A number of recent studies have reported that fetal human neural progenitors, derived from abortuses and expanded in vitro as neurospheres, may terminally differ-entiate and histologically integrate when xenografted to both the prenatal and adult rodent brain *(63,73,74)*. Similarly, v-myc-immortalized human neural stem cells have been shown to differentiate into all three major neural lineages on perinatal engraft-ment into the rodent brain *(75)*. Together, these studies have indicated that neural stem cells may act as such in vivo as well as in vitro, generating multiple lineages in context-dependent fashions. As such, they have tremendously advanced our conception of the potential therapeutic roles of neural stem cells in both structural repair and enzymatic repletion. Nonetheless, because of the possibility of phenotypic degradation attending either immortalization or expansion, it has been unclear whether prolonged mitogen-assisted expansion from single isolated precursors will prove a clinically viable strat-egy for propagating therapeutically sound neural progenitor cells.

On the basis of these studies, we postulated that native progenitor cells might be more likely than their expanded counterparts to generate functionally sound neurons on eventual transplantation. Indeed, we had already found that neurons generated directly from freshly cultured VZ explants exhibited characteristic neuronal responses to both depolarization and excitatory transmitters *(76,77)*. However, the theoretical advantages of using directly harvested progenitor cells had been limited in practice, by our lack of means for specifically identifying and harvesting these cells from donor brain tissues. As a result, relatively large amounts of scarce human fetal tissues have been required to generate enough fetal progenitor cells for engraftment, while no adult tissues have yet yielded progenitor cells in sufficient numbers or purity to allow their direct implantation. To redress this problem of enriching scarce progenitor cells from much larger populations of brain cells, we therefore established a means of identifying and selecting neural progenitor cells on the basis of their expression of fluorescent transgenes driven by cell-specific promoter sequences.

PROMOTER-BASED IDENTIFICATION
ALLOWS PROGENITORS TO BE RECOGNIZED AS SUCH

To recognize live neuronal precursors as such, we chose to use neural promoters to drive the expression of the gene encoding green fluorescent protein (GFP) *(78)*. GFP is a coelenterate protein that fluoresces on blue excitation, with little toxicity; it has evolved into an effective transcriptional reporter in live cells *(79)*. To identify neuronal progenitor cells while still alive, as opposed to in fixed histological sections, we devel-oped constructs of a mutant GFP optimized for human codon usage (hGFP) *(80)*, placed under the control of the early neuronal P/Ta1 tubulin promoter *(81,82)*. In accord with the neuronal specificity of Ta1 tubulin promoter expression *(82)*, P/Ta1 tubulin-driven hGFP was strongly expressed by precursors and young neurons, but not by glia *(83,84)*.

In both fetal and adult-derived cultures, P/Ta1-driven GFP fluorescence was specific to neurons and their committed precursors (dividing as well as postmitotic), and remained bright up to 14 d after transfection *(84)*. This observation established that GFP, when expressed under the control of cell-specific regulatory elements, might be used as a reporter of phenotype in live cells.

PROMOTER-DEFINED RESTRICTION OF GFP PERMITS FLUORESCENCE-ACTIVATED CELL SORTING (FACS) OF NEURAL PROGENITOR CELLS

To separate and harvest native neural progenitor cells directly from brain tissue, we capitalized on the ability of promoters, such as that for Ta1 tubulin, to direct fluorescent gene expression to desired phenotypes. To this end, we first transfected cultured monolayer dissociates of fetal chick and rat VZ cells with P/Ta1:GFP, and then used FACS to extract the P/Ta1:GFP-defined fluorescent neuronal progenitors. This technique allowed both a high degree of enrichment of neuronal progenitor cells, and a virtual abolition of glial contaminants *(84)* (Fig. 4). With the advent of improved methods for dissociating adult forebrain tissue, we then extended this approach by isolating neuronal progenitors from the adult rat brain *(85)*. These P/Ta1:hGFP-sorted progenitors were mitotically competent on initial harvest, yet virtually all matured as antigenically defined neurons when raised in serum-containing media. Together, these results indicated that the use of an early neuron-selective promoter to drive phenotype-specific GFP expression permitted the targeted extraction of neuronal progenitor cells from the adult as well as from the fetal rat brain.

MITOTIC NEURONAL PROGENITOR CELLS CAN BE SELECTED FROM ADULT HUMAN VZ

Based on the successful selection of neuronal progenitor cells from the adult rat ventricular zone using P/Ta1:hGFP-based FACS, we next sought to separate progenitors from the adult human VZ. To this end, the ventricular wall was dissected and dissociated from tissues resected from four adult patients undergoing temporal lobectomy. The cultured cells were transduced with P/Ta1:hGFP plasmid DNA, and the neuronal progenitor cells thereby identified were isolated via GFP-based FACS (Figs. 4 and 5). Within a week after isolation, most P/Ta1:hGFP-isolated cells matured as neurons, which coexpressed bIII-tubulin and MAP-2. Many of these neurons had incorporated bromodeoxyuridine in the days before FACS, indicating their mitogenesis in vitro *(26)* (Fig. 5).

THE NESTIN ENHANCER DIRECTS GFP TO NEURAL PROGENITOR CELLS IN THE ADULT HUMAN VZ

The Ta1 tubulin promoter gave us a means by which to identify and isolate neuronal progenitor cells on the basis of their transcriptional activation. We next sought to identify reagents by which uncommitted neural progenitor and stem cells might be similarly identified and isolated. To this end, we used the neuroepithelial-selective enhancer for the early neural filament protein nestin *(86)*. In brief, the evolutionarily conserved region of the second intron of rat *nestin* gene, which is sufficient to direct gene expression to neuroepithelial progenitors *(86,87)*, was placed 5' to the basal heat shock

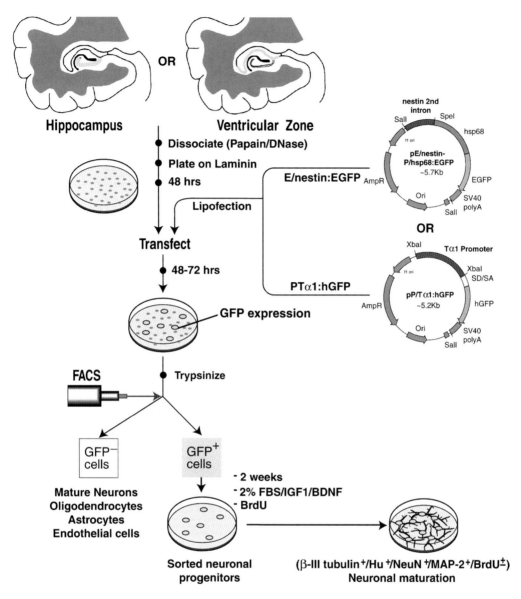

Fig. 4. Separation of neural progenitor cells from the adult human brain via promoter-defined GFP-based FACS. This schematic outlines alternative strategies by which FACS has been used to separate neural progenitor cells from the adult human temporal lobe. Both P/Ta1:hGFP and E/nestin:EGFP selection plasmids have been used to separate neuronal and less-committed neural progenitor cells, respectively, from the adult VZ and hippocampus. Both regions of the brain are outlined, and each selection plasmid is schematized. In addition, white matter derived from these samples has been transfected with DNA encoding hGFP placed under the control of the early oligodendrocytic CNP-2 promoter (*see text*); using essentially the same logic and experimental protocols as employed for isolating the E/nestin and P/Ta1 tubulin-defined progenitor pools, this has allowed the isolation and sorting of P/CNP-2-defined oligodendrocytic progenitor cells from the adult white matter as well. (Adapted from refs. *24* and *25*.)

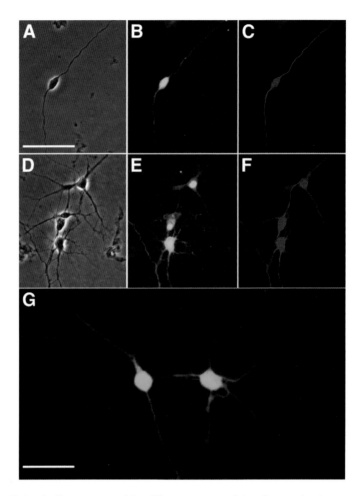

Fig. 5. The Ta1 tubulin promoter identifies neurons arising from mitotic progenitor cells in the adult human VZ. Cultured cells derived from the adult VZ were transfected with pP/Ta1:hGFP after 2 DIV. This plasmid identifies neuronal precursor cells and their young daughters; in vitro, its expression persists during early neuronal maturation. **(A–C)** A young bipolar neuron (**A**, *phase contrast*), that is expressing P/Ta1:hGFP (**B**, *green*) after 5 DIV. The cell coexpressed neuronal bIII-tubulin (**C**, *red*), and incorporated BrdU (**B**, *blue*), indicating its genesis in the days before. **(D–F)** A cluster of neurons (**D**, *phase*) in a matched culture of adult VZ cells, stained for bIII-tubulin (**F**, *red*) at 14 DIV. **(E)** These cells expressed P/Ta1:hGFP (*green*), and each incorporated BrdU (*blue*) to which they were exposed during the first week in culture, indicating their in vitro mitogenesis. **(G)** These more mature neurons were photographed after 14 DIV, 10 d after transfection with P/Ta1:hGFP. Scale = 25 μm. (From ref. *25*.)

promoter (hsp68). P/hsp68 was used because it is expressed only when downstream of a strong enhancer *(88)*. The resultant E/nestin:P/hsp68 unit was then placed 5' to EGFP, yielding a nestin enhancer-defined GFP selection construct. After confirming the neuroepithelial specificity of E/nestin:P/hsp68:EGFP in transgenic mice *(89,90)*, we transfected this selection cassette into both fetal and adult human VZ and hippocampal cell cultures, so as to identify live neural progenitors in these larger pools. In each setting, the E/nestin:P/hsp68 regulatory sequence directed GFP expression in a select fraction of the cell population *(25)*. These E/nestin:EGFP⁺ cells either expressed nestin protein alone, without concurrent neuronal or glial antigenic expression, or concurrently with immature neuronal antigens such as bIII-tubulin. Furthermore, E/nestin:EGFP did not yield GFP fluorescence in cultures of human astrocytes, fibroblasts, or endothelial cells. Thus, the E/nestin:EGFP cassette restricted GFP expression to neural progenitors, and permitted the selective identification and enrichment of neural progenitor cells from the adult human brain. These cells could be propagated as multipotential neurospheres, as has similarly been shown in suspension cultures of both unfractionated *(91)*, and GFAP-sorted human VZ *(23)*. Together, these observations have established the persistence of multipotential neural progenitor cells in the adult human VZ.

DISTRIBUTION AND INCIDENCE OF HUMAN VZ PROGENITORS

These studies established the feasibility of prospectively identifying and isolating viable populations of persistent neural progenitor cells from the adult VZ. Nonetheless, the incidence of these cells in humans remains unclear: Pincus et al. estimated an incidence of 6% of the adult SZ cells of the adult temporal horn expressed musashi *(22)*. Although these likely include the neural progenitor pool in its entirety, these musashi-defined cells may also include subependymal astrocytes of unclear lineage competence, as well as some ependymal cells. Alternatively, E/nestin:GFP-based FACS revealed that roughly 0.2% of human adult VZ cells could be identified by transfection with E/nestin:GFP *(26)*; after correction for transduction efficiency, we can estimate that about 1.5% of the VZ cell dissociate exhibit transcriptional activation of the nestin neuroepithelial enhancer. Yet limiting dilution analysis of human ventricular zone has revealed that even of this small percentage, only a smaller minority still is able to generate neurospheres and exhibit clonal neurogenesis and gliogenesis. Keyoung et al. noted that even in fetal human VZ infected with adenoviruses expressing GFP under musashi and nestin control, less than 10% of the sorted cells generated neurospheres *(92)*. Using a very different sorting strategy, Uchida et al. reported that less than 6% of AC133-isolated human neuroepithelial cells generated multipotential neurospheres *(93)*. In each of these models, the proportionate incidence of VZ neural stem cells active and identifiable as such, whether in the fetal or adult forebrain, was low.

Yet as noted, the incidence of *potential* neural stem cells in the VZ remains unclear. Sanai et al., have reported that the subependymal astrocytes of the lateral ventricles comprise the residual neural stem cell pool, and that VZ cells sorted on the basis of GFAP-driven GFP cells are potentially neurogenic *(23)*. These authors suggest that the incidence of competent stem cells may be higher in the adult human VZ, reflecting the incidence of subependymal astrocytes; If so, then the incidence of potentially neurogenic stem cells may be higher than the incidence of E/nestin:GFP-, musashi- and Hu-defined subependymal cells would suggest. Nonetheless, in the absence of limiting dilution analysis, it is unclear what the incidence is of clonogenic multipotential progenitors within the P/GFAP:GFP-sorted pool, and how that might compare to E/nestin:GFP or P/musashi:GFP-sorted VZ cells.

NEURONAL PROGENITOR CELLS
CAN BE SELECTED FROM THE ADULT HUMAN HIPPOCAMPUS

Past studies have suggested the persistence of neuronal progenitor cells in the dentate gyrus of the adult mammalian hippocampus. Histological evidence of dividing hippocampal progenitor cells has been found in adult animals ranging from chickadees to humans *(94–100)*. In rodents, hippocampal neurogenesis can be modulated by stress *(101)*, enrichment *(102)*, exercise *(103)*, and learning *(104)*. Furthermore, among primates, both adult macaques *(99,105)* and humans *(100)* exhibit histological evidence of neurogenesis in the dentate gyrus. Indeed, the dentate gyrus remains the only site of persistent neurogenesis thus far noted in the adult human brain.

Although postnatal neuronal addition to the frontal neocortex has been noted in both young children *(106,107)* and rhesus monkeys *(42)*, neuronal addition to the normal adult cortex appears rare at best. In culture, neurogenic hippocampal progenitor cells have been found in suspension cultures derived from both adult rats *(108)* and humans *(64)*; these can expand in response to FGF-2, include multipotential founders *(108)*, and are capable of heterotopic integration into other regions of granular neurogenesis, such as the olfactory subependyma *(109)*.

Yet despite the widespread incidence of hippocampal neurogenesis in adult animals, human hippocampal progenitor cells are relatively inaccessible. As a result, no assessment of their abundance, factor-responsiveness, or regenerative capacity has yet been possible. Thus, to identify and extract neuronal progenitors from the adult human hippocampus, we transfected VZ-free dissociates of surgically resected adult human hippocampus with plasmid DNA encoding hGFP, placed under the control of either the early neuronal Ta1 tubulin promoter *(81,82,84)*, or the neuroepithelial nestin enhancer *(46,86)*. These constructs each recognized a population of cells in adult hippocampal dissociates, which divided in vitro, and gave rise to antigenically and functionally appropriate neurons (Fig. 6) *(25)*. In the presence of FGF-2, both the Ta1:hGFP and E/nestin:EGFP-defined cells incorporated BrdU from the culture media, and both matured to express typical neuronal antigens, including bIII-tubulin, MAP-2, Hu, and NeuN. Thus, adult hippocampal cultures harbored a pool of dividing cells, whose progeny became neurons, and which could be identified while alive by the transcriptional activation of the nestin and Ta1 tubulin regulatory sequences.

Using FACS, we then isolated both E/nestin:EGFP$^+$ and P/Ta1:hGFP$^+$ hippocampal cells, enriching each to near-purity. The progenitor cell pools thereby obtained were still able to generate neurons, which matured as such not only morphologically and antigenically, but also physiologically (Fig. 7): Neurons arising in FACS-purified cultures of P/Ta1:hGFP hippocampal cells developed depolarization-induced calcium elevations of >300%, typical of neuronal voltage-gated calcium channels. In addition, patch-clamp analysis reveals that they have fast sodium channels, and respond as neurons with rapid sodium currents to voltage-stepping. Together, these observations indicated that the adult human hippocampus harbors mitotically competent progenitor cells, which can be expanded in vitro to give rise to antigenically appropriate, functionally competent neurons. By using FACS based on GFP expression driven by the Ta1 tubulin promoter and nestin enhancer, these progenitor cells may be specifically targeted and extracted from hippocampal tissue, yielding viable, highly enriched populations of hippocampal progenitor cells *(25)*.

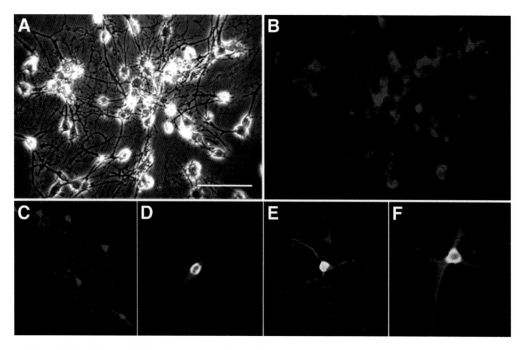

Fig. 6. Adult human hippocampus harbors mitotic neuronal progenitor cells. (**A,B**), A mono-layer dissociate of adult human dentate gyrus, removed from a 33-yr-old man after temporal lobectomy. (**A**) (*phase*) and (**B**) (*fluorescence*) images at 7 DIV of a cluster of adult dentate neurons, labeled with the antineuronal antibody MAP-2 (**B**, *red*). (**C**) A hippocampal culture derived from a 35-yr-old, immunostained for bIII-tubulin. This culture was exposed to BrdU in vitro, then fixed and stained for BrdU as well as bIII-tubulin. (**D–F**) TuJ1$^+$ (*red*)/ BrdU$^+$ (*green*) neurons, generated by mitotic neurogenesis from hippocampal progenitors. Scale: 30 μm. (Adapted from ref. *25*.)

A DISTINCT POOL OF OLIGODENDROCYTE PROGENITORS RESIDES IN ADULT HUMAN WHITE MATTER

Besides the neurogenic progenitor cell populations of the VZ and hippocampal SGZ, a distinct pool of glial progenitors also resides within both the ventricular zone and tissue parenchyma. These adult parenchymal glial progenitors were first isolated as such from adult rodents (*110*), and were found to give rise to both oligodendrocytes and astrocytes in vitro, just as their postnatal counterparts. Retroviral lineage analysis in vivo confirmed that these cells persist in vivo in the adult white matter, and can divide to generate both major glial phenotypes upon demyelinating insult (*111,112*). The role of these parenchymal glial progenitor cells in remyelination, as well as their utility as cellular vectors for induced remyelination, has been extensively reviewed in the past, and is not considered here. Rather, their normal distribution and homeostasis in the adult human brain, and their lineage relationships with both uncommitted and neuronally restricted progenitors of the adult VZ, are of greater import in understanding the contribution of these cells to the cellular composition of the adult brain.

In adult humans, we first identified adult oligodendrocyte progenitor cells in dissociates of adult human white matter, using the early promoter for the oligodendrocyte

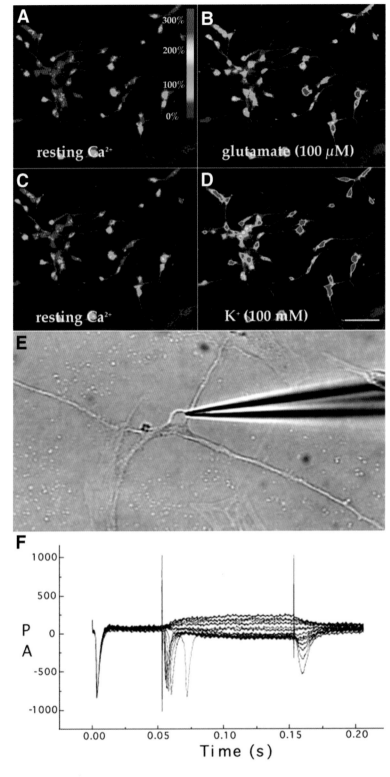

A resting Ca²⁺   300% 200% 100% 0%

B glutamate (100 µM)

C resting Ca²⁺

D K⁺ (100 mM)

E

F

Fig. 7.

protein cyclic nucleotide phosphodiesterase (P/CNP-2) to direct GFP expression. When we transfected P/CNP2:hGFP into dissociates of adult human capsular white matter, we observed that GFP was expressed initially by only a single, morphologically and antigenically discrete class of bipolar cells *(24)*. These cells were mitotically active, and upon initial extraction typically expressed the early oligodendrocytic marker A2B5, but not the more differentiated markers O4, O1, or galactocerebroside. When FACS was used to purify P/CNP-2:hGFP$^+$ cells from adult white matter, most (>90%) were found to mature as oligodendrocytes (see Fig. 10), progressing through a stereotypic sequence of A2B5, O4, O1 and galactocerebroside expression *(24)*, just as in development *(113)*. Remarkably, cytometry first based on P/CNP-2-driven GFP, and later on A2B5 expression, revealed that these oligodendrocyte progenitor cells are not rare, comprising as many as 3% of all cells successfully dissociated from the adult white matter (Fig. 8).

PROGENITOR CELLS OF THE ADULT WHITE MATTER INCLUDE MULTIPOTENTIAL CELLS

Over the past few years, it has become clear that the parenchymal progenitor cells pool of the adult white matter includes a fraction of multipotential parenchymal progenitors, which though nominally glial may generate neurons as well as astrocytes and oligodendrocytes *(24,114–116)*. Specifically, we noted that when adult OPCs were raised in low density and high purity culture after P/CNP2:hGFP-based FACS, some nonoligodendrocytic phenotypes appeared in the sorted cultures: Under these conditions, we noted that within 4 d of FACS, 7.7 ± 4.4% of P/CNP2:hGFP-sorted cells matured into Hu or TuJ1$^+$ neurons in the week after FACS separation, even though no neurons whatsoever—as defined by Hu and bIII-tubulin—had been observed either prior to FACS, or in unsorted control cultures *(24)*. These findings suggested that CNP2-defined white matter progenitors, despite their apparent commitment to become oligodendrocytes in native cultures of adult white matter, were able to generate neurons and astrocytes as well, once sorted to low-density culture apart from other cell types. As such, these cells appeared to retain multilineage potential, and as such resembled precursors isolated from FGF-2-treated rat cortical parenchyma *(56,114,117)*.

Fig. 7. *(previous page)* P/Ta1:GFP-sorted hippocampal cells develop into physiologically mature neurons. P/Ta1:hGFP-sorted progenitors developed neuronal Ca^{2+} responses to depolarization **(A–D)** Images of P/Ta1:hGFP-sorted cells loaded with the calcium indicator dye fluo-3, 10 d after FACS; these have matured uniformly into fiber-bearing cells of neuronal morphology. **(B)** The same field after exposure to glutamate. **(C)** On return to baseline after media wash. **(D)** After exposure to a depolarizing stimulus of 60 mM KCl. The neurons displayed rapid, reversible, >300% elevations in cytosolic calcium in response to K$^+$, consistent with the activity of neuronal voltage-gated calcium channels. Whole cell patch-clamp revealed voltage-gated sodium currents in P/Ta1:hGFP$^+$ dentate neurons. **(E)** A representative cell 14 d after P/Ta1:hGFP-based FACS. Identified visually as a progenitor-derived neuron on the basis of its residual GFP expression, the cell was patch clamped in a voltage-clamped configuration, and its responses to current injection recorded. **(F)** The fast negative deflections noted after depolarized voltage steps are typical of the voltage-gated sodium currents of mature neurons. Scale = 50 µm. (From ref. *26*.)

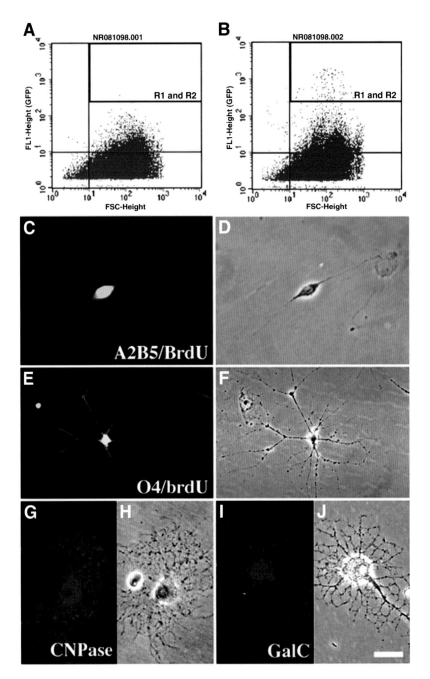

Fig. 8. A distinct pool of oligodendrocyte progenitor cells can be isolated from adult human white matter. **(A,B)** A representative sort of a human white matter sample, derived from the frontal lobe of a 42-yr-old woman during repair of an intracranial aneurysm. This plot shows 50,000 cells (sorting events) with their GFP fluorescence intensity plotted against forward scatter (a measure of cell size). The sort obtained from a nonfluorescent P/hCNP2:*lacZ*-transfected control is shown in **(A)** while **B** indicates the corresponding result from a matched culture transfected with P/hCNP2: hGFP. **(C,D)** A bipolar A2B5[+]/BrdU[+] cell, 48 h after FACS. **(E,F)** By 3 wk post-FACS, P/CNP2: hGFP-sorted cells developed multipolar morphologies, and expressed oligodendrocytic O4 (*red*). These cells often incorporated BrdU, indicating their in vitro origin from replicating A2B5[+] cells. **(G–I)** Matched phase **(G,I)** and immunofluorescent **(H,J)** images of maturing oligodendrocytes, 4 wk after P/CNP2:hGFP-based FACS. These cells expressed both CNP protein **(H)** and galactocerebroside **(J)**, indicating their maturation as oligodendrocytes. Scale bar = 20 μm.

These results argued that the local environment of the adult human brain might serve to restrict the phenotypic potential of its resident progenitors, and that the removal of these cells from their local environment might permit them to pursue alternative avenues of differentiation.

On this basis, we asked whether the white matter progenitor cells of the adult human brain might actually constitute a type of multipotential neural progenitor, or even a parenchymal neural stem cell. We found that white matter progenitor cells (WMPCs), purified by FACS from adult human brain, could indeed generate neurons as well as both astrocytes and oligodendrocytes when raised under conditions of high purity and low density, in which the cells are effectively removed from both paracrine and autocrine influences. Under these conditions, the sorted progenitor cells indeed divided and expanded as multipotential clones, that generated neurons as readily as oligodendrocytes *(115)* (Fig. 9). The sorted WMPCs continued to divide and expand for several months in culture. Moreover, on xenograft to the developing fetal rat forebrain, adult human WMPCs matured into neurons as well as oligodendrocytes and astrocytes in vivo, in a region- and context-dependent manner (Fig. 10). Thus, the nominally glial progenitor cell of the adult human white matter thus appears to constitute a multipotential neural progenitor. These cells appear to be typically restricted by their local brain environment to produce only oligodendrocytes and some astrocytes, in response to local environmental signals whose identities remain to be established. But when removed from the environment of the brain and from other brain cells, these cells proceed to make all brain cell types, including neurons and glia, and remain able to do so for long periods of time in culture.

EPIGENETIC DETERMINATION OF PROGENITOR FATE BY THE ADULT PARENCHYMAL ENVIRONMENT

The latent multipotentiality of nominally glial human progenitor cells has considerable precedent in lower species. Progenitor cells capable of giving rise to multiple lineages, including oligodendrocytes and neurons, have been consistently derived from the cortical and subcortical parenchyma as well as from the VZ of embryos *(118–121)*. Similarly, postnatal rat optic nerve derived O-2A progenitor cells could be "reprogrammed" to multipotential stem cells capable of generating neurons *(116)*. This was achieved by sequential exposure of O-2A progenitors to serum to induce astrocytic differentiation, followed by their expansion in the presence of basic FGF (bFGF) in serum free condition. In addition, other studies have noted that constant mitogenic stimulation of adult rat forebrain parenchymal cells with FGF-2 results in the generation of neurons as well as glia *(16,56)*. Together, these observations of the multilineage potential of CNS glial progenitors suggest that these cells may retain far more lineage plasticity than traditionally appreciated.

Adult subcortical progenitor cells, although individually competent to generate multiple cell types, may thus be restricted to the oligodendrocytic lineage by virtue of an epigenetic bias imparted by their environment before their isolation. A corollary of the environmental restriction of WMPC phenotype is that other, non-white matter-derived neural progenitors might similarly restrict to oligodendrocytic lineage when presented to the environment of the adult white matter. Indeed, several groups have reported that

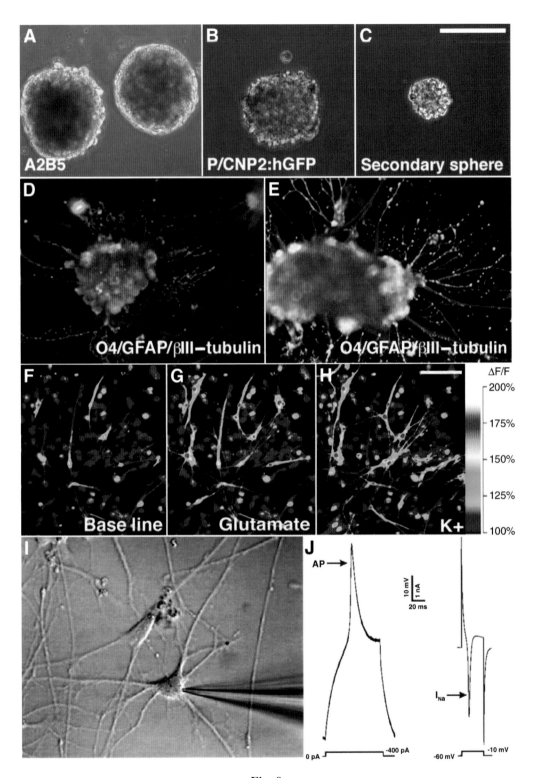

Fig. 9.

epidermal growth factor (EGF)-expanded murine neural stem cells differentiate as oligodendrocytes upon xenograft *(122)*, even though these cells generate few oligodendrocytes in vitro. Similarly, v-myc transformed neural stem cells transplanted to perinatal mice differentiate as oligodendrocytes once recruited to the white matter *(123)*, yet fail to do so in other brain regions, or in vitro.

WHITE MATTER PROGENITOR CELLS ARE ABUNDANT AND WIDESPREAD, BUT OF UNCLEAR HOMOGENEITY

The persistence and sheer abundance of WMPCs in the adult human brain is striking: More than 3% of the white matter cell population may be sorted on the basis of CNP-2:GFP-based FACS, and over half of these cells are mitotically active upon isolation *(24)*. White matter progenitor cells have also been quantified on the basis of their expression of PDGFaR and the A2B5 epitope *(124,125)*, yielding estimates of their incidence that are similar to those achieved with both P/CNP2:GFP- and A2B5-based FACS. In vivo, these cells appear as small, highly ramified cells with thin processes that lack endothelial end-feet or even contact (Fig. 11). Most express nestin and the NG2 chondroitin sulfate proteoglycan, markers of immature neural progenitors, and S100b, a glial marker expressed by immature cells of both the astrocytic and oligodendrocytic lineages; most express neither GFAP nor aquaporin, nor do they transcriptionally activate the GFAP promoter, and hence cannot be readily characterized as astroglial *(29)*.

Despite the seeming uniformity of these descriptive features, the extent to which adult parenchymal progenitor cells comprise a homogeneous pool remains unclear. One must be skeptical about the potential uniformity of this cell population, if for no other reason than because by limiting dilution analysis, only 0.1–0.2% of its cells are multipotential *(28)*. Yet antigenic analyses have failed to discern differences between multipotential founders and neighboring WMPCs cells, and genomic analyses of these phenotypes are now underway in an attempt to define transcriptional identifiers that may distinguish multipotential progenitors. Yet regardless of the relative incidence of

---

Fig. 9. *(previous page)* Adult human WMPCs generate neurons as well as oligodendrocytes and astrocytes. **(A)** First passage spheres generated from A2B5-sorted cells, 2 wk post-sort. **(B)** First passage spheres raised from P/CNP2:hGFP sorted cells, 2 wk. **(C)** Second passage sphere derived from an A2B5-sorted sample, 3 wk. **(D)** Plated onto substrate, primary spheres differentiated as bIII-tubulin+ neurons *(red)*, GFAP+ astrocytes *(blue)*, and O4+ oligodendrocytes *(green)*. **(E)** Neurons *(red)*, astrocytes *(blue)*, and oligodendrocytes *(green)* arose from spheres derived from P/CNP-2:GFP-sorted WMPCs. **(F–H)** WMPC-derived neurons had neuronal Ca^{2+} responses to depolarization. **(F)** WMPC-derived cells loaded with the calcium indicator dye fluo-3, 10 d after plating first passage spheres derived from A2B5-sorted white matter (35 DIV). **(G)** After exposure to 100 μM glutamate. **(H)** After exposure to a depolarizing stimulus of 60 mM KCl. The neurons displayed rapid, reversible, elevations in calcium in response to K+. **(I,J)** Whole cell patch-clamp revealed voltage-gated Na+ currents and action potentials in WMPC-derived neurons. **(I)** At 14 d after plating a WMPC-derived sphere, neurons were identified, patch-clamped, and their responses to current injection noted. **(H)** The fast negative deflections noted after current injection are typical of voltage-gated Na+ currents of mature neurons. Action potentials were noted only at I_{Na} >800 pA. Scale: **(A–E)** = 100 µm; **(F–H)** = 80 µm. (Adapted from ref. *28*.)

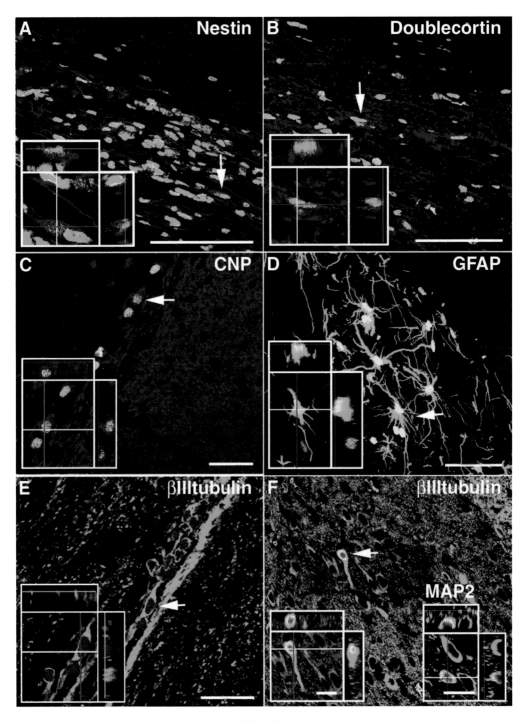

Fig. 10.

multipotential cells within the white matter progenitor cell pool, the very existence of multipotent cells scattered throughout the white matter parenchyma forces us to reconsider our understanding of both the nature and incidence of neural stem cells in the adult brain. At the very least, these observations challenge our conception of the supposed rarity of adult neural progenitor and stem cells. In doing so, they point to an abundant and widespread source of cells, that may be used both as a target for pharmacological induction, and as a cell type appropriate for therapeutic engraftment to the diseased adult brain.

ADULT PROGENITORS MAY BE CATEGORIZED AS DISTINCT POOLS OF TRANSIT-AMPLIFYING CELLS

The neuronal and glial progenitor cells of the adult human brain may considered akin to "transit amplifying cells," which have now been described as such in a variety of solid tissues. As initially defined in the skin and GI mucosae, transit amplifying cells comprise the phenotypically biased, still-mitotic progeny of uncommitted stem cells *(126–129)*. As stem cell progeny depart these localized regions of stem cell expansion, their daughters may commit to more restricted lineages, phenotypically delimited but still mitotic, which comprise the transit-amplifying pools. Although these cells proliferate so as to expand discrete lineages, they do not exhibit unlimited multilineage expansion, as distinct from their parental stem cells.

By this definition, the neuronal and glial progenitor cells of the adult brain may be considered distinct transit-amplifying derivatives of a common ventricular zone stem cell *(29,130)* (Fig. 11). The neuronal progenitor cell of the forebrain subependyma was first proposed as a transit amplifying cell type *(130)*, on the basis of its neuronal bias during concurrent migration and mitotic expansion *(131,132)*. Furthermore, like many transit amplifying pools, it appears capable of replenishing its parental stem cell pool under appropriate mitotic stimulation *(130)*. The subgranular zone progenitors of the dentate gyrus, which may be glial in phenotype *(133)*, similarly continue to divide to generate neurons almost exclusively. These neuronal daughters may still be mitotically competent while migratory within the dentate *(108)*, and as such may also be best considered as transit amplifying intermediates. Most strikingly, even the glial progenitor cell of the adult white matter may now be considered a type of transit-amplifying

Fig. 10. *(previous page)* WMPCs engrafted into fetal rats generated neurons and glia in a site-specific manner. Sections from a rat brain implanted at E17 with A2B5-sorted WMPCs, and killed a month after birth. These cells were maintained in culture for 10 d prior to implant. **(A,B)** Nestin[+] *(red)* progenitors and doublecortin[+] *(red)* migrants, respectively, each coexpressing human nuclear antigen (hNA, *green*) in the hippocampal alvius. **(C)** CNP[+] oligodendrocytes *(red)*, which were found exclusively in the corpus callosum. **(D)** A low-power image of GFAP[+] *(green, stained with anti-human GFAP)* astrocytes along the ventricular wall. **(E)** βIII-Tubulin[+] *(green)*/hNA[+] *(red)* neurons migrating in a chain in the hippocampal alvius. **(F)** βIII-Tubulin[+] and MAP-2[+] *(inset in* **F**) neurons in the striatum, adjacent to the RMS (antigens in *green*; hNA in *red*; *yellow* double-stained human nuclei). **(G)** An Hu[+]/hNA[+] neuron in the septum. **(H)** An hNA[+] *(green)*/GAD-67[+] *(red)* striatal neuron. *Insets* in each figure show orthogonal projections of a high-power confocal image of the identified cell *(arrow)*. Scale: **(A–E)** = 40 μm; **(F–H)** = 20 μm.

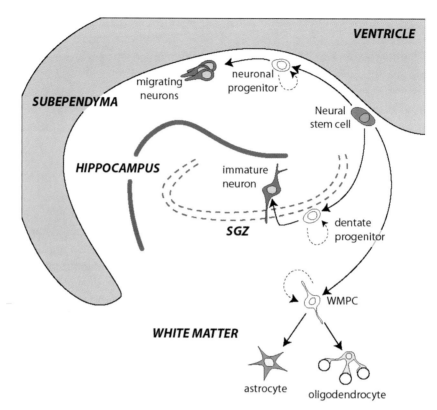

Fig. 11. Progenitors of the adult human brain. This schematic illustrates the identified categories of progenitors in the adult human brain, and their known interrelationships. All derive from VZ neural stem cells, that generate at least three populations of potentially neurogenic transit amplifying progenitors (*yellow*) of both neuronal and glial lineages These include neuronal progenitor cells of the ventricular subependyma, those of the subgranular zone of the dentate gyrus, and the white matter progenitor cells (WMPCs) of the subcortical parenchyma, which although nominally glial remain potentially neurogenic. Parenchymal progenitors may reside in the gray matter as well, although the relationships of parenchymal gray and white matter progenitors have yet to be established. Each transit amplifying pool may give rise to progeny appropriate to their location, including neurons, oligodendrocytes, and parenchymal astrocytes (Adapted from ref. *29.*)

cell; it is able to divide and yield variably restricted daughters, while remaining mitotic but possessed of neither unbiased multipotentiality nor unlimited self-renewal capacity *(115)*.

The nominally glial progenitor cell of the brain parenchyma now appears to comprise by far the most abundant progenitor cell phenotype of the adult brain. In adult humans, in whom the subependymal zone is but a discontiguous monolayer, VZ neural stem cells appear to comprise a relatively scarce pool *(77)*. Similarly, the neuronal progenitor pool of the olfactory subependyma appears to be similarly vestigial in humans *(23)*, although the neuronal progenitors of the adult human hippocampus may be more abundant *(25,100)*. As a result, in adult humans the major transit-amplifying pool would appear to reside within the parenchyma itself, in which large numbers of widely dispersed glial progenitors provide an abundant reservoir of cycling, multipotential progenitors *(134)*, that although restricted to glial phenotype in vivo, are multipotential and neurogenic. These cells may comprise as many as 3% of all cells in the adult white matter, yielding remarkably high estimates for their absolute incidence *(24,115,125)*. Although the incidence of analogous parenchymal progenitor cells in the adult human gray matter has not yet been rigorously evaluated, these cells have already been described as abundant in the gray matter of adult rodents *(114)*, and there is no reason to think that they are any less abundant in humans.

GLIAL PROGENITORS OF THE SUBCORTICAL WHITE MATTER ARE TRANSIT-AMPLIFYING CELLS

Importantly, although the parenchymal progenitor cell seems to be fundamentally multipotential, it is subject to replicative senescence, and does not express measurable telomerase *(115)*. As a result, it typically ceases expansion after 3–4 mo in vitro, spanning no more than 18 population doublings. In light of its lack of telomerase, its self-limited expansion capacity, and its glial bias despite multilineage competence, the parenchymal progenitor cell cannot be considered a stem cell. Rather, this phenotype may best be considered a transit-amplifying progenitor of both astrocytes and oligodendrocytes. Interestingly then, just as the transit amplifying neuronal precursor of the adult rat ventricular zone may revert to a multipotential state in the presence of EGF *(130)*, the dividing glial progenitor of the human white matter is similarly able to revert to a multilineal neurogenic precursor *(115)*. Although this is especially manifest when the cells are expanded in vitro, adult glial progenitor cells may generate neurons as soon as they are removed from the local tissue environment, whether extracted on the basis of CNP promoter activation, A2B5 immunoselection *(115)*, or NG2 expression *(135)*. As noted, when sorted parenchymal progenitors were introduced via transuterine xenograft into the fetal rat brain, all neural phenotypes were found to arise in a context-dependent manner *(115)* (Fig. 10). These observations again argue that glial progenitor cells may need to be removed from the adult tissue environment to manifest their intrinsic yet latent multilineage potential.

NEUROGENIC AND GLIOGENIC NICHES, AND THE INDUCTION OF ENDOGENOUS PROGENITOR CELLS

The parenchymal progenitor pool of the adult brain thus appears to include both multipotential stem cells and their transit-amplifying progeny, at least some of which retain multilineage potential, as well as both neuronal and glial-restricted daughters whose phenotypic restriction may be a function of the local environment (Fig. 11). The relative proportions of neurons, astrocytes and oligodendrocytes generated from resident progenitor cells appears to be both locally and dynamically regulated by the tissue microenvironment, in discrete niches for neurogenesis and gliogenesis *(136–140)*. These observations suggest a hitherto unappreciated degree of cellular plasticity in the adult brain. A salient implication of this work is that with a greater understanding of the necessary and sufficient conditions for establishing gliogenic and neurogenic niches, we might expect to modulate the adult parenchymal environment to encourage the heterotopic production of desired phenotypes from resident progenitors. Indeed, several recent reports have shown that the experimental recapitulation of neurogenic conditions in the adult forebrain ventricular wall restores VZ neurogenesis and neuronal recruitment to the adult striatum *(33,34,38,139,141)*. One might reasonably speculate that new oligodendrocytes may similarly be induced from otherwise astrocyte-biased parenchymal progenitors, and even that neurogenesis might be productively directed from parenchymal glial progenitors. Achieving and then guiding these capabilities to therapeutic endpoints should prove a worthy effort.

CONCLUSION

Neural precursor cells persist within subependymal and dentate granule cell regions of the adult human forebrain, and include distinct populations of neuronal and uncommitted precursors. These may be identified, separated, and enriched from the adult brain, based on their expression of fluorescent transgenes driven by cell-specific promoters. At first glance, these appear to represent distinct cell populations. However, the broadened lineage potential of parenchymal progenitor cells once removed from autocrine and paracrine influences, and the reversion potential of many transit amplifying phenotypes, suggests that each of these progenitor cell types may be relatively plastic in its autonomous lineage potential, and that the fate of these cells and their daughters may rather be dictated by local environmental signals to which they are exposed.

These local signals may be stable in the adult brain, but they are certainly altered by disease and injury, both of which may alter the local environment to expand the range and repertoire of locally permitted cell types. Recent observations of compensatory neurogenesis, in both animal models of subcortical stroke *(142–144)*, and in autopsy tissues derived from Huntington's disease patients *(145)*, suggest that in some subcortical regions, the induction of neurogenesis may be a normal response to injury or degeneration. Although likely insufficient to yield significant structural or functional recovery in most acquired insults, the very existence of compensatory neurogenesis identifies resident neural progenitor cells as feasible targets for therapeutic induction. To be sure, targeted induction of individual progenitors in discrete regions of the brain will require a considerably greater understanding of both the humoral and contact-mediated signals to which resident progenitors respond, as well as the manner of these responses. Yet our ability to now isolate each of the major progenitor cell types of the adult human brain has opened new possibilities for their functional and genomic analysis. By defining the gene expression patterns of different adult progenitor phenotypes, and understanding the ligand–receptor relationships experienced by each, we can now hope to design rational strategies by which endogenous progenitor cells may be induced to regenerate those cells lost to both injury and disease.

ACKNOWLEDGMENTS

I would like to thank my collaborators in these studies, in particular Drs. Neeta Roy, Martha Windrem, H. Michael Keyoung, Marta Nunes, Abdellatif Benraiss, Su Wang, and Maiken Nedergaard. The laboratory's work on human neuronal progenitors has been supported by the NIH, the Mathers Charitable Foundation, the National Multiple Sclerosis Society, the Human Frontiers Scientific Program, the Michael J. Fox Foundation, Christopher Reeve Paralysis Foundation, Project ALS, and by both Aventis Pharmaceuticals and Merck, Inc.

REFERENCES

1. Goldman, S. (1998) Adult neurogenesis: from canaries to the clinic. *J. Neurobiol.* **36,** 267–286.
2. Goldman, S. A. and Luskin, M. B. (1998) Strategies utilized by migrating neurons of the postnatal vertebrate forebrain. *Trends Neurosci.* **21,** 107–114.
3. Goldman, S. A. and Nottebohm, F. (1983) Neuronal production, migration, and differentiation in a vocal control nucleus of the adult female canary brain. *Proc. Natl. Acad. Sci. USA* **80,** 2390–2394.
4. Lois, C. and Alvarez-Buylla, A. (1993) Proliferating subventricular zone cells in the adult mammalian forebrain can differentiate into neurons and glia. *Proc. Natl. Acad. Sci. USA* **90,** 2074–2077.
5. Luskin, M. B. (1993) Restricted proliferation and migration of postnatally generated neurons derived from the forebrain subventricular zone. *Neuron* **11,** 173–189.
6. Kirschenbaum, B., et al. (1994) In vitro neuronal production and differentiation by precursor cells derived from the adult human forebrain. *Cereb. Cortex* **4,** 576–589.
7. Goldman, S. A., Zukhar, A., Barami, K., Mikawa, T., and Niedzwiecki, D. (1996) Ependymal/subependymal zone cells of postnatal and adult songbird brain generate both neurons and nonneuronal siblings in vitro and in vivo. *J. Neurobiol.* **30,** 505–520.
8. Doetsch, F., Caille, I., Lim, D. A., Garcia-Verdugo, J. M., and Alvarez-Buylla, A. (1999) Subventricular zone astrocytes are neural stem cells in the adult mammalian brain. *Cell* **97,** 703–716.
9. Chiasson, B., Tropepe, V., Morshead, C., and van der Kooy, D. (1999) Adult mammalian forebrain ependymal and subependymal cells demonstrate proliferative potential, but only subependymal cells have neural stem cell characteristics. *J. Neurosci.* **19,** 4462–4471.
10. Kirschenbaum, B. and Goldman, S. A. (1995) Brain-derived neurotrophic factor promotes the survival of neurons arising from the adult rat forebrain subependymal zone. *Proc. Natl. Acad. Sci. USA* **92,** 210–214.
11. Doetsch, F. and Alvarez-Buylla, A. (1996) Network of tangential pathways for neuronal migration in the adult mammalian brain. *Proc. Natl. Acad. Sci. USA* **93,** 14895–14900.
12. Bauer-Dantoin, A. C., Weiss, J., and Jameson, J. L. (1996) Gonadotropin-releasing hormone regulation of pituitary follistatin gene expression during the primary follicle-stimulating hormone surge. *Endocrinology* **137,** 1634–1639.
13. Kuhn, G., Dickinson-Anson, H., and Gage, F. (1996) Neurogenesis in the dentate gyrus of the adult rat: Age related decrease of neuronal progenitor proliferation. *J. Neurosci.* **16,** 2027–2033.
14. Goldman, S., Kirschenbaum, B., Harrison-Restelli, C., and Thaler, H. (1997) Neuronal precursor cells of the adult rat ventricular zone persist into senescence, with no change in spatial extent or BDNF response. *J. Neurobiol.* **32,** 554–566.
15. Reynolds, B. A. and Weiss, S. (1992) Generation of neurons and astrocytes from isolated cells of the adult mammalian central nervous system. *Science* **255,** 1707–1710.
16. Richards, L. J., Kilpatrick, T. J., and Bartlett, P. F. (1992) De novo generation of neuronal cells from the adult mouse brain. *Proc. Natl. Acad. Sci. USA* **89,** 8591–8595.
17. Morshead, C. M., et al. (1994) Neural stem cells in the adult mammalian forebrain: a relatively quiescent subpopulation of subependymal cells. *Neuron* **13,** 1071–1082.
18. Johansson, C., et al. (1999) Identification of a neural stem cell in the adult mammalian central nervous system. *Cell* **96,** 25–34.
19. Morshead, C. and van der Kooy, D. (1992) Postmitotic death is the fate of constitutively proliferating cells in the subependymal layer of the adult mouse brain. *J. Neurosci.* **12,** 249–256.
20. Craig, C. G., et al. (1996) In vivo growth factor expansion of endogenous subependymal neural precursor cell populations in the adult mouse brain. *J. Neurosci.* **16,** 2649–2658.

21. Pincus, D. W., et al. (1997) In vitro neurogenesis by adult human epileptic temporal neo-cortex. *Clin. Neurosurg.* **44,** 17–25.
22. Pincus, D. W., et al. (1998) FGF2/BDNF-associated maturation of new neurons generated from adult human subependymal cells. *Ann. Neurol.* **43,** 576–585.
23. Sanai, N., et al. (2004) Unique astrocyte ribbon in adult human brain contains neural stem, cells but lacks chain migration. *Nature* **427,** 740–743.
24. Roy, N. S., et al. (1999) Identification, isolation, and promoter-defined separation of mitotic oligodendrocyte progenitor cells from the adult human subcortical white matter. *J. Neurosci.* **19,** 9986–9995.
25. Roy, N. S., et al. (2000) In vitro neurogenesis by progenitor cells isolated from the adult human hippocampus. *Nat. Med.* **6,** 271–277.
26. Roy, N. S., et al. (2000) Promoter-targeted selection and isolation of neural progenitor cells from the adult human ventricular zone. *J. Neurosci. Res.* **59,** 321–331.
27. Roy, N., Windrem, M., and Goldman, S. A. (2004) Progenitor cells of the adult white matter. In *Myelin Biology and Disorders* (Lazzarini, R., ed.), Elsevier, Amsterdam, pp. 259–287.
28. Nunes, M. C., et al. (2003) Identification and isolation of multipotential neural progenitor cells from the subcortical white matter of the adult human brain. *Nat. Med.* **9,** 439–447.
29. Goldman, S. (2003) Glia as neural progenitor cells. *Trends Neurosci.* **26,** 590–596.
30. Windrem, M. S., et al. (2002) Progenitor cells derived from the adult human subcortical white matter disperse and differentiate as oligodendrocytes within demyelinated lesions of the rat brain. *J. Neurosci. Res.* **69,** 966–975.
31. Windrem, M. S., et al. (2004) Fetal and adult human oligodendrocyte progenitor cell isolates myelinate the congenitally dysmyelinated brain. *Nat. Med.* **10,** 93–97.
32. Svendsen, C., Caldwell, M., and Ostenfeld, T. (1999) Human neural stem cells: Isolation, expansion and transplantation. *Brain Pathol.* **9,** 499–513.
33. Chmielnicki, E., Benraiss, A., Economides, A. N., and Goldman, S. A. (2004) Adenovirally expressed noggin and BDNF cooperate to induce new medium spiny neurons from resident progenitor cells in the adult striatal ventricular zone. *J. Neurosci.* **24,** 2133–2142.
34. Chmielnicki, E. and Goldman, S. A. (2002) Induced neurogenesis by endogenous progenitor cells in the adult mammalian brain. *Prog. Brain Res.* **138,** 451–464.
35. Benraiss, A., Chmielnicki, E., Lerner, K., Roh, D., and Goldman, S. A. (2001) Adenoviral brain-derived neurotrophic factor induces both neostriatal and olfactory neuronal recruitment from endogenous progenitor cells in the adult forebrain. *J. Neurosci.* **21,** 6718–6731.
36. Aberg, M., Aberg, D., Hedbacker, H., Oscarsson, J., and Eriksson, P. (2000) Peripheral infusion of IGF-1 selectively induces neurogenesis in the adult rat hippocampus. *J. Neurosci.* **20,** 2896–2903.
37. Fallon, J., et al. (2000) In vivo induction of massive proliferation, directed migration, and differentiation of neural cells in the adult mammalian brain. *Proc. Natl. Acad. Sci. USA* **97,** 14686–14691.
38. Pencea, V., Bingaman, K. D., Wiegand, S. J., and Luskin, M. B. (2001) Infusion of brain-derived neurotrophic factor into the lateral ventricle of the adult rat leads to new neurons in the parenchyma of the striatum, septum, thalamus, and hypothalamus. *J. Neurosci.* **21,** 6706–6717.
39. Kuhn, H. G., Winkler, J., Kempermann, G., Thal, L. J., and Gage, F. H. (1997) Epidermal growth factor and fibroblast growth factor-2 have different effects on neural progenitors in the adult rat brain. *J. Neurosci.* **17,** 5820–5829.
40. Zigova, T., Pencea, V., Wiegand, S. J., and Luskin, M. B. (1998) Intraventricular administration of BDNF increases the number of newly generated neurons in the adult olfactory bulb. *Mol. Cell. Neurosci.* **11,** 234–245.

41. Kaplan, M. (1983) Proliferation of subependymal cells in the adult primate CNS: differential uptake of thymidine by DNA-labeled precursors. *J. Hirnforsch.* **23**, 23–33.
42. Gould, E., Reeves, A., Graziano, M., and Gross, C. (1999) Neurogenesis in the neocortex of adult primates. *Science* **286**, 548–552.
43. Lois, C. and Alvarez-Buylla, A. (1994) Long-distance neuronal migration in the adult mammalian brain. *Science* **264**, 1145–1148.
44. Barami, K., Kirschenbaum, B., Lemmon, V., and Goldman, S. A. (1994) N-cadherin and Ng-CAM/8D9 are involved serially in the migration of newly generated neurons into the adult songbird brain. *Neuron* **13**, 567–582.
45. Pincus, D. W., Goodman, R. R., Fraser, R. A., Nedergaard, M., and Goldman, S. A. (1998) Neural stem and progenitor cells: a strategy for gene therapy and brain repair. *Neurosurgery* **42**, 858–867; discussion 867–868.
46. Frederiksen, K. and McKay, R. D. (1988) Proliferation and differentiation of rat neuroepithelial precursor cells in vivo. *J. Neurosci.* **8**, 1144–1151.
47. Clark, S., Shetty, A., Bradley, J., and Turner, D. (1994) Reactive astrocytes express the embryonic intermediate neurofilament nestin. *NeuroReport* **5**, 1885–1888.
48. Sakakibara, S., et al. (1996) Mouse-Musashi-1, a neural RNA-binding protein highly enriched in the mammalian CNS stem cell. *Dev. Biol.* **176**, 230–242.
49. Nakamura, M., Okano, H., Blendy, J., and Montell, C. (1994) Musashi, a neural RNA-binding protein required for *Drosophila* adult external sensory organ development. *Neuron* **13**, 67–81.
50. Richter, K., Good, P., and Dawid, I. (1990) A developmentally regulated, nervous system specific gene in Xenopus encodes a putative RNA-binding protein. *New Biologist* **2**, 556–565.
51. Sakakibara, S. and Okano, H. (1997) Expression of neural RNA-binding proteins in the postnatal CNS: implications of their roles in neuronal and glial cell development. *J. Neurosci.* **17**, 8300–8312.
52. Szabo, A., et al. (1991) HuD, a paraneoplastic encephalomyelitis antigen, contains RNA binding domains and is homologous to elav and sex-lethal. *Cell* **67**, 325–333.
53. Marusich, M. and Weston, J. (1992) Identification of early neurogenic cells in the neural crest lineage. *Dev. Biol.* **149**, 295–306.
54. Marusich, M., Furneaux, H., Henion, P., and Weston, J. (1994) Hu neuronal proteins are expressed in proliferating neurogenic cells. *J. Neurobiol.* **25**, 143–155.
55. Barami, K., Iversen, K., Furneaux, H., and Goldman, S. A. (1995) Hu protein as an early marker of neuronal phenotypic differentiation by subependymal zone cells of the adult songbird forebrain. *J. Neurobiol.* **28**, 82–101.
56. Palmer, T. D., Ray, J., and Gage, F. H. (1995) FGF-2-responsive neuronal progenitors reside in proliferative and quiescent regions of the adult rodent brain. *Mol. Cell. Neurosci.* **6**, 474–486.
57. Gritti, A., et al. (1996) Multipotential stem cells from the adult mouse brain proliferate and self-renew in response to basic fibroblast growth factor. *J. Neurosci.* **16**, 1091–1100.
58. Ahmed, S., Reynolds, B. A., and Weiss, S. (1995) BDNF enhances the differentiation but not the survival of CNS stem cell-derived neuronal precursors. *J. Neurosci.* **15**, 5765–5778.
59. Pincus, D., Goodman, R., Fraser, R., Nedergaard, M., and Goldman, S. (1998) Neural stem and progenitor cells: a strategy for gene therapy and brain repair. *Neurosurgery* **42**, 858–868.
60. Vescovi, A. L., Reynolds, B. A., Fraser, D. D., and Weiss, S. (1993) bFGF regulates the proliferative fate of unipotent (neuronal) and bipotent (neuronal/astroglial) EGF-generated CNS progenitor cells. *Neuron* **11**, 951–966.
61. Svendsen, C., et al. (1997) Long-term survival of human central nervous system progenitor cells transplanted into a rat model of Parkinson's disease. *Exp. Neurol.* **148**, 135–146.

62. Carpenter, M., et al. (1999) In vitro expansion of a multipotent population of human neural progenitor cells. *Exp. Neurol.* **158,** 265–278.
63. Vescovi, A. L., Gritti, A., Galli, R., and Parati, E. A. (1999) Isolation and intracerebral grafting of nontransformed multipotential embryonic human CNS stem cells. *J. Neurotrauma* **16,** 689–693.
64. Kukekov, V., et al. (1999) Multipotent stem/progenitor cells with similar properties arise from two neurogenic regions of adult human brain. *Exp. Neurol.* **156,** 333–344.
65. Johe, K. K., Hazel, T. G., Muller, T., Dugich-Djordjevic, M. M., and McKay, R. D. (1996) Single factors direct the differentiation of stem cells from the fetal and adult central nervous system. *Genes Dev.* **10,** 3129–3140.
66. Rao, M. and Mayer-Proschel, M. (1997) Glial-restricted precursors are derived from multipotential neuroepithelial stem cells. *Dev. Biol.* **188,** 48–63.
67. Marmur, R., Kessler, J. A., Zhu, G., Gokhan, S., and Mehler, M. F. (1998) Differentiation of oligodendroglial progenitors derived from cortical multipotent cells requires extrinsic signals including activation of gp130/LIFbeta receptors. *J. Neurosci.* **18,** 9800–9811.
68. Jiang, J., McMurtry, J., Niedzwiecki, D., and Goldman, S. A. (1998) Insulin-like growth factor-1 is a radial cell-associated neurotrophin that promotes neuronal recruitment from the adult songbird ependyma/subependyma. *J. Neurobiol.* **36,** 1–15.
69. Wagner, J., et al. (1999) Induction of a midbrain dopaminergic phenotype in Nurr1-overexpressing neural stem cells by type 1 astrocytes. *Nat. Biotechnol.* **17,** 653–659.
70. Weiss, S., et al. (1996) Is there a neural stem cell in the mammalian forebrain? *Trends Neurosci.* **19,** 387–393.
71. Vescovi, A. L., et al. (1999) Isolation and cloning of multipotential stem cells from the embryonic human CNS and establishment of transplantable human neural stem cell lines by epigenetic stimulation. *Exp. Neurol.* **156,** 71–83.
72. Song, H., Stevens, C. F., and Gage, F. H. (2002) Astroglia induce neurogenesis from adult neural stem cells. *Nature* **417,** 39–44.
73. Brustle, O., et al. (1998) Chimeric brains generated by intraventricular transplantation of fetal human brain cells into embryonic rats. *Nat. Biotech.* **16,** 1040–1044.
74. Fricker, R., et al. (1999) Site-specific migration and neuronal differentiation of human neural progenitor cells after transplantation in the adult rat brain. *J. Neurosci.* **19,** 5990–6005.
75. Flax, J., et al. (1998) Engraftable human neural stem cells respond to developmental cues, replace neurons, and express foreign genes. *Nat. Biotech.* **16,** 1033–1039.
76. Goldman, S. A. and Nedergaard, M. (1992) Newly generated neurons of the adult songbird brain become functionally active in long-term culture. *Dev. Brain Res.* **68,** 217–223.
77. Pincus, D. W., et al. (1998) Fibroblast growth factor-2/brain-derived neurotrophic factor-associated maturation of new neurons generated from adult human subependymal cells. *Ann. Neurol.* **43,** 576–585.
78. Chalfie, M., Tu, Y., Euskirchen, G., Ward, W., and Prasher, D. (1994) Green fluorescent protein as a marker for gene expression. *Science* **263,** 802–805.
79. Cheng, L., Fu, J., Tsukamoto, A., and Hawley, R. (1996) Use of green fluorescent protein variants to monitor gene transfer and expression in mammalian cells. *Nat. Biotech.* **14,** 606–609.
80. Levy, J., Muldoon, R., Zolotukhin, S., and Link, C. (1996) Retroviral transfer and expression of a humanized, red-shifted green fluorescent protein gene into human tumor cells. *Nat. Biotech.* **14,** 610–614.
81. Miller, F., Naus, C., Durand, M., Bloom, F., and Milner, R. (1987) Isotypes of a-tubulin are differentially regulated during neuronal maturation. *J. Cell Biol.* **105,** 3065–3073.
82. Gloster, A., et al. (1994) The Ta1 a-tubulin promoter specifies gene expression as a function of neuronal growth and regeneration in transgenic mice. *J. Neurosci.* **14,** 7319–7330.

83. Goldman, S., et al. (1997) Neural precursors and neuronal production in the adult mammalian forebrain. *Ann. NY Acad. Sci.* **835**, 30–55.
84. Wang, S., et al. (1998) Isolation of neuronal precursors by sorting embryonic forebrain transfected with GFP regulated by the T alpha 1 tubulin promoter. *Nat. Biotechnol.* **16**, 196–201.
85. Wang, S., Roy, N., Benraiss, A., Harrison-Restelli, C., and Goldman, S. (2000) Promoter-based isolation and purification of mitotic neuronal progenitor cells from the adult mammalian ventricular zone. *Dev. Neurosci.* **22**, 167–176.
86. Zimmerman, L., et al. (1994) Independent regulatory elements in the *nestin* gene direct transgene expression to neural stem cells and muscle precursors. *Neuron* **12**, 11–24.
87. Lothian, C. and Lendahl, U. (1997) An evolutionarily conserved region in the second intron of the human *nestin* gene directs gene expression to CNS progenitor cells and to early neural crest cells. *Eur. J. Neurosci.* **9**, 452–462.
88. Rossant, J., Zirngibl, R., Cado, D., Shago, M., and Giguere, V. (1991) Expression of a retinoic acid response element-hsp/lacZ transgene defines specific domains of transcriptional activity during mouse embryogenesis. *Genes Dev.* **5**, 1333–1344.
89. Kawaguchi, A., et al. (2001) Nestin-GFP transgenic mice: visualization of the self-renewal and multipotency of CNS stem cells. *Mol. Cell. Neurosci.* **17**, 259–273.
90. Sawamoto, K., et al. (2001) Generation of dopaminergic neurons in the adult brain from mesencephalic precursor cells labeled with a *nestin-GFP* transgene. *J. Neurosci.* **21**, 3895–3903.
91. Svendsen, C. N., Caldwell, M. A., and Ostenfeld, T. (1999) Human neural stem cells: isolation, expansion and transplantation. *Brain Pathol.* **9**, 499–513.
92. Keyoung, H. M., et al. (2001) High-yield selection and extraction of two promoter-defined phenotypes of neural stem cells from the fetal human brain. *Nat. Biotechnol.* **19**, 843–850.
93. Uchida, N., et al. (2000) Direct isolation of human central nervous system stem cells. *Proc. Natl. Acad. Sci. USA* **97**, 14720–14725.
94. Altman, J. and Das, G. D. (1965) Autoradiographic and histological evidence of postnatal hippocampal neurogenesis in rats. *J. Comp. Neurol.* **124**, 319–335.
95. Kaplan, M. S. and Hinds, J. W. (1977) Neurogenesis in the adult rat: electron microscopic analysis of light radioautographs. *Science* **197**, 1092–1094.
96. Bayer, S., Yackel, J., and Puri, P. (1982) Neurons in the rat dentate gyrus granular layer substantially increase during juvenile and adult life. *Science* **216**, 890–892.
97. Barnea, A. and Nottebohm, F. (1994) Seasonal recruitment of hippocampal neurons in adult free-ranging black-capped chickadees. *Proc. Natl. Acad. Sci. USA* **91**, 11217–11221.
98. Gould, E., McEwen, B., Tanapat, P., Galea, L., and Fuchs, E. (1997) Neurogenesis in the dentate gyrus of the adult tree shrew is regulated by psychosocial stress and NMDA receptor activation. *J. Neurosci.* **17**, 2492–2498.
99. Gould, E., Tanapat, P., McEwen, B., Flugge, G., and Fuchs, E. (1998) Proliferation of granule cell precursors in the dentate gyrus of adult monkeys is diminished by stress. *Proc. Natl. Acad. Sci. USA* **95**, 3168–3171.
100. Eriksson, P. S., et al. (1998) Neurogenesis in the adult human hippocampus. *Nat. Med.* **4**, 1313–1317.
101. Gould, E., Cameron, H., Daniels, D., Wooley, C., and McEwen, B. (1992) Adrenal hormones suppress cell division in the adult rat dentate gyrus. *J. Neurosci.* **12**, 3642–3650.
102. Kempermann, G., Kuhn, H., and Gage, F. (1997) More hippocampal neurons in adult mice living in an enriched environment. *Nature* **386**, 493–495.
103. van Praag, H., Kempermann, G., and Gage, F. (1999) Running increases cell proliferation and neurogenesis in the adult mouse dentate gyrus. *Nat. Neurosci.* **2**, 266–270.
104. Gould, E., Beylin, A., tanapat, P., Reeves, A., and Shors, T. (1999) Learning enhances adult neurogenesis in the adult hippocampal formation. *Nat. Neurosci.* **2**, 260–265.

105. Kornack, D. and Rakic, P. (1999) Continuation of neurogenesis in the hippocampus of the adult macaque monkey. *Proc. Natl. Acad. Sci. USA* **96,** 5768–5773.
106. Shankle, W., et al. (1998) Evidence for a postnatal doubling of neuron number in the developing human cerebral cortex between 15 months and 6 years. *J. Theor. Biol.* **191,** 115–140.
107. Shankle, W., Rafii, M., Landing, B., and Fallon, J. (1999) Approximate doubling of numbers of neurons in postnatal human cerebral cortex and in 35 specific cytoarchitectural areas from birth to 72 months. *Pediatr. Dev. Pathol.* **2,** 244–259.
108. Palmer, T. D., Takahashi, J., and Gage, F. H. (1997) The adult rat hippocampus contains primordial neural stem cells. *Mol. Cell. Neurosci.* **8,** 389–404.
109. Suhonen, J., Peterson, D., Ray, J., and Gage, F. (1996) Differentiation of adult hippocampus-derived progenitors into olfactory neurons in vivo. *Nature* **383,** 624–627.
110. Wolswijk, G. and Noble, M. (1989) Identification of an adult-specific glial progenitor cell. *Development* **105,** 387–400.
111. Gensert, J. M. and Goldman, J. E. (1996) In vivo characterization of endogenous proliferating cells in adult rat subcortical white matter. *Glia* **17,** 39–51.
112. Gensert, J. M. and Goldman, J. E. (1997) Endogenous progenitors remyelinate demyelinated axons in the adult CNS. *Neuron* **19,** 197–203.
113. Noble, M. (1997) The oligodendrocyte-type 2 astrocyte lineage: in vitro and in vivo studies on development, tissue repair and neoplasia. In *Isolation, Characterization and Utilization of CNS Stem Cells* (Gage, F. Y. C., ed.), Springer-Verlag, Berlin, pp. 101–128.
114. Palmer, T. D., Markakis, E. A., Willhoite, A. R., Safar, F., and Gage, F. H. (1999) Fibroblast growth factor-2 activates a latent neurogenic program in neural stem cells from diverse regions of the adult CNS. *J. Neurosci.* **19,** 8487–8497.
115. Nunes, M. C., et al. (2003) Identification and isolation of multipotential neural progenitor cells from the subcortical white matter of the adult human brain. *Nat. Med.* **9,** 439–447.
116. Kondo, T. and Raff, M. (2000) Oligodendrocyte precursor cells reprogrammed to become multipotential CNS stem cells. *Science* **289,** 1754–1757.
117. Marmur, R., et al. (1998) Isolation and developmental characterization of cerebral cortical multipotent progenitors. *Dev. Biol.* **204,** 577–591.
118. Davis, A. A. and Temple, S. (1994) A self-renewing multipotential stem cell in embryonic rat cerebral cortex. *Nature* **372,** 263–266.
119. Qian, X., Davis, A. A., Goderie, S. K., and Temple, S. (1997) FGF2 concentration regulates the generation of neurons and glia from multipotent cortical stem cells. *Neuron* **18,** 81–93.
120. Qian, X., Goderie, S. K., Shen, Q., Stern, J. H., and Temple, S. (1998) Intrinsic programs of patterned cell lineages in isolated vertebrate CNS ventricular zone cells. *Development* **125,** 3143–3152.
121. Williams, B. P., Read, J., and Price, J. (1991) The generation of neurons and oligodendrocytes from a common precursor cell. *Neuron* **7,** 685–693.
122. Mitome, M., et al. (2001) Towards the reconstruction of central nervous system white matter using neural precursor cells. *Brain* **124,** 2147–2161.
123. Yandava, B. D., Billinghurst, L. L., and Snyder, E. Y. (1999) "Global" cell replacement is feasible via neural stem cell transplantation: evidence from the dysmyelinated shiverer mouse brain. *Proc. Natl. Acad. Sci. USA* **96,** 7029–7034.
124. Scolding, N., et al. (1998) Oligodendrocyte progenitors are present in the normal adult human CNS and in the lesions of multiple sclerosis. *Brain* **121,** 2221–2228.
125. Scolding, N. J., Rayner, P. J., and Compston, D. A. (1999) Identification of A2B5-positive putative oligodendrocyte progenitor cells and A2B5-positive astrocytes in adult human white matter. *Neuroscience* **89,** 1–4.
126. Watt, F. M. (2001) Stem cell fate and patterning in mammalian epidermis. *Curr. Opin. Genet. Dev.* **11,** 410–417.

127. Niemann, C. and Watt, F. M. (2002) Designer skin: lineage commitment in postnatal epidermis. *Trends Cell Biol.* **12,** 185–192.
128. Loeffler, M. and Potten, C. S. (1997) Stem cells and cellular pedigrees. In *Stem Cells* (Potten, C. S., ed.), Academic Press, San Diego, pp. 1–28.
129. Potten, C. S. and Loeffler, M. (1990) Stem cells: attributes, cycles, spirals, pitfalls and uncertainties. Lessons for and from the crypt. *Development* **110,** 1001–1020.
130. Doetsch, F., Petreanu, L., Caille, I., Garcia-Verdugo, J., and Alvarez-Buylla, A. (2002) EGF converts transit-amplifying neurogenic precursors in the adult brain into multipotent stem cells. *Neuron* **36,** 1021–1034.
131. Menezes, J. R., Smith, C. M., Nelson, K. C., and Luskin, M. B. (1995) The division of neuronal progenitor cells during migration in the neonatal mammalian forebrain. *Mol. Cell. Neurosci.* **6,** 496–508.
132. Luskin, M. B. (1998) Neuroblasts of the postnatal mammalian forebrain: their phenotype and fate. *J. Neurobiol.* **36,** 221–233.
133. Seri, B., Garcia-Verdugo, J. M., McEwen, B. S., and Alvarez-Buylla, A. (2001) Astrocytes give rise to new neurons in the adult mammalian hippocampus. *J. Neurosci.* **21,** 7153–7160.
134. Arsenijevic, Y., et al. (2001) Isolation of multipotent neural precursors residing in the cortex of the adult human brain. *Exp. Neurol.* **170,** 48–62.
135. Belachew, S., et al. (2003) Postnatal NG2 proteoglycan-expressing progenitor cells are intrinsically multipotent and generate functional neurons. *J. Cell Biol.* **161,** 169–186.
136. Palmer, T., Willhoite, A., and Gage, F. (2000) Vascular niche for adult hippocampal neurogenesis. *J. Comp. Neurol.* **425,** 479–494.
137. Palmer, T. (2002) Adult neurogenesis and the vascular Nietzsche. *Neuron* **34,** 856–858.
138. Louissaint, A., Rao, S., Leventhal, C., and Goldman, S. A. (2002) Coordinated interaction of angiogenesis and neurogenesis in the adult songbird brain. *Neuron* **34,** 945–960.
139. Lim, D. A., et al. (2000) Noggin antagonizes BMP signaling to create a niche for adult neurogenesis. *Neuron* **28,** 713–726.
140. Packer, M., et al. (2003) Nitric oxide negatively regulates mammalian adult neurogenesis. *Proc. Natl. Acad. Sci. USA* **100,** 9566–9571.
141. Benraiss, A., et al. (1999) In vivo transduction of the adult rat ventricular zone with an adenoviral BDNF vector substantially increases neurogenesis and neuronal recruitment to the rat olfactory bulb. *Soc. Neurosci. Abstr.* **25.**
142. Arvidsson, A., Collin, T., Kirik, D., Kokaia, Z., and Lindvall, O. (2002) Neuronal replacement from endogenous precursors in the adult brain after stroke. *Nat. Med.* **8,** 963–970.
143. Nakatomi, H., et al. (2002) Regeneration of hippocampal pyramidal neurons after ischemic brain injury by recruitment of endogenous progenitors. *Cell* **110,** 429–441.
144. Parent, J. M. (2003) Injury-induced neurogenesis in the adult mammalian brain. *Neuroscientist* **9,** 261–272.
145. Curtis, M. A., et al. (2003) Increased cell proliferation and neurogenesis in the adult human Huntington's disease brain. *Proc. Natl. Acad. Sci. USA* **100,** 9023–9027.

13

Embryonic Stem Cells and Neurogenesis

Robin L. Wesselschmidt and John W. McDonald

INTRODUCTION

The convergence of genomic technologies, high-throughput screening techniques, and the availability of pluripotent embryonic stem (ES) cell lines provides an unprecedented opportunity to identify the molecular mechanisms guiding mammalian development, the pathogenesis of disease, and spontaneous regeneration and repair. The isolation and characterization of human ES cells for use in drug discovery programs and as therapeutic agents in degenerative diseases has revitalized interest in the development of methods for stable, perhaps indefinite, culture of ES cells, and methods for predictably driving ES cells to differentiate into specific precursor populations and definitive cell types (Table 1).

The first mouse ES cell lines were reported in 1981 *(1,2)*. Soon afterwards, Robertson and Bradley showed that ES cells could be genetically manipulated in vitro and that, when reintroduced into a mouse blastocyst, they could integrate into the inner cell mass and contribute to all the tissues of the developing chimeric animal, including germ cells *(3,4)*. Since then, ES cell mutagenesis has become the standard method for generating knockout mice containing targeted mutations. Such mice are widely used for exploring gene function in a physiologically relevant manner. In a 2003 review, for example, Zambrowicz and Sands reported the correlation between the phenotypes of knockout mice and the ability of the 100 best-selling drugs to modulate the pathway targeted in each knockout model *(5)*.

The first report of the derivation human ES cell lines in 1998 *(6)* was quickly followed by others *(7–9)*. The most intriguing report to date is that of Hwang, who isolated a human ES cell line from blastocysts generated through nuclear transfer *(10)*.

When the first mouse ES lines were isolated, the genomic tools needed to efficiently dissect the molecular pathways that sustain self-renewal or drive differentiation were not available. Combining genomic methods with genetic and pharmacological manipulation of the in vitro ES cell culture system, researchers can now identify therapeutically relevant pathways and apply this new knowledge to the treatment of disease by using drugs to direct endogenous stem cell differentiation or by transplanting specific ES cell-derived populations.

From: *Neural Development and Stem Cells, Second Edition*
Edited by: M. S. Rao © Humana Press Inc., Totowa, NJ

Table 1
Development of the Embryonic Stem Cells in Neuroscience

Date	Observation	Reference
1981	**Derivation of ES cells from mouse blastocysts**	(1)
	Derivation of ES cells from mouse preimplantation blastocyst. Subcutaneous injection of ES cells into athymic mice produced teratomas containing three germ layers when examined 6 wk later. Culturing whole EBs produced some neuron-like cells over a period of 6 wk.	(2)
1988	**Definitive demonstration of neuronal differentiation from mouse ES cells in culture**. NGF accelerated the generation of neurons (identified by silver staining) from ES cells plated as whole EBs in culture.	(35)
1992	**Methods developed for isolating and culturing mouse ES cell from primordial germ cells (PGCs)**	(100,101)
1994	**Early example of the strength of the in vitro ES cell system for analyzing targeted mutations**. By using in vitro differentiation, this study identified the defect in GATA-1 signaling as a block late in the erythroid lineage. GATA-1 (–/–) mice fail to generate mature erythroid cells but do generate white blood cells. Therefore, the in vitro system was key in determining the stage-specific role of the GATA-1 defect.	(102)
1995	**Derivation of ES cell-like cells from a nonhuman primate (*Rhesus*, Old World Species)**. When ES cells were transplanted into leg muscle or testis of severe combined immunodeficiency (SCID) mice, teratomas formed. They contained cells representing all three germ layers (examined 8–15 wk after transplantation).	(103)
1996	**Transplantation of mouse ES cells into the CNS**. Neurons developed after RA-induced ES cells were transplanted into the quinolinic acid-lesioned striatum.	(47)
1997	**Demonstration of the utility of double allele knockouts in ES cells for studying cell biology**. Neural cells generated from ES cells deprived of both alleles of the *FGF-4* gene exhibited altered growth and survival. FGF-4 (–/–) embryos was arrested shortly after implantation. FGF-4 (–/–) ES cells formed teratomas with neural components 30, 35, 47, and 61 d after subcutaneous transplantation in 129/SvJ mice. Addition of FGF-4 to the culture medium dramatically enhanced the survival of ES cell FGF-4 (–/–) derived cells, which died at higher rates than FGF (+/+) ES cells.	(104)
1998	**Postmitotic neurons and glia were generated after rhesus ES cells were transplanted into muscle of immunocompromised (SCID mice)**. At 5–12 wk post-transplantation, all the teratomas showed neural differentiation. Some aspects of normal differentiation are recapitulated in teratomas from rhesus ES cells.	(105)

Year		Ref.
	Demonstration of genetic selection of lineage-restricted neural progenitors from ES cells. ES cells were engineered using homologous recombination to contain a bifunctional selection marker/reporter gene βgeo integrated into the *Sox2* gene. After induction with RA (4-/4+ protocol), ~50% of the dissociated cultured cells expressed β-galactosidase activity and Sox2 immunoreactivity. Addition of G418 to cultures selected for ~90% expression of β-galactosidase activity and Sox2 immunoreactivity. Further differentiation produced mature neurons. Therefore, genetic selection can be use to obtain pure populations of neural-restricted precursor cells, in this case NRPs.	(37)
1998	**Demonstration of the utility of the double allele-targeted ES cell culture system for analyzing the effects of specific genes on neuronal development.** GD3S (–/–) ESC, with double targeted gene disruption of the GD3 synthase gene, were deficient in GD3S activity, but neurons could still differentiate normally. Therefore, the hypothesis that b-series gangliosides are necessary for neuronal differentiation was disproved.	(106)
	Application of "stem cell selection" using ES cells engineered to express resistance to antibiotic in undifferentiated ES cells. The CGR8 ES cell line was transfected with the *Oct4neofos* construct (*Oct3/4* gene linked to *lacZ/neo*; OKO160). Undifferentiated *Oct4neofos* cells expressed low levels of neomycin phosphotransferase under control of the Oct4 promoter element (stem-cell specific transcription factor Oct4). Differentiated progeny did not express the transgene and therefore were killed by the selection agent G418.	(107)
	Derivation of human ES cell-like cells from human blastocyst. Transplantation of each of five cell lines into SCID mice produced teratomas containing all three germ layers. After 4 mo, the teratomas contained rosettes of neuroepithelium and neural ganglia.	(6)
	Derivation of pluripotent EG cells from human PGCs; cultured PGCs produced cells from all three derivatives of all three embryonic germ layers, including neuroepithelia.	(108)
1999	**Demonstration that ES cell transplantation can enhance recovery of lost functions.** Transplantation of dissociated 4-/4+ RA-stimulated EBs, but not vehicle medium or neocortical cells from adult mice, into the spinal cord 9 d after contusion injury improved functional hindlimb locomotion. ESC-derived neural cells integrated, migrated 1 cm, and differentiated into neurons, oligodendrocytes, and astrocytes.	(79)
2000	**Derivation of human ES cell lines HES1 and HES2 from human blastocyst and the demonstration that neural progenitors can be isolated from human ES and induced to generate mature neurons.** This study showed that hESC express Oct-4, differentiate in vitro, and produce nestin and PS-NCAM-positive neural progenitors when cultured to high density.	(9)

(continued)

301

Table 1 (continued)

Date	Observation	Reference
	Demonstration that human ES cell can be cloned and that the clones maintain normal karyotype after 8 mo of continuous culture. hES cell line H9 was subcloned to generate H9.1 and H9.2, which maintained proliferative capacity, telomerase expression, and their normal karyotype. They formed teratomas when injected into SCID mice.	(109)
	Demonstration that growth factors can induce human ES cell to differentiate. Eight different growth factors were applied to the differentiation protocol of the H1 hES cell line. The line was induced to differentiate through an EB intermediary.	(74)
	Demonstration that human ES cell can be cultured in the absence of a feeder layer set the stage for scale-up production and simplified assays. The hES cell lines H1, H7, H9, and H14 were used. All maintained a normal karyotype, stable proliferation rate, high telomerase activity, and formed teratomas in SCID mice.	(110)
2001	**Derivation of mouse ES cell lines from cloned blastocysts produced by somatic cell nuclear transfer.** Demonstrated that NT-derived mouse ES cell could be isolated and differentiated when derived from cloned mouse embryos.	(111)
2002	**Demonstration that mouse ES cells could be induced to produce specific classes of neurons if treated with factors known to induce specific neuronal subclasses in vivo.** This study indicated that the system can produce specific neuronal subclasses in a predictable fashion despite the apparent lack of an axis of development in the EB system.	(59)
2003	**Demonstration of homologous recombination in human ES cells.** *HPRT* locus was targeted in H1.1 ES cells by electroporation	(78)
	Demonstration that mouse ES cells can be induced to differentiate into neural precursors when grown as a monolayer. May prove to be important to the development of high-throughput screening methods and more predictable differentiation protocols.	(63)
	Demonstration that NT-derived mouse ES cells can differentiate into neural subtypes and, when transplanted into a mouse model of Parkinson's disease, show some therapeutic benefit. Indication of a potential therapeutic application for neurons differentiated from NT-derived ES cell lines.	(112)
2004	**Demonstration that a human ES cell-like cell line can be produced from cloned human blastocysts.** Implications for developing immunopermissive hES cell lines for transplantation.	(10)
	Derivation of 17 human ES cell lines using propagation methods that more closely resemble those used to propagate mouse ES cell lines, including enzymatic dissociation to passage the cells. These lines may prove to be more practically useful than other lines because they the culture methods are simpler.	(7)
	Derivation of human ES cell lines from cryopreserved blastocysts on STO feeders. Technically important in terms of the derivation of new hES cell lines, this method uses embryos at a stage typically frozen for storage in IVF clinics.	(8)

Abbreviations: EBs, Embryoid bodies; ES, embryonic stem; ESC, embryonic stem cell; hESC, human embryonic stem cell; NGF, nerve growth factor; NRPs, neuronal restricted precursors; NSC, neural stem cell; PGCs, primordial germ cells; PS-NCAM, polysialylated neural cell adhesion molecule; RA, retinoic acid; RAR, retinoic acid receptor; SCID, severe combined immunodeficiency; +, positive reactivity; (–/–), double gene allele inactivation; 4/4⁺ RA, induction protocol where EBs are exposed to RA only in the last 4 d of an 8-d protocol.

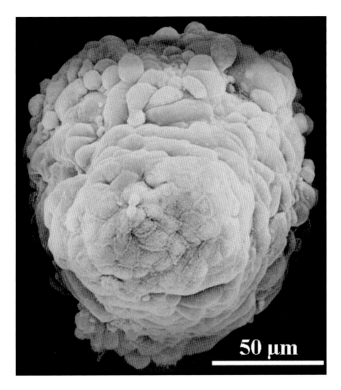

Fig. 1. Scanning EM shows a 4$^-$/4$^+$ stage embryoid body, characterized as floating clusters of undifferentiated cells. The majority of embryoid body cells are NEPs, nestin$^+$, and do not express markers of differentiated neural cells. Scale bar = 50 μm.

This chapter describes work on ES cells and neurogenesis focusing on studies published since our last review of ES cells and neurogenesis in 1999–2000 *(11)*. We describe (1) the in vitro neural differentiation of ES cells, (2) recent studies of transplantation of ES cell-derived neural precursors, and (3) the unique problems that have to be overcome to enable the use of the ES cell system as a tool for scientific discovery towards therapeutics.

THE IN VITRO EMBRYONIC STEM CELL SYSTEM

ES cells are a small population of pluripotent cells, transiently present in the preimplantation embryo from the late morula stage to mid-blastocyst stage. They are characterized by the expression of several transcription factors, including Oct4 and nanog *(12–14)*. After they are isolated from the inner cell mass of the blastocyst, they can be maintained in vitro under conditions that either sustain pluripotency or allow for differentiation *(15)*.

The earliest reports of in vitro differentiation of mouse ES cells were made by Wobus in 1984 and Doetschman in 1985 *(16,17)*. These investigators showed that mouse ES cells spontaneously differentiate into cell types derived from all three germ layers when leukemia inhibitory factor (LIF) is withdrawn from the culture medium. When growing in suspension under these conditions, ES cells aggregate into spherical structures called embryoid bodies (Fig. 1).

The differentiation protocols described by Wobus and Doetschman are dependent on unknown factors found in fetal calf serum *(16,17)*. Thus, the percentage and type of cells produced by this method varies dependent on batch of serum *(18)*. The dominant cell types are mesenteric in origin. They include skeletal myocytes *(19)*, vascular endothelia *(20,21)*, cells of the hematopoietic cell lineage *(16,20,22,23)*, and cardiomyocytes *(24)*. Importantly, when human ES cell lines are induced to differentiate via the same method—suspension culture in the presence of fetal calf serum—they also give rise to recognizable cardiomyocytes and blood islands *(6,9)*.

The embryoid body differentiates in a predictable fashion that recapitulates embryogenesis. Initially, extraembryonic endoderm and primitive ectoderm are established; these layers then differentiate into all three germ layers of the early embryo *(15)*. It is important to note, however, that the embryoid body lacks the axes of development found in vivo. This may impact the ability to efficiently induce the differentiation of some cell types in vitro *(25)*. However, advances in bioengineering and three-dimensional systems may allow this to be overcome as well as more knowledge about the molecular cues that drive the development of specialized cell types.

ES CELLS CAN GIVE RISE
TO ALL THREE PRINCIPAL NEURAL LINEAGES

ES cells can be induced to differentiate into the three principal neural cell types: astrocytes, oligodendrocytes, and neurons *(17,26–35)* (Table 2; Figs. 2–4). Methods for increasing the number of neuronal cells include induction by retinoic acid, application of growth factors, and treatment with neurotrophins. Identifying lineage-restricted transcription factors and using them to induce the differentiation of progenitors and subtype neural populations will increase our ability to regulate the in vitro ES cell system. In general, the transcription factors identified in previous embryonic studies demonstrate similar lineage restriction in the in vitro ES cell system.

Enrichment of specific lineages can be achieved with commonly used selection methods such as fluorescence-activated cell sorting (FACS), immunopanning (which relies on cell surface antigens), and selective survival (which uses selectable markers driven by cell-specific promoters and treatment with pharmacological agents to eliminate populations that do not express the protective protein) *(36–38)*.

In 1995, Bain described an in vitro method that adds retinoic acid to the culture medium after 4 d *(27)*. The $4^-/4^+$ culture method significantly increases the number of neural precursors obtained from embryoid bodies. Under these culture conditions, it is possible to derive neuroepithelial precursors, glial-restricted precursors, neurons, astrocytes, and oligodendrocytes. ES cells can also produce neurons of multiple phenotypes, including γ-aminobutyric acid-ergic (GABAergic), glutamatergic, glycinergic, noradrenergic, and cholinergic neurons (Table 2).

Subtypes of cholinergic motoneurons have also been identified in ES-derived cultures *(32)*, but most of those experiments relied on immunohistologic methods for identity. Recent physiologic studies indicate that ES-derived neurons develop functional synapses, exhibit spontaneous activity, and possess electrophysiological properties remarkably similar to those of neurons in primary culture systems *(26,28,29,34,39–41)* (Table 2).

ES cell-derived neurons express proteins or gene products characteristic of primary neurons: general neuronal functions (β-tubulin III, neurofilament subunits), neuronal surface markers (neural cell adhesion molecule [NCAM]), transmitter synthesizing enzymes (glutamic acid decarboxylase [GAD], tyrosine [TH], choline acetyltransferase [ChAT]), transmitter receptor subunits (GluR, GABA-R), and neurotransmitters (glutamate, GABA). Furthermore, ES cell-derived neurons possess electrophysiological response (e.g., to glutamate and GABA) and intracellular calcium flux properties similar to cells from primary cells (Table 2).

METHODS FOR ISOLATING NEURONAL PRECURSORS FROM ES CELLS

Inductive culture methods which treat embryoid body intermediaries with neural stimulatory factors result in neural precursors. These methods have proven successful in generating cell populations that are predominantly of neural origin. Molecular and mechanical enrichment methods result in very pure populations of progenitors and terminally differentiated cell types *(37,38,42,43)*.

Multiple classes of neural precursor populations have been isolated from mouse ES cells and methods for purifying these populations have been developed. As the molecular events that drive cell specialization and lineage restriction in vivo are identified, the ability to reliably drive ES cell differentiation down specific pathways in vitro will be refined. ES cells are capable of generating all later stage progenitors if the culture system contains the necessary factors and microenvironment. Several key modulators of progenitor cell specialization have been identified, including retinoic acid, sonic hedgehog (Shh), and bone morphogenic protein (BMP) *(27,44–46)*. The derivation of expandable, stable, genetically normal, and lineage-restricted cell populations are necessary for drug discovery and for a transplantable source of cells to treat CNS disease.

Retinoic Acid Induction Protocols

As we noted earlier, one of the first strategies for deriving neural precursors from ES cells involved treatment with retinoic acid *(26–29,34,40,47,48)*; and *see (48)*, Figs. 5 and 6 for a review of molecular mechanisms of retinoic acid induction. When embryoid bodies are exposed to retinoic acid, the overall temporal development of gene and marker expression strongly resembles that of the developing embryo *(27,28,48)*.

Embryoid bodies contain a variety of cell types, but have only a small number of neural cells when the induction protocol lacks retinoic acid *(2,27,47)*. The retinoic acid induction protocol has been shown to produce electrophysiologically active neuronal circuits with functional excitatory and inhibitory synapses *(26,28,34)*. Mouse ES cell studies demonstrate that the 4$^-$/4$^+$ protocol generates embryoid bodies composed primarily of a nestin $^+$ precursor pool. These cells are described as tripotential precursors because they can generate all three primary neural lineages: neurons, oligodendrocytes, and astrocytes *(26,30,40)*.

Many researchers have used the Bain 4$^-$/4$^+$ protocol *(26,30)* to induce neurogenesis in mouse ES cells (Fig. 5). Under this protocol, mouse ES cells are removed from the substratum and cultured in suspension as embryoid bodies in the absence of LIF for 4 d. On d 5, retinoic acid is added to the culture medium and embryoid bodies are allowed to grow in suspension for 4 additional days (Fig. 1). At the end of d 8, the embryoid

Table 2
Published Studies of ES-Derived Neural Cells

Date	Observation	Cell line	RA induction	Neurons	Glia	Reference
1981	**Growth of whole murine EBs in vitro produced some neuron-like cells over a period of 6 wk.** First derivation of ES cells from murine pre-implantation blastocyst. SQ injection of ES cells into athymic mice produced teratomas containing three germ layers when examined 6 wk later.	Murine ICRxSW R/J	No	Neuron-like cells in vitro	NE	(2)
1988	**First demonstration of definitive neuronal differentiation from murine ES cells in vitro.** NGF accelerated the generation of neurons from ES cells plated as whole EBs in vitro. One day after EB plating, 44% of EBs treated with NGF contained neuron-like cells, whereas only 8% of control EBs contained neuron-like cells. NGF treatment also eliminated undifferentiated ES cells by 8 DIV, whereas sham-treated cultures contained undifferentiated ES cells even at 9 DIV.	Murine BLC 6 (129/Sv Gat)	No Whole EBs plated	Silver stain+	NE	(35)
1992	**Neuron-like cells derived from putative bovine ES cell-like cells.** First derivation of bovine ES cell-like cells from blastocysts.	Bovine 2 lines	No	Rare neuron-like cells present after spontaneous differentiation	NE	(113)
	First demonstration of neurons differentiated from mink ES cell-like cells. First derivation of mink ES cells from blastocysts. The same group has since characterized an additional 10 ES cell lines in vitro and in vivo	Mink 10 cell lines: MES1-10	No	Neural cells present in 2/10 lines (MES8 and 9) after 25 DIV NF+	NE	(114)
1993	Derivation of putative ES cell-like cells from rabbit preimplantation embryos. Able to continuously passage (>1 yr), maintain normal karyotype, form EBs, and differentiate into cells characteristic of the three principle germ layers.	Rabbit GM3	No	Neural crest	NE	(115)
	Differentiation of neuron-like cells from porcine and ovine ES cell-like cells.	Porcine, ovine PICM-8, -12, 20	No/yes RA	Neuron-like cells differentiated from ES cells cultured on feeder layers.	NE	(116,117)

Year	Description	Cell type	Neural differentiation	Neurons/markers	Glia	Ref.
1994	**Development of neurons after in vitro differentiation of porcine ES cells.** First establishment of porcine (*Sus scrofa*) "true" ES cells derived from preimplantation embryos and of their ability to develop into normal chimeras.	Porcine	Yes RA	Neurons	NE	(118)
1994	**Demonstration of the strength of the in vitro ES cell neural differentiation system by using double allele inactivation and subsequent "rescue" of the mutant cells.** Demonstration that induction of the *T3Rα* gene is essential for RA stimulation of neuronal development from murine ES cells. Homologous recombination techniques were used to inactivate both *T3Rα* alleles in murine ES cells to evaluate the role of unliganded *T3Rα* in early development and on RA-stimulated neural development. *T3Rα* (−/−) ES cells showed increased basal and RA-induced expression of endogenous RA-responsive genes, RARβ, and alkaline phosphatase. This effect was rescued by cotransfection of T3Rα1 but not the T3Rα variant *c-erbAα2*. It was concluded that T3Rα inhibits the RA response.	Murine CC1.2	Yes RA D1-5	Neurons NFM+	NE	(119)
1995	**Demonstration that RA strongly induces neural cell differentiation in ES cell aggregates.** Neuron-like cells comprised 38% of cells in 4−/4+ RA induced cultures, and about 0% in 4−/4− cultures (2 DIV after dissociation).	Murine D3 CCE	Yes 4−/4+ RA as EB's	β-Tubulin III+, NFM+ RT-PCR: glutamate receptor subunits (GluR1-4,6), Brn-3, GAD67, GAD65 No BF-1, TH expression Physiologic properties: Responses to kainite, NMDA, GABA, glycine	GFAP+ RT-PCR: GFAP	(26)
	First demonstration of functional neurons derived from murine ES cells in vitro, and first demonstration of ESC-derived astrocytes in culture. 4−/4+ RA induced ES cell produced β-tubulin III and NFM+ neurons and cells that expressed gene products for NFL, glutamate receptor subunits (GluR1-4,6), Brn-3, GAD67, GAD65, and GFAP. A noted absence of BF-1 expression suggested that RA may select for hindbrain neural phenotypes since BF-1 is expressed selectively in anterior regions of the CNS. Neurons generated action potentials, expressed TTX-sensitive Na+ channels, voltage gated K+ channels, and Ca2+ channels, and were sensitive to kainate, NMDA, GABA, or glycine.					

(continued)

Table 2 (*continued*)

Date	Observation	Cell line	RA induction	Neurons	Glia	Reference
	Neural tube-like structures developed in rhesus primate ES cell-derived teratomas. First derivation of ES cell-like cells from non-human primate (Rhesus, Old World Species). When ES cells were transplanted into leg muscle or testis of severe combined immunodeficiency (SCID) mice, teratomas formed, with cells representing of all three germ layers (examined 8–15 wk posttransplantation).	Nonhuman primate R278.5	No	Neural tube-like structures	NE	(103)
	First demonstration of ES cell-derived oligodendrocytes in cultures of RA-induced murine ES cells. Demonstrated nestin$^+$ neural precursors in cultured murine ES cell induced with RA (2$^+$/2$^-$ as EBs, then dissociated). The precursors were capable of generating mature neurons (GABAergic and cholinergic) and glia (oligodendrocytes and astrocytes). O4$^+$ cells accounted for <1% of cultured cells. GFAP$^+$ cells were 75% of cultured cells. MAP-2+ neurons were 25% of cultured cells. Voltage-dependent channels observed in voltage clamp studies.	Murine CGR8 (129 Sv)	Yes 2$^+$/2$^-$ RA as EBs	Neuron-like cells NCAM$^+$, Nestin$^+$ GAD$^+$, AChE activity$^+$ MAP2$^+$, MAP5$^+$ NFH$^+$, Synaptophysin$^+$ Physiology: See detail	GFAP$^+$ O4$^+$	(29)
1995	**Demonstration of the value of ES cell-derived in vitro systems for analyzing neuronal function and development at the cellular level.** RA induction for 2 d enhanced neuronal numbers but did not alter their phenotypic fate. Complex electrophysiological and immunocytological properties of postmitotic neurons were evident, and the sequence of expression of voltage-gated and receptor operated ion channels paralleled that observed in previous studies of primary cultures of rat neurons.	Murine BLC6	Yes 4$^-$/2$^+$	Synaptophysin$^+$ Synaptobrevins$^+$ NF-L,M,H$^+$ Synaptic vesicle protein2$^+$, N-CAM$^+$ GAD$^+$ Physiology: Voltage-dependent (K+, Na+, Ca^{2+}) and receptor-operated (GABA$_A$, glycine, AMPA, NMDA) ionic channels Ca^{2+}-dependent GABA release	GFAP$^+$	(34)

Year	Description	Cells	EB/RA	Markers	Glia	Ref
1996	**Demonstration of acquisition of neuronal polarity, synapse formation, and functional synaptic transmission in ES cell-derived neurons in vitro.** Within 14–21 DIV, RA-induced (4/4+) ES cell-derived neurons formed excitatory synapses mediated by glutamate receptors or inhibitory synapses mediated by receptors for GABA or glycine. Both NMDA and non-NMDA receptors contributed to the excitatory postsynaptic responses. Majority of synaptic connections were excitatory ((80%). Only glycinergic inhibitory synapses were observed, and no GABAergic synapses were found. The majority of ES cell-derived neurons displayed spontaneous activity.	Murine D3	Yes 4+/4- RA as EBs	GAP-43+ axons, MAP2+ dendrites, Synaptophysin+, SV2+, Synapsin+, Physiology: See description	NE	(28)
	First study to transplant murine ES cells into the CNS. Development of neurons after transplantation of RA-induced ES cells.	Murine D3 and E14TG2a	Yes 4+ RA	AChE+, GABA+, NSE+, Thy1.2+, III-β-tubulin+	NE	(47)
	RA induction enhances neuronal production and differentiation in culture		Yes 4+	GABA+, GAD+, NF+, III-β-tubulin+, A2B5+	GFAP+	
	Demonstration that RA promotes neural and represses mesodermal gene expression in mouse ES cell in vitro. 4/4+ RA treatment of EBs enhanced expression of NF-L, -M, GAD65, GAD67, Wnt1, and MASH1. EBs not treated with RA (4/4-) did not express these genes except for NF-L, which was expressed weakly. RA downregulated expression of the mesodermal genes Brachyury, cardiac actin, and zeta-globin. During RA treatment, neural genes were activated in the following sequence: Wnt1, then MASH-1, then NFs, then GAD only with the appearance of mature neurons.	Murine D3	Yes 4-/4+	RT-PCR: Enhanced expression with RA treatment: NF-L, -M, GAD65, GAD67, Wnt1, MASH1	NE	(27)
	Murine EG cells. After induction and differentiation protocols similar to those used in previous ES cell experiments, EG-1 cells had the capacity to differentiate into cardiac, skeletal muscle, and neuronal cells in a fashion very analogous to that seen in ES cell differentiation.	Murine EG-1 (129/Sv) D3 ES cell	Hanging drop	NFM+ Neurocan+ RT-PCR: NFM, Neurocan β-tubulin	NE	(120)

(continued)

Table 2 (*continued*)

Date	Observation	Cell line	RA induction	Neurons	Glia	Reference
1996	**Differentiation of neuronal precursors and glia from avian ES cells.** First derivation of "true" ES cells from avian blastocysts. Previous work had shown that similarly isolated cells could produce chimeric offspring in chickens, but the cells were never cultured to verify the other features of ES cells. The chicken ES cells could be cultured long-term, and they exhibited morphology, development, cytokine dependence, and high telomerase activity consistent with ES cells. The ES cells were shown to form cell types from all three major germ layers. Injection of ES cells into host blastocysts produced chimeric chickens. Anti-RA antibody prevented spontaneous differentiation, indicating that ES cells release RA during early differentiation.	Avian CEC QEC	Anti-RA antibody	NCAM$^+$	GFAP$^+$	(121)
	First demonstration that bFGF can be used to select for a highly enriched population of ES cell-derived NEPs. Nestin-immunoreactive cells developed into glia and neurons (multiple neuronal phenotypes) in culture. Moreover, ES cell-derived neurons formed synapses in vitro using TEM and could respond physiologically to glutamate and GABA.	Murine J1 CJ7 R1 D3	No bFGF ITSFn	GABA$^+$, Glutamate$^+$ MAP2$^+$, NF-M$^+$, Synapsin-1$^+$ No ChAT$^+$	GFAP$^+$ O4$^+$	(31)
	When the bFGF, ITSFn induction system was used, >95% cells were nestin+ and >60% were MAP2+.		Yes— RA in B27 suppl.			
	Differentiation of neuron-like cells from cultured EBs derived from fish ES cells. First derivation of ES cell-like cells from fish (medakafish; *Oryzias latipes*) blastocysts. Chimera development not attempted/demonstrated.	Fish MES1-3	Yes RA in EB's	RT-PCR: GAD65, AMPAR, NMDAR1, NMDAR2A,B,D Physiology: Responses to glutamate and GABA Neuron-like cells	NE	(122)
1997	**Characterization of Ca^{2+} channel development in murine ES cell-derived neurons.**	Murine BCL-6	Yes 2$^+$/2$^-$	NF-L$^+$, -M$^+$, -H$^+$ Synaptophysin$^+$	NE	(41)

310

Year	Description	Cell line	hanging drop/ suspension culture	Characterization		Ref
	Development of G protein-mediated Ca^{2+} channel regulation in murine ESC-derived neurons. Somatostatin efficiently suppressed L- and N- type Ca^{2+} channels in immature and mature neurons. In contrast, inhibition of L- and N- type channels by baclofen was rarely observed at the early stage, and it was confined to N-type channels. The findings suggests that specific neurotransmitters such as somatostatin regulate voltage-gated Ca^{2+} channels via G proteins during the early stages of neurogenesis, providing a mechanism for the epigenetic control of neuronal differentiation.			RT-PCR: Synaptophysin, β-tubulin, $G\alpha o1$ $G\alpha o2$ Physiology: Whole cell Ca^{2+} $\{I(Ca)\}$ currents: somatostatin and baclofen reversibly inhibited $I(Ca)$ e.g., GABAergic and glutamatergic		
	Isolation of porcine EG cells (D24–25 embryos) capable of differentiating into neuron-like cells in vitro. EG cells injected into host blastocysts were able to contribute to chimeric piglets.	Porcine PEGC142 PEGC273 PEGC367 PEGC62	Yes	Neuron-like cells and neural rosettes formed in vitro	NE	(123)
1997	**Demonstration of utility of double-allele knockouts in ES cells for studying cell biology.** Neural cells derived from ES cells with both alleles of the *FGF-4* gene deleted showed altered growth and survival. *FGF-4* (-/-) embryos were arrested shortly after implantation. *FGF-4* (-/-) ES cells formed teratomas with neural components 30, 35, 47, 61 d after subcutaneous transplantation in 129/SvJ mice. Adding FGF-4 to the culture medium dramatically enhanced survival of ES *FGF-4* (-/-) derived cells, which otherwise had a higher death rate than *FGF* (+/+) ES cells.	Murine R1(129) & D3 GB3, FD6, HD3, IC3	Yes	Mature neural tissue observed in teratomas created SQ	NE	(104)
	Embryonic intraventricular transplantation of RA-induced ES cells formed neurons, astrocytes, and oligodendrocytes that integrated within host tissues. The temporal appearance of differentiated transplanted cells correlated with the normal postnatal development of each cell type. Four-day-old EBs were plated in culture for 5–12 d in ITSFn medium prior to transplantation.	Murine J1	No	NeuN+, MAP2+ TH+ Neuroepithelium formed in ventricles	CNPase+ Oligos GFAP+	(124)

311

Table 2 (*continued*)

Date	Observation	Cell line	RA induction	Neurons	Glia	Reference
	Demonstration that RA-mediated *Pax6* expression and markedly enriched the yield of neurons and glia from murine ES cells.	Murine R1 MPI-II *Pax6*/lacZ	Yes 4 D RA as EBs	Neuron-like cells NFM$^+$	GFAP$^+$	*(125)*
1998	**Postmitotic neurons and glia were generated and formed teratomas after rhesus ES cells were transplanted into immunocompromised host muscle (SCID mice)**. At 5–12 wk posttransplantation, all teratomas showed neural differentiation: neural tube-like structures, embryonic ganglia, dispersed neurons, and brain-like gray matter. Neurons were NF$^+$. Axon tracts were common in teratomas >6 wk old. Increased astrocyte differentiation (GFAP$^+$) was observed as teratomas aged. Therefore, some aspects of normal differentiation were recapitulated in teratomas from rhesus ES cells. This group has isolated seven Rhesus ES cell lines in total.	Nonhuman primate R278.5	No	Intramuscle teratomas: Neural tube-like structures, embryonic ganglia, neurons, brain-like gray matter. NF$^+$	Intramuscle teratomas: GFAP$^+$	*(126)*
	First demonstration of normal developmental characteristics of neuromuscular junctions from murine ES cells in vitro. Development of colocalization of agrin, synaptophysin, and AChR in mixed muscle/ neurons derived from ES cells. The temporal pattern of expression of striated muscle and neuronal markers closely matched similar expression during in vivo development.	Murine D3 & BLC6	No 5D EBs	Cholinergic cells NF-L$^+$ and synaptophysin (5D+2); NF-M, -H (5D+6); RT-PCR: NF-L,-M and synaptophysin (5D EBs); Neurocan (5D+2); tau (5D+6); NF-H (5D+18)	NE	*(33)*
1998	**First demonstration of genetic selection of lineage-restricted neural progenitors from ES cells.** These ES cells contained a bifunctional selection marker/reporter gene β*geo* that was integrated into the *Sox2* gene by homologous recombination. When induced with RA (4$^-$/4$^+$ protocol), ~50% of the dissociated cultured cells expressed β-galactosidase activity and *Sox-2* immunoreactivity. Further addition of G418 resulted in cultures with >90% expression	Murine E14TG2a CGR8 CCE-Sox2	Yes 4$^-$/4$^+$ RA	GABA$^+$, Glutamate$^+$ β-tubulin III$^+$, MAPs$^+$, Synapsin-1$^+$, NFL$^+$, NFH$^+$ Nestin$^+$	GFAP$^+$	*(37)*

Description	Cells	EB / protocol	Markers		Ref.
of β-galactosidase activity and Sox-2 immunoreactivity. Of the selected cells, 46% were Pax6+, 35% were Pax3+, 24% were Mash1+, 14% were Math4A+, 30% were Delta1+, and 3% were Islet1+. Further differentiation produced mature neurons expressing GABA, glutamate, NF, and MAP immunoreactivity. Therefore, genetic selection can be used to isolate pure populations of neural-restricted precursor cells, in this case NRPs.	Murine J1	Yes 4/4+	NFM+, GAP-43+, MAP-2+	NE	(106)
First demonstration of the utility of double-allele targeted ES cell culture system for analyzing the effects of specific genes on neuronal development. GD3S (-/-) ES cells, with double targeted gene disruptions of the GD3 synthase gene, were deficient in GD3S activity, but neurons could still differentiate normally. Therefore, the hypothesis that b-series gangliosides are necessary for neuronal differentiation was disproved. **Demonstration of the utility of double allele knockouts for studying cellular mechanisms in vitro.** Loss of β1 integrin function accelerated neuronal differentiation. ES cell deprived of both alleles of the β1 integrin gene exhibited accelerated neuronal differentiation (expression of neuron-specific genes and increased numbers of neurons) but retarded neurite outgrowth.	Murine D3, G119(β1+/-), G201, G110(β1-/-)	No and Yes Hanging drop and mass cultures of EB's	Multiple neuronal-specific (NFM+) and glial specific (GFAP+) markers; GABA release; RT-PCR: Expression of NFL and NFM, NFH, synaptophysin, neurocan, tau	GFAP+	(127)
Neuroepithelium and neuroganglia are present in teratomas derived from human ES cell-like cells. For the first time, ES cell-like cells were derived from a human blastocyst. Transplantation of each of five cell lines into SCID-beige mice produced teratomas containing all three germ layers. The teratomas formed rosettes of neuroepithelium and neural ganglia after 4 mo.	human H1, H7, H9, H13, H14	No	Neuroepithelium and neuroganglia in teratomas	NE	(6)
Demonstration of neurons in EBs derived from human EG cells. First isolation of pluripotent EG cells from human PGCs. Cultured PGCs produced cells from all three derivatives of all three embryonic germ layers, including neuroepithelia.	human BF1, KF1, R13, R14, R15, BF2	No	NF+ in cultured EBs	S-100+ in cultured EBs	(108)

(continued)

Table 2 (continued)

Date	Observation	Cell line	RA induction	Neurons	Glia	Reference
1998	**RA induction favors differentiation of ventral CNS neurons.** RA exposure (2-/5+ protocol) generated neurons characteristic of the ventral CNS: somatic (1slet[+]) and cranial (Phox2b[+]) motoneurons and interneurons (islet[−]). RT-PCR demonstrated upregulated expression of GAD, TH, ChAT, *TrkB, TrkC*	Murine CCE	Yes 2-/5+ hanging drops	Somatic MNs and interneurons Nestin+ NPs Pax6[+], few Pax7[+], Islet-1/2[+], Phox2b[+], Lim 1/2[+], Lim3[+], EN1[+], peripherin[+] NFM[+], MAP-2[+] RT-PCR: GAD, TH, ChAT. RA enhanced expression of these, particularly ChAT.		(32)
	Demonstration of a strict temporal differentiation profile for neuroglial cells in RA-induced ES cell in culture. The cell types appeared on the following postplating days: neurons (5), astrocytes and oligodendrocytes (9), microglia (16). First demonstration of microglial differentiation from whole EBs. Therefore, EBs recapitulate the temporal order of neural cell development in the CNS.	Murine BLC6 (129/Sv Gat mouse blastocyst)	Yes RA as EBs	NSE[+] Synaptophysin[+]	GFAP[+] astrocytes O4[+] oligos C56[+] microglia	(128)
1999	**First demonstration that murine ES cells can myelinate in the immature CNS. Development of a procedure to enrich for GRPs from murine ES cells with potential for forming oligodendrocytes and astrocytes.** No RA used for induction. EB growth (4 d), then plated in ITSFn (5 d), then sequential propagation in (i) bFGF, (ii) bFGF and EGF, (iii) bFGF and PDGF. Demonstrated that the GRPs could myelinate axons in the developing nervous system of myelin-deficient mutant rats (spinal cord; 1 wk old; intraventricular at E17).	Murine J1 Cj7	No	NE	A2B5[+] precursors O4[+] CNPase[+] GFAP[+]	(49)
	Demonstration that BMP-4, a TGF-β superfamily member, inhibited RA-induced neural differentiation and enhanced mesodermal differentiation in murine ES cells. The effect of BMP-4 was restricted from d 5–8 of the 4/4[+] EB aggregation protocol. BMP-4 did not alter cell proliferation or death in EBs. As at baseline,	Murine D3	Yes 4-/4+	β-Tubulin III[+] (decreased 5–10-fold by BMP-4) NeuN[+], HNK-1[+]	GFAP[+] (decreased by BMP-4)	(40)

~25% of EB cells (4-/4+ stage at 5–6 d) were TUNEL+, as in earlier observations. Co-incubation with the anti-apoptotic molecule BAF (30–50 μM) reduced TUNEL+ by 35% but did not alter neural differentiation. The effect of BMP-4 could be reversed by coapplication of noggin, a BMP-4 antagonist.

Year	Description	Cell source	Conditions	Markers	Differentiated cells	Ref
1999	**Demonstration of murine ES cell as a source of late embryonic neural precursor cells.** NRPs (E-NCAM+) and GRPs (A2B5+/E-NCAM−) can be immunoderived from ES cell and can differentiate into postmitotic neurons and glia, respectively. ES cells grown as aggregates for 4 d, then plated on fibronectin-coated dishes in NEP basal medium. E-NCAM+ cells expressed early neuronal markers but not GFAP glial markers on differentiation (β-tubulin III+, MAP2+). Immunopanned E-NCAM+ ES cell-derived precursor cells expressed markers for neurons upon differentiation (glutamate, GAD, glycine+). ES cell-derived A2B5-immunoreactive cells differentiated into oligodendrocytes and two types of astrocytes (type I [A2B5−/GFAP+], II [A2B5+/GFAP+] astrocytes).	Murine D3	Yes—RA used for long-term culture PDGF used for long-term glial induction	E-NCAM+ differentiated cells: Glutamate+, GAD+, Glycine+ RT-PCR: ChAT, GAD, Glutaminase A2B5+/E-NCAM− differentiated cells: (−) for markers of differentiated neurons.	E-NCAM+ differentiated cells: no oligo or astrocytes A2B5+/E-NCAM− differentiated cells: Gal-C+ Olig Type I, II astrocytes	(129)
2000	**First demonstration that ES cell transplantation can be used to enhance recovery of lost function.** Transplantation of dissociated 4-/4+ RA-stimulated EBs into the spinal cord 9 days after contusion injury improved functional hindlimb spontaneous locomotion. ES cell-derived cells integrated, migrated 1 cm, and differentiated into neurons, oligodendrocytes and astrocytes.	Murine D3 ROSA26	Yes 4-/4+	NeuN+, EMA+	APC CC-1+ GFAP+	(79)
2000	**Differentiation of neurons from human ES cell-like cells.** Second demonstration of isolation of ES cells from human blastocysts. First demonstration that neural progenitors can be isolated from human ES cells and be induced to generate mature neurons. Two ES cell lines obtained from human blastocyst with demonstration of neuronal differentiation in vitro. The cell lines were able to be passaged 64 (HES-1)	Human HES-1 HES-2	No Yes (7–15 d RA exposure in culture) Hanging-drop	NFL+ NCAM+, Nestin+ RT-PCR: β-Actin, nestin, Pax6 NFH+, MAP2+, AP20+ Synaptophysin+, β-tubulin+ GAD+, Glutamate+ RT-PCR: GABA-ARecα2	NE	(9)

(continued)

Table 2 (*continued*)

Date	Observation	Cell line	RA induction	Neurons	Glia	Reference
	and 44 (HES-2) times, corresponding to a minimum of ~384 and 264 population doublings, respectively. Both lines were successfully recovered from cyropreservation. First demonstration of Oct-4 expression in human ES cells. Oct-4 is a POU domain transcription factor whose expression is limited in the mouse to pluripotent cells, and zygotic expression of Oct-4 is essential for establishing the pluripotent stem population of the inner cell mass. When both lines were transplanted into the testis of SCID mice, teratomas formed that contained derivatives of all three embryonic germ layers (examined 6–7 wk posttransplantation).					
	Demonstration of marked changes in calcium-binding proteins and voltage-dependent Ca^{2+} channel subtypes during in vitro differentiation of murine ES cell-derived neurons, using immunocytochemistry, patch clamp, and videomicroscopy time-lapse techniques. Neuronal maturation proceeded from apolar to bipolar to multipolar morphologies. All Ca^{2+} channel subtypes were expressed; apolar cells had mainly N- and L- type channels in contrast to the predominance of P/Q- and R-type channels in bipolar and multipolar cells. Parvalbumin was present in bipolar cells, while calretinin and calbindin were preferentially found in multipolar cells.	Murine		Parvalbumin$^+$ Calretinin$^+$ Calbindin$^+$ Physiology: N-, L-, P/Q-, R-type Ca^{2+} channel subtypes	NE	*(39)*
2000	**First demonstration that ES cell-derived oligodendrocytes could (1) myelinate axons in culture, (2) myelinate axons in the injured mature nervous system (spinal cord), (3) myelinate axons in the adult myelin mutant *shiverer* mouse**. A simple and rapid method was developed for isolating and purifying oligodendrocyte precursors. It involved an intermediate "oligosphere" step after 4$^-$/4$^+$ RA treated EBs were dissociated.	Murine D3 ROSA26	Yes 4$^-$/4$^+$	β-tubulin III$^+$, NF$^+$	NG2$^+$, O4$^+$, O1$^+$, MBP$^+$, CNPase$^+$ APC CC-1$^+$	*(30)*

Year	Description	Cell line	EB/RA induction	Neuronal markers	Glial markers	Ref
2001	**Demonstration that hES cells could be biased to produce neural progenitors and neurons.** RA- and EB-induction for 4 d, plating and growth in EGF, FGF, PDGF-AA, and replating to allow differentiation into subsets of neural precursors and mature neurons. Subsets of neural progenitors and mature neurons produced by FACS sorting with PS-NCAM and A2B5.	Human H1, H7, H9	Yes 4^+ (10 µM) 10X mESC induction	PS-NCAM$^+$ β-tubulin-III$^+$ MAP-2$^+$	A2B5$^+$ Rare-GFAP$^+$	(42)
	Demonstration that hES cells responded to b-NGF and RA by increasing the number of neural cells they produced. Found that EBs treated with RA (10^{-7} or 10^{-6} M) or β-NGF(100 ng/mL) NF-H$^+$ EBs significantly increased. RA-54% to 76%	Human H9	Yes $4^-/4^+$	NF-H$^+$ dopamine receptor$^+$ serotonin receptor$^+$	NE	(75)
	Demonstration that hES cells could grow as neural spheres in culture and could produce all three neural cell types. Isolated engraftable neural precursors from hES cells by sequential growth factor treatment and differential adhesion of the neural rosettes. Found that neuroepithelial cells lift from the culture dish after shorter exposure to dipase than do undifferentiated ES cells in the culture. In vivo, transplantation of neural spheres into the lateral ventricles of newborn mice resulted in the incorporation of ES cell-derived neurons and glia into various regions of the brain. Few oligodendrocytes were isolated using this differentiation method.	Human H1, H9, H9.1	No 4 d as EB plating, enzymatic removal of neural rosettes, suspension culture in bFGF medium	β-Tubulin III$^+$ NF$^+$ MAP2ab$^+$ TH$^+$	GFAP$^+$ O4$^+$ rare	(76)
	Demonstration that hES cells could grow as neural spheres in culture and could produce all three neural cell types. Derivation of highly enriched and expandable populations of neural progenitors, which could be induced to proliferate into neurons, astrocytes, and some oligodendrocytes. Spheres propagated 10 wk in the presence of bFGF and EGF and then plated in the absence of growth factors for 5 d resulted in 57% β-tubulin$^+$ and 26% GFAP$^+$ cells. In vivo, the neural precursor population differentiated into the three neural lineages when transplanted into the lateral ventricles of newborn mice.	Human HES-1	No Overgrowth of culture, mechanical removal of neural precursors, suspension culture in bFGF+ EGF	β-Tubulin III$^+$ NF$^+$ NSE$^+$ NF-M$^+$ MAP-2ab$^+$ Synaptophysin$^+$ Serotonin$^+$ TH$^+$	GFAP$^+$ O4$^+$	(9)

(continued)

317

Table 2 (*continued*)

Date	Observation	Cell line	RA induction	Neurons	Glia	Reference
2002	**Demonstration that exogenous addition of Shh to RA-treated EBs - shifts the production of neural subtype from midbrain to motor neuron phenotype.** Showed that embryonic patterning signals can be used to induce neuronal specification in vitro using the ES cell system. When motor neuron-enriched EBs were transplanted into chick spinal cord stage 15–17, they repopulated the ventral spinal cord, extended axons into the periphery, and formed synapses with muscle cells.	Murine MM13 W9.5 HBG3—(HB9eGFP transgene derived line)	Yes 2-/5 d+ RA/Shh	ChAT+ Isl1+ NeuN+	NE	(59)
	Induced production of midbrain dopaminergic neurons by constitutively expressing the tissue transcription factor Nurr-1 in mouse ESC. Nurr-1 leads to induction of tyrosine hydroxylase (TH) Resulted in a 4- to 5-fold increase in the proportion of DA neurons. Further increased the number of DA neurons by treatment with Shh, FGF8, and ascorbic acid. Showed that overexpression of transcription factors can drive differentiation down specific pathways.	Murine D3 Nurr-1 tg ESC	No EB induction followed by serum free treatment with bFGF (Okabe)	β-tubulin III+ TH+	NE	(43)
	Tau eGFP lineage selection and transplantation into embryonic day 14.5 Sprague–Dawley rats. Used differentiation protocols aimed at the production of neural progenitors and lineage selection with the tau/GFP knockin to enrich the ES cell-derived neuronal cell population to >90% purity.	Murine J1 tau-eGFP knock in	No EB induction followed by serum free treatment with bFGF (Okabe)	β-Tubulin III+ MAP2+ NeuN+ Synaptophysin+ TH+ Serotonin+	NE	(38)
2003	**NT-derived neurons and application in parkinsonian mice** Developed a protocol that produced ES cell-derived glia and neuronal subtypes by coculturing ES cells with MS5 (a stromal cell line derived from bone marrow) and timed sequential cytokine exposure. Cultures in vitro and in ES cell lines derived from	Murine CJ7 B5 BF1/lacZ-73 ntES cell C15 CT2	No Co-culture with MS5 stromal derived feeder layers	β-Tubulin III+ MAP2+ TH+ DAT+	GFAP+ O4+ O1+ NG2+ MBP+ CNPase+	(88)

nuclear transfer produced embryos. In vivo, transplanted ntES cell-derived dopamine neurons survived and expressed TH 8 wk after transplantation into a parkinsonian mouse model.

Year	Description	Cell line	Induction	In vitro	In vivo	Ref
	(continued)				none	*(45)*
2004	**Demonstration that Hedgehog signaling is required for differentiation of ES cell into neurectoderm.** Showed that ES cell lines mutant for hedgehog signaling were not able to form EBs containing neurectoderm and did not respond to RA or differentiate into neurons or glia. Used gene targeted null mutant ES cell lines: (1) Ptch1/lacZ, (2) ROSA/Smo -/-, (3) Ihh -/- to evaluate specific loss of function in the context of the in vitro ES cell system to dissect early events in neurogenesis.	Murine R1 D3 R1- Ptch1/lacz ROSA- Smo -/- Ihh -/-	Yes 4/4+	None found in -/- ESC lines in vitro	none	*(45)*
	Demonstration that ES cell-derived motor neurons cocultured with myoblasts or transplanted into a NSV-paralyzed rat model are capable of directional growth of axons, formation of neuromuscular junctions, and induction of muscle contraction. Showed that ES cell-derived motor neurons can be induced to extend axons into the peripheral nervous system through the white matter of the spinal cord.	Murine transgenic mouse derived ESC HB9-GFP HBG3	No EB induction 3 d Shh/RA Plated on astrocytes	ChAT+ NF-H+ Synaptophysin+ GFP expressed in axons	NE	*(80)*

Abbreviations: AChE, acetylcholinesterase; AMPAR, AMPA (α-amino-3-hydroxy-5-methyl-4-isoxazoleproprionic acid) receptor; APC CC-1, adenomatous polyposis coli, CC-1 subtype antibody; B27, defined media supplement (with RA); BF-1, brain factor 1; bFGF, fibroblast growth factor 1; BNP-4, bone morphogenic protein 4; ChAT, choline acetyl transferase; CNPase, 2',3'-cyclic nucleotide 3'-phosphodiesterase; D, day; DAT, dopamine transporter; DIV, days in vitro; EBs, embryoid bodies; EG, embryonic germ; EGF, epidermal growth factor; EMA, mouse specific antibody that preferentially recognizes neurons *(123)*; ES, embryonic stem; ESC, embryonic stem cell; FGF, fibroblast growth factor; GABA, gamma amino butyric acid; GAD, glutamic acid decarboxylase; Gal-C, galactocerebroside; GD3S, GD3 synthase; GFAP, glial fibrillary acid protein; GFP, green fluorescent protein; GluR, glutamate receptor; GRPs, glial restricted precursors; Ihh, Indian hedgehog; ITSFn, chemically defined media *(46)*; MAP2, microtubule associated protein 2; MBP, myelin basic protein; MN, motor neuron; N-CAM, neural cell adhesion molecule; N/A, not applicable; NE, not examined; NEP basal medium, neuroepithelial precursor basal media *(109)*; NSC, neural stem cell; NSE, neuron-specific enolase; NeuN, neuron-specific nuclear protein; NF(L,M,H), neurofilament (low, medium, and heavy forms); NG2, NG2 chondroitin sulfate proteoglycan; NGF, nerve growth factor; NMDA, N-methyl-D-aspartate; NPs, neural precursors; NEP, Neuroepithelial precursor; NRPs, neuronal restricted precursors; NSE, neuron specific enolase; O4, pre-oligodendrocyte marker; O1, mature oligodendrocyte marker; Oligo, oligodendrocyte; RA, retinoic acid; RAR, retinoic acid receptor; RT-PCR, reverse transcription polymerase chain reaction; SCID, severe combined immunodeficiency; Shh, sonic hedgehog; SQ, subcutaneous; TEM, transmission electron microscopy; T3Rα, T3 receptor alpha; TH, tyrosine hydroxylase; Trk, tyrosine kinase; TTX, tetrodotoxin; +, positive reactivity; (-), double gene allele inactivation; 4/4+ RA, Induction protocol where EBs are exposed to RA only in the last 4 d of an 8-d protocol.

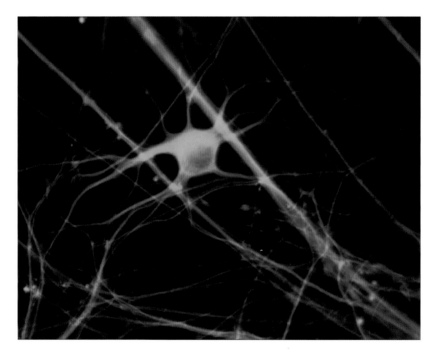

Fig. 2. Mixed neural cell culture derived from mouse ES cells.

bodies are pooled and dissociated with trypsin, plated as monolayers onto adhesive substratum. Neural subtypes are generated by adding neurotrophic factors to the medium which selectively support the survival of primary neural cultures. Growth in neural basal medium supplemented with serum generates mixed cultures containing mostly neurons (about 40%) and astrocytes with a few oligodendrocytes *(26,27)*.

In the original studies, cellular division was inhibited on d 2–4 in vitro by cytosine arabinoside (Ara-C). Ara-C exposure selects against the development of oligodendrocytes, which are highly sensitive to Ara-C-induced death (McDonald et al., *unpublished observations*), whereas omitting Ara-C generates cultures containing large numbers of oligodendrocytes *(30)*. We have also observed that embryoid bodies induced with the $4^-/4^+$ retinoic acid protocol can produce substantial amounts of extracellular matrix when plated. This extracellular matrix markedly reduces the effectiveness of immunocytochemical labeling of cell-surface proteins (McDonald, et al., *unpublished observations*). Because most oligodendrocyte lineage-specific antibodies label cell-surface epitopes, ES cell-derived cultures have to be partially permeabilized before cell labeling can be measured accurately *(30)*. Application of the same type of medium used to enrich for oligodendrocytes in primary central nervous system (CNS) cultures has allowed for enrichment of oligodendrocytes in mouse ES cell-derived cultures, providing useful in vitro models of myelination *(30)*.

Alternative retinoic acid induction protocols have been developed. For example, Strubing et al. *(34)* and Fraichard et al. *(29)* induced differentiation via the embryoid body but exposed cultures to retinoic acid only during the first 2 d of culture. When the resulting cells were plated onto substratum, neurons were observed on d 4–5.

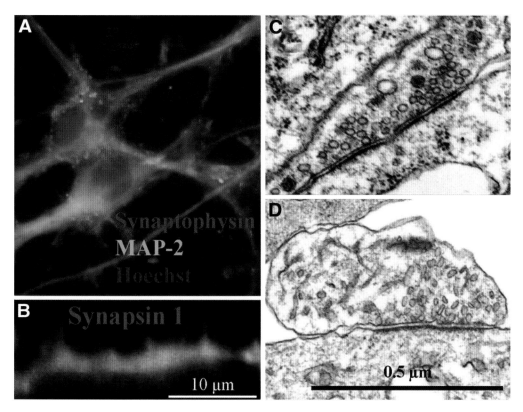

Fig. 3. ES cells that have been induced to become neural precursors spontaneously form thousands of synaptic contacts with each other, creating functional neural networks. ES cells induced with retinoic acid were cultured in defined medium for 9 d and then immunolabeled for receptive dendrites (*green* = MAP-2) and presynaptic markers (*red* = synaptophysin). Panel (**A**) depicts ES cell-derived neurons (*green*) covered with multiple synapses (*red*). Synapses formed not only at cell bodies but also at axons. Panel (**B**) shows a high-power image of a dendrite with presynaptic markers. Panels (**C,D**) demonstrate TEM images of ES cell-derived synapses. (Reproduced with permission from ref. *99*.)

Renoncourt et al. used a $2^-/5^+$ retinoic acid induction protocol to produce neurons with characteristics of the ventral CNS: somatic (Islet$^+$) and cranial (Phox2b$^+$) motoneurons and interneurons (Istet$^-$) *(32)*.

Basic Fibroblast Growth Factor (bFGF) Induction Methods

Retinoic acid-free methods for producing neuronal cells from mouse ES cell cultures have also been developed. These systems take advantage of the development of an embryoid body intermediary in chemically defined medium. The surviving cells are then cultured in medium containing bFGF, which enhances the survival and proliferation of neural progenitors.

To generate nestin$^+$ progenitors and subsequent mixed neural/glial cultures, Okabe et al. *(31)* and Brustle et al. *(49)* made use of bFGF's ability to propagate neural stem cells *(50,51)*. Mouse ES cells were cultured as embryoid bodies for 4 d and then plated on substratum in the presence of bFGF in a defined medium lacking serum *(31)*. Under

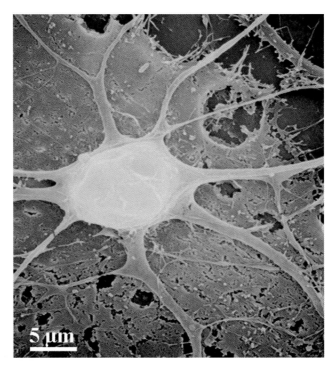

Fig. 4. Scanning EM shows solitary oligodendrocyte in a mixed culture of ES cell-derived neural cells. Scale bar = 5 μm.

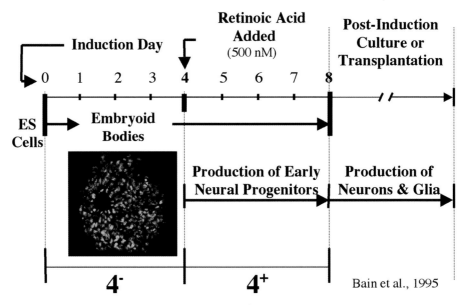

Fig. 5. Schematic comparison of ES cell differentiation and early embryo development. The ES cells we begin with are similar to the cells of the 4-d-old mouse embryo. Day 4 of ES cell differentiation in culture is similar to the time in the embryo when the cells are making fate choices into the three major classes of cells. When ES cells are induced to differentiate into the three principle types of nerve cells in culture, the early rudiments of organs are forming in the human embryo. The recapitulation of development is commonly held as an important feature of successful regeneration such as that we are attempting after spinal cord injury.

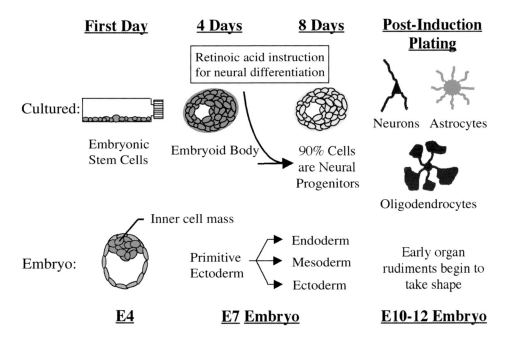

Fig. 6. Schematic description of ES cell differentiation. The method of differentiation used in our studies is outlined as originally developed by Bain et al. ES cells are grown in clusters called embryoid bodies. After 4 d (4⁻), cells are exposed to retinoic acid for 4 d. This process, termed 4⁻/4⁺, protocol instructs the ES cells to become neural lineage cells. At the 4⁻/4⁺ stage cells are plated in culture or transplanted.

those conditions, most of the cells died but the bFGF-sensitive precursor population survived and continued to replicate in the presence of this mitogen. This method selected for nestin⁺/keratin18⁻ neural progenitor cells *(31)*. Withdrawal of bFGF induced the cells to differentiate into neurons and glia. However, some contaminating SSEA1⁺ pluripotent cells and keratin18⁺ ectodermal cells were detected after differentiation under these conditions.

Similar methods of bFGF selection and propagation have been used to isolate uniform populations of mouse ES cell-derived nestin⁺ neural precursors *(52)*, which can be cryopreserved, recovered with good viability, and expanded in culture in the presence of bFGF *(53)*. These cells can later be differentiated into functional neurons.

Induction of Neurogenesis by Sonic Hedgehog

During normal development, motor neurons are among the first neurons to appear. In vertebrates, their induction from the notochord and floorplate is mediated by sonic hedgehog (Shh), a secreted glycoprotein *(54)*. Shh represses *Pax7* expression, giving rise to CNS progenitors. A gradient in Shh activity also regulates *Pax6* expression in progenitor cells and influences the identity of developing neurons, determining whether they become interneurons or motoneurons *(55,56)*. Retinoic acid may also ventralize neuronal development by promoting the generation of neurons characteristic of the ventral spinal cord. This hypothesis comes from the observation that retinoic acid may select for hindbrain neural phenotypes *(57)*.

The application of temporally expressed growth factors to mouse ES-derived progenitor populations has produced specific neuronal subtypes. Much of the focus has been on the BMP and Shh, as these proteins are key dorsal–ventral organizers of the vertebrate notochord and neural tube *(58)*.

Wichterle et al. were able to generate interneurons and motor neurons by exposing retinoic acid-treated mouse embryoid bodies to Shh. The effect depended on the concentration of Shh in the culture medium *(59)*. Maye et al. demonstrated that mouse ES cell lines lacking hedgehog signaling cascade produce embryoid bodies that do not have neuroectoderm. These mutant embryoid bodies do not produce nestin[+] cells in response to retinoic acid treatment. The authors concluded that the developmental progression from ectoderm to neuroectoderm is blocked in absence of hedgehog signaling *(45)*.

The identification of proteins that regulate transcription cascades that direct differentiation down specific pathways will impact our ability to use ES cells as tools of discovery and therapeutics.

Oligodendrocyte Cultures

Oligodendrocytes, the myelinating cells of the CNS, arise from oligodendrocyte precursors (OLP), which develop in a restricted pattern in the neural tube of the embryo. The patterning of the neural tube is established by Shh and BMPs, which are expressed at opposite axes of the tube. Shh is expressed in the ventral floorplate, and BMPs are expressed in the roofplate. The concentration of these proteins and the transcription factors they regulate establish distinct regions within the neural tube that specify the lineages of neural progenitor populations *(58)*.

bFGF has been used to enrich glial precursors from murine ES cells *(30,49)*. Brustle et al. *(49)* produced cultures enriched to about 30% in neural cells, mostly oligodendrocytes, by using a temporal exposure to bFGF and platelet-derived growth factor (PDGF). These methods are extensions of previous studies of oligodendrocyte precursors, neurospheres, and oligospheres *(60,61)*. McKay and colleagues induced differentiation by growing embryoid bodies in suspension for 4 d and then plating them for 5 d in a chemically defined medium adapted from SATO medium, ITSFn *(49,62)*. Transplanting neurosphere-derived cells into embryonic or postnatal rat CNS resulted in differentiation into oligodendrocytes and myelination of host axons.

A simple procedure was developed to highly enrich oligodendrocytes in culture *(30)*. Plating dissociated 4[-]/4[+] retinoic acid-induced murine embryoid bodies into SATO-defined medium produced mixed cultures that included oligodendrocytes capable of myelinating ES-derived neurons. A key point for success was the absence of Ara-C, which limits oligodendrocyte survival.

Further enrichment in oligodendrocytes can be achieved by plating dissociated 4[-]/4[+] retinoic acid-induced embryoid bodies on nonadhesive plates in a chemically defined medium that lacks serum and is supplemented with bFGF. Under these conditions, the cells reaggregate. We term these aggregates oligospheres because, when plated, they produce cultures highly enriched in oligodendrocytes *(30)*. Oligospheres are dissociated after 2 d and replated under similar conditions for another 4 d. Trypsin-dissociated oligospheres can then be plated on adhesive substratum in oligodendrocyte-supporting defined medium to obtain highly enriched cultures of oligodendrocytes. Further enrichment to about 90% can be achieved by plating dissociated oligosphere in conditioned medium *(30)*.

Induction in Monolayer Culture

The most widely used method for inducing ES cell differentiation involves an embryoid body intermediary. Suspended ES cells that have been allowed to aggregate are exposed to mitogens, then dissociated and reattached to a substratum in the presence or absence of mitogens or trophic factors that stimulate proliferation or sustain specific populations.

This method is an effective way to stimulate ES cell differentiation, but it does not permit the development of high-throughput quantitative assays or the systematic evaluation and identification of mechanisms that drive differentiation. Because the multilayered, three-dimensional structure of the embryoid body complicates the interpretation of the effects of mitogens or pharmacological agents on differentiation. It is likely that diffusion gradients are established across the embryoid body, which may contribute to the heterogeneity observed in these systems.

The development of monolayer culture may simplify the experimental process and interpretation of results. One method reported by Ying et al. *(63)* takes advantage of molecular markers to identify neural precursor populations and eliminate nonneural populations. Mouse ES cells were genetically modified at the *Sox1*, the earliest known marker of neuroectoderm in the mouse *(64)*. *Sox1* is not expressed in undifferentiated ES cells, but is up-regulated in neuroectoderm and down-regulated during neuronal and glial differentiation, which makes it a good marker of early neuronal induction. GPF/Puro was knocked into the open reading frame of the *Sox1* locus. The knock-in behaved as expected in vivo and in vitro. In the mouse, GFP was expressed in neuronal tissue at embryonic day 8.5. When this ES cell line was plated on gelatin in the absence of LIF in defined medium (N2B27), more than 60% of the cells expressed GFP by 4 d of monolayer culture *(63)*.

As in all protocols reported to date, neural induction is asynchronous and incomplete. In this case, 10–15% of the cells expressed *Oct4* and remained undifferentiated, and differentiated cells that did not express *Sox1* contaminated the culture. Both populations could be eliminated by FACS or selection with puromycin *(63)*.

Coculture Methods for Enriching ES Cell-Derived Neural Precursors

The development of culture methods that use cells or conditioned medium from the stromal cell line PA6, the hepatoma cell line Hep-G2, and astrocytes have been developed to take advantage of unknown factors and environmental cues that drive ES cells to neurogenesis.

During neurogenesis in the developing embryo, neural progenitor populations, which arise in the neural tube, are specified in response to signaling molecules from adjacent tissues. The dorsal–ventral axis is established through a concentration gradient of Shh from the floor plate and notochord, a structure of mesenteric origin, and of BMP-4 from the roof plate and the overlying surface ectoderm *(25)*.

PA6 Stromal Cells

Kawasaki et al. described stromal cell neural inducing activity (SDIA) derived from bone marrow. SDIA induced neurogenesis of mouse ES cells which were grown on

PA6 cells or in suspension in the presence of PA6-conditioned medium. In this coculture system, 90% of the ES cell became neural cell adhesion molecule positive (NCAM+) and only 2% expressed mesenteric markers. This method efficiently produced TH-expressing neurons. However, it is not a synchronous induction method, and ES cell colonies cultured on the PA6 stromal layer contained both precursor and differentiated neuronal cells. This method may be useful for producing dopaminergic neurons *(65,66)*.

Hep-G2 Cells

Rathjen et al. used conditioned medium (MEDII) from the hepatoma cell line Hep-G2 to produce a nearly homogeneous population of neural precursors that was equivalent to the embryonic neuroectoderm according to tests for known stage-specific expression makers. Embryoid bodies formed a distinctive morphology, resembling neural plate/neural tube. After 9 d in culture, 95% of the cells expressed the NEP markers Sox1, Sox2, nestin, and NCAM. Neurons, glial lineages, and neural crest were formed *(67)*.

Astrocytes

Nakayama et al. used astrocytes and astrocyte-conditioned medium (ACM) to induce neuronal differentiation of mouse and primate ES cells. Entire ES cell colonies were mechanically removed from the fibroblast feeder layer and induced to differentiate by culturing them in suspension in ACM. The cellular spheres formed nestin+ cells on the periphery, but the cells in the center of the sphere expressed Oct4 and remained undifferentiated. When the spheres were plated onto substratum, only neurons were identified; this procedure did not generate glial cells *(68)*.

METHODS FOR SELECTIVELY ENRICHING PRECURSOR POPULATIONS

Cell surface markers and genetic approaches have been used to enrich specific cell lineages. Thus, pure populations of lineage-restricted progenitors and terminally differentiated cells can be isolated. Two successful techniques are immunopanning, which makes use of cell-surface antigens to isolate specific populations, and FACS, which uses fluorescent tags. Enrichment methods requiring genetic manipulation of ES cells and expression of certain proteins with selectable markers such as neomycin- and puromycin-resistance genes can generate highly purified populations.

Immunopanning and FACS

Immunopanning has been used to isolate neural progenitors *(69,70)* and glial restricted precursors *(69–71)* from embryonic rodent spinal cord and murine and human ES cells *(42)*. Mouse neural precursors can be positively selected using E-NCAM, and glial restricted precursors can be selected by first removing the E-NCAM+ precursor cells and then selecting for A2B5+ cells. In the case of human ES-derived neuronal cells, PS-NCAM and A2B5 have been used to enrich for neural precursors *(42)*. In both mouse and human cells, NCAM+ positive progenitor populations are restricted to the neural lineages. However, human ES-derived precursors expressing A2B5 generate cells with neuronal morphology and flat cells, some of which also express GFAP.

On separation, the PS-NCAM population differentiates into neurons, and the A2B5 population differentiates into neurons and astrocytes *(42)*.

Wernig et al. used FACS to isolate a tau-expressing population after inducing differentiation with the method of Okabe *(31,38)*. Tau is a microtubule-binding protein known to be strongly expressed in neurons *(72)*. In brief, eGFP was knocked into the tau locus of a mouse ES cell line by gene targeting. The resulting cells, which expressed eGFP under the control of the *tau* locus, were differentiated through an embryoid body intermediary in defined medium for 4 d. The embryoid bodies were then dissociated and plated in medium containing bFGF. Terminal differentiation was induced by withdrawal of bFGF from the culture medium. The resulting population was 95% neuronal.

Genetic Lineage Selection

In theory, the most efficient and effective method of cell lineage selection is genetic selection. Combinatorial positive and negative selection paradigms can be used simultaneously to enrich and eliminate the cells expressing a given gene. Cell purification methods can then be applied to obtain even greater enrichment.

Nuclear receptor 1 (*Nurr*-1) is required for the specification of ventral neural progenitors to dopaminergic neurons *(43,73)*. The number of TH^+ expressing neurons was increased fivefold when Nurr-1 was overexpressed in neural precursors *(43)*.

ES-derived neural progenitor populations express the NEP markers Sox1, Sox2, and nestin and have the potential to differentiate into both neurons and glia. Sox2 is expressed in the uncommitted dividing stem cell populations in the ICM, epiblast, and germ cells as well as in the precursor cells of the developing CNS *(36)*. Li et al. used gene targeting to knock β-geo into the *Sox2* locus, conferring G-418 resistance to ES cells expressing Sox2 *(37)*. The resulting cells were differentiated, using the $4^-/4^+$ method of Bain *(27)*. After they were plated on substratum, 90% were nestin$^+$. However, only 50% of the nestin$^+$ population expressed Sox2. Through selection with G-418, the nestin$^+$/Sox2-negative population was eliminated from the culture. The remaining G-418-resistant population represented a population of neural precursors expressing both nestin and Sox2 *(37)*.

Ying et al. knocked GFP/Puro into the *Sox1* locus so that neural progenitors expressing Sox1 could be sorted by FACS (because they expressed GFP) or selected with puromycin. Thus, the Sox1-positive population was selected, and nonneural cells were efficiently eliminated from the culture *(63)*.

NEUROGENESIS AND HUMAN EMBRYONIC STEM CELLS

The isolation of human ES cells and the discovery that these cells, like mouse ES cells, have the potential to differentiate into cell types derived from all three germ layers has renewed interest in finding methods for predictably driving differentiation of ES cells down specific lineages.

The differentiation protocols developed for the mouse ES cell system have provided a starting point for developing robust and reliable methods for human ES cell differentiation. Human ES cells can be induced to differentiate spontaneously by removing them from substrata. Growth in suspension culture in the presence of fetal calf serum *(6,9)*. Under these conditions, human ES cells form embryoid bodies composed of an endodermal outer layer and ectodermal inner layer. After 4 d of growth in suspension, Oct4 is down-regulated and cell types from all three germ layers can be identified (9). Schuldiner et al. showed that human ES cell could be induced to produce specific precursor and mature cell types in culture, when growth factors were added to the medium (74). Human ES cells were cultured as embryoid bodies for 5 d, then dissociated and plated in a monolayer that was exposed to growth factors. The resulting cultures were more homogeneous than untreated controls, with up to half of the culture containing just one or two cell types (9,74).

Human ES cells have been shown to produce neuronal cells in response to retinoic acid (42,75). Carpenter et al. enriched for neural precursors in culture by following a modified embryoid body/retinoic acid induction protocol. The cells were then replated into differentiation medium containing neurotrophic factors to enrich for neuronal cell types. Under these conditions, human ES cell differentiated into neural derivatives expressing the lineage-specific cell-surface markers PS-NCAM and A2B5. These markers were used in magnetic bead and immunopanning to further enrich for specific precursor populations. The PS-NCAM-positive cells were restricted into multiple neuronal phenotypes, including a small population of TH-positive, dopamine-responsive neurons. They did not appear to generate astrocytes or oligodendrocytes. The A2B5-expressing cells appeared to differentiate into a mixed population of neurons and astrocytes (42).

In a multistep induction method reported by Zhang et al., embryoid bodies plated in the presence of bFGF attached to the substratum and differentiated to form neural rosettes, which were removed from the dish using selective enzymatic digestion. The rosettes were grown in suspension culture in the presence of bFGF to form neurospheres, which gave rise to neurons, astrocytes, and a few oligodendrocytes when plated (76).

Reubinoff et al. did not use an embryoid body intermediary. By allowing human ES cells to overgrow in culture while attached to the feeder or substratum they obtained spontaneous neural differentiation at the edges of the human ES cell colony. The differentiated cells were removed mechanically from the undifferentiated colonies, then grown in suspension as neurospheres in the presence of bFGF and epidermal growth factor (EGF). Under these conditions, the neural precursor population proliferated and produced neurons, astrocytes, and some oligodendrocytes when plated on appropriate substratum (9,77).

Although some oligodendrocytes have been produced under these culture conditions, their numbers have been very limited. Therefore, experimental protocols for obtaining enriched cultures of myelin-producing cells are required in order to understand the molecular mechanisms that drive oligodendrocyte development.

Zwaka and Thomson showed that human ES cells are capable of homologous recombination at the HPRT1 and Oct4 loci. Human ES cells were electroporated in clumps, not as single cells, and were plated at high density. Using this protocol, homologously targeted clones were isolated. This advance should greatly enhance the utility of human ES cells for drug discovery. For human ES cells to fulfill their potential, however, it will be necessary to develop mechanisms for selecting and modifying progenitor populations as well as eliminating unwanted differentiated and undifferentiated populations (78).

ES CELLS AND TRANSPLANTATION

Since we wrote the chapter on ES cells and neurogenesis in 1999–2000 *(11)*, the rules governing neurogenesis in the ES cell system have become better understood. However, ES cells are just beginning to be exploited for neurotransplantation.

Important early efforts demonstrated that nervous system cells derived from ES cells are largely normal in terms of differentiation, integration, and function. Most of these studies were performed in vitro, but similar functions are now being assessed in vivo *(30,79)*. ES cell transplantation has revealed that neural cells derived from ES cells and transplanted into the injured adult CNS can differentiate into all three principal neural cell types as well as contribute to a large range of neuronal phenotypes *(30,79)*. To date, integration of transplanted cells has been limited largely to anatomy, neuronal circuits, and oligodendrocyte myelination. Functional integration has not been demonstrated. Although some studies have demonstrated electrophysiologic integration in terms of activity, that is far removed from determining the functional importance of such integration *(80,81)*.

An important question is whether neurons or nervous system cells derived from ES cells behave similarly or differently from embryonic, fetal, and adult stem cells. Although this question remains largely unanswered, a growing body of work is beginning to suggest functional differences *(82)*. For example, nervous system cells derived from ES cells appear to differentiate much more quickly than neural stem cells derived from the adult nervous system *(30)*. They also are uniquely able to create extracellular matrix, make metalloproteinases, and remodel the extracellular environment.

Our naive view replacing neuronal elements of the major role of transplantation is giving way to the idea that transplanted stem cells have additional functions. For example, transplanted ES cells can modulate the host environment to make it more hospitable to regeneration. Recent evidence from our laboratories and those of Dr. Jerry Silver demonstrates that ES cell-derived neural stem cells make metalloproteinases that can destroy inhibitory barriers such as those formed by chondroitin sulfates *(unpublished observation)*. ES cell transplantation also directly modulates the immune response: we observed a 50% reduction in the number of macrophages responding to ES cell transplantation compared with sham-transplanted animals. This effect does not appear to result simply from altered proliferation or reduced survival but involves mechanisms that attract macrophages to the nervous system. In addition, ES cells can make a number of proregenerative growth factors, including brain-derived neurotrophic factor and NT3.

To date, ES cells have been shown to differentiate into neurons, astrocytes, and oligodendrocytes when transplanted as neural precursors into the adult injured nervous system *(30,79–81)*. Their transplantation can also produce stable populations or resident pools of progenitor cells.

These initial observations extend data from previous studies that used other sources of cells for transplantation *(83)*. To date, the potential of ES cells as a discovery tool is largely untapped. An exception is the use of ES cells that express GFP, which can therefore be traced after transplantation *(30,84)*. Markers such as GFP also permit neural components such as myelin and axons to be located. Thus, ES cells expressing GFP on neural promoters have proven to be very effective for neuroanatomical tracing of transplanted cells. Using GFP-labeled cells, it has been possible to demonstrate that ES cell-derived oligodendrocytes myelinate appropriately in the nervous system by servicing more than one passing axon. Furthermore, it has been possible to trace the axons and dendrites from growing neurons. Advances in imaging and optics now pave the way for using ES cells to monitor cellular function in real time (real-time imaging).

ES cells with protein production deleted or added have also proved useful. For example, work with ES cells overexpressing Bcl-2 or Bcl-XL has demonstrated that cell survival is enhanced when programmed cell death is inhibited *(85)*. Although interpretation of these studies is complicated, ES cells can serve as tools for many types of transplantation experiments.

The earliest wave of genetic modification focused on nonspecific markers such as GFP. The focus is now shifting to more specific markers, such as GFP fusion proteins with myelin or with synapse-associated proteins such as fusion proteins of GFP with myelin or synapsin in order to track or quantify myelin or synapses *(86)*. Such markers should permit rapid in vivo analysis and greatly improve anatomical delineation.

Transplantation studies promise more than anatomical and molecular markers, however. For example, genetically modified ES cells will allow functional integration to be reversibly tested. By selectively and temporally overexpressing factors that inhibit neuronal function, we will be able to test the hypothesis that transplanted neurons can contribute to novel circuits and to behavioral improvements associated with transplantation. It may be possible to express the antisense RNA to myelin basic protein; producing a dysfunctional oligodendrocyte and thereby testing the importance of replacing oligodendrocytes *(87)*.

ES CELLS OFFER A UNIQUE PATH TO HUMAN TRANSPLANTATION

Numerous political and religious issues surrounding human ES cells have overshadowed the discussion of the scientific challenges that face scientists. To be successful in humans, transplantable cells must meet two important criteria. First, they must contain the same DNA as the recipient. Second, they must be able to differentiate into the cell types normally present in the area of the nervous system being transplanted. Although the nervous system has considerable immunological privilege, histocompatibility will be essential for most nervous system transplant approaches to be successful as many diseases repeatedly break down the blood–brain barrier, making rerejection more likely if transplanted cells differ genetically from the host nervous system cells.

ES cells will allow us to meet both of these important criteria. First, they can differentiate into nervous system cells of multiple lineages. Second, and more importantly, they can obtain the genetic identity of host via nuclear transfer. Specifically, a nucleus from a somatic cell from the transplant recipient can be transferred into an enucleated fertilized egg whose cytoplasm contains the necessary information for replication and generation of an ES cell with host DNA. Recent work demonstrating ES cell derivation from a cloned human embryo suggests that this avenue may be more possible than previously thought *(10)*. Hwang et al. provided an important proof of the principle by creating human ES cells using a somatic cell as a genetic (nuclear) source *(10)*, although only 3.3% of the blastocysts used produced ES cells.

Moreover, the donor somatic cell and oocytes were taken from the same individual, which would mean, in the absence of technical advances that only patients with a supply of healthy oocytes could benefit from therapeutic cloning. Other substantial challenges are reprogramming an egg without inducing abnormalities; inducing and targeting differentiation, controlling stem cell proliferation, and solving the remaining subtle dilemmas or rerejection due to small incompatibilities in major histocompatibility complex (MHC) I and II molecules secondary to reprogramming errors. Nevertheless, the work of Hwang's group in Korea has generated much enthusiasm for research on regenerative medicine, creating a much more favorable climate than in many other countries, including those in North America.

The technique of generating ES cells from somatic cells by nuclear transfer (ntES cells) is relatively new. Studies from mice demonstrate that ntES cells can be established using nuclei from fibroblasts with an efficiency of 10–20%. Cells from donors of either gender and from lines that have never been successfully produced a live cloned animal can be used *(88,89)*. If these results translate to humans, improvements in therapeutic cloning techniques may enable any patient to act as his or own ntES cells donor. It is clear from the mouse studies that success rates for deriving ntES cell lines can be as much as an order of magnitude higher than those for reproductive cloning, reflecting the easier task of creating individual cells in the case of ES cells vs an entire organism in the case of reproductive cloning.

That said, a series of scientific barriers must be overcome before ntES cells can be generated for therapeutic purposes. First, it is clear that we need to better understand the epigenetic and reprogramming that occurs when a nucleus is transferred in order to avoid the developmental abnormalities that are evident in cloned animals *(90)*. Such abnormalities range from placental anomalies to premature aging and mortality of unknown cause, and it is probable that even apparently normal cloned animals have epigenetic defects. Other deficiencies, such as abnormal gene expression patterns and retention of somatic cell-like features have also been reported in cloned animal blastocysts *(91,92)*. These abnormalities have been largely attributed to insufficient reprogramming of donor nuclei, but little is known about reprogramming, even in the normal situation. However, because cloned animals do not appear to pass their abnormalities to their offspring, derivation of germline cells for restorative medicine might not be impossible *(93)*.

At this instance, it is unclear whether cloned blastocysts are inherently different from their natural counterparts or whether such potential differences are artifacts. In contrast, only 10–20% of the few (1–2%) cloned mouse blastocysts that develop to term (the others die soon after implantation) give rise to ntES cells. At a more practical level, the scarcity of human oocytes is a formidable obstacle to using parthenogenesis or oocytes to generate ntES cells. This problem, however, might be addressed by interspecies nuclear transfer or by generating gametes from ES cells. For example, nonhuman oocytes, such as rabbit oocytes, have the potential to reprogram human somatic cell nuclei to establish human ntES cell lines *(94)*. Furthermore, oocytes can be created by in vitro differentiation from ES cells *(95)*. Future studies are required to demonstrate whether oocytes derived from ES cells have the same developmental potential as natural ones and whether the human immune system will tolerate the progeny of ntES cells derived from cross-species oocytes and containing cross-species mitochondrial DNA.

Hopefully, such techniques will some day provide an ample supply of these precious biological resources without the need to obtain oocytes from women. One study has already demonstrated that ntES cells derived from mouse fibroblasts can rescue an immune-deficient phenotype by transplanting progeny cells differentiated into hematopoietic stem cells in vitro *(96)*. Another study involving fibroblast-derived ntES cells showed that neural differentiation could be achieved with higher efficiency than with oocyte-derived ES cells *(88)*. However, successful therapeutic application of ES cells will involve many technically demanding processes. These include nuclear transfer, ntES cells derivation, induction and guidance of differentiation in vitro, and effective delivery of cells to target sites in a patient's body. Parallel advances in these other areas are bringing the global challenge into a more doable range. For example, major efforts are developing percutaneous transplantation methods that can be completed in an outpatient setting, thereby avoiding the large and risky hurdle of intraoperative transplantation.

Although therapeutics often dominate discussions of ES cell potential, it is clear that such cells will make a much greater contribution as tools of scientific discovery, as has been demonstrated by their role in generating transgenic mice, one of the major scientific advances of the past two decades. The revolution in neuroscience caused by the availability of such transgenic mice is advancing to include ES cells in vitro. Whereas transgenic murine fetuses lacking both alleles of an important gene rarely survive, cells can often tolerate such deletions. Moreover, transgenic mice are often produced as a reproducible source of cultured cells, which can now be obtained more efficiently in vitro from ES cells.

RELATIONSHIP BETWEEN NEURAL STEM CELLS DERIVED FROM ES CELLS AND THOSE DERIVED FROM THE CNS

This relationship, which is not well understood, is perhaps one of the most important issues to be addressed before we can consider using ES-derived neural progenitors in drug discovery programs and cell replacement therapies. The major limitations now reflect the limited tools available to identify neural progenitors. These identity systems have initially focused on the absence and presence of immunological cellular epitopes that unfortunately are only partially stage-specific. Advances in genomics and proteomics are offering the prospects for genetic and protein fingerprints of different progenitor cells. Expression of genes and proteins, however, is only one criterion for identification. Additional functional and ultrastructural specifications will prove more pragmatic.

The characteristics used to select and classify stem cells include: (1) stage-specific markers, (2) mitogen/growth factor dependence, and (3) the phenotypes of the cells they produce (neurons, astrocytes, or oligodendrocytes). By comparing native stem cells with stem cells derived from ES cells, we should be able to develop methods for isolating distinct progenitor populations that make use of expression patterns of surface markers and transcription factors. Such methods may lead to protocols for stimulating endogenous neural stem cells to regenerate and repair damaged neural tissue. Moreover, hematopoietic stem cell research may serve as a model because neurogenesis follows the same type of developmentally restrictive pattern: neural stem cells renew themselves and differentiate through asymmetric cell division into cells that are restricted to neural and glial progenitor phenotypes; these partially restricted cells differentiate further into fully restricted cell types of either the neuronal or glial lineage.

Self-renewing neural stem cell populations were discovered only recently in the adult CNS, and it will take much work to understand their roles in homeostasis and disease. By comparing neural stem cells derived from ES cells with those derived from the CNS, we may be able to more quickly identify key factors that regulate the stem cell pool and drive differentiation. The ultimate goal of transplantation is to understand how to harness the potential of similar endogenous stem cells.

THE ES CELL SYSTEM:
ADVANTAGES, LIMITATIONS, AND POTENTIAL

The in vitro ES cell system has great scientific and therapeutic potential, although we are just beginning to tap into the potential and the use of ES cells for transplantation has yet to advance to what has been accomplished with other sources of transplantable cells.

The ES cell system is the only model system that offers sufficient access to the first stages of development for investigating the earliest molecular events of development and repair. It is this in vitro ES cell system that will provide the greatest advances in scientific discovery, mirroring the exponential progress of the transgenic mouse era. The in vitro ES cell system is currently being used in drug discovery and functional genomics to identify the earliest molecular cues that trigger development and disease *(97)*.

Hurdles must be overcome before this potential can be realized. For example, protocols that predictably drive differentiation down desired pathways, while eliminating unwanted cell types, have not yet been developed. Identifying a cohort of cell surface markers and transcription factors expressed in various progenitor populations provide a starting point. Moreover, as more is learned about gene expression patterns in the developing embryo, the temporal application of specific factors will lead to the production and isolation of specific cell types.

The human ES cell system has special advantages in providing a reproducible source of differentiated human cells that are normal. This is in contrast to today's use of immortalized human cell lines. Most of the current protocols for differentiating human ES cells have been adapted from mouse methods. Mouse and human ES cells show similar gene expression patterns and growth characteristics, however they are not identical *(98)*. Thus, we need to identify the developmental pathways and programs that differ between human and mouse ES cell systems. Unique problems also exist in the human ES cell system. Currently there is no gold standard for unambiguous identification of undifferentiated totipotent human ES cells. For ethical reasons, the parallel to the mouse ES cell identification of germline transmission is not possible with the human ES cell system. Accordingly, the molecular fingerprints of undifferentiated ES cells are beginning to be identified using proteomic and genomic strategies.

Unique problems also exist in studying transplantation of human ES cells since early allogenic transplantation is not possible and we must study the transplantation of human ES cells into rodents or nonhuman primates.

We also need to develop culture methods that maintain ES cells in a karyotypically normal state for prolonged periods. This will become a critical issue in the field in the forthcoming years. Protocols for synchronizing ES cell differentiation and eliminating unwanted, undifferentiated cells will be paramount.

Although animal models can be used to approximate the human condition, they are only models and most are not entirely accurate. There are many disorders, unique to humans, where animal models do not even exist. For example, although hepatitis kills millions of afflicted people annually, there are no suitable animal models of this disease because the viruses that cause human hepatitis only infect human cells. The advantages of establishing in vitro model systems, using human ES cells to evaluate such human cell specific diseases, are innumerable.

Also, human ES cell studies will have profound implications for the treatment of human disease. All diseases ultimately involve the death or dysfunction of cells. When disease results from abnormalities in specific cell types, as in Parkinson's disease (dopaminergic neurons), Alzheimer's disease (cholinergic neurons), and juvenile-onset diabetes mellitus (pancreatic β-islet cells), replacement of these specific cell types can be envisioned as a treatment that is potentially lifelong. The therapeutic potential of transplantation has recently expanded beyond element replacement strategies and includes mobilization of endogenous progenitor cells and reprogramming of the host environment to optimize regeneration.

The greatest impedance to moving forward in the ES cell field is not related to science but depends on political and federal decisiveness to invest in this technology. Although limited support exists for use of federal funds to study human ES cells created prior to 9 p.m. on August 9, 2001, this indecisive stand is dramatically impairing progress in the United States (*http://stemcells.nih.gov*). Not surprisingly, the major steps forward in advancing human ES cell technologies are occurring outside the United States. The true effects of these political decisions will not be apparent for decades, reflecting the reduced entry of young scientists into the field of human ES cells work. The solution to the political and ethical problems involved will likely take time and political courage to work out. Advances in nuclear transfer now may circumvent the need for fertilized eggs toward the generation of human ES cells. The proof of principle experiment accomplished in Korea indicates that somatic nuclear transfer can be used to generate human ES cells. Therefore major hurdles of overcoming the requirement for immunosuppression are beginning to fall. Much work is required, but great progress has been made.

Despite limited information, the in vitro ES cell system combined with genomic approaches provides scientists with the means to identify the molecular mechanisms that guide mammalian development, the pathogenesis of disease, and spontaneous regeneration and repair. ES cells have proven to be powerful allies in our quest for scientific discovery and their full potential is only now being realized.

ACKNOWLEDGMENTS

We thank Dr. J. Loring for critical discussions, L. Sage for editing, and T. Steidinger. This work was supported by Primogenix, Inc. (St. Louis, MO), the Barnes-Jewish Hospital Foundation and the NTT Project Group Fund.

REFERENCES

1. Evans, M. J. and Kaufman, M. H. (1981) Establishment in culture of pluripotential cells from mouse embryos. *Nature* **292,** 154–156.
2. Martin, G. R. (1981) Isolation of a pluripotent cell line from early mouse embryos cultured in medium conditioned by teratocarcinoma stem cells. *Proc. Natl. Acad. Sci. USA* **78,** 7634–7638.
3. Bradley, A., Evans, M., Kaufman, M. H., and Robertson, E. (1984) Formation of germline chimaeras from embryo-derived teratocarcinoma cell lines. *Nature* **309,** 255–256.
4. Robertson, E., Bradley, A., Kuehn, M., and Evans, M. (1986) Germ-line transmission of genes introduced into cultured pluripotential cells by retroviral vector. *Nature* **323,** 445–448.
5. Zambrowicz, B. P., Sands, A. T. (2003) Knockouts model the 100 best-selling drugs—will they model the next 100? *Nat. Rev. Drug Discov.* **2,** 38–51.
6. Thomson, J. A., Itskovitz-Eldor, J., Shapiro, S. S., et al. (1998) Embryonic stem cell lines derived from human blastocysts. *Science* **282,** 1145–1147.
7. Cowan, C. A., Klimanskaya, I., McMahon, J., et al. (2004) Derivation of embryonic stem-cell lines from human blastocysts. *N. Engl. J. Med.* **350,** 1353–1356.
8. Park, S. P., Lee, Y. J., Lee, K. S., et al. (2004) Establishment of human embryonic stem cell lines from frozen-thawed blastocysts using STO cell feeder layers. *Hum. Reprod.* **19,** 676–684.
9. Reubinoff, B. E., Pera, M. F., Fong, C. Y., Trounson, A., and Bongso, A. (2000) Embryonic stem cell lines from human blastocysts: somatic differentiation in vitro. *Nat. Biotechnol.* **18,** 399–404.
10. Hwang, W. S., Ryu, Y. J., Park, J. H., et al. (2004) Evidence of a pluripotent human embryonic stem cell line derived from a cloned blastocyst. *Science* **303,** 1669–1674.
11. McDonald, J. W. (2001) In *Stem Cells and CNS Development* (Rao, M. S., ed.), Humana Press, Totowa, NJ, p. 207.
12. Chambers, I., Colby, D., Robertson, M., et al. (2003) Functional expression cloning of Nanog, a pluripotency sustaining factor in embryonic stem cells. *Cell* **113,** 643–655.
13. Mitsui, K., Tokuzawa, Y., Itoh, H., et al. (2003) The homeoprotein Nanog is required for maintenance of pluripotency in mouse epiblast and ES cells. *Cell* **113,** 631–642.
14. Nichols, J., Zevnik, B., Anastassiadis, K., et al. (1998) Formation of pluripotent stem cells in the mammalian embryo depends on the POU transcription factor Oct4. *Cell* **95,** 379–391.
15. Robertson, E. J. (1987) *Teratocarcinomas and Embryonic Stem Cells: A Practical Approach.* IRL Press, Oxford.
16. Doetschman, T. C., Eistetter, H., Katz, M., Schmidt, W., and Kemler, R. (1985) The in vitro development of blastocyst-derived embryonic stem cell lines: formation of visceral yolk sac, blood islands and myocardium. *J. Embryol. Exp. Morphol.* **87,** 27–45.
17. Wobus, A. M., Holzhausen, H., Jakel, P., and Schoneich, J. (1984) Characterization of a pluripotent stem cell line derived from a mouse embryo. *Exp. Cell Res.* **152,** 212–219.
18. Proetzel, G. W. M. V. (2003) In *Methods in Molecular Biology*, Vol. 185 (Turksen, K., ed.), Humana Press, Totowa, NJ.
19. Rohwedel, J., Maltsev, V., Bober, E., Arnold, H. H., Hescheler, J., and Wobus, A. M. (1994) Muscle cell differentiation of embryonic stem cells reflects myogenesis in vivo: developmentally regulated expression of myogenic determination genes and functional expression of ionic currents. *Dev. Biol.* **164,** 87–101.
20. Risau, W., Sariola, H., Zerwes, H. G., et al. (1988) Vasculogenesis and angiogenesis in embryonic-stem-cell-derived embryoid bodies. *Development* **102,** 471–478.
21. Wang, R., Clark, R., and Bautch, V. L. (1992) Embryonic stem cell-derived cystic embryoid bodies form vascular channels: an in vitro model of blood vessel development. *Development* **114,** 303–316.

22. Klug, M. G., Soonpaa, M. H., Koh, G. Y., and Field, L. J. (1996) Genetically selected cardiomyocytes from differentiating embryonic stem cells form stable intracardiac grafts. *J. Clin. Invest.* **98,** 216–224.

23. Wiles, M. V. and Keller, G. (1991) Multiple hematopoietic lineages develop from embryonic stem (ES) cells in culture. *Development* **111,** 259–267.

24. Miller-Hance, W. C., LaCorbiere, M., Fuller, S. J., et al. (1993) In vitro chamber specification during embryonic stem cell cardiogenesis. Expression of the ventricular myosin light chain-2 gene is independent of heart tube formation. *J. Biol. Chem.* **268,** 25244–25252.

25. Lang, K. J., Rathjen, J., Vassilieva, S., and Rathjen, P. D. (2004) Differentiation of embryonic stem cells to a neural fate: a route to re-building the nervous system? *J. Neurosci. Res.* **76,** 184–192.

26. Bain, G., Kitchens, D., Yao, M., Huettner, J. E., and Gottlieb, D. I. (1995) Embryonic stem cells express neuronal properties in vitro. *Dev. Biol.* **168,** 342–357.

27. Bain, G., Ray, W. J., Yao, M., and Gottlieb, D. I. (1996) Retinoic acid promotes neural and represses mesodermal gene expression in mouse embryonic stem cells in culture. *Biochem. Biophys. Res. Commun.* **223,** 691–694.

28. Finley, M. F., Kulkarni, N., and Huettner, J. E. (1996) Synapse formation and establishment of neuronal polarity by P19 embryonic carcinoma cells and embryonic stem cells. *J. Neurosci.* **16,** 1056–1065.

29. Fraichard, A., Chassande, O., Bilbaut, G., Dehay, C., Savatier, P., and Samarut, J. (1995) In vitro differentiation of embryonic stem cells into glial cells and functional neurons. *J. Cell Sci.* **108(Pt 10),** 3181–3188.

30. Liu, S., Qu, Y., Stewart, T. J., et al. (2000) Embryonic stem cells differentiate into oligodendrocytes and myelinate in culture and after spinal cord transplantation. *Proc. Natl. Acad. Sci. USA* **97,** 6126–6131.

31. Okabe, S., Forsberg-Nilsson, K., Spiro, A. C., Segal, M., and McKay, R. D. (1996) Development of neuronal precursor cells and functional postmitotic neurons from embryonic stem cells in vitro. *Mech. Dev.* **59,** 89–102.

32. Renoncourt, Y., Carroll, P., Filippi, P., Arce, V., and Alonso, S. (1998) Neurons derived in vitro from ES cells express homeoproteins characteristic of motoneurons and interneurons. *Mech. Dev.* **79,** 185–197.

33. Rohwedel, J., Kleppisch, T., Pich, U., et al. (1998) Formation of postsynaptic-like membranes during differentiation of embryonic stem cells in vitro. *Exp. Cell Res.* **239,** 214–225.

34. Strubing, C., Ahnert-Hilger, G., Shan, J., Wiedenmann, B., Hescheler, J., and Wobus, A. M. (1995) Differentiation of pluripotent embryonic stem cells into the neuronal lineage in vitro gives rise to mature inhibitory and excitatory neurons. *Mech. Dev.* **53,** 275–287.

35. Wobus, A. M., Grosse, R., and Schoneich, J. (1988) Specific effects of nerve growth factor on the differentiation pattern of mouse embryonic stem cells in vitro. *Biomed. Biochim. Acta* **47,** 965–973.

36. Avilion, A. A., Nicolis, S. K., Pevny, L. H., Perez, L., Vivian, N., and Lovell-Badge, R. (2003) Multipotent cell lineages in early mouse development depend on SOX2 function. *Genes Dev.* **17,** 126–140.

37. Li, M., Pevny, L., Lovell-Badge, R., and Smith, A. (1998) Generation of purified neural precursors from embryonic stem cells by lineage selection. *Curr. Biol.* **8,** 971–974.

38. Wernig, M., Tucker, K. L., Gornik, V., et al. (2002) Tau EGFP embryonic stem cells: an efficient tool for neuronal lineage selection and transplantation. *J. Neurosci. Res.* **69,** 918–924.

39. Arnhold, S., Andressen, C., Angelov, D. N., et al. (2000) Embryonic stem-cell derived neurones express a maturation dependent pattern of voltage-gated calcium channels and calcium-binding proteins. *Int. J. Dev. Neurosci.* **18,** 201–212.

40. Finley, M. F., Devata, S., and Huettner, J. E. (1999) BMP-4 inhibits neural differentiation of murine embryonic stem cells. *J. Neurobiol.* **40,** 271–287.

41. Strubing, C., Rohwedel, J., Ahnert-Hilger, G., Wiedenmann, B., Hescheler, J., and Wobus, A. M. (1997) Development of G protein-mediated Ca^{2+} channel regulation in mouse embryonic stem cell-derived neurons. *Eur. J. Neurosci.* **9,** 824–832.

42. Carpenter, M. K., Inokuma, M. S., Denham, J., Mujtaba, T., Chiu, C. P., and Rao, M. S. (2001) Enrichment of neurons and neural precursors from human embryonic stem cells. *Exp. Neurol.* **172,** 383–397.

43. Chung, S., Sonntag, K. C., Andersson, T., et al. (2002) Genetic engineering of mouse embryonic stem cells by Nurr1 enhances differentiation and maturation into dopaminergic neurons. *Eur. J. Neurosci.* **16,** 1829–1838.

44. Gratsch, T. E. and O'Shea, K. S. (2002) Noggin and chordin have distinct activities in promoting lineage commitment of mouse embryonic stem (ES) cells. *Dev. Biol.* **245,** 83–94.

45. Maye, P., Becker, S., Siemen, H., et al. (2004) Hedgehog signaling is required for the differentiation of ES cells into neurectoderm. *Dev. Biol.* **265,** 276–290.

46. Orentas, D. M., Hayes, J. E., Dyer, K. L., and Miller, R. H. (1999) Sonic hedgehog signaling is required during the appearance of spinal cord oligodendrocyte precursors. *Development* **126,** 2419–2429.

47. Dinsmore, J., Ratliff, J., Deacon, T., et al. (1996) Embryonic stem cells differentiated in vitro as a novel source of cells for transplantation. *Cell Transplant.* **5,** 131–143.

48. Gottlieb, D. I. and Huettner, J. E. (1999) An in vitro pathway from embryonic stem cells to neurons and glia. *Cells Tissues Organs* **165,** 165–172.

49. Brustle, O., Jones, K. N., Learish, R. D., et al. (1999) Embryonic stem cell-derived glial precursors: a source of myelinating transplants. *Science* **285,** 754–756.

50. Gritti, A., Parati, E. A., Cova, L., et al. (1996) Multipotential stem cells from the adult mouse brain proliferate and self-renew in response to basic fibroblast growth factor. *J. Neurosci.* **16,** 1091–1100.

51. Richards, L. J., Kilpatrick, T. J., and Bartlett, P. F. (1992) De novo generation of neuronal cells from the adult mouse brain. *Proc. Natl. Acad. Sci. USA* **89,** 8591–8595.

52. Deng, C., Zhang, P., Harper, J. W., Elledge, S. J., and Leder, P. (1995) Mice lacking p21CIP1/WAF1 undergo normal development, but are defective in G1 checkpoint control. *Cell* **82,** 675–684.

53. Hancock, C. R., Wetherington, J. P., Lambert, N. A., and Condie, B. G. (2000) Neuronal differentiation of cryopreserved neural progenitor cells derived from mouse embryonic stem cells. *Biochem. Biophys. Res. Commun.* **271,** 418–421.

54. Tanabe, Y. and Jessell, T. M. (1996) Diversity and pattern in the developing spinal cord. *Science* **274,** 1115–1123.

55. Ericson, J., Morton, S., Kawakami, A., Roelink, H., and Jessell, T. M. (1996) Two critical periods of Sonic Hedgehog signaling required for the specification of motor neuron identity. *Cell* **87,** 661–673.

56. Ericson, J., Briscoe, J., Rashbass, P., van Heyningen, V., and Jessell, T. M. (1997) Graded sonic hedgehog signaling and the specification of cell fate in the ventral neural tube. *Cold Spring Harb. Symp. Quant. Biol.* **62,** 451–466.

57. Tao, W. and Lai, E. (1992) Telencephalon-restricted expression of BF-1, a new member of the HNF-3/fork head gene family, in the developing rat brain. *Neuron* **8,** 957–966.

58. Rowitch, D. H. (2004) Glial specification in the vertebrate neural tube. *Nat. Rev. Neurosci.* **5,** 409–419.

59. Wichterle, H., Lieberam, I., Porter, J. A., and Jessell, T. M. (2002) Directed differentiation of embryonic stem cells into motor neurons. *Cell* **110,** 385–397.

60. Zhang, S. C., Lipsitz, D., and Duncan, I. D. (1998) Self-renewing canine oligodendroglial progenitor expanded as oligospheres. *J. Neurosci. Res.* **54,** 181–190.

61. Zhang, S. C., Ge, B., and Duncan, I. D. (1999) Adult brain retains the potential to generate oligodendroglial progenitors with extensive myelination capacity. *Proc. Natl. Acad. Sci. USA* **96,** 4089–4094.

62. Bottenstein, J. E. and Sato, G. H. (1979) Growth of a rat neuroblastoma cell line in serumfree supplemented medium. *Proc. Natl. Acad. Sci. USA* **76,** 514–517.

63. Ying, Q. L., Stavridis, M., Griffiths, D., Li, M., and Smith, A. (2003) Conversion of embryonic stem cells into neuroectodermal precursors in adherent monoculture. *Nat. Biotechnol.* **21,** 183–186.

64. Wood, H. B. and Episkopou, V. (1999) Comparative expression of the mouse *Sox1*, *Sox2* and *Sox3* genes from pre-gastrulation to early somite stages. *Mech. Dev.* **86,** 197–201.

65. Kawasaki, H., Mizuseki, K., Nishikawa, S., et al. (2000) Induction of midbrain dopaminergic neurons from ES cells by stromal cell-derived inducing activity. *Neuron* **28,** 31–40.

66. Mizuseki, K., Sakamoto, T., Watanabe, K., et al. (2003) Generation of neural crest-derived peripheral neurons and floor plate cells from mouse and primate embryonic stem cells. *Proc. Natl. Acad. Sci. USA* **100,** 5828–5833.

67. Rathjen, J., Haines, B. P., Hudson, K. M., Nesci, A., Dunn, S., and Rathjen, P. D. (2002) Directed differentiation of pluripotent cells to neural lineages: homogeneous formation and differentiation of a neurectoderm population. *Development* **129,** 2649–2661.

68. Nakayama, T., Momoki-Soga, T., and Inoue, N. (2003) Astrocyte-derived factors instruct differentiation of embryonic stem cells into neurons. *Neurosci. Res.* **46,** 241–249.

69. Kalyani, A. J., Piper, D., Mujtaba, T., Lucero, M. T., and Rao, M. S. (1998) Spinal cord neuronal precursors generate multiple neuronal phenotypes in culture. *J. Neurosci.* **18,** 7856–7868.

70. Mayer-Proschel, M., Kalyani, A. J., Mujtaba, T., and Rao, M. S. (1997) Isolation of lineage-restricted neuronal precursors from multipotent neuroepithelial stem cells. *Neuron* **19,** 773–785.

71. Rao, M. S. and Mayer-Proschel, M. (1997) Glial-restricted precursors are derived from multipotent neuroepithelial stem cells. *Dev. Biol.* **188,** 48–63.

72. Binder, L. I., Frankfurter, A., and Rebhun, L. I. (1985) The distribution of tau in the mammalian central nervous system. *J. Cell Biol.* **101,** 1371–1378.

73. Simon, H. H., Bhatt, L., Gherbassi, D., Sgado, P., and Alberi, L. (2003) Midbrain dopaminergic neurons: determination of their developmental fate by transcription factors. *Ann. NY Acad. Sci.* **991,** 36–47.

74. Schuldiner, M., Yanuka, O., Itskovitz-Eldor, J., Melton, D. A., and Benvenisty, N. (2000) Effects of eight growth factors on the differentiation of cells derived from human embryonic stem cells. *Proc. Natl. Acad. Sci. USA* **97,** 11307–11312.

75. Schuldiner, M., Eiges, R., Eden, A., et al. (2001) Induced neuronal differentiation of human embryonic stem cells. *Brain Res.* **913,** 201–205.

76. Zhang, S. C., Wernig, M., Duncan, I. D., Brustle, O., and Thomson, J. A. (2001) In vitro differentiation of transplantable neural precursors from human embryonic stem cells. *Nat. Biotechnol.* **19,** 1129–1133.

77. Reubinoff, B. E., Itsykson, P., Turetsky, T., et al. (2001) Neural progenitors from human embryonic stem cells. *Nat. Biotechnol.* **19,** 1134–1140.

78. Zwaka, T. P. and Thomson, J. A. (2003) Homologous recombination in human embryonic stem cells. *Nat. Biotechnol.* **21,** 319–321.

79. McDonald, J. W., Liu, X. Z., Qu, Y., et al. (1999) Transplanted embryonic stem cells survive, differentiate and promote recovery in injured rat spinal cord. *Nat. Med.* **5,** 1410–1412.

80. Harper, J. M., Krishnan, C., Darman, J. S., et al. (2004) Axonal growth of embryonic stem cell-derived motoneurons in vitro and in motoneuron-injured adult rats. *Proc. Natl. Acad. Sci. USA* **101,** 7123–7128.

81. Kerr, D. A., Llado, J., Shamblott, M. J., et al. (2003) Human embryonic germ cell derivatives facilitate motor recovery of rats with diffuse motor neuron injury. *J. Neurosci.* **23,** 5131–5140.

82. D'Amour, K. A. and Gage, F. H. (2003) Genetic and functional differences between multipotent neural and pluripotent embryonic stem cells. *Proc. Natl. Acad. Sci. USA* **100(Suppl 1),** 11866–11872.

83. Lo, K. C., Chuang, W. W., and Lamb, D. J. (2003) Stem cell research: the facts, the myths and the promises. *J. Urol.* **170,** 2453–2458.

84. Zhao, W. N., Meng, G. L., and Xue, Y. F. (2003) Labeling of three different mouse ES cell lines with the green fluorescent protein. *Yi. Chuan Xue. Bao.* **30,** 743–749.

85. Shim, J. W., Koh, H. C., Chang, M. Y., et al. (2004) Enhanced in vitro midbrain dopamine neuron differentiation, dopaminergic function, neurite outgrowth, and 1-methyl-4-phenylpyridium resistance in mouse embryonic stem cells overexpressing Bcl-XL. *J. Neurosci.* **24,** 843–852.

86. Zhao, S., Maxwell, S., Jimenez-Beristain, A., et al. (2004) Generation of embryonic stem cells and transgenic mice expressing green fluorescence protein in midbrain dopaminergic neurons. *Eur. J. Neurosci.* **19,** 1133–1140.

87. Davidson, B. L. and Paulson, H. L. (2004) Molecular medicine for the brain: silencing of disease genes with RNA interference. *Lancet Neurol.* **3,** 145–149.

88. Barberi, T., Klivenyi, P., Calingasan, N. Y., et al. (2003) Neural subtype specification of fertilization and nuclear transfer embryonic stem cells and application in parkinsonian mice. *Nat. Biotechnol.* **21,** 1200–1207.

89. Wakayama, T., Rodriguez, I., Perry, A. C., Yanagimachi, R., and Mombaerts, P. (1999) Mice cloned from embryonic stem cells. *Proc. Natl. Acad. Sci. USA* **96,** 14984–14989.

90. Humpherys, D., Eggan, K., Akutsu, H., et al. (2002) Abnormal gene expression in cloned mice derived from embryonic stem cell and cumulus cell nuclei. *Proc. Natl. Acad. Sci. USA* **99,** 12889–12894.

91. Bortvin, A., Eggan, K., Skaletsky, H., et al. (2003) Incomplete reactivation of Oct4-related genes in mouse embryos cloned from somatic nuclei. *Development* **130,** 1673–1680.

92. Gao, S., McGarry, M., Priddle, H., et al. (2003) Effects of donor oocytes and culture conditions on development of cloned mice embryos. *Mol. Reprod. Dev.* **66,** 126–133.

93. Tamashiro, K. L., Wakayama, T., Akutsu, H., et al. (2002) Cloned mice have an obese phenotype not transmitted to their offspring. *Nat. Med.* **8,** 262–267.

94. Chen, Y., He, Z. X., Liu, A., et al. (2003) Embryonic stem cells generated by nuclear transfer of human somatic nuclei into rabbit oocytes. *Cell Res.* **13,** 251–263.

95. Hubner, K., Fuhrmann, G., Christenson, L. K., et al. (2003) Derivation of oocytes from mouse embryonic stem cells. *Science* **300,** 1251–1256.

96. Rideout, W. M., III, Hochedlinger, K., Kyba, M., Daley, G. Q., and Jaenisch, R. (2002) Correction of a genetic defect by nuclear transplantation and combined cell and gene therapy. *Cell* **109,** 17–27.

97. McNeish, J. (2004) Embryonic stem cells in drug discovery. *Nat. Rev. Drug Discov.* **3,** 70–80.

98. Ginis, I., Luo, Y., Miura, T., et al. (2004) Differences between human and mouse embryonic stem cells. *Dev. Biol.* **269,** 360–380.

99. Becker, D., Sadowsky, C. L., and McDonald, J. W. (2003) Restoring function after spinal cord injury. *Neurologist* **9,** 1–15.

100. Matsui, Y., Zsebo, K., and Hogan, B. L. (1992) Derivation of pluripotential embryonic stem cells from murine primordial germ cells in culture. *Cell* **70,** 841–847.

101. Resnick, J. L., Bixler, L. S., Cheng, L., and Donovan, P. J. (1992) Long-term proliferation of mouse primordial germ cells in culture. *Nature* **359,** 550–551.

102. Weiss, M. J., Keller, G., and Orkin, S. H. (1994) Novel insights into erythroid development revealed through in vitro differentiation of GATA-1 embryonic stem cells. *Genes Dev.* **8,** 1184–1197.
103. Thomson, J. A., Kalishman, J., Golos, T. G., et al. (1995) Isolation of a primate embryonic stem cell line. *Proc. Natl. Acad. Sci. USA* **92,** 7844–7848.
104. Wilder, P. J., Kelly, D., Brigman, K., et al. (1997) Inactivation of the FGF-4 gene in embryonic stem cells alters the growth and/or the survival of their early differentiated progeny. *Dev. Biol.* **192,** 614–629.
105. Thomson, J. A., Marshall, V. S., and Trojanowski, J. Q. (1998) Neural differentiation of rhesus embryonic stem cells. *APMIS* **106,** 149–156.
106. Kawai, H., Sango, K., Mullin, K. A., and Proia, R. L. (1998) Embryonic stem cells with a disrupted GD3 synthase gene undergo neuronal differentiation in the absence of b-series gangliosides. *J. Biol. Chem.* **273,** 19634–19638.
107. Mountford, P., Nichols, J., Zevnik, B., O'Brien, C., and Smith, A. (1998) Maintenance of pluripotential embryonic stem cells by stem cell selection. *Reprod. Fertil. Dev.* **10,** 527–533.
108. Shamblott, M. J., Axelman, J., Wang, S., et al. (1998) Derivation of pluripotent stem cells from cultured human primordial germ cells. *Proc. Natl. Acad. Sci. USA* **95,** 13726–13731.
109. Amit, M., Carpenter, M. K., Inokuma, M. S., et al. (2000) Clonally derived human embryonic stem cell lines maintain pluripotency and proliferative potential for prolonged periods of culture. *Dev. Biol.* **227,** 271–278.
110. Xu, C., Inokuma, M. S., Denham, J., et al. (2001) Feeder-free growth of undifferentiated human embryonic stem cells. *Nat. Biotechnol.* **19,** 971–974.
111. Wakayama, T., Tabar, V., Rodriguez, I., Perry, A. C., Studer, L., and Mombaerts, P. (2001) Differentiation of embryonic stem cell lines generated from adult somatic cells by nuclear transfer. *Science* **292,** 740–743.
112. McKay, R. (1997) Stem cells in the central nervous system. *Science* **276,** 66–71.
113. Saito, S., et al. (1992) Bovine embryonic stem cell-like cell lines cultured over several passages. *Roux Arch. Dev. Biol.* **201,** 134–141.
114. Sukoyan, M. A., Golubitsa, A. N., Zhelezova, A. I., et al. (1992) Isolation and cultivation of blastocyst-derived stem cell lines from American mink (*Mustela vison*). *Mol. Reprod. Dev.* **33,** 418–431.
115. Graves, K. H. and Moreadith, R. W. (1993) Derivation and characterization of putative pluripotential embryonic stem cells from preimplantation rabbit embryos. *Mol. Reprod. Dev.* **36,** 424–433.
116. Talbot, N. C., Rexroad, C. E., Jr., Pursel, V. G., and Powell, A. M. (1993) Alkaline phosphatase staining of pig and sheep epiblast cells in culture. *Mol. Reprod. Dev.* **36,** 139–147.
117. Talbot, N. C., Rexroad, C. E., Jr., Pursel, V. G., Powell, A. M., and Nel, N. D. (1993) Culturing the epiblast cells of the pig blastocyst. *In Vitro Cell Dev. Biol. Anim.* **29A,** 543–554.
118. Wheeler, M. B. (1994) Development and validation of swine embryonic stem cells: a review. *Reprod. Fertil. Dev.* **6,** 563–568.
119. Lee, L. R., Mortensen, R. M., Larson, C. A., and Brent, G. A. (1994) Thyroid hormone receptor-alpha inhibits retinoic acid-responsive gene expression and modulates retinoic acid-stimulated neural differentiation in mouse embryonic stem cells. *Mol. Endocrinol.* **8,** 746–756.
120. Rohwedel, J., Sehlmeyer, U., Shan, J., Meister, A., and Wobus, A. M. (1996) Primordial germ cell-derived mouse embryonic germ (EG) cells in vitro resemble undifferentiated stem cells with respect to differentiation capacity and cell cycle distribution. *Cell Biol. Int.* **20,** 579–587.

121. Pain, B., Clark, M. E., Shen, M., et al. (1996) Long-term in vitro culture and characterisation of avian embryonic stem cells with multiple morphogenetic potentialities. *Development* **122,** 2339–2348.

122. Hong, Y., Winkler, C., and Schartl, M. (1996) Pluripotency and differentiation of embryonic stem cell lines from the medakafish (*Oryzias latipes*). *Mech. Dev.* **60,** 33–44.

123. Shim, H., Gutierrez-Adan, A., Chen, L. R., BonDurant, R. H., Behboodi, E., and Anderson, G. B. (1997) Isolation of pluripotent stem cells from cultured porcine primordial germ cells. *Biol. Reprod.* **57,** 1089–1095.

124. Brustle, O., Spiro, A. C., Karram, K., Choudhary, K., Okabe, S., and McKay, R. D. (1997) In vitro-generated neural precursors participate in mammalian brain development. *Proc. Natl. Acad. Sci. USA* **94,** 14809–14814.

125. Gajovic, S., St Onge, L., Yokota, Y., and Gruss, P. (1997) Retinoic acid mediates *Pax6* expression during in vitro differentiation of embryonic stem cells. *Differentiation* **62,** 187–192.

126. Thomson, J. A. and Marshall, V. S. (1998) Primate embryonic stem cells. *Curr. Top. Dev. Biol.* **38,** 133–165.

127. Rohwedel, J., Guan, K., Zuschratter, W., et al. (1998) Loss of beta1 integrin function results in a retardation of myogenic, but an acceleration of neuronal, differentiation of embryonic stem cells in vitro. *Dev. Biol.* **201,** 167–184.

128. Angelov, D. N., Arnhold, S., Andressen, C., et al. (1998) Temporospatial relationships between macroglia and microglia during in vitro differentiation of murine stem cells. *Dev. Neurosci.* **20,** 42–51.

129. Mujtaba, T., Piper, D. R., Kalyani, A., Groves, A. K., Lucero, M. T., and Rao, M. S. (1999) Lineage-restricted neural precursors can be isolated from both the mouse neural tube and cultured ES cells. *Dev. Biol.* **214,** 113–127.

14

Mobilization of Neural Precursors in the Adult Central Nervous System

Theo D. Palmer and Fred H. Gage

In spite of our increased knowledge of adult neurogenesis, Cajal's dogma of no new neurons is still fundamentally correct when viewed in the context of the brain's intrinsic repair mechanisms. In the embryo, neurogenesis operates with extraordinary dynamics to generate all of the basic brain structures and circuitry that will be used for the remainder of an individual's life. At birth, all areas of the brain down-regulate neurogenesis and, in the adult, most areas have stopped producing neurons altogether (at least within the current limits of detection). The last 50 yr, however, have provided evidence for persistent neurogenesis within several anatomically distinct loci in the adult brain. In rodents, the unambiguous exceptions to Cajal's rule are the hippocampus and olfactory bulb. Ongoing studies indicate that this process may extend to other areas of the primate forebrain (1–7) and injury may trigger an abortive neurogenesis in many brain regions (8–13). In spite of this increasingly liberal view of neurogenesis in the adult, the paucity of neuron replacement following disease or injury leaves the dogma relatively intact. Looking forward, it seems clear that the successful therapeutic mobilization of neural progenitor cells will depend on the precise modulation of local signaling that spans from the recruitment of endogenous stem cells to the fine functional tuning of mature neurons and glia that are inserted into the preexisting circuitry of the adult brain.

CHALLENGING THE DOGMA OF "NO-NEW-NEURONS"

Monitoring Mitosis In Vivo

Neurogenesis is the process of adding new neurons by the proliferative expansion of a neuronal precursor cell. In the late 1950s, the earliest evidence for neurogenesis in the adult was observed following the systemic injection of radiolabeled thymidine ([^{3}H]Tdr). Endogenous nucleoside pools become substituted with the labeled nucleoside and newly synthesized DNA incorporates analog in proportion to its relative systemic concentration. The α-particle emissions can be visualized by autoradiography (14–17). Because the number of silver grains developed in the photographic emulsion is dependent on the amount of [^{3}H]Tdr incorporated, grain counts associated with each nucleus can provide reliable quantitative information on whether a cell has

From: *Neural Development and Stem Cells, Second Edition*
Edited by: M. S. Rao © Humana Press Inc., Totowa, NJ

completed an entire S phase or how many times a cell transits S phase during a labeling period *(18)*.

More recently, antibodies that recognize nonradioactive thymidine analogs such as bromodeoxyuridine (BrdU) have been used in lieu of autoradiography *(2,3)*. In contrast to [³H]Tdr, nonradioactive analogs can be immunologically detected in any thickness of tissue that can be penetrated by the detecting antibody and, by combining antibodies to BrdU with those that recognize lineage-specific epitopes, it is possible to identify unambiguously the phenotype of newborn cells (Fig. 1).

Technical Caveats

Unfortunately, the remarkable sensitivity of immunodetection comes at a price. In the context of neurogenesis in the adult, it is known that the small amounts of nucleoside analog incorporated into neuronal nuclei during DNA repair may introduce false positives, although it is thought that careful accounting for this process can avoid confusion *(19)*. Other caveats should also be considered. High substitution rates with thymidine analogs can significantly influence cell behavior. At moderate substitution levels, BrdU can be mutagenic *(20,21)* and is known to alter gene expression patterns *(22–25)*. Subsequent changes in physiology may directly impact proliferative activity. For example, BrdU is known to elevate adrenal glucocorticoid levels in rats *(26,27)* and adrenal steroids are known to suppress the proliferative activity of neural progenitors in the adult hippocampus *(28)*. At higher concentrations, both [³H]Tdr and BrdU become directly cytotoxic, an effect that can potentially lead to the ablation of the population being evaluated *(29)* (Fig. 2). Even now, it is possible to argue that labeling a cell may change its fate or make a nonneuronal cell inappropriately express phenotypic attributes of neurons but current evidence for the addition of functional neurons in the adult is not entirely based on nucleoside incorporation and the data collected to date provide extensive evidence that neurogenesis plays an important role in the adult.

The concept of DNA repair in preexisting mature neurons can be countered with the fact that BrdU labeling does not initially mark mature neurons but instead marks an immature progenitor cell that does not express neuronal markers. With time, these cells begin to express neuronal markers and ultimately take on the phenotypes of postmitotic neurons *(19,30,31)*. In addition, in areas suspected of neurogenesis, the number of new neurons actually increases over the life of the organism *(32)*. Ultrastructural analysis adds confidence that these new projecting cells display the intracellular architecture of neurons *(33,34)*. Furthermore, viral vectors that infect only dividing cells have unambiguously shown that progenitors in the ventricular zone migrate to the olfactory bulb where they differentiate into new periglomerular and granule cell interneurons *(35,36)*. Within the hippocampus, retrograde tracing of marked neurons shows that most newborn neurons project appropriately to the CA3 region of the hippocampus *(2,37–39)* and recordings from newborn hippocampal granule layer neurons demonstrate that the newly generated neurons undergo a development-like progression of electrophysiological characteristics and ultimately become fully integrated as active and mature granule cell neurons *(40)*.

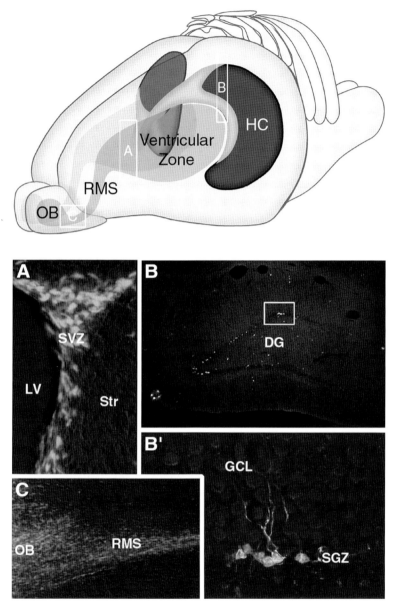

Fig. 1. After 1 wk of treatment with BrdU, dividing neural progenitors are readily observed within the adult rat anterior subventricular zone (SVZ, **A**) and subgranular zone (SGZ, **B**) of the hippocampal dentate gyrus (DG). Cells that proliferate in the SVZ adjacent to the lateral ventricle (LV) migrate along the surface of the striatum (Str) and converge in a rostral migratory stream (RMS) leading to the olfactory bulb (OB) (**C**). Within the SGZ, cells proliferate in clusters and then migrate short distances to become disseminated throughout the GCL. Type IIIβ-tubulin is an early intermediate filament marker for the neuronal lineage that is expressed by migrating cells within the RMS and the SGZ. Immunoreactivity for type IIIβ-tubulin and BrdU have been combined in **B′** to show an individual neuroblast within a small cluster of BrdU-labeled progenitors.

345

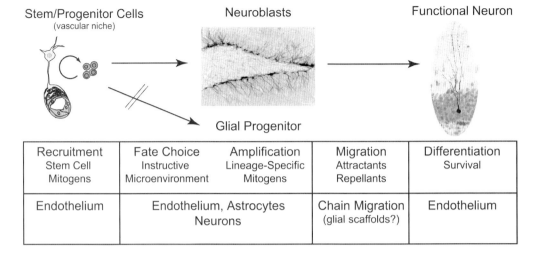

Recruitment	Fate Choice	Amplification	Migration	Differentiation
Stem Cell Mitogens	Instructive Microenvironment	Lineage-Specific Mitogens	Attractants Repellants	Survival
Endothelium	Endothelium, Astrocytes Neurons		Chain Migration (glial scaffolds?)	Endothelium

Fig. 2. Mobilization of neural progenitor for neuronal replacement or augmentation may require the manipulation of progenitors at numerous points along a complex regulatory pathway. First, stem cells must be recruited into the cycle and then influenced to adopt a neuronal fate in regions that may normally produce only glia. The neuroblasts must then be amplified and instructed to migrate along routes that may not naturally exist within the adult brain. The newborn neurons may then require additional instructions that direct the appropriate connectivity and transmitter phenotype. The hippocampal subgranular zone provides insights into the cellular participants that may make up the SGZ's unique neurogenic niche. Dividing progenitor cells are focally recruited within the perivascular space. Interactions between endothelium, astrocytes, and neurons are all known to influence progenitor cell behavior. It remains to be determined whether there are single or multiple influences provided by each instructive cell types and where, along the phenotypic and temporal progression of differentiation, each of these influences has the most impact for mobilizing progenitors for repair.

The Evidence for Stem Cells

In development, stem cells are defined as an undifferentiated progenitor that can divide to give rise to an identical progenitor (self-renewal) as well as progeny that go on to differentiate into one or more terminal phenotypes (as reviewed in refs. *41–43*). In the adult CNS, the strongest evidence for the presence of stem-like cells in the adult brain has been generated in primary cultures isolated from the ventricular zone or hippocampus. Progenitors from the adult germinal zones can be stimulated to proliferate in vitro using epidermal growth factor (EGF) and/or basic fibroblast growth factor (FGF-2). The cultures contain a mixture of cell phenotypes similar to that seen in vivo, with only a minor population of cells displaying definitive markers for mature neurons or glia *(41,44–48)*. By isolating or marking single cells in vitro, it has been shown that the entire array of cell phenotypes can originate from a small population of multipotent stem-like cells within the relatively heterogeneous population of dividing progenitors *(29,48–51)*.

Dividing cells in the adult brain generate both neurons and glia but there is little direct in vivo evidence for a naturally occurring self-renewing stem cell that actively gives rise to both neurons and glia. Chemotoxic ablation of the proliferative cells of the ventricular zone and hippocampus shows that the entire proliferative zones can be repopulated from the progeny of a small number of relatively quiescent cells *(29,52)*. If these progenitor cells are marked with an inheritable genetic marker (i.e., a retroviral vector), it can be shown that both neurons and glia are generated from this responding population *(52)*. But again, a clonal analysis of the type used to demonstrate multilineage potential in developmental models has not been performed in vivo in adult animals *(53,54)*. Indeed, there is well founded skepticism that the "stem cell" phenotype of concurrent tri-lineage production (i.e., production of neurons, astrocytes and oligodendrocytes) is an artifact of in vitro culture and that authentic programs of cell genesis in vivo do not invoke this potential *(55)*. Developmental progenitor cell programs are temporally and spatially separated, and attempts to mobilize stem cells for repair/replacement should maintain a clear awareness that both temporal and spatial sequencing may be important when manipulating progenitor cells toward a defined outcome.

THE ANATOMY OF NEUROGENESIS: A NEUROGENIC MICRONICHE UNVEILED IN THE HIPPOCAMPAL SUBGRANULAR ZONE

Neural Progenitor Cells in Nonneurogenic Brain Regions

Given the excitement about neurogenesis in the adult, it is easy to be distracted from the fact that an abundant population of dividing neural progenitors leave the ventricular zone and become distributed throughout the adult brain. These cells remain competent to divide and play the important role of generating oligodendrocytes and astrocytes in prodigious numbers (thousands of oligodendrocytes per cubic millimeter of white matter each month) *(56)*. Although these cells are more sparsely scattered than those of the ventricular zone, they do proliferate *in situ* and when taken as a whole they numerically eclipse the neurogenic zones, representing as much as 70% of all dividing cells in the adult central nervous system (CNS) *(57,58)*. Several lines of evidence suggest that these progenitor cells may not be intrinsically restricted to a glial fate and as such may represent an important premobilized target population for therapy.

In situ, the most immature glial progenitor cells express A2B5 antigen, platelet-derived growth factor receptor-α (PDGFR-α) and NKx2.2 *(59)*. As they transit into the oligodendrocyte differentiation program they up-regulate markers such as NG2, proteolipid protein (PLP), and O4 *(57,60)*. Those cells that exit the cell cycle down-regulate NG2 and begin to express mature oligodendrocyte proteins *(61)*; however, most NG2-expressing cells that are marked with BrdU remain as preoligodendrocytes (reviewed in refs. *62* and *63*). In vivo, the natural fate of these cells is fixed and there is no evidence to date that a glial restricted precursors produce neurons in vivo. However, there is abundant evidence that progenitor cells from brain regions that generate only glia will readily switch to a multilineage program and immediately begin producing neurons in primary culture.

Isolation of progenitor cells from the adult brain by bouyancy fractionation or by sorting for markers such as A2B5, NG2, or O4 allows one to acutely isolate glial precursor cells in primary culture. After a brief exposure to bFGF-2, the cultures begin to produce neurons *(64–66)*. Furthermore, when FGF-2 stimulated progenitor cells (isolated from either neurogenic zones or nonneurogenic parenchyma) are transplanted into the normal hippocampus or ventricular zone, they readily respond to the local neurogenic signals and begin producing neurons of the exact phenotype specified by each location, regardless of their origin (i.e., granule layer neurons in the hippocampus and periglomerular and granule layer interneurons in the olfactory bulb) *(41,67)*. It may be possible that cells displaying a number of similar, yet distinct phenotypes are all able to display stem-like properties under appropriate conditions. Regardless of the exact identity(s) of the stem cell, the presence of an immature stem-like cell in the adult provides the underpinnings for most working hypotheses regarding adult neurogenesis.

Progenitor Cells in the Hippocampus

The competence of progenitors to generate neurons in culture but their failure to do so in many brain regions suggests that neurogenesis is restricted by local signaling in the adult. The local anatomy of neurogenic regions provides the first clues as to how the adult may regulate the production of new neurons. As elegantly described by Lim and Alvarez-Buylla in Chapter 2, the dividing cells of the adult that give rise to neurons are not themselves neurons but immature progenitors similar to those seen in the developing brain. As in development *(68,69)*, progenitor cells in the adult may retain radial glia-like attributes, such as the expression of glial fibrillary acidic protein (GFAP) and nestin *(70,71)*. Within the hippocampus, these cells are found within a laminar zone of proliferation that is located at the margin between the hilus and granule cell layer proper, or subgranular zone (SGZ) *(2,3)*. Within this lamina, progenitors cycle relatively rapidly, completing one cell cycle every 20–24 h *(18)*. However, the majority of cells produced eventually differentiate into neurons *(1,19,30,31,34,36,47)*.

Chemical ablation of mitotic cells within the SGZ results in the transient depletion of the actively dividing progenitors and a relatively quiescent subpopulation of progenitors subsequently repopulate the SGZ. Viral marking indicates that the earliest repopulating cells are nestin-positive and also expresses GFAP *(72)*. These cells then give rise to immature neuronal precursors that express type IIIβ-tubulin, polysialylated (PSA) neural cell adhesion molecule (NCAM), and doublecortin. Using BrdU to mark cells in S phase, it becomes clear that at any given point in time, a small portion of the cells transiting S phase belong to the nestin-GFAP immunoreactive class and a much larger fraction (up to 60%) divide as doublecortin-positive transient amplifying neuroblasts *(71)*. These dividing cells initially accumulate in small clusters reminiscent of a local clonal expansion and within days of their last division, postmitotic progeny have migrated away from the tightly packed cluster to become distributed as maturing neurons within the adjacent granule cell layer *(19,31)*.

The Vascular Niche

A closer look at clusters of dividing cells shows that they are very closely juxtaposed to small capillaries within the SGZ. Endothelial cells also divide in the neighboring vessel, suggesting that progenitor recruitment may be accompanied by a simultaneous and colocalized angiogenic stimulus *(19)*. This focal clustering of proliferative progenitors within the perivascular niche is such a striking hallmark of the SGZ that it is attractive to speculate that the vascular niche is somehow instructive or permissive for neurogenesis.

Although the evidence for angiogenic influences in mammalian neurogenesis remains hypothetical, there are elegant data demonstrating a role for angiogenesis in the production of higher vocal center neurons in canaries *(73)* and the peripheral infusion of angiogenic factors such as vascular endothelial growth factor (VEGF), FGF-2, and insulin-like growth factor-1 (IGF-1) up-regulates neurogenesis in rodents *(74–77)*. Not only might angiogenic factors stimulate a change in signaling within the vascular microenvironment, but neural progenitors themselves share strikingly similar mitogen responsiveness to endothelial cells, suggesting that the local mitogenic stimulus may involve a common molecule(s) that acts on both endothelium and neural progenitor cells.

The two most widely used mitogens for neural progenitor culture are EGF *(46,78–80)* and FGF-2 *(41,44,81,82)*. In vivo, the known endothelial cell mitogens sonic hedgehog, EGF, FGF-2, VEGF, and IGF-1 all induce proliferation within the SGZ. Viral delivery of sonic hedgehog to the hippocampus stimulates a robust increase in neurogenesis *(83)*. When injected into the lateral ventricle, recombinant EGF stimulates a dramatic proliferation of the ventricular zone progenitors with smaller, yet measurable effects in the SGZ *(84,85)*. Recombinant FGF-2 administered in the ventricle shows similar effects on SGZ progenitors but is not able to diffuse into the parenchyma and has little effect on hippocampal neurogenesis *(85,86)*. However, peripheral injection of FGF-2 in neonatal animals does have striking effects on hippocampal neurogenesis *(75,76)*, but only during the first few postnatal weeks, suggesting that FGF-2 can access progenitors in the SGZ only until the blood–brain barrier becomes complete. In contrast, peripheral injections of IGF-1 induce a twofold increase in the number of dividing cell within the adult SGZ *(77)*, and VEGF peripheral administration also potently stimulates neurogenesis *(74)*. Presumably, this activity is due to delivery via the vascular system, indicating that some circulating factors may have considerable influences on progenitors resident within the parenchyma. This may be via a direct action or by altering the cells that make up the progenitor cells local microenvironment.

CELLS OF THE NEUROGENIC NICHE

Within the neuroangiogenic context, there are numerous cell types that could influence progenitor cell fate including vascular endothelium or smooth muscle, astrocytes that form the blood–brain barrier and, of course, neurons of the adjacent granule cell layer and hilus. Surprisingly, a potential role in neurogenesis has been identified for all but smooth muscle cells, perhaps only because smooth muscle remains unstudied in this context.

Endothelial Cells

The endothelial cell becomes an increasingly interesting instructive cell in a number of developmental paradigms *(87,88)*, and recent work has demonstrated that endothelium can have potent influences on neural progenitor cells in both the adult and developing animal. As in the avian model of adult neurogenesis *(73)*, endothelium from the rodent brain can provide potent trophic support for newborn neurons via the VEGF-stimulated elaboration of brain derived neurotrophic factor (BDNF) *(89)*. In development, endothelial cells may also influence neurogenesis by stimulating additional self-renewing divisions of cortical progenitor cells *(90)*.

Astroctyes

At present, there is no evidence that the blood–brain barrier is compromised in the hippocampal SGZ and this implies that astrocytic end feet must be present within the space that separates the dividing neural progenitor cells from the neighboring endothelium. In an interesting comparison of astrocytes from different regions of the CNS, it has been shown that hippocampal astrocytes are unique in their ability to promote neurogenesis when placed in coculture with neural progenitor cells *(91)*. The molecules that mediate this effect are not yet known, but surprisingly the astroctyes do not need to be alive to provide this influence, as ethanol fixed cell substrates are equally effective. This implicates a contact-mediated phenomenon rather than the elaboration of an actively secreted soluble factor, perhaps further strengthening the concept that close cellular communication within the neurogenic niche is an essential element of neurogenesis.

Neurons

Neural precursors within the SGZ reside at the hilar margin of the granule cell layer (GCL), a location exceptionally rich in granule layer axonal projections. Recent work has examined progenitor cells from the hippocampus for their ability to sense "activity" within these neighboring neurons by coculturing progenitors with primary neuron cultures from neonatal hippocampal formations. Precursor cells were found to be responsive to depolarizing stimuli in coculture and dramatically increased their production of neurons *(92)*. However, in a startling observation, killing the neuron culture with an ethanol fixation did not eliminate the response to *N*-methyl-D-aspartate (NMDA) or potassium. Interestingly, the neural precursor cells them selves were found to express NMDA receptors and L-type calcium channels and were able to respond directly to "activity" stimuli of the types that should be present within the SGZ. Neurons may also produce soluble factors, and one candidate in the context of hippocampal neurogenesis is the axonal delivery of sonic hedgehog by medial septal neurons that innervate the hippocampus *(83)*. In this sense, neural progenitor cells can integrate information presented by neuron-intrinsic circuitry and respond dynamically to demand placed on the circuit itself.

Unique Attributes of the Neuroangiogenic Niche

Obviously, the SGZ is not the only place in the brain where capillaries, astrocytes, and neurons coexist. Just as patterning in the developing brain regulates regional cell fate choice, the adult brain must also establish subtle distinctions in gene expression patterns within an otherwise ubiquitously distributed instructive cell population. The one attribute that appears to be unique is the evidence for angiogenic stimulation of the local vasculature that accompanies the focal mitogenic recruitment of progenitor cells.

Local neuronal activity heightens the metabolic demand placed on vasculature and astrocytes. This may stimulate a unique activated status for cells in the local microenvironment and one mechanism for inducing a change in vascular function might be via the activity-dependent action of hypoxia-inducible factor 1 α *(93)*. Parallel activity-dependent activation of nitric oxide (NO) synthase in neurons as well as local glia and endothelium also leads to increased circulation. Part of the vascular response to NO is up-regulation of BDNF and erythropoietin *(73,94,95)*. When neuronal activity is artificially increased (seizures or electroshock therapy *[96–98]*) or if NO is directly manipulated *(99)*, the result is a significant increase in neurogenesis. The unique activation of astrocytes and vascular cells is integral to this activity-dependent signaling network and this unique "activated status" may provide the context-specific cues that define where neurogenesis is to occur.

INJURY-INDUCED NEUROGENESIS AND GROWTH FACTOR MANIPULATION OF NEURAL PROGENITOR BEHAVIOR

Injury-Induced Neurogenic Niche

Brain injury of virtually any sort is accompanied by a local increases in excititory stimuli, activation of astrocytes, an angiogenic response, and the local mitogenic recruitment of progenitor cells. In light of the activated vascular niche hypothesis, it is not surprising that recent reports are indeed suggesting that injury evokes a neurogenic response in areas where neurogenesis is not normally detected. For example, discrete photoablation of corticothalamic projecting neurons within the cortex is followed over the next several weeks by the proliferative replacement of neurons within the damaged cortical lamina *(11)*. Similarly, focal ischemia is also accompanied by a fleeting neurogenic response *(13)*. In both instances very few neurons are produced, and only a tiny fraction (if any) of these survive to become mature neurons.

This intriguingly supports the "activated cell status" hypothesis but even this injury-induced response appears to be extremely fleeting and context specific. Focal ischemia triggers angiogenic and astrocytic responses in the affected striatum and overlying cortex yet abortive neurogenesis is observed only within the striatum *(13)*. Similarly, mild global hypoxic/ischemic insults result in the selective loss of hippocampal CA1 neurons but while the hippocampal CA1 region activates astrocytes and vasculature, it does not natively replace neurons (although the neighboring granule cell layer does respond with increased neurogenesis) *(10)*. Amazingly, the neurogenic failure in CA1 can be overcome if recombinant FGF and EGF are infused into the ventricle following ischemia *(12)*. Similar robust recruitment of neurogenic progenitor cells into the striatal parenchyma is observed following infusion of BDNF or transforming growth factor-α (TGF-α) *(100,101)*.

Inflammation

One obvious distinction between the native neurogenic niche of the hippocampus and the niche created by injury is the inflammatory response to injury. Although there is clear potential for inflammatory cells and cytokines to influence neural progenitor cell fate, only recently has the full extent of this influence been realized in the context of adult neurogenesis. Cranial irradiation of the sort used to treat brain tumors results in a complete and permanent loss of hippocampal neurogenesis, even though the doses given do not appear to ablate all progenitor cells *(102)*. The radiation-induced inflammatory response is unusually persistent, and recent work indicates that the presence of activated microglia and proinflammatory cytokines inhibits the production of neurons and impairs newborn neuron survival *(102)*. The same mechanisms appear to be true in seizure-induced hippocampal injury *(103)*, and in both instances, modulation of the inflammatory response with nonsteroidal antiinflammatory drugs is surprisingly effective in restoring neurogenesis. This indicates that neuroinflammation may be the single most important impediment to mobilizing endogenous progenitor cells for repair *(104)* in the context of injury or disease, as virtually all known injury and disease processes are accompanied by a surprisingly persistent microglial response. Specific intervention in one or more components of neuroinflammatory signaling may significantly enhance the native neurogenic response to injury, for example, growth factor infusions as used in stimulating CA1 neurogenesis *(12)* or the use of nonsteroidal drugs that modulate the inflammatory response *(103–105)*. Importantly, the traditional use of steroidal antiinflammatory drugs may be the wrong choice in the specific context of neurogenesis given the potent antineurogenic effects of corticosteroids on adult neurogenesis *(106,107)*.

Continuing Controversy

It is important to be aware that the field has not reached a consensus on whether all reports of neurogenesis are well substantiated. A particularly troublesome problem is encountered when fleetingly rare newborn neurons are scored within a region suffused with both glial and immune cell proliferation. When one of the abundant nonneuronal nuclei lies directly over a neuron, the juxtaposition of markers misleads the observer into believing that a nucleus belongs to the underlying neuron. High resolution confocal microscopy can reduce these errors but this is surprisingly inadequate unless a detailed three-dimensional reconstruction of the rare candidate cell is performed. A large component of the dividing cells consists of oligodendrocyte precursors that are so tightly coupled to neurons that they reside within shallow indentations of the neuron cell body. These "satellite" cells can easily be mistaken for neurons and many observations of neurogenesis are still disputed (e.g., *see* refs. *108* and *109*). Another source of ambiguity is the accumulating evidence from bone marrow transplant studies that immune cells, which invade an area of injury, can fuse with neurons *(110,111)*. This suggests that a neuron can in fact become "labeled" but not due to neurogenesis. In addition, there are the continuing issues of DNA repair following injury (as mentioned earlier). These technical illusions are very difficult to control and until a more effective means of evaluating neurogenesis is developed, it will be difficult to reach a consensus on where and under what circumstances the adult brain can or cannot support neurogenesis. To an extreme, it might be argued that the only undisputed regions of adult neurogenesis in rodents are the hippocampal SGZ and olfactory SVZ.

LESSONS FROM THE PHYSIOLOGICAL MODULATION OF NEUROGENESIS IN THE HIPPOCAMPUS

The stem/progenitor cell niche of the hippocampal SGZ is a "cellular integrator" of complex physiological stimuli, and future studies can draw on the known architecture of this zone to understand more fully the cellular and molecular interactions that regulate neural progenitor activity and fate. Neurogenesis in the adult dentate gyrus is a dynamic process that responds to numerous intrinsic and extrinsic influences (Table 1). Each of these would be integrated via the unique cellular neuroangiogenic microenvironment of the SGZ.

Table 1
Regulators of Neural Progenitor Activity in the Hippocampal SGZ

	Effects	Context	References
Genetic	Changes in proliferation	Unknown loci	(116)
	Number of new neurons	Unknown loci	(116)
Environmental enrichment	Increased number of new neurons in the hippocampus	Population cage, food treats, toys, running wheel	(4,112,118; see also 119–121)
	Absence of effect in SVZ and olfactory bulb		(122)
Physical exercise	Increases in proliferation and number of new neurons in the hippocampus	Running wheel	(114,115)
Learning	Increased number of new neurons	Water maze, eye-blink conditioning	(113)
Stress and other hormones	Increased proliferation	Adrenalectomy, estrogen,	(28,189)
	Reduced proliferation	Glucocorticoids, predator/psychosocial stress	(28,106,124)
Neurotransmitters	Increased proliferation	NMDA antagonists, serotonin, norepinephrine, and dopamine signaling	(127–129,131,132,190)
	Reduced proliferation	NMDA agonists, serotonin receptor antagonists, depletion of 5-hydroxytryptamine, antidepressants	(129–133,190)
Growth factors/mitogens	Increased proliferation and number of neurons	FGF-2, EGF, IGF-1, VEGF, Shh, TGF-α	(74–77,83–85,101)

The concept that new granule cell neurons are important for processing novel information has gained support by the results of several studies showing that progenitor cell activity and the net number of new neurons generated correlates well with performance in learning and memory-related tasks *(4,112–115)*. This correlation extends well beyond any potential variation between species or even differences between individuals, as neurogenesis in any given group of individuals can be dramatically influenced by environmental, physical, psychological, and cognitive processes. This intrinsic modulation and its apparent correlation with learning and memory make hippocampal neurogenesis an excellent platform for unraveling the molecular basis of neurogenesis and, eventually, understanding how stimulating ectopic neurogenesis might positively or negatively effect cognition following attempts to repair the CNS (Table 2).

Genetic Factors

We all may have wondered, when faced with the dizzying array of intellect in a typical kindergarten class or recent faculty meeting, how the relative contributions of genetics vs environment dictate cognitive ability. In the context of hippocampal neurogenesis, it seems clear that both genetics and experience have a significant impact on the number of new neurons that are generated. For example, different strains of the common laboratory mouse show striking differences in baseline neurogenesis when housed under identical conditions *(116)*. Differences can be seen in both the size of the proliferative progenitor pool as well as on the fraction of newborn cells that survive and differentiate into neurons. The allelic variations that control this modulation can be divided into loci that influence proliferative activity vs. those that influence survival of newborn cells. Using a strategy to map attributes to chromosomal loci in different strains, it has been possible to show that major determinants of natural proliferative activity and subsequent retention of new neurons may map to separate but surprisingly few loci *(116,117)*.

Environmental Enrichment

For each genetic makeup, neurogenesis is modulated further by numerous influences. For example, animals housed under standard laboratory conditions (several animals in a single cage with nothing interesting to do) can be compared to those placed in large population cages containing toys, edible treats, and numerous social cohorts *(4,118)*. The differences this nondeprived ("enriched") environment makes in hippocampal neurogenesis are striking. Those in the enriched environment (also see refs. *119–121*) generate roughly two times more neurons than their underprivileged compatriots. This increase is generated in the absence of any increases in proliferation, suggesting that enrichment induces more of the newborn cells to differentiate and survive as neurons. Although this enrichment yields robust experience-related changes in neurogenesis within the hippocampus, there is little effect on the neurogenesis in the SVZ and olfactory bulb *(122)*. This dissociation of influences suggests that physiological approaches to augmenting native repair may require a region-specific approach.

Physical Exercise

One element of the enriched environment was access to running wheels and subsequent studies have shown that physical exercise alone can increase both the size of the

Table 2
Regulators of Stem Cell Activity In Vitro

	Effectors	Effect	Reference
Proliferation	FGF-2	Mitogenic, recruits stem cells into cycle and may reprogram cells to have broader fate potential than displayed in vivo	(41,44–46,80–82,191,192)
	FGF-1, -4, -7, -8	Mitogenic, can substitute for FGF-2 to maintain rat neural progenitors in cycle	(193,194)
	EGF	Mitogenic, recruits mouse stem cells but also stimulates increased gliogenesis	(46,47,51,78,80)
	PDGF	Mitogen for glial precursors	(136,137)
Differentiation	Retinoic acid	Increase in neuronal differentiation. Upregulation of Trk receptors.	(64,178,187)
	Cyclic AMP	Increase in neuronal differentiation.	(64,178,187)
	Neurotrophins: NGF, BDNF, NT-3	Increase in neuronal differentiation. Neuronal types include those that express TH, GABA, acetyl cholinesterase, NP-Y and calbindin	(45,48,49,51,80,82,178)
	CNTF	Glial differentiation	(195)
Transmitter phenotype	Nurr1	Direct activation of tyrosine hydroxylase expression	(187)
	Nurr1 + glial cofactors	Increased differentiation of dopaminergic neurons	(188)
	Neurotrophins: NGF, BDNF, NT-3	Pleiotropic effects: promote maturation of several neuronal phenotypes including TH, GABA, cholinesterase, NP-Y and calbindin-expressing neurons.	(48,78–80,178)
Instructive cell types of the local microenvironment	Astrocytes, neurons, endothelium	Pleiotropic effects including enhanced neuron production/ survival and, enhanced self-renewing progenitor divisions (endothelium)	(89,91,92)

proliferative progenitor pool and the number of new neurons that survive and become integrated into the GCL *(114,115)*. When given the opportunity to run, individual animals will clock more than 10,000 revolutions per night on a running wheel (3–5 miles). One would anticipate numerous physiological changes in both the CNS and periphery. These would include increased blood flow and changes in oxygen and glucose metabolism and, within the CNS alone, the propagation of numerous motor and cognitive patterns, some of which may feed back into the neurogenic regulatory cascade via specific neuronal activity patterns. Indeed, several studies do indicate that there are distinct peripheral and central influences that contribute to neurogenic regulation in the hippocampus. Running induces IGF-1 and VEGF production in the periphery and blockade of the circulating factors by infusion or in vivo production of antagonizing molecules can completely abrogate the influence of running indicating that both molecules are necessary for a somatically derived signal that potently regulates neurogenesis *(77,123)*. Interestingly, blockade of peripheral VEGF has no impact on baseline neurogenesis in a nonrunning animal, suggesting that its influence can be entirely separated from a CNS-intrinsic "central" regulator of neurogenesis.

Learning

Even the act of learning a spatial task appears to trigger an increase in the number of the newborn progenitors that survive and differentiate into neurons *(113)*. When animals housed under standard laboratory conditions are placed in a water maze, those animals that have the opportunity to learn the position of a submerged platform retain more newborn neurons than those that are simply asked to swim for the same amount of time. The extent to which purely cerebral activities influence neurogenesis may be subtly embedded within other regulatory influences. For example, similar learning paradigms do not seem to have a measurable effect and the absence of increased neurogenesis following swimming (a form of physical exercise) seems to contradict the running data *(114,115)*. However, the very brief swimming periods may not be equivalent to the extended periods of exercise provided by a wheel. In addition, swimming is not an activity a rat would normally choose and the psychological stress of swimming may actually counteract any neurogenic stimuli.

Stress, Glucocorticoids, Neurotransmitters, and Antidepressants

Stress induced in a number of paradigms can rapidly influence neural progenitor proliferation in the hippocampus. Within 24 h of being placed in an environment of psychosocial stress, for example, the odor of a predator, rodents show a significant decrease in the number of dividing cells in the subgranular zone *(106,124)*. Artificial modulation of stress-related hormones by adrenalectomy or exogenous administration of adrenal steroids shows that at least some of this neurogenic suppression is moderated via circulating corticosteroids *(28,106,125)*. However, steroids may in part impact neurogenesis via changes in neurotransmitter signaling, as blockade of NMDA receptor activation with MK-801 can counteract the effects of stress on proliferation while amplification of glutamate signaling via NMDA receptor agonists mimics the suppression seen in the stress *(28,126)*. The recent observations that progenitors themselves can sense circuit activity also draws attention to the progenitor-intrinsic action of NMDA or L-type calcium channel modulators in vivo *(92)*.

In addition to NMDA receptors, perturbations in several other transmitter systems also influence proliferation in the SGZ. Reduction in serotonin is accompanied by decreased neurogenesis while augmentation increases the number of new neurons *(127,128)*. Similar changes are seen following manipulation of norepinephrine and dopamine systems, each of which are also modulated following physical exercise. The extensive correlations seem to indicate a additional role for monoamine signaling in modulating neurogenesis *(129–132)*. A particularly interesting linkage between depression and attenuated hippocampal neurogenesis has also uncovered the potential utility of traditional antidepressants in promoting neurogenesis within the neurogenic niche of the SGZ *(133)*. When taken together, these somatic and CNS-intrinsic modulatory mechanisms indicate that neurogenesis in the hippocampus responds dynamically to a complex set of overlapping cues. Leveraging these physiological cues within nonneurogenic regions might provide the means for a more successful mobilization of stem cells for repair.

KEY QUESTIONS FOR THE FUTURE

In retrospect, the last 10 yr of research has brought neurosciences from the well-deserved perception of the brain as an immutable collection of cells to our present healthy skepticism that the neuronal and glial precursors and/or stem-like progenitors of the adult brain may retain the dynamic capacity to overturn Cajal's dogma, but only through aggressive intervention. There are several key issues that may represent restriction points in any attempt to direct repair.

Fate Choice

Although it is not directly proven that a neuron-glia fate choice event is intrinsic to neurogenesis, the fact that glial precursor cells may represent a potentially useful substrate for local neuron replacement demands that this concept be explored. In this context, the lineage of progeny generated in vivo is likely regulated by both instructive and selective cues. For example, mitogens may themselves influence the fate potential of neural stem cells. In the embryo, FGF-2 can trigger a multilineage differentiation program (both neurons and glia) at a time when progenitors normally generate only neurons *(134)*. In the adult, precursors that generate only glia can also be switched to a multilineage fate under the influence of FGF-2 *(65,135)*. Other growth factors appear to be more selective in their action. Intraventricular injection of BDNF increases the number of neurons produced by SVZ progenitors *(89,100)*. Progenitors that select a glial fate can be amplified by platelet-derived growth factor (PDGF) *(136–138)* and serum appears to favor the accumulation of astrocytes in cultures initially established from multipotent progenitors *(48)*.

The cues that modulate the fate-choice outcome of mitogenic amplification are not known in the adult but it seems likely that elements of developmentally relevant signaling pathways may be retained. Early in development, factors such as the bone morphogen proteins (BMPs) are instrumental in determining peripheral vs central fates *(42,139,140)* and within the CNS further choices to adopt neuronal or glial fates may be regulated via a balance of instructive, selective and inhibitory cues, the later being typified by the Notch–Delta complex *(141–144)* in addition to antagonists of BMP signaling such as Noggin, which when introduced along with progenitor cells in an ectopic graft can actually promote neurogenesis *(145)*. Because progenitors from nonneurogenic areas do generate neurons after they are removed from their local environment, it is possible that progenitors may simply be prevented from differentiating into neurons in areas where neurogenesis does not occur. Antibodies to several members of the Notch family do recognize related epitopes in the postnatal brain but the role of notch and BMP signaling in the adult remains to be determined *(146–148)*.

Migration

In the adult SVZ and SGZ, newborn neurons migrate from their site of proliferation to a final destination, acquire region-specific transmitter phenotypes, and then send projections into the surrounding parenchyma to establish functional synaptic interactions within the local circuitry. As in development, getting to the right place, becoming the correct cell type and connecting to the appropriate targets must involve a complex cascade of patterning as well as attractive and/or repulsive signals. To a large extent, these signals are unknown in the adult but some insights are being gained within the SVZ. Progenitors within the SVZ migrate in unique self-assembling chains along tracts rich in PSA NCAM *(34,149)*. It is unlikely that chemoattractants are produced by the olfactory bulb, as removal of the olfactory bulb itself has little effect on migration *(150)*. Instead, repulsive proteins related to the Slit family members may drive rostral migration. The evidence for Slit involvement is still correlative but two reports show that septum and choroid plexus produce repulsive factors that act on progenitors in the anterior SVZ *(151)* and both tissues express Slit. In vitro, Slit can repel SVZ progenitors and migration within the rostral migratory stream can be inhibited by a soluble form of Robo, the receptor for Slit proteins *(152)*. Once in the olfactory bulb, progenitors must uncouple from the chain-migration and enter radially into the parenchyma. Recent work suggests that this is mediated, in part, by tenascin-R within the olfactory bulb and that ectopic expression of tenascin-R can re-route neuroblast migration *(153)*.

Slit family members are also expressed in the developing and postnatal hippocampus and expression patterns are consistent with a role in guiding migration by repulsion. However, most studies in the hippocampus have focused on Slit effects on axonal extension rather than cell migration *(154)*. Deficits in the migration of granule cells in development may provide some insight into the molecules active in the adult. For example, Reelin, a large extracellular matrix protein highly expressed by Cajal-Retzius cells *(155–159)*, may provide cues defining where specific neuronal lamina should form by inducing migrating cells to stop *(159–161)*. The combination of repulsion, attraction, and stop signals provided by the Slits and Reelins likely act in concert with other extracellular matrix proteins expressed in the dentate gyrus (such as F-spondin *[162]*, Mindin *[162]*, and PSA-NCAM *[163–165]*) to establish the precisely defined migration patterns of progenitors in the adult brain. Although the guidance signals that normally target cells to a particular location are likely to be somewhat complex, it may not be necessary to perturb each individual element in turn if more global effectors could be identified. For example, ventricular infusion of brain-derived neurotrophic factor amplifies neurogenesis in the SVZ and induces some newborn neuron to migrate tangentially into the overlying striatum *(100)*. These relatively non-specific stimuli might eventually be refined as the relevance of individual guidance proteins become more apparent in the adult.

Axonal Pathfinding

Newborn neurons appear to elaborate axons and dendrites quite rapidly after their last division. In the adult hippocampus, newborn granule cells project to CA3 within a few days of incorporating BrdU *(39)* and receive afferent connections sometime in the following weeks *(38)*. In development, neurites are directed to their final targets by a variety of cues found in the environment through which they are navigating. Within the postnatal hippocampus, Slit proteins may provide some of the repulsive cues that initiate projection away from the granule cell layer. Slit-2 is expressed by cells within the developing and postnatal dentate and may be one of the signals that tell the growth cone to migrate away from the GCL. The fact that exogenously applied Slit-2 is able to repel the axons emanating from dentate explants *(154)* seems to support this possibility; however, Slit-1 and Slit-2 are also expressed in the CA3 target field. If the Slit-responsive axons emanating from dentate explants are in fact those that normally project to CA3 in vivo, then Slits or Slit-like repellants may both initiate extension and help refine the topography of synapse formation by acting at short distances within the target field.

Although we have used the Slit interactions as examples in the preceding, connectivity is ultimately modulated by multiple arrays of repulsive, attractive and stop signals. In addition to Slit, Semaphorin–Neuropilin interactions provide repellent cues within the developing hippocampus and genetic removal of the Neuropilin-2 receptor results in aberrant mossy fiber targeting *(166–171)*. Additional modulation thorough Eph receptor signaling *(172–176)* provides yet further patterning that may be relevant to establishing connections for the newborn dentate granule cells in the adult. Reeler mice also display subtle defects in axon targeting and synaptogenesis within the dentate gyrus, which may suggest a role for Reelin, which is independent of its participation in guidance of cell body migrations. Even the cues that stimulate axonal fasciculation may influence patterns of connectivity since disruption of NCAM *(164)* or LAMP-mediated signaling *(177)* results in improper pathfinding the mossy fiber axons within the pyramidal layers.

Neuronal Subtype Specification

In addition to directing cell fate, final location and connectivity, local cues also instruct progenitors to consolidate location-specific transmitter phenotypes. The numerous transmitter phenotypes generated by adult-derived stem cells in vitro suggest that it may be possible to trigger specific transcriptional programs to produce a wider range of neuronal types than naturally generated in vivo. For example, the simple act of removing mitogen and stimulating cultured stem cells with retinoic acid dramatically up-regulates Trk A, B, and C receptor expression. Subsequent application of neurotrophic factors can promote cells to acquire attributes of dopaminergic, cholinergic, or γ-aminobutyric acid-ergic (GABAergic) neurons *(178)*. If relatively generic "differentiate" signals such as this are combined with the specific manipulation of key transcription factors, it may be possible to precisely direct a specific neuronal fate. An example of how this might be done can be seen in the experimental manipulation of stem cells to generate dopaminergic neurons, the cells at risk in Parkinson's disease.

Dopaminergic neurons are developmentally generated under the influence of a partially defined signaling cascade. Sonic hedgehog protein (Shh) and FGF-8 expression are known to intersect in regions of the developing CNS that become induction sites for dopaminergic neurons in the midbrain and forebrain *(179–181)*. Downstream and independent of Shh signaling, are additional factors, such as Nurr1, that act in concert to implement the gene expression patterns of a midbrain dopaminergic neuron *(182–186)*. In culture, the combination of genetic manipulation (ectopic expression of Nurr1) and exposure to Shh or glial feeder layers can induce cells to acquire many of the dopaminergic cells' phenotypes, the most important of which is the ability to generate dopamine *(187,188)*. Because the adult brain does generate new tyrosine-hydroxylase positive neurons within the olfactory bulb, the ability to recapitulate dopamine production in vitro might not be unexpected but it remains to be determined how broadly the range of neuronal phenotypes can be expanded as similar cascades are identified for other neuronal populations.

CONCLUSIONS

Native neurogenesis appears to involve the local control of neural progenitors that are widely distributed throughout the adult brain. Within each anatomical context, local microenvironments dictate the fate of these progenitors. Additional local cues control migration, connectivity, neuronal phenotype, and ultimately long-term survival and function. Although a number of candidate molecules have been identified for some of these steps, there are still a considerable number of unknowns. It is not known how the decision to generate neurons vs glia is made in the adult. With few exceptions, the cues that direct migration or the projection of neurites in the adult are entirely unknown and, for the vast majority of neuronal types, the transcriptional regulators that control transmitter phenotype remain anonymous.

Perhaps the single largest uncertainty relates to the longstanding fact that evolutionary pressures have unambiguously selected for the absence of global reconstruction in the mammalian brain. It seems likely that the evolutionary "advantages" provided by the absence of large-scale regeneration may ultimately provide one of the more difficult obstacles in repair if the cognitive repercussions of generating new neurons outweigh the anticipated ability to replace lost neurons and glia. Perhaps the first emphasis in exploring the therapeutic potential of mobilizing stem cells should be a careful evaluation of how ectopic neurogenesis in the intact CNS affects behavior and cognition.

REFERENCES

1. Luskin, M. B. and Boone, M. S. (1994) Rate and pattern of migration of lineally-related olfactory bulb interneurons generated postnatally in the subventricular zone of the rat. *Chem. Senses* **19,** 695–714.
2. Gould, E., et al. (1999) Hippocampal neurogenesis in adult Old World primates. *Proc. Natl. Acad. Sci. USA* **96,** 5263–5267.
3. Kuhn, H. G., Dickinson-Anson, H., and Gage, F. H. (1996) Neurogenesis in the dentate gyrus of the adult rat: age-related decrease of neuronal progenitor proliferation. *J. Neurosci.* **16,** 2027–2033.
4. Kempermann, G., Kuhn, H. G., and Gage, F. H. (1997) More hippocampal neurons in adult mice living in an enriched environment. *Nature* **386,** 493–495.
5. Cameron, H. A. and McKay, R. (1998) Stem cells and neurogenesis in the adult brain. *Curr. Opin. Neurobiol.* **8,** 677–680.
6. Gould, E., Reeves, A. J., Graziano, M. S., and Gross, C. G. (1999) Neurogenesis in the neocortex of adult primates. *Science* **286,** 548–552.

7. Bernier, P. J., Bedard, A., Vinet, J., Levesque, M., and Parent, A. (2002) Newly generated neurons in the amygdala and adjoining cortex of adult primates. *Proc. Natl. Acad. Sci. USA* **99,** 11464–11469.

8. Parent, J. M., Janumpalli, S., McNamara, J. O., and Lowenstein, D. H. (1998) Increased dentate granule cell neurogenesis following amygdala kindling in the adult rat. *Neurosci. Lett.* **247,** 9–12.

9. Parent, J. M., et al. (1997) Dentate granule cell neurogenesis is increased by seizures and contributes to aberrant network reorganization in the adult rat hippocampus. *J. Neurosci.* **17,** 3727–3738.

10. Liu, J., Solway, K., Messing, R. O., and Sharp, F. R. (1998) Increased neurogenesis in the dentate gyrus after transient global ischemia in gerbils. *J. Neurosci.* **18,** 7768–7778.

11. Magavi, S. S., Leavitt, B. R., and Macklis, J. D. (2000) Induction of neurogenesis in the neocortex of adult mice. *Nature* **405,** 951–955.

12. Nakatomi, H., et al. (2002) Regeneration of hippocampal pyramidal neurons after ischemic brain injury by recruitment of endogenous neural progenitors. *Cell* **110,** 429.

13. Arvidsson, A., Collin, T., Kirik, D., Kokaia, Z., and Lindvall, O. (2002) Neuronal replacement from endogenous precursors in the adult brain after stroke. *Nat. Med.* **8,** 963–970.

14. Altman, J. and Das, G. D. (1965) Post-natal origin of microneurones in the rat brain. *Nature* **207,** 953–956.

15. Altman, J. and Das, G. D. (1965) Autoradiographic and histological evidence of postnatal hippocampal neurogenesis in rats. *J. Comp Neurol.* **124,** 319–335.

16. Altman, J. and Bayer, S. A. (1990) Migration and distribution of two populations of hippocampal granule cell precursors during the perinatal and postnatal periods. *J. Comp Neurol.* **301,** 365–381.

17. Altman, J. and Bayer, S. A. (1990) Mosaic organization of the hippocampal neuroepithelium and the multiple germinal sources of dentate granule cells. *J. Comp Neurol.* **301,** 325–342.

18. Nowakowski, R. S. and Lewin, S. B. (1989) Bromodeoxyuridine immunohistochemical determination of the lengths of the cell cycle and the DNA-synthetic phase for an anatomically defined population. *J. Neurocytol.* **18,** 311–318.

19. Palmer, T. D., Willhoite, A. R., and Gage, F. H. (2000) Vascular niche for adult hippocampal neurogenesis. *J. Comp Neurol.* **425,** 479–494.

20. Anisimov, V. N. (1995) Carcinogenesis induced by neonatal exposure to various doses of 5-bromo-2'-deoxyuridine in rats. *Cancer Lett.* **91,** 63–71.

21. Ashman, C. R., Reddy, G. P., and Davidson, R. L. (1981) Bromodeoxyuridine mutagenesis, ribonucleotide reductase activity, and deoxyribonucleotide pools in hydroxyurea-resistant mutants. *Somatic. Cell Genet.* **7,** 751–768.

22. Comi, P., et al. (1986) Bromodeoxyuridine treatment of normal adult erythroid colonies: an in vitro model for reactivation of human fetal globin genes. *Blood* **68,** 1036–1041.

23. Keoffler, H. P., Yen, J., and Carlson, J. (1983) The study of human myeloid differentiation using bromodeoxyuridine (BrdU). *J. Cell Physiol.* **116,** 111–117.

24. Kinoshita, Y., Makita, A., and Takeuchi, T. (1982) Bromodeoxyuridine-induced molecular species conversion of sialic acids of gangliosides and the alteration of cellular phenotypic expression in B16 mouse melanoma cells. *J. Biochem.* **92,** 801–808.

25. Ashman, C. R. and Davidson, R. L. (1980) Inhibition of Friend erythroleukemic cell differentiation by bromodeoxyuridine: correlation with the amount of bromodeoxyuridine in DNA. *J. Cell Physiol.* **102,** 45–50.

26. Malendowicz, L. K., Rebuffat, P., Andreis, P. G., Nussdorfer, G. G., and Nowak, M. (1997) Different mechanisms mediate the in vivo aldosterone and corticosterone responses to 5-bromo-2'-deoxyuridine in rats. *Exp. Clin. Endocrinol. Diabetes* **105,** 277–281.

27. Malendowicz, L. K. and Nussdorfer, G. G. (1996) 5-Bromo-2'-deoxyuridine stimulates the pituitary-adrenal axis in the rat: an effect blocked partially by endothelin-receptor antagonists. *J. Int. Med. Res.* **24,** 363–368.

28. Cameron, H. A., Tanapat, P., and Gould, E. (1998) Adrenal steroids and *N*-methyl-D-aspartate receptor activation regulate neurogenesis in the dentate gyrus of adult rats through a common pathway. *Neuroscience* **82,** 349–354.

29. Morshead, C. M., et al. (1994) Neural stem cells in the adult mammalian forebrain: a relatively quiescent subpopulation of subependymal cells. *Neuron* **13,** 1071–1082.

30. Brown, J. P., et al. (2003) Transient expression of doublecortin during adult neurogenesis. *J. Comp Neurol.* **467,** 1–10.

31. Kempermann, G., Gast, D., Kronenberg, G., Yamaguchi, M., and Gage, F. H. (2003) Early determination and long-term persistence of adult-generated new neurons in the hippocampus of mice. *Development* **130,** 391–399.

32. Bayer, S. A. (1985) Neuron production in the hippocampus and olfactory bulb of the adult rat brain: addition or replacement? *Ann. NY Acad. Sci.* **457,** 163–172.

33. Kaplan, M. S. and Hinds, J. W. (1977) Neurogenesis in the adult rat: electron microscopic analysis of light radioautographs. *Science* **197,** 1092–1094.

34. Doetsch, F., Garcia-Verdugo, J. M., and Alvarez-Buylla, A. (1997) Cellular composition and three-dimensional organization of the subventricular germinal zone in the adult mammalian brain. *J. Neurosci.* **17,** 5046–5061.

35. Betarbet, R., Zigova, T., Bakay, R. A., and Luskin, M. B. (1996) Dopaminergic and GABAergic interneurons of the olfactory bulb are derived from the neonatal subventricular zone. *Int. J. Dev. Neurosci.* **14,** 921–930.

36. Craig, C. G., D'sa, R., Morshead, C. M., Roach, A., and van der, K. D. (1999) Migrational analysis of the constitutively proliferating subependyma population in adult mouse forebrain. *Neuroscience* **93,** 1197–1206.

37. Stanfield, B. B. and Trice, J. E. (1988) Evidence that granule cells generated in the dentate gyrus of adult rats extend axonal projections. *Exp. Brain Res.* **72,** 399–406.

38. Markakis, E. A. and Gage, F. H. (1999) Adult-generated neurons in the dentate gyrus send axonal projections to field CA3 and are surrounded by synaptic vesicles. *J. Comp. Neurol.* **406,** 449–460.

39. Hastings, N. B. and Gould, E. (1999) Rapid extension of axons into the CA3 region by adult-generated granule cells (published erratum appears in *J. Comp. Neurol.* [1999] **415,** 144). *J. Comp. Neurol.* **413,** 146–154.

40. van Praag, H., et al. (2002) Functional neurogenesis in the adult hippocampus. *Nature* **415,** 1030–1034.

41. Gage, F. H., et al. (1995) Survival and differentiation of adult neuronal progenitor cells transplanted to the adult brain. *Proc. Natl. Acad. Sci. USA* **92,** 11879–11883.

42. Morrison, S. J., Shah, N. M., and Anderson, D. J. (1997) Regulatory mechanisms in stem cell biology. *Cell* **88,** 287–298.

43. Temple, S. and Alvarez-Buylla, A. (1999) Stem cells in the adult mammalian central nervous system. *Curr. Opin. Neurobiol.* **9,** 135–141.

44. Kilpatrick, T. J. and Bartlett, P. F. (1995) Cloned multipotential precursors from the mouse cerebrum require FGF-2, whereas glial restricted precursors are stimulated with either FGF-2 or EGF. *J. Neurosci.* **15,** 3653–3661.

45. Gritti, A., et al. (1999) Epidermal and fibroblast growth factors behave as mitogenic regulators for a single multipotent stem cell-like population from the subventricular region of the adult mouse forebrain. *J. Neurosci.* **19,** 3287–3297.

46. Ciccolini, F. and Svendsen, C. N. (1998) Fibroblast growth factor 2 (FGF-2) promotes acquisition of epidermal growth factor (EGF) responsiveness in mouse striatal precursor cells: identification of neural precursors responding to both EGF and FGF-2. *J. Neurosci.* **18,** 7869–7880.

47. Pincus, D. W., et al. (1997) In vitro neurogenesis by adult human epileptic temporal neocortex. *Clin. Neurosurg.* **44,** 17–25.

48. Palmer, T. D., Takahashi, J., and Gage, F. H. (1997) The adult rat hippocampus contains primordial neural stem cells. *Mol. Cell Neurosci.* **8,** 389–404.

49. Gritti, A., et al. (1996) Multipotential stem cells from the adult mouse brain proliferate and self-renew in response to basic fibroblast growth factor. *J. Neurosci.* **16,** 1091–1100.

50. Chiasson, B. J., Tropepe, V., Morshead, C. M., and van der, K. D. (1999) Adult mammalian forebrain ependymal and subependymal cells demonstrate proliferative potential, but only subependymal cells have neural stem cell characteristics. *J. Neurosci.* **19,** 4462–4471.

51. Tropepe, V., et al. (1999) Distinct neural stem cells proliferate in response to EGF and FGF in the developing mouse telencephalon. *Dev. Biol.* **208,** 166–188.

52. Doetsch, F., Caille, I., Lim, D. A., Garcia-Verdugo, J. M., and Alvarez-Buylla, A. (1999) Subventricular zone astrocytes are neural stem cells in the adult mammalian brain. *Cell* **97,** 703–716.

53. Cepko, C., Ryder, E. F., Austin, C. P., Walsh, C., and Fekete, D. M. (1995) Lineage analysis using retrovirus vectors. *Methods Enzymol.* **254,** 387–419.

54. Levison, S. W. and Goldman, J. E. (1997) Multipotential and lineage restricted precursors coexist in the mammalian perinatal subventricular zone. *J. Neurosci. Res.* **48,** 83–94.

55. Gabay, L., Lowell, S., Rubin, L. L., and Anderson, D. J. (2003) Deregulation of dorsoventral patterning by FGF confers trilineage differentiation capacity on CNS stem cells in vitro. *Neuron* **40,** 485–499.

56. Horner, P. J., et al. (2000) Proliferation and differentiation of progenitor cells throughout the intact adult rat spinal cord [In Process Citation]. *J. Neurosci.* **20,** 2218–2228.

57. Levine, J. M., Stincone, F., and Lee, Y. S. (1993) Development and differentiation of glial precursor cells in the rat cerebellum. *Glia* **7,** 307–321.

58. Horner, P. J., et al. (2000) Proliferation and differentiation of progenitor cells throughout the intact adult rat spinal cord. *J. Neurosci.* **20,** 2218–2228.

59. Rogister, B., Ben Hur, T., and Dubois-Dalcq, M. (1999) From neural stem cells to myelinating oligodendrocytes. *Mol. Cell. Neurosci.* **14,** 287–300.

60. Levine, J. M. and Nishiyama, A. (1996) The NG2 chondroitin sulfate proteoglycan: a multifunctional proteoglycan associated with immature cells. *Perspect. Dev. Neurobiol.* **3,** 245–259.

61. Horner, P. J., Thallmair, M., and Gage, F. H. (2002) Defining the NG2 cell of the adult central nervous system. *J. Neurocytol.* **31,** 469–480.

62. Lipson, A. C. and Horner, P. J. (2002) Potent possibilities: endogenous stem cells in the adult spinal cord. *Spinal Cord Trauma Regen. Neural Repair Funct. Recov.* **137,** 283–297.

63. Dawson, M. R. L., Levine, J. M., and Reynolds, R. (2000) NG2-Expressing cells in the central nervous system: Are they oligodendroglial progenitors? *J. Neurosci. Res.* **61,** 471–479.

64. Palmer, T. D., Ray, J., and Gage, F. H. (1995) FGF-2-responsive neuronal progenitors reside in proliferative and quiescent regions of the adult rodent brain. *Mol. Cell Neurosci.* **6,** 474–486.

65. Kondo, T. and Raff, M. (2000) Oligodendrocyte precursor cells reprogrammed to become multipotential CNS stem cells (see comments). *Science* **289,** 1754–1757.

66. Nunes, M. C., et al. (2003) Identification and isolation of multipotential neural progenitor cells from the subcortical white matter of the adult human brain. *Nat. Med.* **9,** 439–447.

67. Shihabuddin, L. S., Horner, P. J., Ray, J., and Gage, F. H. (2000) Adult spinal cord stem cells generate neurons after transplantation in the adult dentate gyrus. *J. Neurosci.* **20,** 8727–8735.

68. Noctor, S. C., et al. (2002) Dividing precursor cells of the embryonic cortical ventricular zone have morphological and molecular characteristics of radial glia. *J. Neurosci.* **22,** 3161–3173.

69. Noctor, S. C., Flint, A. C., Weissman, T. A., Dammerman, R. S., and Kriegstein, A. R. (2001) Neurons derived from radial glial cells establish radial units in neocortex. *Nature* **409,** 714–720.

70. Tramontin, A. D., Garcia-Verdugo, J. M., Lim, D. A., and Alvarez-Buylla, A. (2003) Postnatal development of radial glia and the ventricular zone (VZ): a continuum of the neural stem cell compartment. *Cereb. Cortex* **13,** 580–587.

71. Filippov, V., et al. (2003) Subpopulation of nestin-expressing progenitor cells in the adult murine hippocampus shows electrophysiological and morphological characteristics of astrocytes. *Mol. Cell Neurosci.* **23,** 373–382.

72. Seri, B., Garcia-Verdugo, J. M., McEwen, B. S., and Alvarez-Buylla, A. (2001) Astrocytes give rise to new neurons in the adult mammalian hippocampus. *J. Neurosci.* **21,** 7153–7160.

73. Louissaint, A., Jr., Rao, S., Leventhal, C., and Goldman, S. A. (2002) Coordinated interaction of neurogenesis and angiogenesis in the adult songbird brain. *Neuron* **34,** 945–960.

74. Jin, K., et al. (2002) Vascular endothelial growth factor (VEGF) stimulates neurogenesis in vitro and in vivo. *Proc. Natl. Acad. Sci. USA* **99,** 11946–11950.

75. Wagner, J. P., Black, I. B., and DiCicco-Bloom, E. (1999) Stimulation of neonatal and adult brain neurogenesis by subcutaneous injection of basic fibroblast growth factor. *J. Neurosci.* **19,** 6006–6016.

76. Tao, Y., Black, I. B., and DiCicco-Bloom, E. (1996) Neurogenesis in neonatal rat brain is regulated by peripheral injection of basic fibroblast growth factor (bFGF). *J. Comp Neurol.* **376,** 653–663.

77. Aberg, M. A., Aberg, N. D., Hedbacker, H., Oscarsson, J., and Eriksson, P. S. (2000) Peripheral infusion of IGF-I selectively induces neurogenesis in the adult rat hippocampus. *J. Neurosci.* **20,** 2896–2903.

78. Reynolds, B. A., Tetzlaff, W., and Weiss, S. (1992) A multipotent EGF-responsive striatal embryonic progenitor cell produces neurons and astrocytes. *J. Neurosci.* **12,** 4565–4574.

79. Reynolds, B. A. and Weiss, S. (1992) Generation of neurons and astrocytes from isolated cells of the adult mammalian central nervous system [see comments]. *Science* **255,** 1707–1710.

80. Vescovi, A. L., Reynolds, B. A., Fraser, D. D., and Weiss, S. (1993) bFGF regulates the proliferative fate of unipotent (neuronal) and bipotent (neuronal/astroglial) EGF-generated CNS progenitor cells. *Neuron* **11,** 951–966.

81. Bartlett, P. F., Dutton, R., Likiardopoulos, V., and Brooker, G. (1994) Regulation of neurogenesis in the embryonic and adult brain by fibroblast growth factors. *Alcohol Alcohol Suppl.* **2,** 387–394.

82. Cameron, H. A., Hazel, T. G., and McKay, R. D. (1998) Regulation of neurogenesis by growth factors and neurotransmitters. *J. Neurobiol.* **36,** 287–306.

83. Lai, K., Kaspar, B. K., Gage, F. H., and Schaffer, D. V. (2003) Sonic hedgehog regulates adult neural progenitor proliferation in vitro and in vivo. *Nat. Neurosci.* **6,** 21–27.

84. Craig, C. G., et al. (1996) In vivo growth factor expansion of endogenous subependymal neural precursor cell populations in the adult mouse brain. *J. Neurosci.* **16,** 2649–2658.

85. Kuhn, H. G., Winkler, J., Kempermann, G., Thal, L. J., and Gage, F. H. (1997) Epidermal growth factor and fibroblast growth factor-2 have different effects on neural progenitors in the adult rat brain. *J. Neurosci.* **17,** 5820–5829.

86. Gonzalez, A. M., et al. (1994) Storage, metabolism, and processing of ^{125}I-fibroblast growth factor-2 after intracerebral injection. *Brain Res.* **665,** 285–292.

87. Matsumoto, K., Yoshitomi, H., Rossant, J., and Zaret, K. S. (2001) Liver organogenesis promoted by endothelial cells prior to vascular function. *Science* **294,** 559–563.

88. Lammert, E., Cleaver, O., and Melton, D. (2001) Induction of pancreatic differentiation by signals from blood vessels. *Science* **294,** 564–567.

89. Leventhal, C., Rafii, S., Rafii, D., Shahar, A., and Goldman, S. A. (1999) Endothelial trophic support of neuronal production and recruitment from the adult mammalian subependyma. *Mol. Cell Neurosci.* **13,** 450–464.

90. Shen, Q., et al. (2004) Endothelial cells stimulate self-renewal and expand neurogenesis of neural stem cells. *Science* **304,** 1338–1340.

91. Song, H., Stevens, C. F., and Gage, F. H. (2002) Astroglia induce neurogenesis from adult neural stem cells. *Nature* **417,** 39–44.

92. Deisseroth, K., et al. (2004) Excitation-neurogenesis coupling in adult neural stem/progenitor cells. *Neuron* **42,** 535–552.

93. Guillemin, K. and Krasnow, M. A. (1997) The hypoxic response: huffing and HIFing. *Cell* **89,** 9–12.

94. Cheng, A., Wang, S., Cai, J., Rao, M. S., and Mattson, M. P. (2003) Nitric oxide acts in a positive feedback loop with BDNF to regulate neural progenitor cell proliferation and differentiation in the mammalian brain. *Dev. Biol.* **258,** 319–333.

95. Shingo, T., Sorokan, S. T., Shimazaki, T., and Weiss, S. (2001) Erythropoietin regulates the in vitro and in vivo production of neuronal progenitors by mammalian forebrain neural stem cells. *J. Neurosci.* **21,** 9733–9743.

96. Parent, J. M. (2002) The role of seizure-induced neurogenesis in epileptogenesis and brain repair. *Epilepsy Res.* **50,** 179–189.

97. Madsen, T. M., et al. (2000) Increased neurogenesis in a model of electroconvulsive therapy. *Biol. Psychiatry* **47,** 1043–1049.

98. Coyle, J. T. and Duman, R. S. (2003) Finding the intracellular signaling pathways affected by mood disorder treatments. *Neuron* **38,** 157–160.

99. Cheng, A., Wang, S., Cai, J., Rao, M. S., and Mattson, M. P. (2003) Nitric oxide acts in a positive feedback loop with BDNF to regulate neural progenitor cell proliferation and differentiation in the mammalian brain. *Dev. Biol.* **258,** 319–333.

100. Zigova, T., Pencea, V., Wiegand, S. J., and Luskin, M. B. (1998) Intraventricular administration of BDNF increases the number of newly generated neurons in the adult olfactory bulb. *Mol. Cell. Neurosci.* **11,** 234–245.

101. Fallon, J., et al. (2000) In vivo induction of massive proliferation, directed migration, and differentiation of neural cells in the adult mammalian brain. *Proc. Natl. Acad. Sci. USA* **97,** 14686–14691.

102. Monje, M. L., Mizumatsu, S., Fike, J. R., and Palmer, T. D. (2002) Irradiation induces neural precursor-cell dysfunction. *Nat. Med.* **8,** 955–962.

103. Ekdahl, C. T., Classen, J. H., Bonde, S., Kokaia, Z., and Lindvall, O. (2003) Inflammation is detrimental for neurogenesis in adult brain. *Proc. Natl. Acad. Sci. USA* **100,** 13632–13637.

104. Monje, M. L., Toda, H., and Palmer, T. D. (2003) Inflammatory Blockade Restores Adult Hippocampal Neurogenesis. *Science*.

105. Monje, M. L. and Palmer, T. (2003) Radiation injury and neurogenesis. *Curr. Opin. Neurol.* **16,** 129–134.

106. Tanapat, P., Galea, L. A., and Gould, E. (1998) Stress inhibits the proliferation of granule cell precursors in the developing dentate gyrus. *Int. J. Dev. Neurosci.* **16,** 235–239.

107. McEwen, B. S., et al. (1993) Adrenal steroids and plasticity of hippocampal neurons: toward an understanding of underlying cellular and molecular mechanisms. *Cell Mol. Neurobiol.* **13,** 457–482.

108. Zhao, M., et al. (2003) Evidence for neurogenesis in the adult mammalian substantia nigra. *Proc. Natl. Acad. Sci. USA* **100,** 7925–7930.

109. Lie, D. C., et al. (2002) The adult substantia nigra contains progenitor cells with neurogenic potential. *J. Neurosci.* **22,** 6639–6649.

110. Brazelton, T. R., Rossi, F. M., Keshet, G. I., and Blau, H. M. (2000) From marrow to brain: expression of neuronal phenotypes in adult mice. *Science* **290,** 1775–1779.

111. Weimann, J. M., Charlton, C. A., Brazelton, T. R., Hackman, R. C., and Blau, H. M. (2003) Contribution of transplanted bone marrow cells to Purkinje neurons in human adult brains. *Proc. Natl. Acad. Sci. USA* **100,** 2088–2093.

112. Kempermann, G., Kuhn, H. G., and Gage, F. H. (1998) Experience-induced neurogenesis in the senescent dentate gyrus. *J. Neurosci.* **18**, 3206–3212.

113. Gould, E., Beylin, A., Tanapat, P., Reeves, A., and Shors, T. J. (1999) Learning enhances adult neurogenesis in the hippocampal formation (see comments). *Nat. Neurosci.* **2**, 260–265.

114. van Praag, H., Kempermann, G., and Gage, F. H. (1999) Running increases cell proliferation and neurogenesis in the adult mouse dentate gyrus (see comments). *Nat. Neurosci.* **2**, 266–270.

115. van Praag, H., Christie, B. R., Sejnowski, T. J., and Gage, F. H. (1999) Running enhances neurogenesis, learning, and long-term potentiation in mice. *Proc. Natl. Acad. Sci. USA* **96**, 13427–13431.

116. Kempermann, G., Kuhn, H. G., and Gage, F. H. (1997) Genetic influence on neurogenesis in the dentate gyrus of adult mice. *Proc. Natl. Acad. Sci. USA* **94**, 10409–10414.

117. Kempermann, G. and Gage, F. H. (2002) Genetic determinants of adult hippocampal neurogenesis correlate with acquisition, but not probe trial performance, in the water maze task. *Eur. J. Neurosci.* **16**, 129–136.

118. Eriksson, P. S., et al. (1998) Neurogenesis in the adult human hippocampus [see comments]. *Nat. Med.* **4**, 1313–1317.

119. Greenough, W. T., Cohen, N. J., and Juraska, J. M. (1999) New neurons in old brains: learning to survive? [news; comment]. *Nat. Neurosci.* **2**, 203–205.

120. Diamond, M. C., Rosenzweig, M. R., Bennett, E. L., Lindner, B., and Lyon, L. (1972) Effects of environmental enrichment and impoverishment on rat cerebral cortex. *J. Neurobiol.* **3**, 47–64.

121. Diamond, M. C., Ingham, C. A., Johnson, R. E., Bennett, E. L., and Rosenzweig, M. R. (1976) Effects of environment on morphology of rat cerebral cortex and hippocampus. *J. Neurobiol.* **7**, 75–85.

122. Brown, J., et al. (2003) Enriched environment and physical activity stimulate hippocampal but not olfactory bulb neurogenesis. *Eur. J. Neurosci.* **17**, 2042–2046.

123. Fabel, K., et al. (2003) VEGF is necessary for exercise-induced adult hippocampal neurogenesis. *Eur. J. Neurosci.* **18**, 2803–2812.

124. Gould, E., McEwen, B. S., Tanapat, P., Galea, L. A., and Fuchs, E. (1997) Neurogenesis in the dentate gyrus of the adult tree shrew is regulated by psychosocial stress and NMDA receptor activation. *J. Neurosci.* **17**, 2492–2498.

125. McEwen, B. S. (1999) Stress and hippocampal plasticity. *Annu. Rev. Neurosci.* **22**, 105–122.

126. Cameron, H. A., McEwen, B. S., and Gould, E. (1995) Regulation of adult neurogenesis by excitatory input and NMDA receptor activation in the dentate gyrus. *J. Neurosci.* **15**, 4687–4692.

127. Brezun, J. M. and Daszuta, A. (2000) Serotonin may stimulate granule cell proliferation in the adult hippocampus, as observed in rats grafted with foetal raphe neurons. *Eur. J. Neurosci.* **12**, 391–396.

128. Brezun, J. M. and Daszuta, A. (1999) Depletion in serotonin decreases neurogenesis in the dentate gyrus and the subventricular zone of adult rats. *Neuroscience* **89**, 999–1002.

129. Dawirs, R. R., Hildebrandt, K., and Teuchert-Noodt, G. (1998) Adult treatment with haloperidol increases dentate granule cell proliferation in the gerbil hippocampus. *J. Neural Transm.* **105**, 317–327.

130. Hildebrandt, K., Teuchert-Noodt, G., and Dawirs, R. R. (1999) A single neonatal dose of methamphetamine suppresses dentate granule cell proliferation in adult gerbils which is restored to control values by acute doses of haloperidol. *J. Neural Transm.* **106**, 549–558.

131. Jacobs, B. L. and Fornal, C. A. (1999) Activity of serotonergic neurons in behaving animals. *Neuropsychopharmacology* **21**, 9S–15S.

132. Duman, R. S., Malberg, J., and Thome, J. (1999) Neural plasticity to stress and antidepressant treatment. *Biol. Psychiatry* **46**, 1181–1191.

133. Santarelli, L., et al. (2003) Requirement of hippocampal neurogenesis for the behavioral effects of antidepressants. *Science* **301**, 805–809.
134. Stemple, D. L. and Mahanthappa, N. K. (1997) Neural stem cells are blasting off. *Neuron* **18**, 1–4.
135. Palmer, T. D., Markakis, E. A., Willhoite, A. R., Safar, F., and Gage, F. H. (1999) Fibroblast growth factor-2 activates a latent neurogenic program in neural stem cells from diverse regions of the adult CNS. *J. Neurosci.* **19**, 8487–8497.
136. Barres, B. A., Schmid, R., Sendnter, M., and Raff, M. C. (1993) Multiple extracellular signals are required for long-term oligodendrocyte survival. *Development* **118**, 283–295.
137. Wolswijk, G. and Noble, M. (1992) Cooperation between PDGF and FGF converts slowly dividing O-2Aadult progenitor cells to rapidly dividing cells with characteristics of O-2Aperinatal progenitor cells. *J. Cell Biol.* **118**, 889–900.
138. Wolswijk, G., Riddle, P. N., and Noble, M. (1991) Platelet-derived growth factor is mitogenic for O-2Aadult progenitor cells. *Glia* **4**, 495–503.
139. Mujtaba, T., Mayer-Proschel, M., and Rao, M. S. (1998) A common neural progenitor for the CNS and PNS. *Dev. Biol.* **200**, 1–15.
140. Kalyani, A. J. and Rao, M. S. (1998) Cell lineage in the developing neural tube. *Biochem. Cell Biol.* **76**, 1051–1068.
141. Lindsell, C. E., Boulter, J., diSibio, G., Gossler, A., and Weinmaster, G. (1996) Expression patterns of Jagged, Delta1, Notch1, Notch2, and Notch3 genes identify ligand-receptor pairs that may function in neural development. *Mol. Cell. Neurosci.* **8**, 14–27.
142. Zhong, W., Jiang, M. M., Weinmaster, G., Jan, L. Y., and Jan, Y. N. (1997) Differential expression of mammalian Numb, Numblike and Notch1 suggests distinct roles during mouse cortical neurogenesis. *Development* **124**, 1887–1897.
143. Chenn, A. and McConnell, S. K. (1995) Cleavage orientation and the asymmetric inheritance of Notch1 immunoreactivity in mammalian neurogenesis. *Cell* **82**, 631–641.
144. Temple, S. and Qian, X. (1996) Vertebrate neural progenitor cells: subtypes and regulation. *Curr. Opin. Neurobiol.* **6**, 11–17.
145. Lim, D. A., et al. (2000) Noggin antagonizes BMP signaling to create a niche for adult neurogenesis. *Neuron* **28**, 713–726.
146. Allen, T. and Lobe, C. G. (1999) A comparison of Notch, Hes and Grg expression during murine embryonic and post-natal development. *Cell Mol. Biol.* **45**, 687–708.
147. Tanaka, M., Kadokawa, Y., Hamada, Y., and Marunouchi, T. (1999) Notch2 expression negatively correlates with glial differentiation in the postnatal mouse brain. *J. Neurobiol.* **41**, 524–539.
148. Higuchi, M., Kiyama, H., Hayakawa, T., Hamada, Y., and Tsujimoto, Y. (1995) Differential expression of Notch1 and Notch2 in developing and adult mouse brain. *Brain Res. Mol. Brain Res.* **29**, 263–272.
149. Lois, C., Garcia-Verdugo, J. M., and Alvarez-Buylla, A. (1996) Chain migration of neuronal precursors. *Science* **271**, 978–981.
150. Kirschenbaum, B., Doetsch, F., Lois, C., and Alvarez-Buylla, A. (1999) Adult subventricular zone neuronal precursors continue to proliferate and migrate in the absence of the olfactory bulb. *J. Neurosci.* **19**, 2171–2180.
151. Hu, H. (1999) Chemorepulsion of neuronal migration by Slit2 in the developing mammalian forebrain. *Neuron* **23**, 703–711.
152. Wu, W., et al. (1999) Directional guidance of neuronal migration in the olfactory system by the protein Slit (see comments). *Nature* **400**, 331–336.
153. Saghatelyan, A., De, C. A., Schachner, M., and Lledo, P. M. (2004) Tenascin-R mediates activity-dependent recruitment of neuroblasts in the adult mouse forebrain. *Nat. Neurosci.* **7**, 347–356.
154. Nguyen Ba-Charvet, K. T., et al. (1999) Slit2-Mediated chemorepulsion and collapse of developing forebrain axons. *Neuron* **22**, 463–473.

155. Borrell, V., Ruiz, M., Del Rio, J. A., and Soriano, E. (1999) Development of commissural connections in the hippocampus of reeler mice: evidence of an inhibitory influence of Cajal-Retzius cells. *Exp. Neurol.* **156,** 268–282.
156. Borrell, V., et al. (1999) Reelin regulates the development and synaptogenesis of the layer-specific entorhino-hippocampal connections. *J. Neurosci.* **19,** 1345–1358.
157. Del Rio, J. A., et al. (1997) A role for Cajal-Retzius cells and reelin in the development of hippocampal connections (see comments). *Nature* **385,** 70–74.
158. Deller, T., Drakew, A., and Frotscher, M. (1999) Different primary target cells are important for fiber lamination in the fascia dentata: a lesson from reeler mutant mice. *Exp. Neurol.* **156,** 239–253.
159. Frotscher, M. (1998) Cajal-Retzius cells, Reelin, and the formation of layers. *Curr. Opin. Neurobiol.* **8,** 570–575.
160. Nakajima, K., Mikoshiba, K., Miyata, T., Kudo, C., and Ogawa, M. (1997) Disruption of hippocampal development in vivo by CR-50 mAb against reelin. *Proc. Natl. Acad. Sci. USA* **94,** 8196–8201.
161. Frotscher, M. (1997) Dual role of Cajal-Retzius cells and reelin in cortical development. *Cell Tissue Res.* **290,** 315–322.
162. Feinstein, Y., et al. (1999) F-spondin and mindin: two structurally and functionally related genes expressed in the hippocampus that promote outgrowth of embryonic hippocampal neurons. *Development* **126,** 3637–3648.
163. Aubert, I., Ridet, J. L., Schachner, M., Rougon, G., and Gage, F. H. (1998) Expression of L1 and PSA during sprouting and regeneration in the adult hippocampal formation. *J. Comp Neurol.* **399,** 1–19.
164. Cremer, H., Chazal, G., Goridis, C., and Represa, A. (1997) NCAM is essential for axonal growth and fasciculation in the hippocampus. *Mol. Cell Neurosci.* **8,** 323–335.
165. Chazal, G., Durbec, P., Jankovski, A., Rougon, G., and Cremer, H. (2000) Consequences of neural cell adhesion molecule deficiency on cell migration in the rostral migratory stream of the mouse. *J. Neurosci.* **20,** 1446–1457.
166. Chedotal, A., et al. (1998) Semaphorins III and IV repel hippocampal axons via two distinct receptors. *Development* **125,** 4313–4323.
167. Steup, A., et al. (2000) Sema3C and netrin-1 differentially affect axon growth in the hippocampal formation. *Mol. Cell. Neurosci.* **15,** 141–155.
168. Steup, A., et al. (1999) Semaphorin D acts as a repulsive factor for entorhinal and hippocampal neurons. *Eur. J. Neurosci.* **11,** 729–734.
169. Chen, H., et al. (2000) Neuropilin-2 regulates the development of selective cranial and sensory nerves and hippocampal mossy fiber projections. *Neuron* **25,** 43–56.
170. Chen, H., He, Z., and Tessier-Lavigne, M. (1998) Axon guidance mechanisms: semaphorins as simultaneous repellents and anti-repellents (news; comment). *Nat. Neurosci.* **1,** 436–439.
171. Giger, R. J., et al. (2000) Neuropilin-2 is required in vivo for selective axon guidance responses to secreted semaphorins. *Neuron* **25,** 29–41.
172. Holder, N. and Klein, R. (1999) Eph receptors and ephrins: effectors of morphogenesis. *Development* **126,** 2033–2044.
173. Zhang, J. H., Cerretti, D. P., Yu, T., Flanagan, J. G., and Zhou, R. (1996) Detection of ligands in regions anatomically connected to neurons expressing the Eph receptor Bsk: potential roles in neuron-target interaction. *J. Neurosci.* **16,** 7182–7192.
174. Gao, P. P., et al. (1996) Regulation of topographic projection in the brain: Elf-1 in the hippocamposeptal system. *Proc. Natl. Acad. Sci. USA* **93,** 11161–11166.
175. Gao, P. P., Yue, Y., Cerretti, D. P., Dreyfus, C., and Zhou, R. (1999) Ephrin-dependent growth and pruning of hippocampal axons. *Proc. Natl. Acad. Sci. USA* **96,** 4073–4077.
176. Stein, E., et al. (1999) A role for the Eph ligand ephrin-A3 in entorhino-hippocampal axon targeting. *J. Neurosci.* **19,** 8885–8893.

177. Pimenta, A. F., et al. (1995) The limbic system-associated membrane protein is an Ig superfamily member that mediates selective neuronal growth and axon targeting. *Neuron* **15,** 287–297.
178. Takahashi, J., Palmer, T. D., and Gage, F. H. (1999) Retinoic acid and neurotrophins collaborate to regulate neurogenesis in adult-derived neural stem cell cultures. *J. Neurobiol.* **38,** 65–81.
179. Hynes, M., et al. (1995) Induction of midbrain dopaminergic neurons by Sonic Hedgehog. *Neuron* **15,** 35–44.
180. Murone, M., Rosenthal, A., and de Sauvage, F. J. (1999) Sonic hedgehog signaling by the patched-smoothened receptor complex. *Curr. Biol.* **9,** 76–84.
181. Ye, W., Shimamura, K., Rubenstein, J. L., Hynes, M. A., and Rosenthal, A. (1998) FGF and Shh signals control dopaminergic and serotonergic cell fate in the anterior neural plate. *Cell* **93,** 755–766.
182. Law, S. W., Conneely, O. M., DeMayo, F. J., and O'Malley, B. W. (1992) Identification of a new brain-specific transcription factor, NURR1. *Mol. Endocrinol.* **6,** 2129–2135.
183. Zetterstrom, R. H., Williams, R., Perlmann, T., and Olson, L. (1996) Cellular expression of the immediate early transcription factors Nurr1 and NGFI-B suggests a gene regulatory role in several brain regions including the nigrostriatal dopamine system. *Brain Res. Mol. Brain Res.* **41,** 111–120.
184. Zetterstrom, R. H., et al. (1997) Dopamine neuron agenesis in Nurr1-deficient mice [see comments]. *Science* **276,** 248–250.
185. Saucedo-Cardenas, O., et al. (1998) Nurr1 is essential for the induction of the dopaminergic phenotype and the survival of ventral mesencephalic late dopaminergic precursor neurons. *Proc. Natl. Acad. Sci. USA* **95,** 4013–4018.
186. Castillo, S. O., et al. (1998) Dopamine biosynthesis is selectively abolished in substantia nigra/ventral tegmental area but not in hypothalamic neurons in mice with targeted disruption of the Nurr1 gene. *Mol. Cell Neurosci.* **11,** 36–46.
187. Sakurada, K., Ohshima-Sakurada, M., Palmer, T. D., and Gage, F. H. (1999) Nurr1, an orphan nuclear receptor, is a transcriptional activator of endogenous tyrosine hydroxylase in neural progenitor cells derived from the adult brain. *Development* **126,** 4017–4026.
188. Wagner, J., et al. (1999) Induction of a midbrain dopaminergic phenotype in Nurr1-overexpressing neural stem cells by type 1 astrocytes [see comments]. *Nat. Biotechnol.* **17,** 653–659.
189. Tanapat, P., Hastings, N. B., Reeves, A. J., and Gould, E. (1999) Estrogen stimulates a transient increase in the number of new neurons in the dentate gyrus of the adult female rat. *J. Neurosci.* **19,** 5792–5801.
190. Brezun, J. M. and Daszuta, A. (2000) Serotonergic reinnervation reverses lesion-induced decreases in PSA-NCAM labeling and proliferation of hippocampal cells in adult rats [In Process Citation]. *Hippocampus* **10,** 37–46.
191. Bartlett, P. F., et al. (1995) Factors regulating the differentiation of neural precursors in the forebrain. *Ciba Found. Symp.* **193,** 85–99.
192. Svendsen, C. N., Caldwell, M. A., and Ostenfeld, T. (1999) Human neural stem cells: isolation, expansion and transplantation. *Brain Pathol.* **9,** 499–513.
193. DeHamer, M. K., Guevara, J. L., Hannon, K., Olwin, B. B., and Calof, A. L. (1994) Genesis of olfactory receptor neurons in vitro: regulation of progenitor cell divisions by fibroblast growth factors. *Neuron* **13,** 1083–1097.
194. Ray, J., Baird, A., and Gage, F. H. (1997) A 10-amino acid sequence of fibroblast growth factor 2 is sufficient for its mitogenic activity on neural progenitor cells. *Proc. Natl. Acad. Sci. USA* **94,** 7047–7052.
195. Bonni, A., et al. (1997) Regulation of gliogenesis in the central nervous system by the JAK-STAT signaling pathway. *Science* **278,** 477–483.

15

Neural Stem Cells and Transplant Therapy

Intrinsic Programs and Clinical Applications

Jaime Imitola, Yang D. Teng, Vaclav Ourednik, Kook In Park, Richard L. Sidman, and Evan Y. Snyder

INTRODUCTION

Approximately two decades ago, it became evident that the developing and adult mammalian central nervous system (CNS) contained a population of neural stem cells (NSCs). These immature, undifferentiated, multipotent cells could be isolated, expanded, and used as cellular vectors for the treatment of neurodegenerative and demyelinating diseases. Their potential as therapeutic agents in a wide range of CNS and peripheral nervous system (PNS) disorders is beginning to be understood. NSCs may give rise to more committed progenitors, such as oligodendrocyte progenitor cells (OPCs), that may also be used as reparative cells. As the "repair" mechanisms by which NSCs act begin to be better elucidated, new therapies may emerge.

One of the crucial questions in neurodegenerative medicine is the source of the cells for repair, whether they be endogenous or exogenous NSCs. In the CNS, several studies that have examined the spontaneous behavior of endogenous progenitors in the intact and injured adult mammalian brain have found neuron replacement to be small *(1)*, if present at all, very restricted, and short-lived. Several strategies have been proposed to expand the pool of neuron-yielding endogenous progenitors *(2–8)*. Their success in practice remains to be determined. However, even if endogenous stem cells could be recruited, induced to reenter the cell cycle, and coaxed to yield relevant neurons, several challenges remain, such as generating adequate numbers of the proper phenotypes in their correct distributions, and properly integrated. The most effective therapies will likely entail mobilized endogenous cells supplemented by exogenous cells in particular differentiation states. Therefore, transplantation is always likely to have a role in regenerative medicine.

In this chapter, we review the intrinsic properties of NSCs and neural progenitor cells that may be critical for clinical use. We then review current evidence for the response of exogenous NSCs and other progenitors to a neurodegenerative environment and the experimental use of exogenous NSCs in a variety of neurodegenerative models, followed by a discussion of the current challenges and limitations to moving forward to the bedside. Finally we review evidence for the reciprocal interactions

From: *Neural Development and Stem Cells, Second Edition*
Edited by: M. S. Rao © Humana Press Inc., Totowa, NJ

between exogenous NSCs and the host and the therapeutical relevance of such "cross-talk." We believe study of the intrinsic properties of NSCs and the biological basis of host–NSC interactions is of critical importance when thinking about future clinical applications of NSCs.

INTRINSIC PROPERTIES OF NSCs CRITICAL FOR CLINICAL USE

Definition and Characterization

Although several potential markers have been suggested, the most rigorous definition of an NSC still relies on "operational" criteria rather than on a set of molecular markers alone. NSCs are cells from the CNS and PNS that are multipotent and self-renewing *(9)* (Fig. 1A). Multipotency is the ability of a single cell clone to give rise to the three major types of cells in the CNS—neurons, oligodendrocytes, and astrocytes—throughout the nervous system at all stages of life, as well as to repopulate those regions when depleted of cells. The term "self-renewal" is used to define the capacity of a clone to generate new stem cells with identical properties from generation to generation. It is this characteristic of NSCs that makes them valuable transplantation material. NSCs proliferate in response to certain cytokines such as epidermal growth factor (EGF) and basic fibroblast growth factor (bFGF), although the number of such factors seems to be growing *(9)*.

"Progenitor cells" are a step further along than NSCs in the differentiation process; they have committed to a particular lineage (neuronal or glial) and have begun to express lineage-specific markers. How irreversible or invariant such commitment is remains an area of speculation and investigation. Progenitor cells such as OPCs may, under certain circumstances in vitro, exhibit "stemness" in that they can be "coaxed" to be multipotent *(10–12)*. Adult ependymal cells when cultured in vitro or when monitored in vivo have been reported to give rise to both neurons and glia *(4)*, although controversy exists about their real multipotency. Other investigators suggest that subventricular zone (SVZ) astrocytes, rather than ependymal cells, are the true stem cells in that periventricular region. Rietze et al. *(13)* found nestin-positive pluripotent stem cells in both the subventricular and the ependymal area. Interestingly, these cells

---

Fig. 1. *(opposite page)* One method for isolating neural stem cells (NSCs). **(A)** Adult NSCs may be isolated by dissection of the subventricular zone. A single cell suspension contains some proliferative multipotent cells in FGF and EGF; these cells give rise to a "primary neurosphere" that contains NSCs and more differentiated cells. When plated one cell per well, the true NSCs give rise to cells with identical multipotentiality (in this case, defined as a "secondary neurosphere") in order to be deemed as "self-renewing." NSCs exhibit multipotency when cultured in medium containing serum: they give rise to neuronal and glial progenitors and subsequently more mature and terminally differentiated cells. **(B)** Confocal laser microscopy of BrdU incorporation by cells in the SVZ of adult mice demonstrating proliferation of SVZ precursor cells. Bar = 100 μm. **(C)** Representation of the types of cellular architecture in the SVZ. The ependymal cell layer (EP) lines the ventricles; Although controversial, some have regarded these cells as NSCs. The SVZ is composed of a heterogeneous population of cells: neuronal precursors; astrocytes or type B cells that may also be stem-like; type C multipotent precursor cells that exhibit NSC properties in vivo and in vitro; and adult OPCs (in *red*). Reproduced from ref. *196* and *197* with permission.

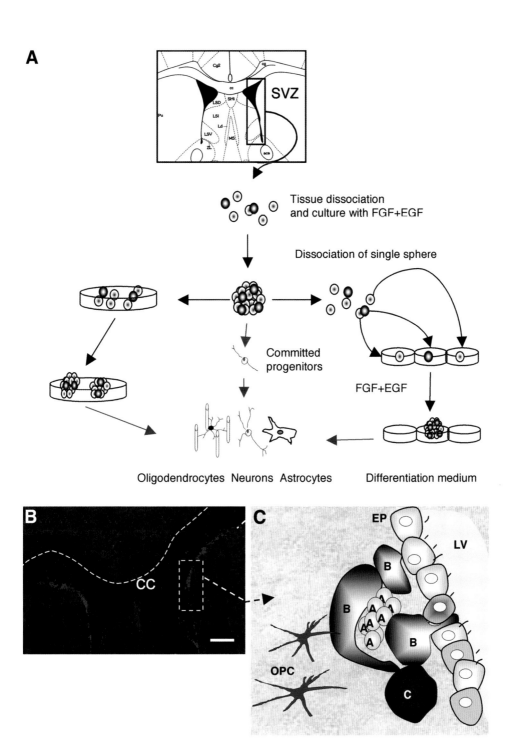

A

SVZ

Tissue dissociation
and culture with FGF+EGF

Dissociation of single sphere

Committed
progenitors

FGF+EGF

Oligodendrocytes Neurons Astrocytes

Differentiation medium

B

CC

C

EP

LV

B

B

A A
A A
A
A

B

OPC

C

Fig. 1.

were glial fibrillary (GFAP)-negative, suggesting heterogeneity of NSCs *(13–16)*. Other investigators have found stem-like cells within a supposedly committed "glial" population extracted from the postnatal and adult cortex, adult substantia nigra, as well as the adult optic nerve; such immature "glia" give rise to neurons as well as mature oligodendrocytes and astrocytes *(15,17,18)*. It remains unclear what this heterogeneity of progenitor populations implies—a true biological phenomenon or a limitation in our ability to provide cell-specific unambiguous defining markers.

There are specific germinative zones in the embryonic and adult mammalian CNS *(19)* that can be considered as sources of NSCs. These zones include the ventricular zone (VZ), the SVZ, the external germinal layer of the cerebellum, the subgranular zone of the dendate gyrus, and possibly the ependymal layer or other cells in the central canal of the spinal cord *(20)*. During the earliest stages of cerebrogenesis, neurons and glia are born in the VZ from NSCs that become progenitors and migrate out using the radial glia as a scaffold to reach the cortex. In addition, radial glia themselves may be multipotent neural precursors with stem cell properties *(21–24)*. These same NSCs give rise to secondary germinal zones, including the SVZ, that contain a reservoir of undifferentiated, uncommitted NSCs that persist into adulthood *(25)*. In the adult mammalian CNS, NSCs can be isolated from the SVZ, striatum, cortex, and the rostral extension of the olfactory bulb *(26)*. Adult neurogenesis from hippocampus has been observed in humans and rodents during normal and abnormal conditions *(27,28)* but the exact cells giving rise to new neurons are still under investigation. Previous studies have suggested that neurogenesis in the adult hippocampus arises from NSCs *(28,29)*, and that astrocytes from hippocampus are capable of regulating neurogenesis by instructing the stem cells to adopt a neuronal fate *(30)*. Furthemore, these adult hippocampal NSCs are able to generate functional neurons *(31)*. However, these findings have recently been challenged; Seaberg et al. showed that the dentate gyrus contains multipotent neural stem cells during development and until birth, but these cells become restricted neuronal progenitors during adulthood *(32)*. These results would suggest that what were thought to be adult NSCs from hippocampus were actually contaminating cells from the periventricular region that persist near the adult dentate gyrus, and that neuronal restricted progenitors and not NSCs are the source of newly generated dentate gyrus neurons throughout adulthood.

The adult SVZ *(33)* is a heterogeneous complex of several layers of cells adjacent to the ependyma, surrounding the lateral ventricles. So far, four different types of cells have been identified in the SVZ (Fig. 1B,C): type A migrating neuronal precursors that migrate to the olfactory bulb; type B nestin-positive, GFAP-positive astrocytes that exhibit NSC properties; type C nestin-positive multipotent progenitors cells *(34)*; and ependymal cells that line the ventricles and the spinal cord and that may have stem-like qualities as well *(4,35,36)*. Current evidence suggests that in the adult SVZ, NSCs express GFAP *(37)*. The developmental origin of these cells is unclear. It has been suggested that these cells may evolve directly from radial glia, which are multipotent precursor cells that participate in neurogenesis as an anchor for tangential chain migration of neuroblasts as well as radial migration *(14–16,35)*. Another possibility is that adult neural stem cells are indeed radial glia that adopt an adult developmental expression of GFAP *(37)*. In the adult CNS, NSCs of the SVZ divide symmetrically, yielding two NSCs, one of which dies by apoptosis, leaving the other to maintain the NSC pool during the life span of the individual *(38)*. During development or when external triggering occurs (such as injury), NSCs proliferate either by symmetric division, where each cell divides into two new NSCs, or by asymmetric division, where the NSC gives rise to one new NSC and a progenitor cell. When asymmetric division predominates, a great number of rapidly proliferating progenitors are generated that migrate out to their final destination. In the songbird *(39)*, NSCs in the adult participate in the neurogenesis responsible for seasonal changes of the song. Although neurogenesis has been found to exist in adult mammalian brain, including humans, it is unclear what role NSCs play there, although they do seem to become integrated into neuronal circuitry of the hippocampus, possibly participating in neural plasticity *(28,40,41)* and learning; targeting the proliferation of endogenous dentate precursors affects behavioral learning *(42,43)*. Whether there is ongoing neurogenesis in the human other than in hippocampus remains unresolved and controversial. This widespread heterogeneity of location and "stemness" makes the selection of a particular NSC for all neurodegenerative disorders difficult; it is more likely that several sources of NSCs will be required in human disorders.

Several biological markers have been investigated and tested for sensitivity and specificity. Nestin, an intermediate filament protein, has been useful in the study of NSCs *(44,45)*. Nestin, however, although sensitive, is not specific; it is expressed by a variety of cells that include reactive astrocytes, endothelial cells, SVZ neuronal progenitor cells, and ependymal cells *(46,47)* as well as NSCs. It can also be expressed by nonneural stem cells, such as embryonic stem cells *(48,49)* and pancreatic progenitors *(50)*. Some investigators have used the low expression of peanut agglutinin (PNA)-binding and heat-stable antigen (HSA) to identify a nestin-positive pluripotent neural stem cell from the adult SVZ in mice with the phenotype nestin$^+$ PNA^{lo} HSA^{lo} *(13)*. Multipotent neural progenitor cells from the SVZ may also express the intermediate filament vimentin, the polysialic form of neural cell adhesion molecule (PS-NCAM), and the transcription factor mushashi *(51,52)*. Another proposed marker is the carbohydrated Lewis X expressed on embryonic pluripotent stem cells, and found in 4% of the adult SVZ, but not in the ependymal region. These Lex positive populations possess stem cell characteristics, allowing consideration of many areas of the brain as potential sources of neural stem and progenitor cells *(53)*.

Some studies have identified and isolated populations of NSC based on flow cytometric characteristics in response to uptake of the DNA dye Hoechst—both red and blue wavelengths, similar to studies done in other stem cells *(54,55)*. The isolation is based on the differential efflux of the dye by a multidrug transporter. The population isolated in this way is called "the side population" or "SP" fraction because the cells segregate to a tiny bin that looks like a small "hook" of cells branching off from the main accumulation of cells after fluorescence-activated cell sorting (FACS). Floating clusters of cells in serum-free medium from dissociated neural cultures (known as "neurospheres") may segregate to this SP population *(56)*.

The hematopoietic stem cell marker CD133 has been used to define a population of human neural precursors cells that exhibit a CD133$^+$CD34$^-$CD45$^-$ phenotype *(57)*. Neural crest stem cells (NCSCs), have been prospectively isolated from fetal mouse sciatic nerve using cell surface antigens such as p75, the low-affinity neurotrophin receptor, and P_0, a peripheral myelin protein: these cells exhibit a $p75^+P_0^-$ phenotype and are capable of self-renewal and the generation of neurons and glia *(58)*.

It is most likely that a battery of markers will be needed to define a genuine stem cell. Future work will involve defining the molecular profile or fingerprint of a NSC, much as has been derived for the hematopoietic stem cell.

Self-Renewal and Multipotency of NSCs

NSCs will proliferate in response to EGF and/or bFGF. This proliferative response can be used as a first level screen to isolate and expand stem-like cells from the CNS. Any proliferative cell grown in serum-free medium without a substrate will form a floating cluster of cells. When such clusters are obtained from primary dissociated neural cultures (e.g., from the SVZ or embryonic forebrain), they may contain and help select for cells with stem-like features. Some investigators who employ this technique have termed this a "neurosphere" assay. When plated on an adherent substrate with serum-containing medium, neurons, astrocytes, oligodendrocytes, as well as undifferentiated cells may appear. It should be emphasized that a single cluster does *not* equal a clone unless it has been proven to derive from a single isolated cell in an isolated well *(4,14,38,45,59–62)*. (Furthermore, the ability to form a neurosphere is, in and of itself, not sufficient to define a stem cell.) Self-renewal can be implied if a single cell can give rise to differentiated cells as well as to other undifferentiated cells that can be similarly placed into an isolated well and give rise to all differentiated and undifferentiated progeny. The above-mentioned maneuvers constitute that part of an "operational" definition of a stem cell that deals with self-renewal and multipotence. This biological property is of great value for clinical use because it allows for expansion of clonal derived cells. Recently two genes involved in transcriptional regulation—*bmi* and *N-cor*—have been implicated in controlling the self-renewal capacity of NSCs *(63,64)*.

Another critical property of clinical value is the differentiation ability of NSCs. "Multipotence," the ability to give rise to all cells of a given organ system—in this case, the nervous system—is an obligate part of the NSC definition. The term "pluripotency" refers to the capacity of stem cells to give rise to the *full range* of cells and tissues in an organism including non-neural cells. This most extensive potential is thought to be a property of embryonic stem (ES) cells alone. Several controversial observations, however, have suggested that other stem cells, including NSCs, may have such potential under extraordinary nonphysiological circumstances. NSCs have been reported to give rise to mature nonneural cells *(65)*. Adult murine NSCs have been claimed to become hematopoietic cells after injection into an irradiated host, and to express such T-cell markers as CD3 *(66)*. Others have shown that, when injected into early-stage mice and chick embryos, adult NSCs may differentiate into cells of the gastrointestinal tract, heart, and kidney, expressing markers typically found in these tissues in a nontumorogenic manner *(61)*. NSCs have been claimed to produce skeletal myotubes both in vitro and in vivo *(67)*. The opposite type of transdifferentiation, non-neural stem cells into neural cells, has also been reported. For example, bone marrow derived stem cells after intravenous injection in mice may travel to the CNS, express neural markers, and yield an astroglial phenotype *(5,68)*. These transdifferentiation experiments remain very controversial. The purity of the NSC populations used in these experiments as well as the specificity of the markers used to define specific neural and nonneural cell types remain issues of ongoing investigation and inquiry in such experiments. Other groups have failed to reproduce these findings; recently Morshead et al. transplanted 128 host animals with NSCs and they could not confirm a contribution to hematopoiesis *(69)*. An alternative explanation to the Bjornson experiment is that fusion rather than true transdifferentiation may explain some of the extraordinary claims of pluripotency of NSCs *(70,71)*. In support of this explanation is the recent observation of bone marrow derived cells fused to Purkinje neurons and other post-mitotic neural cells after bone marrow transplantation *(72–76)*.

Regardless of how confirmatory experiments for the above-cited studies turn out, the differentiation potential of stem cells, including NSCs, remains quite extraordinary even if restricted to their orthotypic organ. Their ability to differentiate in response to specific environmental clues suggests a critical role for cytokines and cell-to-cell contact signals. The transcription factor *Oct-4* is associated with pluripotency and self-renewal of ES cells *(73)*. It is down-regulated when ES cells change to nestin-positive neural stem cells *(49)*. Terminal differentiation likely depends on the spatiotemporal expression and interactions of multiple cytokines with their receptors on the NSC surface that activate specific transcriptional programs *(7,74)*.

Alternative sources of NSCs and protocols for differentiation are being explored other than from ES cells or the fetus. In humans cells residing in the periventricular areas may behave as NSCs and can be isolated from individuals by biopsies *(77)*. Others have shown that neural progenitors can be safely isolated from adult cadavers *(2,78)*. It is currently unknown whether these cells may be a viable source for transplantation in humans.

Oligodendrocyte Progenitor Cells (OPCs)

Progenitor cells represent one stage further advanced beyond the stem cell in terms of restriction of potential and lineage commitment. Although they are regarded as having had their fate narrowed to a subset of cell types, they nevertheless have potential therapeutic utility. OPCs have emerged as a viable source of cells for transplants *(10,79)*. Oligodendrocytes are terminally differentiated cells. New oligodendrocytes seem to originate from OPCs and NSCs *(80)* as there is production of new oligodedrocytes even in the adult forebrain *(81)* and spinal cord *(82)*. OPCs can be identified by several markers: the ganglioside GD3, the cell surface marker A2B5, the O4 antigen, 14F7 monoclonal antibody *(83)*, the glycoprotein AN2 *(84)*, the spliced form of 2', 3'-cyclic nucleotide 3'-phosphohydrolase (CNPase) *(85)*, the transcription factors Olig1 Olig2, NKx2., Dlx2 *(86,87)*, and the integral membrane proteoglycan NG2 *(88,89)*. Although NG2 may be expressed by macrophages and endothelial cells, the pattern of staining and the complex morphology of OPCs help to make the distinction *(90,91)* (Fig. 2A,B). Using these markers, OPCs have been detected in the adult CNS *(92)*.

OPCs undergo several maturational stages determined by specific antigenic expression and developmental potential. In the initial stages of development, OPCs exhibit the $NG2^+$, $PDGFR\text{-}\alpha^+$ $O4^-$ phenotype. These cells give rise to more advanced progenitors expressing O4 which, in turn, generate premyelinating oligodendrocytes that lose the expression of NG2 and gain the expression of proteolipid protein (PLP), and, finally, to mature oligodendrocytes expressing myelin basic protein (MBP) and CNPase *(93)*. Expression of O4 is a first step into terminal oligodendrocyte differentiation *(94)* and indicates a more committed stage with less proliferative potential *(95)*. Gal-C expression is associated with terminal differentiation and is followed by MBP, PLP, and myelin/oligodendroglial glycoprotein (MOG) expression *(96)*.

Some of the above-described precursors persist as adult OPCs. These OPCs differ from their perinatal counterparts in several respects: They divide, migrate, and differentiate three or four times more slowly than perinatal OPCs. These differences are likely to be cell intrinsic, but the exact mechanism of the progressive change of potential from perinatal OPCs to adult OPCs is unknown. The cell cycle inhibitor P27kip1 accumulates as these cells divide, and has been proposed as one of the mechanisms leading to the change in proliferation potential *(97)*. In addition, the levels of cdk2 and cyclin are diminished in adult OPCs compared to perinatal cells; this may account for the proliferative state of adult OPCs *(98)*. However, cell intrinsic mechanisms are not sufficient to explain the dormancy of adult OPCs in vivo; Horner et al., found that fewer than 1% of OPCs divide and exhibit a prolonged cell cycle *(82)* (Fig. 2C). It is possible that environmental cues absent in the adult brain but present in the myelinating brain, or molecules enriched in the adult brain may influence this behavior: molecules such as Notch and Jagged have been shown to inhibit OPC differentiation *(99)*. Moreover, OPCs are regionally heterogeneous in their ability to differentiate; for example, cortical OPCs isolated from P7 rats exhibit a slow differentiation behavior when compared with optic nerve derived cells *(100)*. Despite the biological difference, adult OPCs also share many of the characteristics of the perinatal OPCs such as response to growth factors, the triiodothyronine (T3)-dependent timing for differentiation, and maintenance of their self-renewing capacity. Adult OPCs, which can yield mature oligodendrocytes in the adult brain, express NG2, the platelet-derived growth factor-α (PDGF-α) receptor, O4, and the FGF receptor *(101)*. They also express *c-kit*, a marker for hematopoietic stem cells that is lost when they differentiate into postmitotic oligodendrocyte *(102)*.

Adult OPCs are maintained in a quiescent state by a mechanism that involves the α-amino-3-hydroxy-5-methyl-4-isoxatzole propionic acid (AMPA) receptor *(103)*, the cell cycle inhibitor p27Kip1 *(104)*, and Notch. Activation of the Notch receptor on OPCs blocks their oligodendrocyte differentiation in the developing optic nerve *(99)*. Owing to their abundance in the CNS and the fact that their processes contact the nodes of Ranvier *(105)*, it has been suggested that OPCs subserve synaptic remodeling and plasticity in the adult CNS *(106,107)*. Recent data, however, point to a broader differentiation potential and replication capacity of OPC; depending on the cytokine milieu, they may exhibit actual neural stem-like characteristics *(10,17,108)* that make them an attractive source of reparative cells.

OPCs have been isolated from brains of healthy humans and of diseased patients, and express the p75 [NTR] (neurotrophin receptor) that is implicated in oligodendrocyte survival and apoptosis *(109)*. In vitro oligodendroglial development can be recapitulated from NSCs: Zhang et al. demonstrated that human oligodendrocytes appear from neurospheres and express the PDGF-α receptor. The proliferation of these human OPCs was augmented by coculture with neurons and astrocytes *(110)*. Furthermore, human neurospheres increase their yield of oligodendrocyte production when cultured with T_3 *(111)*. Finally, control of the timing of OPC differentiation requires extracellular signals such as PDGF-α and T_3 *(112)*. Recent work has shown that human OPCs can be

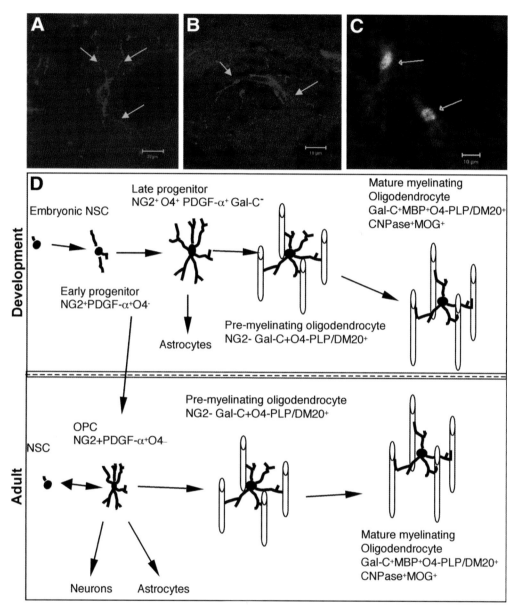

Fig. 2. Oligodendrocytes developmental lineage and morphology. NG2-positive (*red*) adult OPCs from the corpus callosum can exhibit multipolar (**A**) and bipolar morphology (**B**). Symmetrical cell division is shown in (**C**) two young OPCs (*red*) with incorporated BRDU (*green*) indicative of cell division and showing typical morphology with radially oriented processes in the adult mice spinal cord. The arrows in (**A**) and (**B**) point to OPC processes and in (**C**) to BRDU positive nucleus. Scale bar = 10 μm. (**D**) Developmental stages of oligodendrocytes from an NSC are shown. CNPase, 2,3-Cyclic nucleotide 3-phosphohydrolase; Gal-C, galacto-cerebrosidase; MBP, myelin basic protein; MOG, myelin oligodendrocyte glycoprotein; PDGF, platelet-derived growth factor; PLP, proteolipid protein. Modified from ref. *197* with permission of the American Physiological Society.

isolated, expanded, and used in experimental settings, suggesting that is possible to obtain cells able to replace oligodendrocytes in vivo *(79,113–115)*.

CURRENT EXPERIMENTAL EVIDENCE
OF THE ABILITY OF TRANSPLANTED NSCs
TO AMELIORATE NEUROLOGICAL DISORDERS

We review some of the work in models of diseases of the nervous system for which transplanted stem cells have been demonstrated to have positive effects. The disorders include genetic or inheritable metabolic and deficiency diseases, infectious or inflammatory diseases, and age-related degeneration. These diseases have in common widespread neural cell loss and/or dysfunction. The widespread nature of these diseases makes them difficult to treat by conventional transplantation approaches, in which a limited number of cells can be delivered to a restricted area. Because NSCs will migrate to distant, multiple, and extensive regions of the nervous system, they can be useful in multifocal degeneration, in which all or most of the nervous system is affected. Examples of such disorders include myelin deficiencies and leukodystrophies. NSCs are also valuable therapeutic agents in the face of more limited damage to the CNS or PNS. In diseases such as Parkinson's, Huntington's, or specific degeneration of cerebellar neurons, transplantation may be restricted to a region of the CNS. Stroke and CNS or spinal injury also represent situations of a restricted area of damage. However, in these types of disorders, multiple neural cells types must be replaced. The multipotency of NSCs provides the mechanism by which multiple cells can be regenerated; but the molecular mediators that trigger migration, site-specific differentiation, and survival of NSCs remains to be discovered.

Besides the self-renewing capacity and multipotency of NCSs, perhaps the most critical biological property of NSCs is their extraordinary mobilization toward injury *(59,116–119)*, although the mechanisms of such migratory capacity are not well known. The migratory nature of NSCs makes them potent vehicles for gene therapy. NSCs can carry copies of normal genes into tissue with missing or dysfunctional genes. NSCs will migrate, integrate, and produce normal gene products in normal amounts. Because they will differentiate into both neurons and glia, they can carry either neuronal or glial genes into host tissue. In addition, NSCs can be engineered to express a variety of other genes from all organisms including humans. Another property that is critical in a clinical setting is the ability to endogenously produce growth factors that may help to modulate the environment and promote beneficial effects in the host *(120,121)*. These aspects are reviewed in the next sections.

Acute Degeneration

Stroke, CNS injury, and spinal injury represent additional disorders that may be successfully treated by NSC transplantation. Here, damage is restricted to a circumscribed region (both in space and in time), but multiple neural cell types must be replaced. The multipotency of NSCs provides the mechanism to reconstruct damaged neural tissue. In early work *(122)*, an experimental model of neurodegeneration was produced, and the potency of a clonal line of NSCs to repopulate the brain was examined. Apoptosis was induced in adult mouse brain, resulting in degeneration of cortical neurons in a circumscribed region. NSCs implanted into the brains engrafted and differentiated into neurons only within that "niche," although differentiation of engrafted cells in normal adult brain (including outside the "niche" in these lesioned brains) is limited to glia. This experiment actually constituted the first demonstration of a neurogenic niche for stem cells, at least as created by a pathological condition. Further work extended investigation to include an examination of the fate of NSCs transplanted into brains that were subjected to ischemic and hypoxic injury. In a study by Park et al. *(123)*, the right common carotid artery of a 1-wk-old mouse was ligated, and the animal was exposed to 8% ambient oxygen. The combination of ischemia and hypoxia resulted in extensive injury to the ipsilateral hemisphere. Following transplantation into the ventricles or directly into the infarct cavity, NSCs migrated to and throughout the infarct cavity and engrafted and differentiated into all major neural cell types *(123)*. Recently, these observations were extended to an injury model with extensive parenchymal loss by providing a three-dimensional template for neural stem cells. NSCs seeded onto a biodegradable polymer scaffold implanted into infarction cavities established reciprocal interactions with the damaged brain with a reduction of parenchyma loss, an increase in directed neurite outgrowth, and a reduction in glial scarring *(124)*.

Another study examining functional and structural repair of adult ischemic brain with stem cells is that by Fukunaga et al. *(125)*. Adult male spontaneous hypertensive rats were given middle cerebral artery occlusion (MCAO) followed by reperfusion. Embryonic tissue was implanted into the ischemic striatum. Several weeks later the grafted animals were found to have improved performance in the Morris water maze task, and neurons were seen within the graft. In animal models of lower motor neuron degeneration, a percentage of NSCs differentiated into cells morphologically consistent with lower motor neurons *(123)* as if responding somewhat to an "altered niche" in the spinal cord, as well. Therefore, it appears that NSCs are capable of repopulating and reconstituting areas of injury in the CNS. In addition, it appears that degenerating brain tissue may elicit elaborate signals that draw stem cells to the area and alter the fate of the donor cell.

Ischemia models present another example of the potential of NSCs to be agents of gene delivery, as seen in the work of Andsberg et al. *(126)*. Rat NSCs engineered to overexpress nerve growth factor (NGF) were transplanted into the brains of rats that had been subjected to MCAO. MCAO results in ischemia-induced cell death in the rat striatum. Forty-eight hours after the insult, NGF-secreting NSCs had migrated through the area of infarct, and the loss of striatal neurons was less in animals that had received transplants. Others have reported additional benefits from NSCs implantation in stroke such as improvement of impaired spatial learning in a water maze test *(127)*.

Several groups have extended the observation that NSCs can be beneficial in models of acute injury in the forebrain and the spinal cord. Riess et al. used controlled cortical impact brain injury in mice to study the effects of NSCs. Injured animals that received NSC transplants showed significantly improved motor and neuronal and glial differentiation. NSCs survive for as long as 13 wk after transplantation and were detected in the hippocampus and cortical areas adjacent to the injury cavity *(128)*.

Integration and reconstruction of circuitry is an important goal for NSCs transplants during injury. Several groups have shown that in vitro-expanded CNS precursors, following transplantation into the brains of rats, form electrically active and functionally connected neurons *(129,130)* and integrate into host cortical circuitry *(131)*. Results from our group show that during a model of ischemic injury, NSCs shows proper integration and connectivity *(124)*.

The spinal cord presents an enormous challenge because it ostensibly has fewer neurogenic niches than the forebrain *(132)*. Neural progenitor cells from the spinal cord may harbor neuronal capabilities, but activation of the notch pathway during spinal cord injury may limit their neuronal regenerative potential *(132)*. Others have found that during spinal cord injury, neural progenitor cells integrate along axons surrounding the lesion site. These cells differentiate only into astro- and oligodendroglial lineages, supporting the notion that the adult spinal cord provides molecular cues for glial, but not for neuronal, differentiation *(133)*. Nevertheless transplantation of NSCs after spinal cord injury has shown several benefits; for example, a combination of stem cell transplantation and gene therapy may be the most successful approach to the treatment of acute injury, especially when using the cells to promote a regenerative environment. For instance, after genetically modified NSCs were transplanted into spinal cord engineered to express neurotrophin-3 (NT-3), the cells migrated long distances, differentiated into neurons and glia, and continued to express NT-3 *(121)*. In addition, others have combined growth factor support and transplantation of NSCs. The coadministration of sonic hedgehog (Shh) and transplantation of oligodendrocyte precursors results in improved function and white matter sparing in the spinal cords of adult rats after contusion *(134)*. Using a similar approach, Schumn et al. showed that transplanting cells able to produce growth factors (such as chromaffin cells) along with NSCs may protect and extend the survival of the transplanted neural progenitors cells without changing their differentiation potential *(135,136)*. NSCs may be working as cell replacements, but there is good evidence that an additional benefit may be related to a chaperone effect that improves the survival of host cells after experimental contusion in rats and other models of injury *(137,138)*. This chaperone effect is due to the secretion of bioactive substances by transplanted NSCs. NSCs have been found to constitutively secrete significant quantities of several neurotrophic factors, including nerve growth factor (NGF), brain-derived neurotrophic factor (BDNF), and glial cell line derived neurotrophic factor (GDNF). When grafted to cystic dorsal column lesions in the cervical spinal cord of adult rats, NSCs supported extensive growth of host axons of known sensitivity to these growth factors. When NSCs were genetically modified to produce NT-3, this significantly expanded the effects of NSC on host axons though the proportions of axon type shifted *(139)*. This ability to secrete growth factor and neurotransmitters may have additional clinical applications. Secretion of serotonin by serotonergic precursor cells has been proven to be beneficial for modulating central pain caused by hyperexcitability of dorsal neurons after spinal cord injury *(140)*. Furthermore, using the same tissue engineering paradigm in a model of spinal cord injury, Teng et al. showed that implantation of a scaffold NSC unit into an adult rat hemisection model of spinal cord injury promoted long-term improvement in function. Histology and immunocytochemical analysis suggested that this recovery might be attributable partly to a reduction in tissue loss from secondary injury processes as well as diminished glial scarring. Tract tracing demonstrated host corticospinal tract fibers passing through the injury epicenter and enhanced local GAP-43 expression suggestive of regeneration *(141)*.

Chronic and Age-Related Degeneration

Progressive neurodegenerative diseases such as Parkinson's, Huntington's, and Alzheimer's, as well as normal aging, are associated with progressive cell loss in the CNS. These diseases, as well as aging, represent perhaps the greatest challenge to stem cell therapy. They require the replacement of all neural cell types in large brain regions (in the case of Alzheimer's disease), in the face of ongoing degeneration and possibly the presence of toxic molecules. Thus, the multipotency of stem cells, their ability to migrate over long distances, and their ability to express foreign genes may all be called into play. In a disorder such as Alzheimer's disease (AD) NSCs may have a coadjutant rather that a primary role. Future therapy of AD must focus on the underlying neurobiology of the disease, namely buildup of Aβ and the neuronal dysfunction that occurs. Aβ transgenic animals have an impairment of neurogenesis due to deleterious effects of Aβ on neural progenitors *(142)*. NSCs may deliver genes that impede Aβ build-up, decrease inflammation, or protect host neurons. At the same time, the NSCs must avoid being affected themselves. Neuronal replacement at this time is difficult to envision.

Parkinson's disease (PD) represents the CNS disorder in which transplantation therapy has a long history. Fetal tissue grafts have been used in rodent and primate models of PD *(143)* as well as in clinical trials *(144,145)*. However, short graft survival and limited integration of the grafts appeared to reduce the usefulness of fetal tissue. Cells derived from the fetal midbrain can modify the course of the disease, but they are an inadequate source of dopamine-synthesizing neurons because their ability to generate these neurons is unstable.

More recently, animal models of PD were given grafts of stem cells, and the behavioral and neurochemical outcomes were assessed. An immortalized rodent neuroprogenitor cell line was transplanted into primate and rodent PD models, with resultant increases in tyrosine hydroxylase (TH) in the brains of transplanted animals *(146)*. Lundberg et al. *(147)* transduced astrocytes to produce TH and thus to secrete L-3,4-dihydroxyphenylalanine (L-DOPA). Transplantation of these cells into the striatum of rats with unilateral 6-hydroxydopamine (6-OHDA) lesions resulted in a reduction in behavioral symptoms and the presence of TH-positive cells in the lesioned area. Zigova et al. *(148)* transplanted neuronal progenitor cells derived from neonatal rat SVZ into the striatum of adult rats 1 mo after unilateral 6-OHDA lesions. Animals were examined 1 wk, 2–3 wk, and 5 mo postimplant. The donor cells survived and migrated, and many differentiated into neurons. Cells were still present 5 mo after transplantation. The stem cells, therefore, appear to be far superior to fetal tissue grafts.

Embryonic (11–13) mesencephalic progenitors have been successfully used in models of PD. It was shown that location and number of implants enhanced the beneficial effect. After transplants were implanted into the striatum only (single graft) or the substantia nigra (SN) and the striatum (double grafts), it was found that double grafts of mesencephalic progenitors had more potent effects on rotational behavior than single grafts *(149)*. The adult or 6-OHDA-lesioned brain contains intrinsic cues sufficient to direct the specific expression of dopaminergic traits in immature multipotential NSCs. In addition, NSCs transplanted into the intact or 6-OHDA-lesioned striatum, withdrawn from the cell cycle, migrate extensively in the host striatum and express markers associated with neuronal but not glial differentiation. After 5 wk postgrafting, in the majority of these transplants, nearly all engrafted cells express the dopamine-synthesizing enzymes TH and aromatic L-amino acid decarboxylase, sometimes resulting in changes in motor behavior. In contrast, no NSCs stain for dopamine-β-hydroxylase, choline acetyltransferase, glutamic acid decarboxylase, or serotonin *(150)*. Other investigators have shown that using a three-dimensional cell differentiation system, E12 rat ventral mesencephalon precursors survive intrastriatal transplantation, differentiate into dopaminergic neurons, and induce functional recovery in hemiparkinsonian rats *(151)*. In addition, the use of growth factors such as Sonic Hedgehog facilitates differentiation into dopaminergic neurons in cocultures of E11 rat mesencephalon *(152)*. Preliminary studies by Redmond, Sladek, Teng, Bjugstad, and Snyder suggest that human NSCs may restore homeostasis to the nigrostriatal system of Parkinsonian monkey by not only differentiating into dopaminergic neurons (a minor effect) but by preserving host cells and circuitry *(152a)*.

One source of stem cells that has shown great promise are ES cells, which proliferate extensively and can generate dopamine neurons. In vitro, an enriched population of midbrain NSCs can be derived from mouse ES cells; the dopamine neurons generated by these stem cells show electrophysiological and behavioral properties expected of neurons from the midbrain *(154)*. In addition, the discovery of a stromal cell-derived inducing activity (SDIA) that promotes neural differentiation of mouse ES cells provides a powerful tool to improve the number of dopaminergic neurons from ES cells. SDIA induces efficient neuronal differentiation of cocultured ES cells in serum-free conditions without the use of either retinoic acid or embryoid bodies. A high proportion of TH-positive neurons producing dopamine are obtained from SDIA-treated ES cells. When transplanted, SDIA-induced dopaminergic neurons integrate into the mouse striatum and remain positive for TH expression *(155,156)*; others have shown that human neural progenitor differentiate into a small number of neurons that expressed TH and were sufficient to partially ameliorate lesion-induced behavioral deficits in some animals *(157)*.

NSCs were also shown to be of value following transplantation into a rodent model of Huntington's disease *(158)*. Rats given intrastriatal injections of quinolinic acid show large areas of degeneration in the striatum. Transplantation of stem cells derived from transgenic animals overexpressing hNGF reduced the lesion size, with sparing of host striatal neurons. Delivery of hNGF by transplanted stem cells appeared to prevent degeneration of host striatal neurons. These data demonstrate an important aspect of stem cell transplantation therapy, that donor cells may not only replace host cells but may also help to prevent loss of host tissue, by secretion of either endogenous factors or transgene products.

Aged rats demonstrate cognitive deficits, which are associated with atrophy of forebrain cholinergic neurons. In a study by Martinez-Serrano and Bjorklund *(159)* middle-aged rats with no cognitive deficits were given grafts of neural progenitor cells engineered to express NGF. The animals were examined during the next 9 mo for cognitive decline. At the end of the 9-mo period, age-matched control rats showed significant behavioral impairment when compared with grafted animals. The transplanted animals maintained cognitive performance at a level similar to that of younger adult animals. In addition, age-related atrophy of cholinergic neurons was not present in transplanted animals. Transplanted cells were integrated into the host tissue and continued to produce the transgenic product up to 9 mo postgrafting. These results support the use of genetically engineered stem cells in transplantation therapy of age-related neurodegeneration.

Demyelination Disorders

Myelination disorders are mainly of two classes: disorders in which endogenous myelinating cells are genetically impaired and fail to myelinate during development and disorders that result from loss/failure of remyelination in the adult (e.g., multiple sclerosis [MS], allergic encephalomyelitis, and injury). MS is the most commonly diagnosed neurological disease in young adults *(160)*. Demyelination, axonal degeneration, and neuronal dysfunction *(161,162)* are key features in MS pathology; current evidence suggests that remyelination to some extent also occurs spontaneously *(163,164)*. This chronic debilitating disease represents a high cost to society in terms of both productivity and chronic health care resources *(165)*. The current treatment of MS relies on immunological interventions. However, it is becoming clear that repair should be considered as a goal for treatment.

The prospect of using transplants of NSCs and progenitors during demyelination requires an understanding of the behavior of these cells in experimental models. This would provide information about the interaction between the damaged host and the NSCs *(25,122)*. Several groups have used this approach to show that NSCs and OPCs can differentiate into mature oligodendrocytes. For instance, injection of murine NSC in the neonatal SVZ of dysmyelinated shiverer (*shi*) mice results in widespread oligodendrocyte differentiation with myelination of 40% of the host neuronal process in regions of engraftment with evident clinical improvement *(166)*. EGF responsive NSCs also have shown efficacy and oligodendrocyte differentiation when transplanted into the thoracolumbar region of *md* rats *(167)* and the shaking (*Sh*) pup canine myelin mutant *(167,168)*. Nestin-positive human neural precursor cells removed from surgical specimens have been used to induce repair in rat spinal cord with extensive remyelination *(169)*. Even ES cells differentiate into oligodendrocytes and myelinate in culture and after spinal cord transplantation in *shi* mice *(48)* and *md* rat *(170)*.

Transplanted OPCs were able to repair focal demyelinated areas in the neonatal and adult canine mutant *(171)*. In the *md* mutant rat carrying a mutation in myelin PLP, injected OPCs result in myelin formation in a wide distribution in the host parenchyma *(172)*; these cells can be isolated from the rat SVZ as well and produce robust myelin after transplantation *(173)*. Some progenitors isolated from the SVZ require in vitro preinduction to an oligodendroglial lineage to achieve myelination in vivo *(174)*. Other cells such as olfactory ensheating cells (OECs) and Schwann cells have been proposed as useful cells for myelin repair. Purified populations of human OECs have extremely high viability in tissue culture, and are capable of remyelinating persistently demyelinated CNS axons and of induction of axonal regeneration *(175)* following transplantation into experimentally induced demyelinating lesions in the rat spinal cord *(176,177)*. In addition, Schwann cells have been used for transplantation into demyelinated areas, Schwann cells derived from human sural nerve were transplanted into the X-irradiation/ethidium bromide-lesioned dorsal columns of rats showing extensive remyelination, engraftment, and improved conduction velocity by electrophysiology analysis several weeks postransplant *(178)*. These results indicate that several types of progenitors and even Schwann cells may be used for therapy and that they receive environmental cues that drive their migration and differentiation toward oligodendrocyte lineage *(179)*. However, the selection of a particular cell type will require extensive experimentation and careful consideration of other factors such as source of isolation, in vitro manipulation, and ethical issues. Finally the use of immature multipotent progenitors may be more beneficial considering that NSCs cannot only replace neurons and oligodendrocytes but also serve as modulators of the microenvironment by their ability to release growth factors even without transgenic manipulation *(120)*. In humans, neural progenitor cells have been isolated from adult white matter; these multipotent cells form neurospheres that might generate functional neurons and oligodendrocytes *(79)*. Using a similar selection protocol, Windrem et al. isolated human OPCS that myelinated shiverer mouse brain. Adult OPCs myelinated more rapidly than their fetal counterparts, generated oligodendrocytes more efficiently than fetal OPCs, and ensheathed more host axons per donor cell than fetal cells *(113)*. These results suggest that OPCs can be isolated from humans and the demyelinating microenvironment may be able to engage exogenous progenitor cells to become effectively myelinating cells. However, more information on the behavior of the exogenous NSCs and OPCs in a deleterious environment such as experimental autoimmune encephalomyelitis (EAE) is needed.

Cerebellar Degeneration

NSCs may assume a specialized neuronal phenotype when transplanted into brains with a specific loss of neurons. Rosario et al. *(180)* transplanted NSCs into newborn meander tail mice *(mea)*, which are characterized by the lack of development of granule cells in the anterior cerebellar lobe. Transplanted cells preferentially differentiated into granule neurons, suggesting that once transplanted into host animals, NSCs will compensate for the specific cell loss characteristic of a disorder. Similar shifts in fate were observed in mouse models of glial dysfunction *(166)*.

Metabolic Diseases

A number of metabolic diseases affect the CNS. These diseases represent a second class of disorders for which stem cells offer a powerful approach to therapy. Stem cells can provide therapeutic molecules whose entry into the brain may normally be restricted by the blood–brain barrier. Stem cells can provide these molecules either because they normally produce them or because they have been genetically engineered to do so. Our laboratory demonstrated the successful use of NSCs in a metabolic disorder a number of years ago by cross-correcting a mouse model of the lysosomal storage disease, mucopolysaccharidosis VII (Sly disease). MPS VII mice have a deficiency of the enzyme β-glucuronidase (GUSB), which results in a lysosomal accumulation of glycosaminoglycans in the brain and other tissues. The result is a progressive degenerative disorder, with mental retardation and eventually death. Transplantation of NSCs engineered to express the human GUSB enzyme into the ventricles of neonatal MPS VII mice resulted in expression of GUSB throughout the brain and widespread correction of lysosomal storage in neurons and glia. Grafted animals had significant enzymatic activity up to at least 8 mo posttransplantation *(181)*.

A second example of the use of NSCs in a model of a lysosomal storage disease is the work of Lacorazza et al. *(182)*. In this study, NSCs were engineered to express the human form of the β-hexosaminidase α-subunit. This enzyme is defective in Tay–Sachs disease, a severe neurodegenerative disorder that results from the accumulation of G_{m2} ganglioside in the CNS. The engineered cells were transplanted into fetal and neonatal normal mouse brain. Engrafted brains produced high levels of the human protein. This work demonstrated that engrafted cells can migrate throughout the brain and, once integrated into host tissue, continue to produce transgenes. This approach has been extended by Lee and Snyder to the use of human neural and embryonic stem cells in another gangliosidosis, Sandhoff Disease. Torchiana et al. *(183)* presented additional evidence for the use of stem cells in the treatment of a lysosomal storage disease, Krabbe disease, by demonstrating that retroviral packing cell lines can be used to transduce immortalized neural progenitor cells to produce the lysosomal enzyme galactocerebrosidase (Galc). These studies provide evidence of the feasibility of stem cell transplantation to aid in the treatment of lysosomal storage diseases, an example of disorders characterized by dysfunction or absence of specific gene products. Stem cells can be both a producer and a delivery vehicle of missing and/or abnormal gene products. Human neural stem cells also have shown this capacity as well; transplanted human NSCs were found to integrate and migrate in the host brain and to produce large amounts of β-glucuronidase. Brain contents of the substrates of β-glucuronidase were reduced to nearly normal levels, and widespread clearing of lysosomal storage was observed in the MPS VII mouse brain *(184)*.

Other Neurological Disorders

Transplantation of NSCs has been attempted in mouse cochleae injured by cisplatin. Fetal mouse NSCs expressing green fluorescence protein (GFP) were injected into the modiolus of cisplatin-treated cochleae of mice. The majority of grafted NSCs differentiated into glial cells and few into neurons *(185)*. In addition, NSCs have been used in a model of induced apoptotic retinal ganglion cell death in neonatal and adult mice. Donor cells stably integrated; however, most grafted cells did not express retinal-specific markers, although occasional donor cells were immunopositive for β-III tubulin; thus targeted rapid RGC depletion increased cell incorporation of NSCs into the damaged retina, but grafted NSCs did not appear to differentiate into a retinal ganglion cell phenotype *(186)*. We have demonstrated that NSCs exhibit extensive homing to brain tumors *(59)*, and several groups have exploited this extraordinary homing capacity to attempt to modulate glioma growth by injecting modified NSCs. Ehtesham et al. used NSCs secreting tumor necrosis factor-related apoptosis-inducing ligand (TRAIL) and demonstrated glioma apoptosis and growth reduction. Furthermore, using interleukin-12 (IL-12)-secreting NSC therapy they have shown enhanced T-cell infiltration and long-term antitumor immunity *(187,188)*. Other NSCs secreting cytokines have shown efficacy. When followed by magnetic resonance imaging, IL-4 secreting NSCs have been shown to improve the survival of glioma-bearing mice and reduce tumor size *(189)*. K. I. Park in our group has shown similar efficacy using human neural stem cells.

CHALLENGES AND LIMITATIONS OF EXOGENOUS NSC THERAPY

In thinking about the practical application of NSC biology to clinical situations, it is instructive to remember that study of the NSC emerged as the unanticipated byproduct of investigations by developmental neurobiologists into fundamental aspects of neural determination, commitment, and plasticity and this relationship is quite central to the understanding and application of NSC translational biology. NSC behavior is ultimately an expression of developmental principles, a fascinating vestige from the more plastic and generative stages of organogenesis. In attempting to apply NSC biology therapeutically, it is instructive always to bear in mind what role the stem cell plays in development and to what cues it was "designed" to respond in trying to understand the "logic" behind its behavior (both what investigators or clinicians want to see and what they do not want to see). Furthermore, in transplantation paradigms, the interaction between engrafted NSCs and recipient hosts is a dynamic, complex, ongoing reciprocal interaction in which both entities are constantly in flux.

Clinical Rationale for a Prospective Neural Therapy: Type of Disease

NSCs have been successfully isolated *(190,191)*, genetically manipulated, and transplanted in order to replace cells and introduce genes in models of neurodegenerative disease in mice *(2,180–182,192)*. Several authors have shown that NSCs survive and differentiate in diverse disease models. NSCs are able to differentiate into the three major cell types in the mammalian CNS; thus they offer promising strategies for transplant as well as gene therapy protocols *(182)*. However, it remains to be determined whether a particular CNS disease will benefit from NSC transplantation *(193)*. The chances for success seem best in those diseases in which clinical efficacy is determined ostensibly by a single biological mechanism, for example, a single gene defect in lysosomal storage diseases. Parkinson's and Huntington's diseases might fit into that category—that is, requiring the replacement of a single neuronal cell type in a circumscribed region. MS and AD have always represented major therapeutic challenges because their pathologies are so widespread, affecting multiple sites in the CNS, impairing neuronal as well as glial function. While targeting localized lesions that cause great disability can be envisioned, addressing multiple lesions that extend throughout the CNS remains a daunting prospect, even with extensively migratory NSCs. Careful strategic planning and extensive animal testing will be required before clinical studies can be considered. Clinical judgment of reparative therapy with NSCs must be seen in concert with other traditional therapies that aim to ameliorate degeneration and promote neuroprotection, although we need to learn the extent to which an inflammatory and neurodegenerative microenvironment may be a trigger for NSC to function as well as whether long-term inflammation may be inimical to the survival of NSCs *(142,194–197)*. Today, it remains unclear whether the best strategy for repair will entail promoting cell replacement by endogenous progenitors or transplanting in new exogenous progenitors. Much depends on a better understanding not only of the fundamental biological properties of stem/progenitor cells but also of the fundamental pathophysiological processes underlying neurodegenerative diseases and the cross-talk between NSCs and a neurodegenerative environment.

Autografts of immunologically compatible and less ethically problematic adult stem cells are often proclaimed as being useful for such neurodegenerative diseases. However, if the etiology for disease progression resides in the host genome (e.g., abnormal lifespan, excessive vulnerability to stress, diminished self-renewal capacity) or a genetic defect such as in Huntington and amyotrophic lateral sclerosis (ALS), or in AD, then endogenous progenitors will also be flawed and will not represent a good source for repair and may not be optimal for genetically based diseases, because differentiated progeny will have the same genetic defect with the same susceptibility to degeneration *(9,198–200)*. If the process is non-cell-autonomous, then implanting exogenous cells may be problematic unless they have been engineered to be resistant to the environment that caused the injury. In many neurodegenerative disorders, it is likely that both scenarios are implicated and a combined strategy may be needed. Either way, exploiting the biological properties of precursors and promoting their differentiation in desired directions (e.g., to neurons and remyelinating oligodendrocytes) requires a better understanding of the molecular pathways governing the response of NSC and progenitors pools during disease. Thus we need to understand the biology and nature of NSC–host interactions.

On the other hand it is not clear whether NSCs cellular therapies may need to be augmented or optimized by adjunctive molecular therapies. For example, it has been demonstrated that the intraventricular injection of transforming growth factor-α (TGF-α) in an animal model of PD induces a massive proliferation of forebrain cells and their migration to the striatum; this may be accompanied by clinical improvement *(201)*. Cannella et al. showed that the neuregulin GGF2 induced clinical improvement and remyelination in EAE, a model for multiple sclerosis. One of the potential mechanisms of recovery could be mediated by the effects of GGF2 on OPC *(202,203)*. The continuous local infusion of exogenous cytokines may have positive effects on recruiting endogenous progenitors. In vivo infusion of EGF and FGF results in proliferation and differentiation of progenitor cells *(204)*. In a model of hippocampal injury the infusion of EGF restored the architecture and neurogenesis by recruitment of endogenous progenitors *(27)*. It is not clear, however, how long such manipulations are required in the clinical setting to induce an effect; on the other hand, a continuous infusion may induce SVZ hyperplasia, raising questions about the tumorigenic potential of such manipulations *(205)*. It is important to remember that trophic factors have pleiotrophic effects on the brain—while some may be desirable, others may be undesirable and may, in fact, work at cross-purposes to each other. Indeed, administering the trophic factors via cellular vehicles (such as via neural stem/progenitor cells that have genetically engineered ex vivo) may actually be an optimal delivery system because the factors are provided in a site-specific and regulated manner. In addition, because many factors are intrinsically made by such neural-derived cells, potential down-regulation of a foreign transgene may be compensated for.

Source of Human NSCs

Since, in the CNS, the progenitor or stem cell population to be isolated for transplant is small, questions remain about the best sources of stem cells and the most efficacious methods to generate them. Self-renewing pluripotent ES cells may provide an unlimited supply of rapidly dividing cells that can differentiate into any cells; however, with ES cells, we must be certain to direct them down a given lineage and to create safeguards against the appearance of inappropriate nonneural cells, such as conversion to teratocarcinomas or the emergence of autonomous organs. In addition, isolating neural progenitors has its limitations. Human somatic stem cells are often slow to expand and, unless genetically augmented, may senesce. Furthermore, autograft paradigms particularly could be technically problematic owing to the need to isolate, expand, and characterize the NSCs for each individual cases. This procedure may not be a good strategy for acute injury when the success for transplantation may be more optimal in the acute or subacute period of injury. Nevertheless, autologous neural progenitor cells still may prove useful for trauma-based or acquired deficits. Here too, however, circumspection is warranted. Grafting a patient's own cells might circumvent ethical and immunological concerns, but the practical hurdles could be daunting. With each new patient, the healthcare team would be confronted with prospective isolation, expansion, decontamination, characterization, and directed differentiation that will cost time, resources, and personnel, and with potential variability between preparations, patients, and institutions. If one is to contemplate using nonneural adult stem cells for neural purposes, a low-efficiency transdifferentiation event (if it exists at all) must be scaled up to a clinically relevant level, which presupposes a knowledge of the signals involved and an ability to provide them in a controlled way—a goal far from realized.

An alternative to autografts is the use of established, somatic stem or progenitor cell lines. These have the appeal of being homogeneous, well characterized and maintained under good manufacturing practices, readily available in limitless quantities for the acute phases of an injury or disease, and documented to be safe. Their downside, of course, is the possibility of immune incompatibility (which might be addressed through additional engineering or immunosuppressive agents) and the fact that the best source for such universal lines may be the embryo or the fetus, in which various immunogenic markers are less prevalent, rather than the adult. Another concern that must be addressed whenever any expanded or passaged cell—whether propagated by chronic exposure to mitogens or by genetic enhancement—is placed in the body is the risk of producing neoplasms.

In this regard our group has shown that all paradigms of neural stem cell therapy can be achieved safely with NSCs in which a stemness gene (e.g., myc) has been over-expressed but is constitutively self-regulated by the cell itself. Over the years these cells have been used by a great number of investigators and have contributed to our understanding of NSC behavior and therapy during neurodegeneration *(25,59, 122,137,139,147,150,166,181,182,196,206,207)*. Recently Roy et al. extended this observations to human cells, showing that the retroviral overexpression of human telomerase reverse transcriptase (hTERT) can propagate neural progenitors from the human fetal spinal cord *(6,208)*. They showed these cells can yield, among a number of cell lines, some that appear to be restricted to a neuronal lineage both in vitro and in vivo. In vitro, these cells seem to express some molecules consistent with a ventral spinal neuronal phenotype. The cells could be passaged without evidence of senescence, karyotypic abnormality, or loss of normal growth control. After transplantation into developing rat fetal telencephalon or spinal cord, no neoplasms formed, and neuronal markers persisted in vivo with an absence of glial markers *(6,208)*. These data help to debunk the notion that gene-based methods for generation of NSCs clones are inherently dangerous and must be avoided *a priori*. But the expression of certain transgenes—for example, the gene encoding myc or TERT, which is not a foreign gene—may be modulated by the cell's intrinsic regulatory mechanisms or may blunt senescence and stabilize the phenotype. Of course, more extensive research is required to satisfy that they are not prone to form tumors or aberrant connections, and that they will differentiate appropriately in neurodegenerative disorders, standards that have been achieved with mouse NSCs *(25,59,122,137,139,147,150,166,181,182,196,206,207)*.

Human NSCs are been more frequently isolated by different techniques, making possible the preclinical and clinical testing of clones of NSCs. Several laboratories have now isolated multipotent NSCs from fetal and adult sources *(2,77–79,113)*. Preclinical testing has shown the ability of human NSCs to differentiate and migrate. NSCs have been isolated from fetal brain tissue using the cell surface markers, e.g., CD133$^+$CD34$^-$CD45$^-$. Neurosphere cells transplanted into neonatal immuno-deficient mice proliferated, migrated, and differentiated in a site-specific manner *(8)*. To enrich for a specific neuronal population, in vitro priming procedures have been used to generate purer populations of neurons in adult rat CNS, for example, a cholinergic phenotype in a region-specific manner *(209)*. Others have shown that in vitro propagated human NSCs transplanted into neurogenic regions in the adult rat brain (the subventricular zone and hippocampus) migrated specifically along routes normally taken by the endogenous neuronal precursors: along the rostral migratory stream to the olfactory bulb and within the subgranular zone in the dentate gyrus, and exhibited site-specific neuronal differentiation in the granular and periglomerular layers of the bulb and in the dentate granular cell layer. The cells exhibited substantial migration also within a nonneurogenic region, the striatum, and showed differentiation into both neuronal and glial phenotypes *(2,25,210,211)*. Secretory products from human NSCs have corrected a prototypical genetic metabolic defect in neurons and glia *(2)*. Recently it has been found that, similar to the rodent CNS, SVZ astrocytes of the adult human brain proliferate in vivo and behave as multipotent progenitor cells in vitro, providing a prospective source of human cells for repair *(77)*. Interestingly, they do not seem to track along the rostral migratory stream in the same way as in rodents.

Practical Considerations for Preclinical Application of NSC Therapy

Several practical aspects deserve consideration. For instance, the development of methods for noninvasive monitoring of neural stem transplant is required. Magnetic resonance imaging (MRI) tracking of neural progenitors has been developed and tested in several models; some rely on the use of the transferrin receptor as an efficient intracellular delivery device for magnetic nanoparticles. Transplanted tagged oligodendrocyte progenitor cells injected into the spinal cord of myelin-deficient rats showed a close correlation between the areas of contrast enhancement and the achieved extent of myelination *(212,213)* and an EAE model showed good anatomical correlation between histological lesion and imaging *(214)*. MRI has been also applied to following NSCs during stroke, using gadolinium–rhodamine dextran, which allows imaging and fluorescent microcopy analysis *(215)*. Other have used NSCs stably transfected with firefly luciferase and implanted and followed during cerebral infarcts, using biolumi-nescence imaging. These studies show that NSC recruitment to an infarct can be assessed noninvasively by serial in vivo imaging with good correlation between histology and imaging. This study showed NSC migrate mainly along the corpus callosum within 7 d of transplantation with extensive repopulation of the peri-lesion area by 14 d following implantation *(216)*. MRI can be used to track NSCs migrating to gliomas. NSCs migrate toward the tumor bed through the corpus callosum, first detected at 1 wk, with maximal density at the tumor site 2–3 wk after implantation *(207)*.

The survival of transplanted NSCs in a potentially toxic environment remains another critical consideration. There are some encouraging data on migration and proliferation of transplanted OPCs *(116)* and multipotent neural progenitors in the EAE model *(217)*. Recently, injection of adult neurosphere-forming cells (presumably neural stem/progenitors cells), either intravenously or intracerebroventricularly, resulted in significant numbers of donor cells entering into demyelinating areas of the CNS and differentiating into mature brain cells. Within these areas, oligodendrocyte progenitors markedly increased, with many of them being of donor origin and actively remyelinating axons *(120)*. Replication of these results and more research in relevant models of immune demyelinating disease are needed, especially in order to investigate the relationship of exogenous repair with the clinico-pathological features of MS such as relapses and remissions, axonal damage, sustained oxidative injury, and immune cell infiltrates. For instance, suppression of microglia activation was shown to be beneficial for the survival of transplanted progenitors *(218)*. Furthermore, the implantation procedure itself induces a local injury and opening of the blood–brain barrier for several weeks *(219)*. It is unknown whether the amount of injury inflicted may trigger a worsening of the local inflammation in an already diseased brain, which could lead to infiltration of immune cells in the region of injection and decreased survival of exogenous progenitors cells *(218)*. These results and the recent observations that microglia induces a decrease in neurogenesis *(195)* point to an important challenge to NSCs biology: the potential deleterious effects of the inflammatory environment by innate or adaptive immunity to the long-term survival of NSCs *(194)*.

It is likely that the inflammatory microenvironment may have both positive and negative influences on transplanted NSCs *(197)*. We have shown that NSCs may possess an intrinsic program for responding to an inflammatory environment by the expression of functional molecules with immunological capacity *(196)*.

Other cells that may modulate the integration of NSCs are astrocyte. NSCs transplanted into animals that lack GFAP integrated robustly into the host retina with distinct neuronal identity and appropriate neuronal projections *(220)*. Others have found that astrocytes from the hippocampus enhanced neurogenic differentiation from NSCs *(30)*.

NSCs may be a better source of transplants than other progenitor cells including OPCs *(200)*. They seem to possess a greater ability than the more differentiated OPCs for widespread migration toward sites of pathology *(59,166)*. NSCs may also be easier to use because they can be obtained in great numbers theoretically without the need to predifferentiate them in vitro, allowing environmental cues present at the transplantation site to drive their differentiation *(122)*. Indeed, Yandava et al. found that an environment deficient in functioning oligodendrocytes forced multipotent NSCs to shift their differentiation fate and yield an even greater proportion of that cell type *(166)*. Whether priming NSCs toward an oligodendrocyte lineage *ex vivo* would optimize their efficacy remains an important area of investigation. Finally, NSCs may inherently, or after *ex vivo* manipulation, provide additional neurotrophic factors to repair axonal and neuronal abnormalities present in neurodegenerative disorders *(221)*. For many diseases, reconstruction of the damaged milieu may require replacement of multiple cell types and multiple proteins—the cells that have died are not only neurons, but also support cells that detoxify the environment, myelinate the axons and dendrites, supply ongoing trophic and matrix support, and provide reservoirs for ongoing cell replenishment. The neural progenitor cell inherently expresses genes that are capable of signaling, instructing, remodeling, and protecting the host CNS, suggesting another mechanism by which therapeutic outcomes might be achieved: an inherent capacity of neural progenitor cells (without genetic engineering) to create host environments sufficiently rich in trophic and/or neuroprotective support to rescue endogenous cells.

THE RECIPROCAL INTERACTION
OF TRANSPLANTED NSCs AND THE HOST:
EVIDENCE OF PROGRAMS AND CLINICAL VALUE

In the final section, we examine the evidence that interaction between the NSC and the injured brain is a dynamic, complex, ongoing reciprocal set of interactions in which both entities are constantly in flux and the notion of the biological interactions is of critical importance for therapy. We suggest that this interaction can be viewed in a "systems biology" approach and may have broader implications to the future use of NSCs in clinical settings. Our data and those from other laboratories allow us to view this stem cell behavior as part of an innate regenerative program. The reciprocal interactions and behavior of NSCs may be seen as part of this program.

We have somewhat arbitrarily delineated three categories of programs. We call the first classification "Macro Programs." In such programs, NSCs that emanate from primary germinal zones participate in *organogenesis*. However, in our view, organogenesis entails not only "putting the nervous system together," that is, creating the structures, regions, and cytoarchitectonics of the brain, but also establishing "reservoirs" for maintaining homeostasis throughout life. These reservoirs are typically secondary germinal zones that persist throughout life. Evidence for such programs was evident when NSCs implanted during primate development self-distributed into two subpopulations: one contributed to corticogenesis by migrating along radial glia toward the cortical plate, terminating at temporally appropriate layers, and differentiating into lamina-appropriate neurons or glia; the other subpopulation remained undifferentiated and contributed to a secondary germinal zone (the SVZ) with occasional members interspersed throughout brain parenchyma *(25)*. These findings suggested the existence of a unitary embryonic neurogenetic program allocating the progeny of NSCs either for immediate use in organogenesis or to quiescent pools for later use in the "postdevelopmental" (including adult) brain for maintaining homeostasis and/or subserving self-repair. If true, then the prediction would be that, in the face of a perturbation, without specific instruction, induction, or nonphysiological manipulations, this developmental pattern (and the secondary stem/progenitor cell pool that constitutes it) should shift constitutively in the face of a dysequilibrating force toward an attempted reestablishment of equipoise.

The second category of programs we call "System Programs," that is, programs that constitutively unfold and allow the structure (or indeed the entire organism) to respond to perturbations. Such perturbations may be those that occur during the remainder of the complex yet precise process of development, or the "minor" perturbations that occur "day-to-day" throughout the lifespan of an organism in the "wild," or the "extreme" perturbations that often are encountered (e.g., ischemia, trauma, toxins). Compensation for the latter perturbations is often insufficient to reattain baseline, leaving the organism with a persistent handicap. Also, failure of these programs to respond to the more routine perturbations of daily life may be the essence of some slowly progressive degenerative neuropathological processes. The "system" invoked by some programs may entail the mobilization of stem cells from secondary germinal zones and the redistribution (in time and/or space) of the expression of molecular cues. Evidence for such programs is emerging from our studies and others in which endogenous stem cells seem to be activated by injury as well as exogenous NSCs *(59,120,198,217,222)*.

We term the third class of programs "Micro Programs." These are programs that direct the process by which cell type and functional diversity spontaneously emerge within a given region of CNS. Some of these programs appear to allow the multiple progeny of a single stem cell to self-assemble in an autonomous manner, spontaneously allocating various neural cell type identities to these progeny such that they interweave with each other to form the "fabric" of a given region of nervous system.

We suggest that a better understanding of these fundamental developmental "programs" will ultimately yield not only a better understanding of development but also how best to exploit NSC biology for therapy. For example, it might lend insight into the heretofore unclear teleology of "secondary" germinal zones and "vestigial" stem cells in the "postdevelopmental" or adult CNS. It may also pinpoint and elucidate those developmentally programmed compensatory mechanisms that need to be reinvoked and/or exploited for purposes of repair.

Interestingly, the exploration of some of these fundamental processes may actually be abetted by the use of exogenous NSCs—not as simply therapeutic vehicles—although their utility in that regard will become obvious—but as biological "tools." In other words, we introduce the notion of the NSC as a "reporter cell"—by way of analogy, at the cellular level, to a reporter gene as used in molecular biology—to reflect (or signal) when a particular process has occurred. Such exogenous stem cells can "interrogate" the environment and track (i.e., "report on") the behavior of endogenous CNS progenitor/stem cells that are otherwise "invisible" to such monitoring, too few to track reliably, and whose clonal relationships and degree of homogeneity may be less certain.

The Injured CNS Interacts Reciprocally with NSCs to Reconstitute Lost Tissue

As a part of such programs we have accumulated evidence of the cross-talk between host and neural stem cells. Using exogenous NSCs to "interrogate" the environment and using HI brain injury as a prototype for insults to the CNS characterized by extensive tissue loss, we were able to confirm that a reciprocal dynamic indeed occurs between NSCs and degenerating neural tissue. Seeding NSCs onto a biosynthetic scaffold that is subsequently implanted into the large infarction cavities of mouse brains injured by HI not only provided a template for bridging extensive cystic lesions and guiding restructuring, but also served to "fix" NSCs in space as well as to "fix" and prolong the effects of (1) molecules emanating from the injured brain and (2) molecules emanating from the NSCs (Fig. 3). In so doing, we were permitted to observe—in a manner heretofore unavailable—the multiple robust reciprocal interactions that spontaneously ensue between NSCs and the extensively damaged brain. NSCs grew exuberantly into a lattice of neurons and glia, parenchymal loss was dramatically reduced, an intricate meshwork of many highly arborized neurites of both host- and donor-derived neurons emerged, and some anatomical connections were reconstituted.

The exogenous NSCs, nestled within the necrotic host parenchyma, altered the trajectory and complexity of host cortical neurites, promoting their entrance into the matrix. In a reciprocal manner, tract tracing demonstrated donor-derived neurons extending processes into host parenchyma as far as the opposite hemisphere. Of interest was the degree to which these neurons were capable of seemingly directed, target-appropriate neurite outgrowth *without* specific external instructive guidance cues, induction, or genetic manipulation of host brain or donor cells. These NSC/scaffold complexes, these "biobridges," appeared to unveil and/or augment a constitutive reparative response by facilitating a series of reciprocal interactions between NSC and host CNS tissue (both injured and intact), including promoting neuronal differentiation, enhancing the ingrowth/outgrowth of neural processes, fostering the reformation of cortical tissue, and promoting connectivity following brain injury. Inflammation and scarring were also reduced, facilitating reconstitution *(124)*.

That certain reciprocal interactions spontaneously unfold between transplanted NSCs and an injured host—as if "preprogrammed"—suggests that NSCs might influence the fate of host cells as profoundly as the fate of the NSC itself is changed. The power and implications of this underrecognized axis of influence are discussed in the following section.

NSCs Display an Inherent Mechanism for Rescuing Dysfunctional Neurons and Axons

The notion that stem cells—as exemplified by NSCs—may actually possess an *intrinsic* capacity to "rescue" dysfunctional host neurons and their connections was first confirmed in two very different situations: the brains of aged mice *(137)* (Fig. 4) and the injured spinal cords of adult rats *(141)* (Fig. 5).

The first of these studies focused on a neuronal cell type with stereotypical projections that is commonly compromised in the aged brain—the dopaminergic (DA) neuron *(137)* (Fig. 4). The DA-selective neurotoxin (and complex I inhibitor) 1-methyl-4-phenyl-1,2,3,6-tetrahydropyridine (MPTP) was administered systemically to intensify and accelerate permanent impairment of these neurons bilaterally (an experimental lesion that emulates Parkinson's disease). Unilateral implantation of murine NSCs into the midbrains of these aged Parkinsonian mice promoted reconstitution of the mesostriatal system, an impressive outcome supported by both histological and functional assays. The recovery of DA activity mirrored the spatiotemporal distribution of donor-derived cells. Although the spontaneous conversion of some donor NSCs into replacement DA neurons contributed to nigral reconstitution in DA-depleted areas, the *majority* of DA neurons in the mesostriatal system were actually "rescued" *host* cells. Pools of undifferentiated donor NSCs in and adjacent to the mesostriatal nuclei appeared to have mediated this "rescue." That these pools spontaneously expressed such neuroprotective substances as GDNF provided (in part) a plausible molecular basis for this phenomenon. This unexpected and novel observation suggested that host structures may benefit not only from NSC-derived replacement of lost neurons but also from the "chaperone" effect of other NSC-derived progeny. This process—dominant in this Parkinson's disease model—likely represents a mechanism of NSC action for a range of neurodegenerative disorders and provides insight into the broader use of stem cells

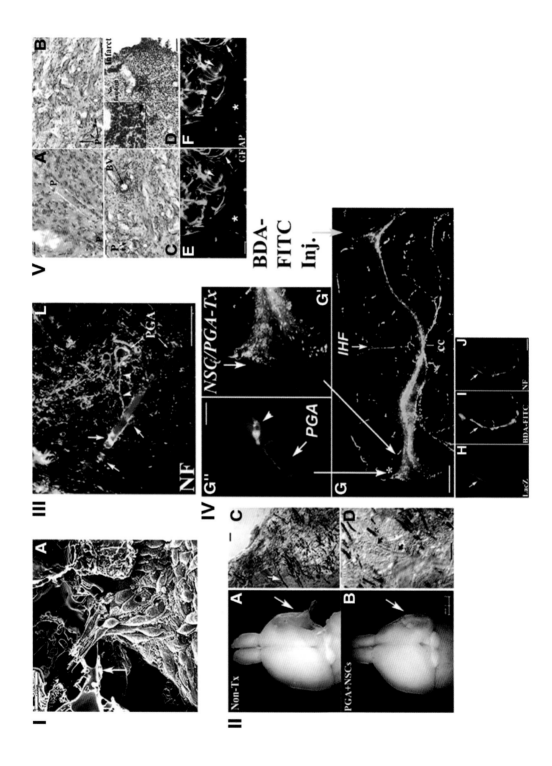

Fig. 3. The injured brain interacts reciprocally with neural stem cells supported by scaffolds to reconstitute lost tissue—evidence from hypoxic–ischemic (HI) injury. (Modified from ref. *124*.) **I.** Characterization of NSCs in vitro when seeded on a PGA scaffold. Cells, seen with scanning electron microscopy at 5 d after seeding, were able to attach to, impregnate, and migrate throughout a highly porous PGA matrix (*arrow*). The NSCs differentiated primarily into neurons (>90%) that sent out long, complex processes that adhered to, enwrapped, and interconnected the PGA fibers. **II.** Implantation of NSC/PGA complexes into a region of cavity formation following extensive HI brain injury and necrosis. **(A)** Brain of an untransplanted ("non-Tx") mouse subjected to right HI injury with extensive infarction and cavitation of the ipsilateral right cortex, striatum, thalamus, and hippocampus (*arrow*). Contrast with **(B)**, the brain of a similarly injured mouse implanted with an NSC/PGA complex ("PGA+NSCs") (generated in vitro as per **(I.)**) into the infarction cavity 7 d after the induction of HI (*arrow*) (*n* = 60). At maturity (age-matched to the animal pictured in **(A)**, the NSC/scaffold complex appears, in this whole-mount, to have filled the cavity (*arrow*) and become incorporated into the infarcted cerebrum. Representative coronal sections through that region are seen at higher magnification in **(C,D)** in which parenchyma appears to have filled in spaces between the dissolving black polymer fibers (*white arrow* in **C**) and, as seen in **(D)**, even to support neovascularization by host tissues (blood vessel indicated by closed black arrow in **D**; *open arrow* in **D** points to degrading black polymer fiber). Scale bars: **(C,D)** = 100 mm. **III.** Characterization in vivo of the neural composition of NSC–PGA complexes within the HI injured brain. At 2 wk following transplantation of the NSC–PGA complex into the infarction cavity, donor-derived cells showed robust engraftment within the injured region. An intricate network of multiple long, branching NF⁺ (*green*) processes were present within the NSC–PGA complex and its parenchyma enwrapping the PGA fibers (*orange autofluorescent tube-like structures under a Texas Red filter*), adherent to and running along the length of the fibers (*arrows*), often interconnecting and bridging the fibers (*arrowheads*). Those NF⁺ processes were of both host- and donor-derivation. In other words, not only were donor-derived neural cells present, but also host-derived cells seemed to have entered the NSC–PGA complex, migrating along and becoming adherent to the PGA matrix. In a reciprocal manner, donor-derived (*lacZ⁺*) neurons (NF⁺ cells) within the complex appeared to send processes along the PGA fibers out of the matrix into host parenchyma as seen in **(IV.)** Scale bars = 100 μm. **IV.** Long-distance neuronal connections extend from the transplanted NSC–PGA complexes in the HI-injured brain toward presumptive target regions in the intact contralateral hemisphere. By 6 wk following engraftment, donor-derived *lacZ⁺* cells appeared to extend many exceedingly long, complex NF⁺ processes along the length of the disappearing matrix apparently extending into host parenchyma. To confirm the suggestion that long-distance processes projected from the injured cortex into host parenchyma, a series of tract tracing studies were performed. **(G–G″)** BDA-FITC was injected **(G)** into the contralateral intact cortex and external capsule (*green arrow*) at 8 wk following implantation of the NSC–PGA complex into the infarction cavity ("NSC/PGA-Tx"). Axonal projections (labeled *green* with fluorescein under an FITC filter) are visualized (via the retrograde transport of BDA) leading back to (across the interhemispheric fissure ["IHF"] via the corpus callosum ["cc"]) and emanating from cells in the NSC/PGA complex within the damaged contralateral cortex and penumbra (seen at progressively higher magnification in **G′** (region indicated by arrow to **G**) and **G″** (region indicated by *arrow* and asterisk (*) in **G**). In **(G″)**, the retrogradely BDA-FITC-labeled perikaryon of a representative neuron adherent to a dissolving PGA fiber is well visualized. That such cells are neurons of donor derivation is supported by their triple-labeling **(H–J)** for *lacZ* **(H)** (bgal), BDA-FITC **(I)**, and the neuronal marker NF **(J)**; *arrow* in **(H–J)** indicates same cell in all three panels. Such neuronal clusters were never seen under control conditions—that is, in untransplanted cases or when vehicle or even an NSC suspension *unsupported* by scaffolds was injected into the infarction cavity. Scale bars = **(G)**, 500 mm; **(G″)**, 20 mm; **(H–J)**, 30 mm. *(Figure 3 caption is continued on the next page).*

Fig. 3. (*continued from previous page*) **V.** Adverse secondary events that typically follow injury (e.g., monocyte infiltration and astroglial scar formation) are minimized by and within the NSC–PGA complex. (**A–D**) Photomicrographs of H&E-stained sections prepared to visualize the degree of monocyte infiltration in relation to the NSC–PGA complex and the injured cortex 3 wk following implantation into the infarction cavity. Monocytes are classically recognized under H&E as very small cells with small round nuclei and scanty cytoplasm (e.g., inset in **D**, *arrowhead*). While some very localized monocyte infiltration was present immediately surrounding a blood vessel ("BV" in **C**, *arrow*) that grew into the NSC–PGA complex from the host parenchyma, there was little or no monocyte infiltration either in the center of the NSC–PGA complex (**B**) or at the interface between the NSC–PGA complex and host cortical penumbra (**A**)—in stark contrast to the excessive monocyte infiltration seen in an untransplanted infarct of equal duration, age, and extent (**D**), the typical histopathologic picture otherwise seen following HI brain injury (see *inset*, a higher magnification of the region indicated by the *arrowhead*). While neural cells (nuclei of which are seen in **A–C**) adhere exuberantly to the many polymer fibers ("P" in **A–C**), monocyte infiltration was minimal compared to that in (**D**). (**E,F**) Astroglial scarring (another pathological condition confounding recovery from ischemic CNS injury) is also much constrained and diminished following implantation of the NSC–PGA complex. While GFAP⁺ cells (astrocytes) were among the cell types into which NSCs differentiated when in contact with the PGA fibers, *away* from the fibers (*) there was minimal astroglial presence either of donor or host origin. (**E**) GFAP immunostaining recognized by a fluorescein-conjugated secondary antibody (*green*) is observed. Note little scarring in the regions indicated by the *asterisk* (*). Under a Texas red filter (**F**) (merged with the fluorescein filter image), the tube-like PGA fibers (*arrowhead* in both panels) becomes evident (as an *autofluorescent orange*), and most of the donor-derived astrocytes (*arrows*) (*yellow* because of their dual *lacZ* and GFAP immunoreactivity) are seen to be associated with these fibers, again leaving most regions of the infarct (*asterisk* [*]) astroglial scar-free (*arrows* in **E** and **F** point to the same cells). Far from creating a barrier to the migration of host- or donor-origin cells or to the ingrowth/outgrowth of axons of host- or donor-origin neurons (as per **III** and **IV**), NSC-derived astrocytes may actually have helped provide a facilitating bridge. Scale bars = (**A**), 10 mm; (**C,D**) and (**E,F**), 20 mm. Reproduced by permission of The Royal Society of London.

398

from and for other organ systems. Human NSCs in monkey Parkinsonian models may have a similar effect *(152a)*.

A similar mechanism played a pivotal and equally unanticipated role in a model of acquired neural impairment, spinal cord injury (Fig. 5). Murine NSCs were implanted into the extensive injury site that results when the spinal cords of adult rats are subjected to a hemiresection between thoracic level 9 and 10 (T9–10) *(141)*. (As described for the extensive cerebral ischemic lesions detailed earlier *(124)*, these NSCs, too, were supported by a biodegradable synthetic scaffold in order to fix them in space.) Hindlimb deficits were evaluated weekly for up to a year. By 2–3 mo postimplant, engrafted rats exhibited coordinated weight-bearing stepping while the lesion-control group failed to ambulate even months following injury (see Movie 1, *www.pnas.org*). Improvement persisted for at least a year (when the study was terminated). Histology, immuno-cytochemistry (including for expression of GAP-43, a marker of regeneration) and tract-tracing all suggested that the long-term reduction in functional deficits resulted *not* from replacement of neural fibers by the NSCs but rather from their role in providing trophic support, reducing scar formation, increasing the amount of preserved host tissue (including neuronal) by mitigating secondary cell death, promoting host fiber regrowth through the lesion epicenter, and catalyzing regeneration of damaged host tissue. Indeed, the NSCs themselves remained largely immature nestin-expressing cells—*not* differentiating into neurons but also not becoming astrocytes that might contribute to the glial scar (which, in fact, was significantly diminished). As noted earlier for neurodegenerative diseases, it appeared that NSCs in their nonneuronal state, within the traumatized CNS, also produced growth factors, antiinflammatory factors, angiogenic factors, and differentiation factors—to a degree not witnessed if they had become neuronally committed. Indeed, NSCs in this state may be superior tools for promoting repair in some acquired conditions (e.g., trauma, ischemia, toxins)—via their promotion of host axonal regeneration and/or preservation.

Suspecting that NSCs may constitutively express these factors as part of their fundamental biology, we began to explore the possibility that their natural production of neurotrophic agents (particularly those known to promote sensory and motor axon growth) might be used intentionally to promote regeneration. To examine in vivo the effects of NSCs on host axonal regeneration (in collaboration with Mark Tuszynski), adult rats underwent lesions of the cervical (C3) spinal cord with a microwire knife *(139)*. This cervical lesion transects the dorsal columns bilaterally, thereby disrupting both descending motor corticospinal projections and ascending dorsal column proprioceptive pathways. Murine NSCs were injected into the lesion cavity immediately postlesioning. NSCs survived well in vivo after grafting, filling the lesion site, becoming well vascularized. Their extension stopped at the borders of the injury; there was no deformation of the spinal cord or tumor formation. In this model, the NSCs remained undifferentiated, labeling for nestin but not for neuronal, astroglial, or oligodendroglial markers. Despite the absence of NSC differentiation, or possibly because of it, axons were observed penetrating the grafts directly from the host SC (to a significantly greater extent than control fibroblasts grafts). Furthermore, specific classes of host axons grew extensively within the grafts: motor axons labeled with choline acetyltransferase (ChAT), and sensory axons labeled with CGRP or p75. These findings further suggested that NSCs can inherently provide permissive substrates and factors to promote

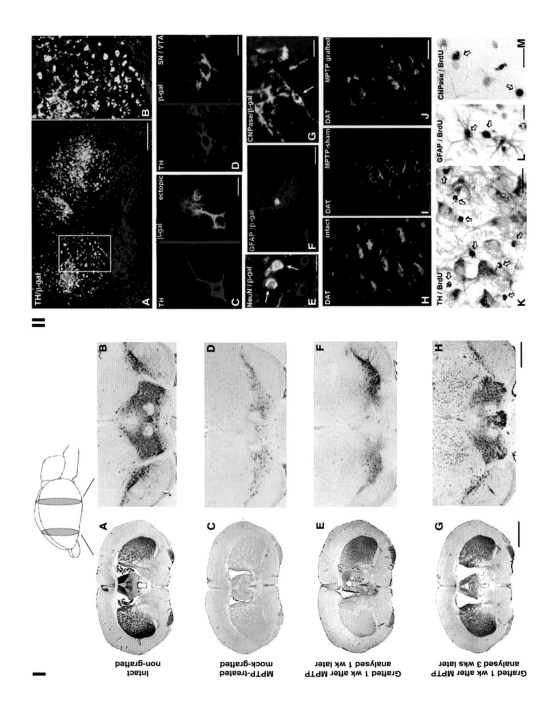

Fig. 4. NSCs possess an inherent mechanism for rescuing dysfunctional neurons: evidence from the effects of NSCs in the restoration of mesencephalic dopaminergic function. (Modified from ref. *137*). **I.** TH expression in mesencephalon and striatum of aged mice following MPTP lesioning and unilateral NSC engraftment into the substantia nigra/ventral tegmental area (SN/VTA). A model that emulates the slow dysfunction of aging dopaminergic neurons in substantia nigra (SN) was generated by giving aged mice repeated high doses of MPTP. Schematic on *top* indicates the levels of the analyzed transverse sections along the rostrocaudal axis of the mouse brain. Representative coronal sections through the striatum are presented in the *left column* (**[a],[c],[e],[g]**) and through the SN/VTA area in the *right column* (**[b],[d],[f],[h]**)[a,b] Immunodetection of TH (*black cells*) shows the normal distribution of DA-producing TH+ neurons in coronal sections in the intact SN/VTA (**b**) and their projections to the striatum (**a**). (**c,d**) Within 1 wk, MPTP treatment caused extensive and permanent bilateral loss of TH immunoreactivity in both the mesostriatal nuclei (**c**) and the striatum (**d**), which lasted life long. Shown in this example, and matching the time point in (**g,h**), is the situation in a mock-grafted animal 4 wk after MPTP treatment (**e,f**) Unilateral (*right side*) stereotactic injection of NSCs into the nigra is associated, within 1 wk after grafting, with substantial recovery of TH synthesis within the ipsilateral DA nuclei (**f**) and their ipsilateral striatal projections (**e**). By 3 wk posttransplant, however (**g,h**), the asymmetric distribution of TH expression disappeared, giving rise to TH immunoreactivity in the midbrain (**h**) and striatum (**g**) of both hemispheres that approached that of intact controls (**a,b**) and gave the appearance of mesostriatal restoration. Similar observations were made when NSCs were injected 4 wk after MPTP treatment (not shown). Bars: 2 mm (*left*), 1 mm (*right*). Note the ectopically placed TH+ cells in [H]. These are analyzed in greater detail, along with the entire SN in (**II**). **II.** Immunohistochemical analyses of TH-, DAT-, and BrdU-positive cells in MPTP-treated and grafted mouse brains. The presumption was initially that the NSCs had replaced the dysfunctional TH neurons. However, examination of the reconstituted SN with dual βgal (*green*) and TH (*red*) ICC showed that (**A,C**) 90% of the TH+ cells in the SN were host-derived cells that had been rescued and only 10% donor-derived (**D**). Most NSC-derived TH+ cells were actually just above the SN ectopically (*blocked area* in [A], enlarged in [B]). These photomicrographs were taken from immunostained brain sections from aged mice exposed to MPTP, transplanted 1 wk later with NSCs, and killed after 3 wk. The following combinations of markers were evaluated: TH (*red*) with bgal (*green*) (**a–d**); NeuN (*red*) with βgal (*green*) (**e**); GFAP (*red*) with bgal (*green*) (**f**); CNPase (*green*) with bgal (*red*) (**g**); as well as TH (*brown*) and BrdU (*black*) (**k**): GFAP (*brown*) with BrdU (*black*) (**l**); and CNPase (*brown*) with BrdU (*black*) (**m**). Anti-DAT-stained areas are revealed in *green* in the SN of intact (**h**), mock-grafted (**i**), and NSC-grafted (**j**) brains. Three different fluorescence filters specific for Alexa Fluor 488 (*green*), Texas Red (*red*), and a double-filter for both types of fluorochromes (*yellow*) were used to visualize specific antibody binding; (**c**), (**d**), and (**h–j**) are single-filter exposures; (**a**), (**b**), (**e–g**) are double-filter exposures. (**a**) shows a low-power overview of the SN+VTA of both hemispheres, similar to the image in **Fig. 5h**. The majority of TH+ cells (*red* cells in [a]) within the nigra are actually of host-origin (~90%) with a much smaller proportion there being of donor-derivation (*green cells*) (~10%) (representative close-up of such a donor-derived TH+ cell in **d**). Although a significant proportion of NSCs did differentiate into TH+ neurons, many of these actually resided ectopically, dorsal to the SN—(*boxed area* in **a**, enlarged in **b**; high-power view of donor-derived (*green*) cell that was also TH+ (*red*) in **c**)—where the ratio of donor-to-host cells was inverted: ~90% donor-derived compared with ~10% host-derived. Note the almost complete absence of a green βgal-specific signal in the SN+VTA while, ectopically, many of the TH+ cells were double-labeled and thus NSC-derived (appearing *yellow-orange* in higher power under a *red/green double-filter* in panel **b**). (**c–g**) NSC-derived non-TH neurons (NeuN+) (**e**, *arrow*), astrocytes (GFAP+) (**f**), and oligodendrocytes (CNPase+) (**g**, *arrow*) were also seen, both within the mesencephalic nuclei and dorsal to them.
(Figure 4 caption is continued on the next page).

401

Fig. 4. (*continued from previous page*) (**h–j**) The green DAT-specific signal in (**j**) suggests that the reconstituted mesencephalic nuclei in the NSC-grafted mice (as in **I–h**) were functional DA neurons comparable to those seen in intact nuclei (**h**) but not in MPTP-lesioned sham-engrafted controls (**i**). This further suggests that the TH[+] mesostriatal DA neurons effected by MPTP are, indeed, functionally impaired. (Note that sham-grafted animals [**i**] contain only punctate residual DAT staining within their dysfunctional fibers, while DAT staining in normal [**h**] and, similarly, in engrafted [**j**] animals was normally and robustly distributed both within processes and throughout their cell bodies.) (**k–m**) Any proliferative BrdU[+] cells after MPTP insult and/or grafting were confined to glial cells while the TH[+] neurons [**k**] were BrdU[-]. This finding suggested that the reappearance of TH[+] host cells was not the result of neurogenesis but rather the recovery of extant host TH[+] neurons. Bars = 90 μm (**a**); 20 μm (**c–e**); 30 μm (**f**); 10 μm (**g**); 20 μm (**h–j**); 25 μm, (**k**); 10 μm, (**l**); and 20 μm (**m**). Used with permission of The Royal Society of London.

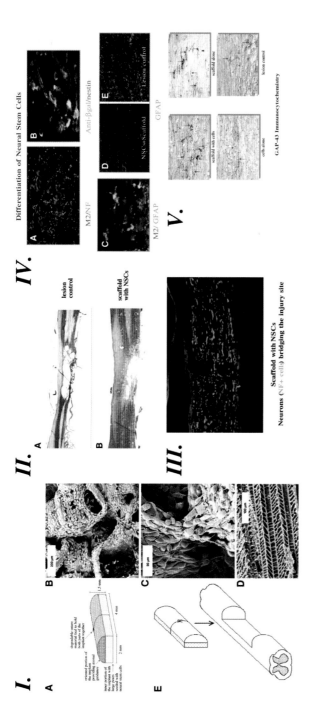

Fig. 5. Functional recovery following traumatic spinal cord injury mediated by a unique polymer scaffold seeded with neural stem cells. (Modified from ref. *141.*) **I.** Schematics of scaffold design showing inner and outer portions. (**B,C**) Inner scaffold seeded with NSCs. Outer scaffold created to have long, axially oriented pores for axonal guidance and radial pores to allow fluid transport and inhibit ingrowth of cells. (**E**) Schematic of surgical insertion of implant into SC. **II.** Based on Basso-Bresnahan-Beatie (BBB) open-field walking scores, the "scaffold+NSCs" group showed significant improvement in open-field locomotion compared with "lesion-control" groups (*P* < 0.007). Histology (H&E) of longitudinal sections from (**A**) lesioned untreated group and from (**B**) "scaffold+cells" groups was revealing. Note greater integrity of parenchyma in the latter. **III.** Examination of composition of the tissue at the lesion site demonstrated numerous NF⁺ cells and processes. However, as illustrated in (**IV**), the neurons were host and not donor NSC-derived. **IV.** The neurons were neither NF⁺ (**A**) nor even GFAP⁺, the latter finding suggesting that they did not contribute to the glial scar. In fact, glial scarring was *diminished* in "NSC+scaffold" SCs (**D**) compared to "lesion control" SCs (**E**) based on GFAP immunoreactivity. Most mNSCs remained undifferentiated nestin⁺ cells (**B**). **V.** "Scaffold+NSC" implantation significantly increased the presence of GAP-43⁺ fibers relative to other controls, a marker for regenerating neurites. Following administration of BDA for antegrade tracing, BDA⁺ axons (not shown, but see ref. *141*) were coursed through the lesion epicenter (as in **III**) to reach areas caudal to the lesion in the scaffold containing groups, suggesting an anatomical substrate for the functional improvement seen in those animals (a mean of 14 on the 21 point BBB scale). Reproduced with permission of The Royal Society of London.

403

growth of host axons in vivo. Indeed, attempting to intervene in the natural expression of the various neurotrophic factors in their various proportions through genetic manipulation actually appeared to throw the system into somewhat of an imbalance *(139)*. For example, in the above-described experiments, enhancing expression of NT-3 in a given clone of NSCs actually extinguished its expression of GDNF, obliterating its promotion of *motor* axonal ingrowth which instead became supplanted by the enhanced ingrowth of *sensory* axons. In other words, manipulating one aspect of a delicately balanced natural system may yield desirable affects if the consequences are understood, but may also yield unanticipated and undesirable effects if the system and its "logic" from the "viewpoint" of the NSC are not. The molecular mechanism underlying all of these above-described observations, we believe, constitutes the normal constitutive expression of yet another developmental program—one we term a "Micro Program"—and is discussed in the next section.

Reciprocal Signaling: Expression of a Broader Developmental Scheme— A "Micro" Program

It was determined via enzyme-linked immunosorbent assay (ELISA), Western blots, and immunocytochemistry that murine and human NSCs constitutively produce a broad range of peptide neurotrophic and neurite outgrowth-promoting factors that function appropriately in appropriate bioassays (e.g., the promotion of motor neuron outgrowth from organotypic spinal explants). Conditioned medium from NSCs contained significant quantities of NGF (7.5 ± 2.5 pg/10^6 cells/d), BDNF (7.1 ± 0.1 pg/10^6 cells/d), GDNF (70 ± 1 pg/10^6 cells/d) *(139)*, and others. Fibroblasts expressed no detectable levels. Of the various factors, GDNF was of particular interest because of its known neuroprotective and outgrowth-promoting effect on such ventralized neural cell types as nigral DA neurons and spinal anterior horn motor neurons—cell types we had established to be impacted in vivo by NSCs *(137,139,141)*. We elected, in preliminary studies, to use GDNF as an index neurotrophic agent and explore the NSC's regulation of its intrinsic GDNF expression to help reveal what we believed was a little recognized but pervasive NSC developmental mechanism with powerful therapeutic possibilities. In pilot studies, using motor neuron axon outgrowth from spinal explants as a quantifiable bioassay, it was determined that NSCs could mimic the effect of exogenously administered GDNF peptide; GDNF antisense or a soluble "scavenger" GDNF receptor was sufficient to blunt NSC-induced neurite outgrowth while SC explants obtained from the *ret* (GDNF-receptor)-null mouse, when used in this bioassay, elaborated dramatically fewer axons toward the NSCs. Of interest was the observation that, when the progeny of a given NSC clone existed in a non-neuronal (undifferentiated or glial) state, intrinsic GDNF expression was robust. Curiously, however, the cell in that state could not respond to the GDNF it had just produced because it did not bear a GDNF (*ret*) receptor. On the other hand, when the same clonal progeny were induced to differentiate into neurons, GDNF production diminished virtually to nil, but gave way to expression of a functional *ret*-receptor, one that could be appropriately phosphorylated by GDNF. This dynamic suggested a developmental program—a "micro" program, if you will—by which a single "mother" NSC gives rise to progeny that, in a symbiotic fashion, provide reciprocal support for each other—serving as "chaperones," so to speak.

Using subclones of NSCs that contained various neural cell type-specific promoters driving green fluorescent protein (GFP) expression to signal when various fate decisions were made by various equipotent members of a given clone, we began to amass preliminary evidence that pointed to an "autonomous CNS self-assembly program" pursued constitutively by NSCs. Key to that model was the observation that NSCs that have become neuronally committed (seemingly their default differentiation pathway) appear to actively promote the nonneuronal differentiation of their equipotent sister cells via a membrane-associated mechanism. In brief, within a clone of equipotent sister NSCs, when the first cell exits the cell cycle and commits to a neuronal phenotype (either stochastically, by default, or by instruction) it then actively inhibits the neuronal differentiation of its equipotent sister cells that subsequently exit the cell cycle (even under conditions that would ordinarily propel them toward a neuronal lineage). It effects this inhibition, we believe, based on pilot studies, via membrane-associated factors that exert their influence by direct cell–cell contact. Interestingly, these factors appear to be independent of Notch–Delta or BMP signaling. Membranes from sister cells that differ only in that they have *not* made such a neuronal commitment do not have this effect.

Such an autonomous self-assembly developmental scheme establishes a network independent of external instruction wherein a neuron is always flanked by nonneurons (often astroglia). One can envision the entire fabric of the brain being spontaneously woven based on this scheme starting with a few multipotent NSCs. A possible biological "rationale" for the existence of such a developmental "program" is provided by taking into account our recent observations (described earlier) of GDNF peptide and receptor expression by various differentiation states of the same NSC. The nonneurons are forced to be "chaperones" for—and by—their sibling neuron, providing the trophic support needed by the neuron. Such a developmental scheme for NSC-mediated CNS self-assembly, cell-type determination, and "division of labor," based on intercellular communication between members of a single NSC clone insures that each neuron is surrounded by cells that can vouchsafe its survival. Although GDNF may be "intended" by non-neuronal "chaperones" for support of their juxtaposed neuronal clonal members, this factor likely has a broader sphere of influence, including support and/or neuroprotection of "bystander" host neurons. In other words, when one transplants NSCs into a diseased recipient, host cells—as "bystanders" of this developmental program—become the indirect beneficiaries of this trophic factor production.

It is further significant to realize that the GDNF is not produced by the NSCs tonically but seems to be released in a sporadic, pulsatile manner. In attempting to dissect the signal transduction pathway mediating GDNF expression and the type of production observed, inhibitors of either the MEK pathway were employed vs inhibitors of the PI3 kinase pathway—the former pathway broadly subserving more permanent changes in neural progenitors (e.g., differentiation, apoptosis, etc.), the latter pathway subserving responses that are more transient adjustments to environmental influences (e.g., proliferation, stress, etc.). Such preliminary experiments suggested that it was the PI3 kinase pathway that mediated the GDNF response. Nitric oxide donor molecules— simulating environmental stress—increased GDNF expression.

Such evidence that GDNF (presumably representative of other neurotrophic agents) is expressed in a regulated, stimulus-appropriate, region- and cell type-specific manner supports a view that NSCs may serve as gene delivery vehicles better than nonneural cells or noncellular vectors because the production of neural-relevant gene products by NSCs is part of their fundamental biology. This point was reinforced in a recent experiment *(223)* in which the ability of NT-3 to rescue neurons in Clarke's nucleus following axotomy was explored. Rescue was found to be greater when NT-3 was delivered from engrafted NT-3-expressing NSCs than by administering the peptide alone. The suggestion was that the NSCs may provide additional factors, or provide more physiological, regulated concentrations of the factors, or act as a target or bridge that supports regenerating axons. This observation gets to the heart of some of the advantages of NSCs—whether unmanipulated or genetically engineered—in CNS dysfunction. We believe that trophic support is best supplied by cellular vehicles of neural origin—specifically NSCs—because, as suggested earlier, these molecules can be released in a regulated fashion, targeted in a site-specific manner from members of the parenchyma, with less concern for transgene down-regulation (given their intrinsic basal expression by the NSC) while simultaneously providing the possibility of cellular replacement.

Whether one chooses to use transplanted NSCs or attempts to manipulate endogenous NSCs, an understanding of the reciprocal interactions between genes and NSC biology, between differentiation state and gene expression, and between injured host and NSC will be critical. Their use must be dictated by a greater knowledge of NSC biology and of how various neurotrophic agents interact within the NSC and with the degenerating host environment. Isolated, well-characterized, homogenous clones of NSCs may make such study more easily observed and controlled.

Modulation of NSCs to Enhancing Neuronal Differentiation

In preliminary studies, when exogenous NSCs are transplanted into brains of young mice subjected (as described earlier) to unilateral HI injury (optimally within 3–7 d), donor-derived cells migrate preferentially to and integrate extensively within the large ischemic areas that typically span the injured ipsilateral hemisphere. Even donor cells implanted in more distant locations (including the contralateral hemisphere) migrate toward the regions of HI injury (emulating what endogenous progenitors appear to do). (Waiting 5 wk post-HI yields virtually no engraftment, suggesting a "window" for this phenomenon.) A subpopulation of donor NSCs, particularly in the penumbra, "shift" their differentiation fate towards neurons (5%) and oligodendrocytes, the neural cell types typically damaged following asphyxia/stroke although no neurons and few oligodendrocytes are derived from NSCs in intact postnatal neocortex. Clearly, as in the targeted apoptosis model described earlier *(122)*, novel signals appear to be transiently elaborated to which NSCs respond.

Because engrafted NSCs continue to express their *lac*Z reporter transgene, it appeared feasible that desired differentiation of both host and donor-derived cells might be enhanced if donor NSCs were genetically manipulated *ex vivo* to (over)express certain bioactive transgenes, for example, the neuron-inducing factor, NT-3, a neurotrophic factor it expresses at baseline low amounts. In pilot studies, a subclone of the NSCs was transduced with a retroviral vector encoding NT-3. The engineered NSCs produced large amounts of NT-3 in vitro *(121,223)*. We determined that both the parent clone and its NT-3-producing subclone expressed trkC receptors, that these receptors were appropriately tyrosine-phosphorylated in response to exogenous NT-3, that this phosphorylation could be blocked by K252a, and that the signal was appropriately transduced via MAP kinase. Therefore, it appeared that this engineered NSC subclone could not only secrete excess NT-3, but could also respond to NT-3 in an autocrine/paracrine fashion. In culture, NT-3-overexpressing NSCs, like the parent clone, still differentiate into neurons, astrocytes, and oligodendrocytes. However, unlike the parent clone whose percent of neurons falls as new cells are born, the percentage of this NT-3-overexpressing subclone that remained neuronal in vitro was approx 95%. Therefore, pilot studies were performed in which NT-3-overexpressing NSCs were implanted into the infarct. NT-3 expression remained robust in vivo. The percentage of donor-derived neurons was increased from 5% (in the above-described experiments) to 20% in the infarct and to >80% in the penumbra. Many of the neurons became cholinergic, glutamatergic, or GABAergic. NT-3 was also likely acting on host—as well as donor—cells in an a paracrine fashion to enhance their neuronal differentiation. Now, it is quite plausible that the original yield of 5% new neurons was actually the correct ratio and that 80% neurons is actually a "prescription for dysfunction"; we have come to adopt the aphorism that even the "dumbest stem cell is smarter than the smartest neurobiologist." However, the NT-3 experiment served as a proof-of-concept: the observations suggest that, when a molecular mechanism underlying a naturally occurring NSC-based process in a degenerative environment is known, it can be augmented via genetic engineering. It also enunciated the potential use of migratory NSCs for simultaneous gene therapy *and* cell replacement during the same procedure in the same recipient using the same cells, an intriguing NSC ability. This work constitutes a paradigm for using NSCs to express other trophic factors in other instances, such as spinal cord injury. Indeed, we have evidence that the same parent NSC clone can be variously engineered to express a range of gene products serving a variety of therapeutic ends, including NT-4/5, GDNF, BDNF, NGF, L1, *sonic hedgehog*, *wnt-1*, *wnt-3a*, as well as a variety of biosynthetic and metabolic enzymes. Hence, implantation of genetically engineered NSCs expressing bioactive transgenes—when used in a thoughtful manner—might enhance neuronal differentiation, neurite outgrowth, and proper connectivity.

CONCLUSIONS AND FUTURE DIRECTIONS

We have attempted to provide a conceptual framework for the clinical application of exogenous neural stem cells to neurodegenerative diseases. Our knowledge of neural stem cell biology is based on observing the behavior of such cells in vivo during development or injury. We need to comprehend the molecular basis of these phenomena and the molecular programs that underlie intrinsic NSC properties: NSC, self-renewal, differentiation, migration, and secretion of neurotrophic substance. We have attempted to frame our observations in the context of biological programs. This framework we believe, will be of value when thinking about clinical applications. We need to learn more about the neurodegenerative environment and the intrinsic properties of NSCs before we can formulate potential therapies. To realize fully the therapeutic potential of NSCs, clinicians and neuroscientists face many challenges: how to direct such NSCs to different CNS regions to yield cells of the right type(s) without making aberrant connections, and how to shield NSCs from potential deleterious effects of the environment. This has to be accompanied by clinical judgment, choosing which disease may realistically benefit from NSC transplants. NSCs will likely be used in combination with other therapeutic strategies, again based on a judicious assessment of the biologies of both the cells and the disease. This judgment might vary from disease to disease and likely has to be determined empirically over the next decade.

ACKNOWLEDGMENTS

Portions of this chapter were expanded and updated from an earlier review by the authors, *Phil. Trans. R. Soc. Lond.* 359:823–837 (2004) and ref. *197* with permission from the publishers. We would like to thank numerous members of the Snyder laboratory, whose work has been reviewed in this chapter. The work from our laboratory reviewed here was supported in part by grants from the Charles H. Hood Foundation; the Late Onset Tay-Sachs Foundation; a Mental Retardation Research Center grant from NIH (HD18655); the National Institute of Neurological Disorders and Stroke (NS07264, NS24707, NS34247, and NS33852); the Paralyzed Veterans of America; Project ALS; the Research Service of the Department of Veterans Affairs; the A-T Children's Project, Children's Neurobiological Solutions, and GMP Companies, Inc.

REFERENCES

1. Magavi, S. S., Leavitt, B. R., and Macklis, J. D. (2000) Induction of neurogenesis in the neocortex of adult mice [see comments]. *Nature* **405,** 951–955.
2. Flax, J. D., Aurora, S., Yang, C., et al. (1998) Engraftable human neural stem cells respond to developmental cues, replace neurons, and express foreign genes. *Nat. Biotechnol.* **16,** 1033–1039.
3. Gokhan, S., Song, Q., and Mehler, M. F. (1998) Generation and regulation of developing immortalized neural cell lines. *Methods* **16,** 345–358.
4. Johansson, C. B., Momma, S., Clarke, D. L., Risling, M., Lendahl, U., and Frisen, J. (1999) Identification of a neural stem cell in the adult mammalian central nervous system. *Cell* **96,** 25–34.
5. Mezey, E., Chandross, K. J., Harta, G., Maki, R. A., and McKercher, S. R. (2000) Turning blood into brain: cells bearing neuronal antigens generated in vivo from bone marrow [In Process Citation]. *Science* **290,** 1779–1782.
6. Roy, N. S., Nakano, T., Keyoung, H. M., et al. (2004) Telomerase immortalization of neuronally restricted progenitor cells derived from the human fetal spinal cord. *Nat. Biotechnol.* **22,** 297–305.
7. Schuldiner, M., Yanuka, O., Itskovitz-Eldor, J., Melton, D. A., and Benvenisty, N. (2000) From the cover: effects of eight growth factors on the differentiation of cells derived from human embryonic stem cells. *Proc. Natl. Acad. Sci. USA* **97,** 11307–11312.
8. Tamaki, S., Eckert, K., He, D., et al. (2002) Engraftment of sorted/expanded human central nervous system stem cells from fetal brain. *J. Neurosci. Res.* **69,** 976–986.
9. Gage, F. H. (2000) Mammalian neural stem cells. *Science* **287,** 1433–1438.
10. Kondo, T. and Raff, M. (2000) Oligodendrocyte precursor cells reprogrammed to become multipotential CNS stem cells. *Science* **289,** 1754–1757.
11. Marmur, R., Mabie, P. C., Gokhan, S., Song, Q., Kessler, J. A., and Mehler, M. F. (1998) Isolation and developmental characterization of cerebral cortical multipotent progenitors. *Dev. Biol.* **204,** 577–591.
12. Ben-Hur, T., Rogister, B., Murray, K., Rougon, G., and Dubois-Dalcq, M. (1998) Growth and fate of PSA-NCAM+ precursors of the postnatal brain. *J. Neurosci.* **18,** 5777–5788.
13. Rietze, R. L., Valcanis, H., Brooker, G. F., Thomas, T., Voss, A. K., and Bartlett, P. F. (2001) Purification of a pluripotent neural stem cell from the adult mouse brain. *Nature* **412,** 736–739.

14. Doetsch, F., Caille, I., Lim, D. A., Garcia-Verdugo, J. M., and Alvarez-Buylla, A. (1999) Subventricular zone astrocytes are neural stem cells in the adult mammalian brain. *Cell* **97,** 703–716.

15. Laywell, E. D., Rakic, P., Kukekov, V. G., Holland, E. C., and Steindler, D. A. (2000) Identification of a multipotent astrocytic stem cell in the immature and adult mouse brain. *Proc. Natl. Acad. Sci. USA* **97,** 13883–13888.

16. Suslov, O. N., Kukekov, V. G., Ignatova, T. N., and Steindler, D. A. (2002) Neural stem cell heterogeneity demonstrated by molecular phenotyping of clonal neurospheres. *Proc. Natl. Acad. Sci. USA* **99,** 14506–14511.

17. Palmer, T. D., Markakis, E. A., Willhoite, A. R., Safar, F., and Gage, F. H. (1999) Fibroblast growth factor-2 activates a latent neurogenic program in neural stem cells from diverse regions of the adult CNS. *J. Neurosci.* **19,** 8487–8497.

18. Lie, D. C., Dziewczapolski, G., Willhoite, A. R., Kaspar, B. K., Shults, C. W., and Gage, F. H. (2002) The adult substantia nigra contains progenitor cells with neurogenic potential. *J. Neurosci.* **22,** 6639–6649.

19. Alvarez-Buylla, A., and Temple, S. (1998) Stem cells in the developing and adult nervous system. *J. Neurobiol.* **36,** 105–110.

20. Gage, F. H., Kempermann, G., Palmer, T. D., Peterson, D. A., and Ray, J. (1998) Multipotent progenitor cells in the adult dentate gyrus. *J. Neurobiol.* **36,** 249–266.

21. Hunter-Schaedle, K. E. (1997) Radial glial cell development and transformation are disturbed in reeler forebrain. *J. Neurobiol.* **33,** 459–472.

22. Morshead, C. M., Craig, C. G., and van der Kooy, D. (1998) In vivo clonal analyses reveal the properties of endogenous neural stem cell proliferation in the adult mammalian forebrain. *Development* **125,** 2251–2261.

23. Goldman, J. E., Zerlin, M., Newman, S., Zhang, L., and Gensert, J. (1997) Fate determination and migration of progenitors in the postnatal mammalian CNS. *Dev. Neurosci.* **19,** 42–48.

24. Levison, S. W. and Goldman, J. E. (1993) Both oligodendrocytes and astrocytes develop from progenitors in the subventricular zone of postnatal rat forebrain. *Neuron* **10,** 201–212.

25. Ourednik, V., Ourednik, J., Flax, J. D., et al. (2001) Segregation of human neural stem cells in the developing primate forebrain. *Science* **293,** 1820–1824.

26. Gritti, A., Bonfanti, L., Doetsch, F., et al. (2002) Multipotent neural stem cells reside into the rostral extension and olfactory bulb of adult rodents. *J. Neurosci.* **22,** 437–445.

27. Nakatomi, H., Kuriu, T., Okabe, S., et al. (2002) Regeneration of hippocampal pyramidal neurons after ischemic brain injury by recruitment of endogenous neural progenitors. *Cell* **110,** 429–441.

28. Eriksson, P. S., Perfilieva, E., Bjork-Eriksson, T., et al. (1998) Neurogenesis in the adult human hippocampus [see comments]. *Nat. Med.* **4,** 1313–1317.

29. van Praag, H., Schinder, A. F., Christie, B. R., Toni, N., Palmer, T. D., and Gage, F. H. (2002) Functional neurogenesis in the adult hippocampus. *Nature* **415,** 1030–1034.

30. Song, H., Stevens, C. F., and Gage, F. H. (2002) Astroglia induce neurogenesis from adult neural stem cells. *Nature* **417,** 39–44.

31. Song, H. J., Stevens, C. F., and Gage, F. H. (2002) Neural stem cells from adult hippocampus develop essential properties of functional CNS neurons. *Nat. Neurosci.* **5,** 438–445.

32. Seaberg, R. M. and van der Kooy, D. (2002) Adult rodent neurogenic regions: the ventricular subependyma contains neural stem cells, but the dentate gyrus contains restricted progenitors. *J. Neurosci.* **22,** 1784–1793.

33. Lois, C. and Alvarez-Buylla, A. (1993) Proliferating subventricular zone cells in the adult mammalian forebrain can differentiate into neurons and glia. *Proc. Natl. Acad. Sci. USA* **90,** 2074–2077.

34. Doetsch, F., Petreanu, L., Caille, I., Garcia-Verdugo, J. M., and Alvarez-Buylla, A. (2002) EGF converts transit-amplifying neurogenic precursors in the adult brain into multipotent stem cells. *Neuron* **36,** 1021–1034.

35. Doetsch, F., Garcia-Verdugo, J. M., and Alvarez-Buylla, A. (1997) Cellular composition and three-dimensional organization of the subventricular germinal zone in the adult mammalian brain. *J. Neurosci.* **17,** 5046–5061.

36. Levison, S. W. and Goldman, J. E. (1997) Multipotential and lineage restricted precursors coexist in the mammalian perinatal subventricular zone. *J. Neurosci. Res.* **48,** 83–94.

37. Imura, T., Kornblum, H. I., and Sofroniew, M. V. (2003) The predominant neural stem cell isolated from postnatal and adult forebrain but not early embryonic forebrain expresses GFAP. *J. Neurosci.* **23,** 2824–2832.

38. Morshead, C. M., Reynolds, B. A., Craig, C. G., et al. (1994) Neural stem cells in the adult mammalian forebrain: a relatively quiescent subpopulation of subependymal cells. *Neuron* **13,** 1071–1082.

39. Kirn, J. R., Fishman, Y., Sasportas, K., Alvarez-Buylla, A., and Nottebohm, F. (1999) Fate of new neurons in adult canary high vocal center during the first 30 days after their formation. *J. Comp. Neurol.* **411,** 487–494.

40. van Praag, H., Christie, B. R., Sejnowski, T. J., and Gage, F. H. (1999) Running enhances neurogenesis, learning, and long-term potentiation in mice. *Proc. Natl. Acad. Sci. USA* **96,** 13427–13431.

41. van Praag, H., Kempermann, G., and Gage, F. H. (1999) Running increases cell proliferation and neurogenesis in the adult mouse dentate gyrus. *Nat. Neurosci.* **2,** 266–270.

42. Shors, T. J., Miesegaes, G., Beylin, A., Zhao, M., Rydel, T., and Gould, E. (2001) Neurogenesis in the adult is involved in the formation of trace memories. *Nature* **410,** 372–376.

43. Shors, T. J., Townsend, D. A., Zhao, M., Kozorovitskiy, Y., and Gould, E. (2002) Neurogenesis may relate to some but not all types of hippocampal-dependent learning. *Hippocampus* **12,** 578–584.

44. Lendahl, U., Zimmerman, L. B., and McKay, R. D. (1990) CNS stem cells express a new class of intermediate filament protein. *Cell* **60,** 585–595.

45. Villa, A., Snyder, E. Y., Vescovi, A., and Martinez-Serrano, A. (2000) Establishment and properties of a growth factor-dependent, perpetual neural stem cell line from the human CNS. *Exp. Neurol.* **161,** 67–84.

46. Lin, R. C. S., Matesic, D. F., Marvin, M., McKay, R. D., and Brustle, O. (1995) Re-expression of the intermediate filament nestin in reactive astrocytes. *Neurobiol. Dis.* **2,** 79–85.

47. Messam, C. A., Hou, J., and Major, E. O. (2000) Coexpression of nestin in neural and glial cells in the developing human CNS defined by a human-specific anti-nestin antibody. *Exp. Neurol.* **161,** 585–596.

48. Liu, S., Qu, Y., Stewart, T. J., et al. (2000) Embryonic stem cells differentiate into oligodendrocytes and myelinate in culture and after spinal cord transplantation. *Proc. Natl. Acad. Sci. USA* **97,** 6126–6131.

49. Lumelsky, N., Blondel, O., Laeng, P., Velasco, I., Ravin, R., and McKay, R. (2001) Differentiation of embryonic stem cells to insulin-secreting structures similar to pancreatic islets. *Science* **292,** 1389–1394.

50. Zulewski, H., Abraham, E. J., Gerlach, M. J., et al. (2001) Multipotential nestin-positive stem cells isolated from adult pancreatic islets differentiate ex vivo into pancreatic endocrine, exocrine, and hepatic phenotypes. *Diabetes* **50,** 521–533.

51. Shihabuddin, L. S., Ray, J., and Gage, F. H. (1997) FGF-2 is sufficient to isolate progenitors found in the adult mammalian spinal cord. *Exp. Neurol.* **148,** 577–586.

52. Zerlin, M., Levison, S. W., and Goldman, J. E. (1995) Early patterns of migration, morphogenesis, and intermediate filament expression of subventricular zone cells in the postnatal rat forebrain. *J. Neurosci.* **15,** 7238–7249.

53. Capela, A. and Temple, S. (2002) LeX/ssea-1 is expressed by adult mouse CNS stem cells, identifying them as nonependymal. *Neuron* **35,** 865–875.

54. Goodell, M. A., Brose, K., Paradis, G., Conner, A. S., and Mulligan, R. C. (1996) Isolation and functional properties of murine hematopoietic stem cells that are replicating in vivo. *J. Exp. Med.* **183**, 1797–1806.

55. Goodell, M. A., Rosenzweig, M., Kim, H., et al. (1997) Dye efflux studies suggest that hematopoietic stem cells expressing low or undetectable levels of CD34 antigen exist in multiple species. *Nat. Med.* **3**, 1337–1345.

56. Hulspas, R. and Quesenberry, P. J. (2000) Characterization of neurosphere cell phenotypes by flow cytometry. *Cytometry* **40**, 245–250.

57. Uchida, N., Buck, D. W., He, D., et al. (2000) Direct isolation of human central nervous system stem cells [In Process Citation]. *Proc. Natl. Acad. Sci. USA* **97**, 14720–14725.

58. Morrison, S. J., White, P. M., Zock, C., and Anderson, D. J. (1999) Prospective identification, isolation by flow cytometry, and in vivo self-renewal of multipotent mammalian neural crest stem cells. *Cell* **96**, 737–749.

59. Aboody, K. S., Brown, A., Rainov, N. G., et al. (2000) From the cover: neural stem cells display extensive tropism for pathology in adult brain: evidence from intracranial gliomas [In Process Citation]. *Proc. Natl. Acad. Sci. USA* **97**, 12846–12851.

60. Chiasson, B. J., Tropepe, V., Morshead, C. M., and van der Kooy, D. (1999) Adult mammalian forebrain ependymal and subependymal cells demonstrate proliferative potential, but only subependymal cells have neural stem cell characteristics. *J. Neurosci.* **19**, 4462–4471.

61. Clarke, D. L., Johansson, C. B., Wilbertz, J., et al. (2000) Generalized potential of adult neural stem cells. *Science* **288**, 1660–1663.

62. McLaren, F. H., Svendsen, C. N., Van der Meide, P., and Joly, E. (2001) Analysis of neural stem cells by flow cytometry: cellular differentiation modifies patterns of MHC expression. *J. Neuroimmunol.* **112**, 35–46.

63. Hermanson, O., Jepsen, K., and Rosenfeld, M. G. (2002) N-CoR controls differentiation of neural stem cells into astrocytes. *Nature* **419**, 934–939.

64. Molofsky, A. V., Pardal, R., Iwashita, T., Park, I. K., Clarke, M. F., and Morrison, S. J. (2003) Bmi-1 dependence distinguishes neural stem cell self-renewal from progenitor proliferation. *Nature* **425**, 962–967.

65. Snyder, E. Y. and Vescovi, A. L. (2000) The possibilities/perplexities of stem cells [news]. *Nat. Biotechnol.* **18**, 827–828.

66. Bjornson, C. R., Rietze, R. L., Reynolds, B. A., Magli, M. C., and Vescovi, A. L. (1999) Turning brain into blood: a hematopoietic fate adopted by adult neural stem cells in vivo [see comments]. *Science* **283**, 534–537.

67. Galli, R., Borello, U., Gritti, A., et al. (2000) Skeletal myogenic potential of human and mouse neural stem cells. *Nat. Neurosci.* **3**, 986–991.

68. Brazelton, T. R., Rossi, F. M., Keshet, G. I., and Blau, H. M. (2000) From marrow to brain: expression of neuronal phenotypes in adult mice [In Process Citation]. *Science* **290**, 1775–1779.

69. Morshead, C. M., Benveniste, P., Iscove, N. N., and van der Kooy, D. (2002) Hematopoietic competence is a rare property of neural stem cells that may depend on genetic and epigenetic alterations. *Nat. Med.* **8**, 268–273.

70. Terada, N., Hamazaki, T., Oka, M., et al. (2002) Bone marrow cells adopt the phenotype of other cells by spontaneous cell fusion. *Nature* **416**, 542–545.

71. Ying, Q. L., Nichols, J., Evans, E. P., and Smith, A. G. (2002) Changing potency by spontaneous fusion. *Nature* **416**, 545–548.

72. Weimann, J. M., Charlton, C. A., Brazelton, T. R., Hackman, R. C., and Blau, H. M. (2003) Contribution of transplanted bone marrow cells to Purkinje neurons in human adult brains. *Proc. Natl. Acad. Sci. USA* **100**, 2088–2093.

73. Niwa, H., Miyazaki, J., and Smith, A. G. (2000) Quantitative expression of Oct-3/4 defines differentiation, dedifferentiation or self-renewal of ES cells. *Nat Genet* **24**, 372–376.

74. Tsai, R. Y. and McKay, R. D. (2000) Cell contact regulates fate choice by cortical stem cells. *J. Neurosci.* **20**, 3725–3735.
75. Wagers, A. J., Sherwood, R. I., Christensen, J. L., and Weissman, I. L. (2002) Little evidence for developmental plasticity of adult hematopoietic stem cells. *Science* **297**, 2256–2259.
76. Alvarez-Dolado, M., Pardal, R., Garcia-Verdugo, J. M., et al. (2003) Fusion of bone-marrow-derived cells with Purkinje neurons, cardiomyocytes and hepatocytes. *Nature* **425**, 968–973.
77. Sanai, N., Tramontin, A. D., Quinones-Hinojosa, A., et al. (2004) Unique astrocyte ribbon in adult human brain contains neural stem cells but lacks chain migration. *Nature* **427**, 740–744.
78. Palmer, T. D., Schwartz, P. H., Taupin, P., et al. (2001) Cell culture. Progenitor cells from human brain after death. *Nature* **411**, 42–43.
79. Nunes, M. C., Roy, N. S., Keyoung, H. M., et al. (2003) Identification and isolation of multipotential neural progenitor cells from the subcortical white matter of the adult human brain. *Nat. Med.* **9**, 439–447.
80. Hardy, R. and Reynolds, R. (1991) Proliferation and differentiation potential of rat fore-brain oligodendroglial progenitors both in vitro and in vivo. *Development* **111**, 1061–1080.
81. Wu, H. Y., Dawson, M. R., Reynolds, R., and Hardy, R. J. (2001) Expression of QKI proteins and MAP1B identifies actively myelinating oligodendrocytes in adult rat brain. *Mol. Cell. Neurosci.* **17**, 292–302.
82. Horner, P. J., Power, A. E., Kempermann, G., et al. (2000) Proliferation and differentiation of progenitor cells throughout the intact adult rat spinal cord. *J. Neurosci.* **20**, 2218–2228.
83. Yoshimura, K., Sakurai, Y., Nishimura, D., et al. (1998) Monoclonal antibody 14F7, which recognizes a stage-specific immature oligodendrocyte surface molecule, inhibits oligodendrocyte differentiation mediated in co-culture with astrocytes. *J. Neurosci. Res.* **54**, 79–96.
84. Niehaus, A., Stegmuller, J., Diers-Fenger, M., and Trotter, J. (1999) Cell-surface glyco-protein of oligodendrocyte progenitors involved in migration. *J. Neurosci.* **19**, 4948–4961.
85. Yu, W. P., Collarini, E. J., Pringle, N. P., and Richardson, W. D. (1994) Embryonic expression of myelin genes: evidence for a focal source of oligodendrocyte precursors in the ventricular zone of the neural tube. *Neuron* **12**, 1353–1362.
86. Rakic, S. and Zecevic, N. (2003) Early oligodendrocyte progenitor cells in the human fetal telencephalon. *Glia* **41**, 117–127.
87. Lu, Q. R., Yuk, D., Alberta, J. A., et al. (2000) Sonic hedgehog–regulated oligodendro-cyte lineage genes encoding bHLH proteins in the mammalian central nervous system. *Neuron* **25**, 317–329.
88. Nishiyama, A., Chang, A., and Trapp, B. D. (1999) NG2+ glial cells: a novel glial cell population in the adult brain. *J. Neuropathol. Exp. Neurol.* **58**, 1113–1124.
89. Levine, J. M., Stincone, F., and Lee, Y. S. (1993) Development and differentiation of glial precursor cells in the rat cerebellum. *Glia* **7**, 307–321.
90. Pouly, S., Prat, A., Blain, M., Olivier, A., and Antel, J. (2001) NG2 immunoreactivity on human brain endothelial cells. *Acta Neuropathol. (Berl.)* **102**, 313–320.
91. Jones, L. L., Yamaguchi, Y., Stallcup, W. B., and Tuszynski, M. H. (2002) NG2 is a major chondroitin sulfate proteoglycan produced after spinal cord injury and is expressed by macrophages and oligodendrocyte progenitors. *J. Neurosci.* **22**, 2792–2803.
92. Reynolds, R. and Hardy, R. (1997) Oligodendroglial progenitors labeled with the O4 antibody persist in the adult rat cerebral cortex in vivo. *J. Neurosci. Res.* **47**, 455–470.
93. Espinosa de los Monteros, A., Zhang, M., and De Vellis, J. (1993) O2A progenitor cells transplanted into the neonatal rat brain develop into oligodendrocytes but not astrocytes. *Proc. Natl. Acad. Sci. USA* **90**, 50–54.

94. Gard, A. L. and Pfeiffer, S. E. (1990) Two proliferative stages of the oligodendrocyte lineage (A2B5+O4- and O4+GalC-) under different mitogenic control. *Neuron* **5,** 615–625.

95. Warrington, A. E., Barbarese, E., and Pfeiffer, S. E. (1993) Differential myelinogenic capacity of specific developmental stages of the oligodendrocyte lineage upon transplantation into hypomyelinating hosts. *J. Neurosci. Res.* **34,** 1–13.

96. Scolding, N. J., Frith, S., Linington, C., Morgan, B. P., Campbell, A. K., and Compston, D. A. (1989) Myelin-oligodendrocyte glycoprotein (MOG) is a surface marker of oligodendrocyte maturation. *J. Neuroimmunol.* **22,** 169–176.

97. Shi, J., Marinovich, A., and Barres, B. A. (1998) Purification and characterization of adult oligodendrocyte precursor cells from the rat optic nerve. *J. Neurosci.* **18,** 4627–4636.

98. Belachew, S., Aguirre, A. A., Wang, H., et al. (2002) Cyclin-dependent kinase-2 controls oligodendrocyte progenitor cell cycle progression and is downregulated in adult oligodendrocyte progenitors. *J. Neurosci.* **22,** 8553–8562.

99. Wang, S., Sdrulla, A. D., diSibio, G., et al. (1998) Notch receptor activation inhibits oligodendrocyte differentiation. *Neuron* **21,** 63–75.

100. Power, J., Mayer-Proschel, M., Smith, J., and Noble, M. (2002) Oligodendrocyte precursor cells from different brain regions express divergent properties consistent with the differing time courses of myelination in these regions. *Dev. Biol.* **245,** 362–375.

101. Levison, S. W., Young, G. M., and Goldman, J. E. (1999) Cycling cells in the adult rat neocortex preferentially generate oligodendroglia. *J. Neurosci. Res.* **57,** 435–446.

102. Ida, J. A., Jr., Dubois-Dalcq, M., and McKinnon, R. D. (1993) Expression of the receptor tyrosine kinase c-kit in oligodendrocyte progenitor cells. *J. Neurosci. Res.* **36,** 596–606.

103. Patneau, D. K., Wright, P. W., Winters, C., Mayer, M. L., and Gallo, V. (1994) Glial cells of the oligodendrocyte lineage express both kainate- and AMPA-preferring subtypes of glutamate receptor. *Neuron* **12,** 357–371.

104. Casaccia-Bonnefil, P., Hardy, R. J., Teng, K. K., Levine, J. M., Koff, A., and Chao, M. V. (1999) Loss of p27Kip1 function results in increased proliferative capacity of oligodendrocyte progenitors but unaltered timing of differentiation. *Development* **126,** 4027–4037.

105. Bergles, D. E., Roberts, J. D., Somogyi, P., and Jahr, C. E. (2000) Glutamatergic synapses on oligodendrocyte precursor cells in the hippocampus. *Nature* **405,** 187–191.

106. Wren, D., Wolswijk, G., and Noble, M. (1992) In vitro analysis of the origin and maintenance of O-2Aadult progenitor cells. *J. Cell Biol.* **116,** 167–176.

107. Noble, M., Wren, D., and Wolswijk, G. (1992) The O-2A(adult) progenitor cell: a glial stem cell of the adult central nervous system. *Semin. Cell Biol.* **3,** 413–422.

108. Tang, D. G., Tokumoto, Y. M., Apperly, J. A., Lloyd, A. C., and Raff, M. C. (2001) Lack of replicative senescence in cultured rat oligodendrocyte precursor cells. *Science* **291,** 868–871.

109. Yoon, S. O., Casaccia-Bonnefil, P., Carter, B., and Chao, M. V. (1998) Competitive signaling between TrkA and p75 nerve growth factor receptors determines cell survival. *J. Neurosci.* **18,** 3273–3281.

110. Zhang, S. C., Ge, B., and Duncan, I. D. (2000) Tracing human oligodendroglial development in vitro. *J. Neurosci. Res.* **59,** 421–429.

111. Murray, K. and Dubois-Dalcq, M. (1997) Emergence of oligodendrocytes from human neural spheres. *J. Neurosci. Res.* **50,** 146–156.

112. Durand, B. and Raff, M. (2000) A cell-intrinsic timer that operates during oligodendrocyte development. *Bioessays* **22,** 64–71.

113. Windrem, M. S., Nunes, M. C., Rashbaum, W. K., et al. (2004) Fetal and adult human oligodendrocyte progenitor cell isolates myelinate the congenitally dysmyelinated brain. *Nat. Med.* **10,** 93–97.

114. Roy, N. S., Wang, S., Jiang, L., et al. (2000) In vitro neurogenesis by progenitor cells isolated from the adult human hippocampus. *Nat. Med.* **6,** 271–277.

115. Piper, D. R., Mujtaba, T., Keyoung, H., et al. (2001) Identification and characterization of neuronal precursors and their progeny from human fetal tissue. *J. Neurosci. Res.* **66,** 356–368.
116. Tourbah, A., Linnington, C., Bachelin, C., Avellana-Adalid, V., Wekerle, H., and Baron-Van Evercooren, A. (1997) Inflammation promotes survival and migration of the CG4 oligodendrocyte progenitors transplanted in the spinal cord of both inflammatory and demyelinated EAE rats. *J. Neurosci. Res.* **50,** 853–861.
117. Nait-Oumesmar, B., Decker, L., Lachapelle, F., Avellana-Adalid, V., Bachelin, C., and Van Evercooren, A. B. (1999) Progenitor cells of the adult mouse subventricular zone proliferate, migrate and differentiate into oligodendrocytes after demyelination. *Eur. J. Neurosci.* **11,** 4357–4366.
118. Conover, J. C., Doetsch, F., Garcia-Verdugo, J. M., Gale, N. W., Yancopoulos, G. D., and Alvarez-Buylla, A. (2000) Disruption of Eph/ephrin signaling affects migration and proliferation in the adult subventricular zone. *Nat. Neurosci.* **3,** 1091–1097.
119. Forsberg-Nilsson, K., Behar, T. N., Afrakhte, M., Barker, J. L., and McKay, R. D. (1998) Platelet-derived growth factor induces chemotaxis of neuroepithelial stem cells. *J. Neurosci. Res.* **53,** 521–530.
120. Pluchino, S., Quattrini, A., Brambilla, E., et al. (2003) Injection of adult neurospheres induces recovery in a chronic model of multiple sclerosis. *Nature* **422,** 688–694.
121. Liu, Y., Himes, B. T., Solowska, J., et al. (1999) Intraspinal delivery of neurotrophin-3 using neural stem cells genetically modified by recombinant retrovirus. *Exp. Neurol.* **158,** 9–26.
122. Snyder, E. Y., Yoon, C., Flax, J. D., and Macklis, J. D. (1997) Multipotent neural precursors can differentiate toward replacement of neurons undergoing targeted apoptotic degeneration in adult mouse neocortex. *Proc. Natl. Acad. Sci. USA* **94,** 11663–11668.
123. Park, K. I., Liu, S., Flax, J. D., Nissim, S., Stieg, P. E., and Snyder, E. Y. (1999) Transplantation of neural progenitor and stem cells: developmental insights may suggest new therapies for spinal cord and other CNS dysfunction. *J. Neurotrauma* **16,** 675–687.
124. Park, K. I., Teng, Y. D., and Snyder, E. Y. (2002) The injured brain interacts reciprocally with neural stem cells supported by scaffolds to reconstitute lost tissue. *Nat. Biotechnol.* **20,** 1111–1117.
125. Fukunaga, A., Uchida, K., Hara, K., Kuroshima, Y., and Kawase, T. (1999) Differentiation and angiogenesis of central nervous system stem cells implanted with mesenchyme into ischemic rat brain. *Cell Transplant.* **8,** 435–441.
126. Andsberg, G., Kokaia, Z., Bjorklund, A., Lindvall, O., and Martinez-Serrano, A. (1998) Amelioration of ischaemia-induced neuronal death in the rat striatum by NGF-secreting neural stem cells. *Eur. J. Neurosci.* **10,** 2026–2036.
127. Toda, H., Takahashi, J., Iwakami, N., et al. (2001) Grafting neural stem cells improved the impaired spatial recognition in ischemic rats. *Neurosci. Lett.* **316,** 9–12.
128. Riess, P., Zhang, C., Saatman, K. E., et al. (2002) Transplanted neural stem cells survive, differentiate, and improve neurological motor function after experimental traumatic brain injury. *Neurosurgery* **51,** 1043–1052; discussion 1052–1044.
129. Auerbach, J. M., Eiden, M. V., and McKay, R. D. (2000) Transplanted CNS stem cells form functional synapses in vivo. *Eur. J. Neurosci.* **12,** 1696–1704.
130. Song, H. J., Stevens, C. F., and Gage, F. H. (2002) Neural stem cells from adult hippocampus develop essential properties of functional CNS neurons. *Nat. Neurosci.* **5,** 438–445.
131. Lundberg, C., Englund, U., Trono, D., Bjorklund, A., and Wictorin, K. (2002) Differentiation of the RN33B cell line into forebrain projection neurons after transplantation into the neonatal rat brain. *Exp. Neurol.* **175,** 370–387.
132. Yamamoto, S., Nagao, M., Sugimori, M., et al. (2001) Transcription factor expression and Notch-dependent regulation of neural progenitors in the adult rat spinal cord. *J. Neurosci.* **21,** 9814–9823.

133. Vroemen, M., Aigner, L., Winkler, J., and Weidner, N. (2003) Adult neural progenitor cell grafts survive after acute spinal cord injury and integrate along axonal pathways. *Eur. J. Neurosci.* **18,** 743–751.

134. Bambakidis, N. C. and Miller, R. H. (2004) Transplantation of oligodendrocyte precursors and sonic hedgehog results in improved function and white matter sparing in the spinal cords of adult rats after contusion. *Spine J.* **4,** 16–26.

135. Schumm, M. A., Castellanos, D. A., Frydel, B. R., and Sagen, J. (2004) Improved neural progenitor cell survival when cografted with chromaffin cells in the rat striatum. *Exp. Neurol.* **185,** 133–142.

136. Schumm, M. A., Castellanos, D. A., Frydel, B. R., and Sagen, J. (2003) Direct cell-cell contact required for neurotrophic effect of chromaffin cells on neural progenitor cells. *Brain Res. Dev. Brain Res.* **146,** 1–13.

137. Ourednik, J., Ourednik, V., Lynch, W. P., Schachner, M., and Snyder, E. Y. (2002) Neural stem cells display an inherent mechanism for rescuing dysfunctional neurons. *Nat. Biotechnol.* **20,** 1103–1110.

138. Hagan, M., Wennersten, A., Meijer, X., Holmin, S., Wahlberg, L., and Mathiesen, T. (2003) Neuroprotection by human neural progenitor cells after experimental contusion in rats. *Neurosci. Lett.* **351,** 149–152.

139. Lu, P., Jones, L. L., Snyder, E. Y., and Tuszynski, M. H. (2003) Neural stem cells constitutively secrete neurotrophic factors and promote extensive host axonal growth after spinal cord injury. *Exp. Neurol.* **181,** 115–129.

140. Hains, B. C., Johnson, K. M., Eaton, M. J., Willis, W. D., and Hulsebosch, C. E. (2003) Serotonergic neural precursor cell grafts attenuate bilateral hyperexcitability of dorsal horn neurons after spinal hemisection in rat. *Neuroscience* **116,** 1097–1110.

141. Teng, Y. D., Lavik, E. B., Qu, X., et al. (2002) Functional recovery following traumatic spinal cord injury mediated by a unique polymer scaffold seeded with neural stem cells. *Proc. Natl. Acad. Sci. USA* **99,** 3024–3029.

142. Haughey, N. J., Nath, A., Chan, S. L., Borchard, A. C., Rao, M. S., and Mattson, M. P. (2002) Disruption of neurogenesis by amyloid beta-peptide, and perturbed neural progenitor cell homeostasis, in models of Alzheimer's disease. *J. Neurochem.* **83,** 1509–1524.

143. Mehta, V., Hong, M., Spears, J., and Mendez, I. (1998) Enhancement of graft survival and sensorimotor behavioral recovery in rats undergoing transplantation with dopaminergic cells exposed to glial cell line-derived neurotrophic factor. *J. Neurosurg.* **88,** 1088–1095.

144. Lindvall, O. (2000) Neural transplantation in Parkinson's disease. *Novartis Found. Symp.* **231,** 110–123; discussion 123–118, 145–117.

145. Piccini, P., Lindvall, O., Bjorklund, A., et al. (2000) Delayed recovery of movement-related cortical function in Parkinson's disease after striatal dopaminergic grafts. *Ann. Neurol.* **48,** 689–695.

146. Anton, R., Kordower, J. H., Maidment, N. T., et al. (1994) Neural-targeted gene therapy for rodent and primate hemiparkinsonism. *Exp. Neurol.* **127,** 207–218.

147. Lundberg, C., Field, P. M., Ajayi, Y. O., Raisman, G., and Bjorklund, A. (1996) Conditionally immortalized neural progenitor cell lines integrate and differentiate after grafting to the adult rat striatum. A combined autoradiographic and electron microscopic study. *Brain Res.* **737,** 295–300.

148. Zigova, T., Pencea, V., Betarbet, R., et al. (1998) Neuronal progenitor cells of the neonatal subventricular zone differentiate and disperse following transplantation into the adult rat striatum. *Cell Transplant.* **7,** 137–156.

149. Sun, Z. H., Lai, Y. L., Zeng, W. W., et al. (2003) Mesencephalic progenitors can improve rotational behavior and reconstruct nigrostriatal pathway in PD rats. *Acta Neurochir. Suppl.* **87,** 175–180.

150. Yang, M., Stull, N. D., Berk, M. A., Snyder, E. Y., and Iacovitti, L. (2002) Neural stem cells spontaneously express dopaminergic traits after transplantation into the intact or 6-hydroxydopamine-lesioned rat. *Exp. Neurol.* **177,** 50–60.
151. Studer, L., Tabar, V., and McKay, R. D. (1998) Transplantation of expanded mesencephalic precursors leads to recovery in parkinsonian rats. *Nat. Neurosci.* **1,** 290–295.
152. Matsuura, N., Lie, D. C., Hoshimaru, M., et al. (2001) Sonic hedgehog facilitates dopamine differentiation in the presence of a mesencephalic glial cell line. *J. Neurosci.* **21,** 4326–4335.
152a. Bjugstad, K. B., Redmond, D. E., Teng, Y. D., Elsworth, J. D., Roth, R. H., Blanchard, B. C., Snyder, E. Y., Sledek, J. R. Neural stem cells implanted into MPTP-treated monkeys increases the size of endogenous tyrosine-hydroxylase-positive cells found in the caudate. *Cell Transplantation* (in press).
153. Dziewczapolski, G., Lie, D. C., Ray, J., Gage, F. H., and Shults, C. W. (2003) Survival and differentiation of adult rat-derived neural progenitor cells transplanted to the striatum of hemiparkinsonian rats. *Exp. Neurol.* **183,** 653–664.
154. Kim, J. H., Auerbach, J. M., Rodriguez-Gomez, J. A., et al. (2002) Dopamine neurons derived from embryonic stem cells function in an animal model of Parkinson's disease. *Nature* **418,** 50–56.
155. Kawasaki, H., Suemori, H., Mizuseki, K., et al. (2002) Generation of dopaminergic neurons and pigmented epithelia from primate ES cells by stromal cell-derived inducing activity. *Proc. Natl. Acad. Sci. USA* **99,** 1580–1585.
156. Kawasaki, H., Mizuseki, K., Nishikawa, S., et al. (2000) Induction of midbrain dopaminergic neurons from ES cells by stromal cell-derived inducing activity. *Neuron* **28,** 31–40.
157. Svendsen, C. N., Caldwell, M. A., Shen, J., et al. (1997) Long-term survival of human central nervous system progenitor cells transplanted into a rat model of Parkinson's disease. *Exp. Neurol.* **148,** 135–146.
158. Kordower, J. H., Chen, E. Y., Winkler, C., et al. (1997) Grafts of EGF-responsive neural stem cells derived from GFAP-hNGF transgenic mice: trophic and tropic effects in a rodent model of Huntington's disease. *J. Comp. Neurol.* **387,** 96–113.
159. Martinez-Serrano, A., Fischer, W., and Bjorklund, A. (1995) Reversal of age-dependent cognitive impairments and cholinergic neuron atrophy by NGF-secreting neural progenitors grafted to the basal forebrain. *Neuron* **15,** 473–484.
160. Noseworthy, J. H., Lucchinetti, C., Rodriguez, M., and Weinshenker, B. G. (2000) Multiple sclerosis. *N. Engl. J. Med.* **343,** 938–952.
161. De Stefano, N., Narayanan, S., Francis, G. S., et al. (2001) Evidence of axonal damage in the early stages of multiple sclerosis and its relevance to disability. *Arch. Neurol.* **58,** 65–70.
162. Lucchinetti, C., Bruck, W., Parisi, J., Scheithauer, B., Rodriguez, M., and Lassmann, H. (2000) Heterogeneity of multiple sclerosis lesions: implications for the pathogenesis of demyelination. *Ann. Neurol.* **47,** 707–717.
163. Scolding, N. J., Rayner, P. J., and Compston, D. A. (1999) Identification of A2B5-positive putative oligodendrocyte progenitor cells and A2B5-positive astrocytes in adult human white matter. *Neuroscience* **89,** 1–4.
164. Scolding, N., Franklin, R., Stevens, S., Heldin, C. H., Compston, A., and Newcombe, J. (1998) Oligodendrocyte progenitors are present in the normal adult human CNS and in the lesions of multiple sclerosis. *Brain* **121,** 2221–2228.
165. Catanzaro, M. and Weinert, C. (1992) Economic status of families living with multiple sclerosis. *Int. J. Rehabil. Res.* **15,** 209–218.
166. Yandava, B. D., Billinghurst, L. L., and Snyder, E. Y. (1999) "Global" cell replacement is feasible via neural stem cell transplantation: evidence from the dysmyelinated shiverer mouse brain. *Proc. Natl. Acad. Sci. USA* **96,** 7029–7034.
167. Hammang, J. P., Archer, D. R., and Duncan, I. D. (1997) Myelination following transplantation of EGF-responsive neural stem cells into a myelin-deficient environment. *Exp. Neurol.* **147,** 84–95.

168. Milward, E. A., Lundberg, C. G., Ge, B., Lipsitz, D., Zhao, M., and Duncan, I. D. (1997) Isolation and transplantation of multipotential populations of epidermal growth factor-responsive, neural progenitor cells from the canine brain. *J. Neurosci. Res.* **50,** 862–871.

169. Akiyama, Y., Honmou, O., Kato, T., Uede, T., Hashi, K., and Kocsis, J. D. (2001) Transplantation of clonal neural precursor cells derived from adult human brain establishes functional peripheral myelin in the rat spinal cord. *Exp. Neurol.* **167,** 27–39.

170. Brustle, O., Jones, K. N., Learish, R. D., et al. (1999) Embryonic stem cell-derived glial precursors: a source of myelinating transplants. *Science* **285,** 754–756.

171. Archer, D. R., Cuddon, P. A., Lipsitz, D., and Duncan, L. D. (1997) Myelination of the canine central nervous system by glial cell transplantation: a model for repair of human myelin disease. *Nat. Med.* **3,** 54–59.

172. Espinosa de los Monteros, A., Zhao, P., Huang, C., et al. (1997) Transplantation of CG4 oligodendrocyte progenitor cells in the myelin-deficient rat brain results in myelination of axons and enhanced oligodendroglial markers. *J. Neurosci. Res.* **50,** 872–887.

173. Zhang, S. C., Ge, B., and Duncan, I. D. (1999) Adult brain retains the potential to generate oligodendroglial progenitors with extensive myelination capacity. *Proc. Natl. Acad. Sci. USA* **96,** 4089–4094.

174. Smith, P. M. and Blakemore, W. F. (2000) Porcine neural progenitors require commitment to the oligodendrocyte lineage prior to transplantation in order to achieve significant remyelination of demyelinated lesions in the adult CNS. *Eur. J. Neurosci.* **12,** 2414–2424.

175. Imaizumi, T., Lankford, K. L., Burton, W. V., Fodor, W. L., and Kocsis, J. D. (2000) Xenotransplantation of transgenic pig olfactory ensheathing cells promotes axonal regeneration in rat spinal cord. *Nat. Biotechnol.* **18,** 949–953.

176. Kato, T., Honmou, O., Uede, T., Hashi, K., and Kocsis, J. D. (2000) Transplantation of human olfactory ensheathing cells elicits remyelination of demyelinated rat spinal cord. *Glia* **30,** 209–218.

177. Barnett, S. C., Alexander, C. L., Iwashita, Y., et al. (2000) Identification of a human olfactory ensheathing cell that can effect transplant-mediated remyelination of demyelinated CNS axons. *Brain* **123(Pt 8),** 1581–1588.

178. Kohama, I., Lankford, K. L., Preiningerova, J., White, F. A., Vollmer, T. L., and Kocsis, J. D. (2001) Transplantation of cryopreserved adult human Schwann cells enhances axonal conduction in demyelinated spinal cord. *J. Neurosci.* **21,** 944–950.

179. Franklin, R. J. and Blakemore, W. F. 1997) Transplanting oligodendrocyte progenitors into the adult CNS. *J. Anat.* **190,** 23–33.

180. Rosario, C. M., Yandava, B. D., Kosaras, B., Zurakowski, D., Sidman, R. L., and Snyder, E. Y. (1997) Differentiation of engrafted multipotent neural progenitors towards replacement of missing granule neurons in meander tail cerebellum may help determine the locus of mutant gene action. *Development* **124,** 4213–4224.

181. Snyder, E. Y., Taylor, R. M., and Wolfe, J. H. (1995) Neural progenitor cell engraftment corrects lysosomal storage throughout the MPS VII mouse brain. *Nature* **374,** 367–370.

182. Lacorazza, H. D., Flax, J. D., Snyder, E. Y., and Jendoubi, M. (1996) Expression of human beta-hexosaminidase alpha-subunit gene (the gene defect of Tay-Sachs disease) in mouse brains upon engraftment of transduced progenitor cells. *Nat. Med.* **2,** 424–429.

183. Torchiana, E., Lulli, L., Cattaneo, E., et al. (1998) Retroviral-mediated transfer of the galactocerebrosidase gene in neural progenitor cells. *NeuroReport* **9,** 3823–3827.

184. Meng, X. L., Shen, J. S., Ohashi, T., Maeda, H., Kim, S. U., and Eto, Y. (2003) Brain transplantation of genetically engineered human neural stem cells globally corrects brain lesions in the mucopolysaccharidosis type VII mouse. *J. Neurosci. Res.* **74,** 266–277.

185. Tamura, T., Nakagawa, T., Iguchi, F., et al. (2004) Transplantation of neural stem cells into the modiolus of mouse cochleae injured by cisplatin. *Acta Otolaryngol. Suppl.* 65–68.

186. Mellough, C. B., Cui, Q., Spalding, K. L., et al. (2004) Fate of multipotent neural precursor cells transplanted into mouse retina selectively depleted of retinal ganglion cells. *Exp. Neurol.* **186,** 6–19.

187. Ehtesham, M., Kabos, P., Gutierrez, M. A., et al. (2002) Induction of glioblastoma apoptosis using neural stem cell-mediated delivery of tumor necrosis factor-related apoptosis-inducing ligand. *Cancer Res.* **62,** 7170–7174.

188. Ehtesham, M., Kabos, P., Kabosova, A., Neuman, T., Black, K. L., and Yu, J. S. (2002) The use of interleukin 12-secreting neural stem cells for the treatment of intracranial glioma. *Cancer Res.* **62,** 5657–5663.

189. Benedetti, S., Pirola, B., Pollo, B., et al. (2000) Gene therapy of experimental brain tumors using neural progenitor cells. *Nat. Med.* **6,** 447–450.

190. Nakafuku, M. and Nakamura, S. (1995) Establishment and characterization of a multipotential neural cell line that can conditionally generate neurons, astrocytes, and oligodendrocytes in vitro. *J. Neurosci. Res.* **41,** 153–168.

191. Hulspas, R., Tiarks, C., Reilly, J., Hsieh, C. C., Recht, L., and Quesenberry, P. J. (1997) In vitro cell density-dependent clonal growth of EGF-responsive murine neural progenitor cells under serum-free conditions. *Exp. Neurol.* **148,** 147–156.

192. Ryder, E. F., Snyder, E. Y., and Cepko, C. L. (1990) Establishment and characterization of multipotent neural cell lines using retrovirus vector-mediated oncogene transfer. *J. Neurobiol.* **21,** 356–375.

193. Bjorklund, A. and Lindvall, O. (2000) Cell replacement therapies for central nervous system disorders. *Nat. Neurosci.* **3,** 537–544.

194. Monje, M. L., Mizumatsu, S., Fike, J. R., and Palmer, T. D. (2002) Irradiation induces neural precursor-cell dysfunction. *Nat. Med.* **8,** 955–962.

195. Monje, M. L., Toda, H., and Palmer, T. D. (2003) Inflammatory blockade restores adult hippocampal neurogenesis. *Science* **302,** 1760–1765.

196. Imitola, J., Comabella, M., Chandraker, A. K., et al. (2004) Neural stem/progenitor cells express costimulatory molecules that are differentially regulated by inflammatory and apoptotic stimuli. *Am. J. Pathol.* **164,** 1615–1625.

197. Imitola, J., Snyder, E. Y., and Khoury, S. J. (2003) Genetic programs and responses of neural stem/progenitor cells during demyelination: potential insights into repair mechanisms in multiple sclerosis. *Physiol. Genom.* **14,** 171–197.

198. Gensert, J. M. and Goldman, J. E. (1997) Endogenous progenitors remyelinate demyelinated axons in the adult CNS. *Neuron* **19,** 197–203.

199. Wolswijk, G. (1998) Chronic stage multiple sclerosis lesions contain a relatively quiescent population of oligodendrocyte precursor cells. *J. Neurosci.* **18,** 601–609.

200. Rogister, B., Ben-Hur, T., and Dubois-Dalcq, M. (1999) From neural stem cells to myelinating oligodendrocytes. *Mol. Cell. Neurosci.* **14,** 287–300.

201. Fallon, J., Reid, S., Kinyamu, R., et al. (2000) In vivo induction of massive proliferation, directed migration, and differentiation of neural cells in the adult mammalian brain [In Process Citation]. *Proc. Natl. Acad. Sci. USA* **97,** 14686–14691.

202. Cannella, B., Hoban, C. J., Gao, Y. L., et al. (1998) The neuregulin, glial growth factor 2, diminishes autoimmune demyelination and enhances remyelination in a chronic relapsing model for multiple sclerosis. *Proc. Natl. Acad. Sci. USA* **95,** 10100–10105.

203. Cannella, B., Pitt, D., Marchionni, M., and Raine, C. S. (1999) Neuregulin and erbB receptor expression in normal and diseased human white matter. *J. Neuroimmunol.* **100,** 233–242.

204. Martens, D. J., Seaberg, R. M., and van der Kooy, D. (2002) In vivo infusions of exogenous growth factors into the fourth ventricle of the adult mouse brain increase the proliferation of neural progenitors around the fourth ventricle and the central canal of the spinal cord. *Eur. J. Neurosci.* **16,** 1045–1057.

205. Kuhn, H. G., Winkler, J., Kempermann, G., Thal, L. J., and Gage, F. H. (1997) Epidermal growth factor and fibroblast growth factor-2 have different effects on neural progenitors in the adult rat brain. *J. Neurosci.* **17,** 5820–5829.

206. Snyder, E. Y., Deitcher, D. L., Walsh, C., Arnold-Aldea, S., Hartwieg, E. A., and Cepko, C. L. (1992) Multipotent neural cell lines can engraft and participate in development of mouse cerebellum. *Cell* **68,** 33–51.
207. Tang, Y., Shah, K., Messerli, S. M., Snyder, E., Breakefield, X., and Weissleder, R. (2003) In vivo tracking of neural progenitor cell migration to glioblastomas. *Hum. Gene Ther.* **14,** 1247–1254.
208. Rothstein, J. D. and Snyder, E. Y. (2004) Reality and immortality—neural stem cells for therapies. *Nat. Biotechnol.* **22,** 283–285.
209. Wu, P., Tarasenko, Y. I., Gu, Y., Huang, L. Y., Coggeshall, R. E., and Yu, Y. (2002) Region-specific generation of cholinergic neurons from fetal human neural stem cells grafted in adult rat. *Nat. Neurosci.* **5,** 1271–1278.
210. Fricker, R. A., Carpenter, M. K., Winkler, C., Greco, C., Gates, M. A., and Bjorklund, A. (1999) Site-specific migration and neuronal differentiation of human neural progenitor cells after transplantation in the adult rat brain. *J. Neurosci.* **19,** 5990–6005.
211. Brustle, O., Choudhary, K., Karram, K., et al. (1998) Chimeric brains generated by intraventricular transplantation of fetal human brain cells into embryonic rats. *Nat. Biotechnol.* **16,** 1040–1044.
212. Bulte, J. W., Douglas, T., Witwer, B., et al. (2001) Magnetodendrimers allow endosomal magnetic labeling and in vivo tracking of stem cells. *Nat. Biotechnol.* **19,** 1141–1147.
213. Bulte, J. W., Zhang, S., van Gelderen, P., et al. (1999) Neurotransplantation of magnetically labeled oligodendrocyte progenitors: magnetic resonance tracking of cell migration and myelination. *Proc. Natl. Acad. Sci. USA* **96,** 15256–15261.
214. Bulte, J. W., Ben-Hur, T., Miller, B. R., et al. (2003) MR microscopy of magnetically labeled neurospheres transplanted into the Lewis EAE rat brain. *Magn. Reson. Med.* **50,** 201–205.
215. Modo, M., Mellodew, K., Cash, D., et al. (2004) Mapping transplanted stem cell migration after a stroke: a serial, in vivo magnetic resonance imaging study. *Neuroimage* **21,** 311–317.
216. Kim, D. E., Schellingerhout, D., Ishii, K., Shah, K., and Weissleder, R. (2004) Imaging of stem cell recruitment to ischemic infarcts in a murine model. *Stroke* **35,** 952–957.
217. Ben-Hur, T., Einstein, O., Mizrachi-Kol, R., et al. (2003) Transplanted multipotential neural precursor cells migrate into the inflamed white matter in response to experimental autoimmune encephalomyelitis. *Glia* **41,** 73–80.
218. Zhang, S. C., Goetz, B. D., and Duncan, I. D. (2003) Suppression of activated microglia promotes survival and function of transplanted oligodendroglial progenitors. *Glia* **41,** 191–198.
219. Isenmann, S., Brandner, S., Kuhne, G., Boner, J., and Aguzzi, A. (1996) Comparative in vivo and pathological analysis of the blood-brain barrier in mouse telencephalic transplants. *Neuropathol. Appl. Neurobiol.* **22,** 118–128.
220. Kinouchi, R., Takeda, M., Yang, L., et al. (2003) Robust neural integration from retinal transplants in mice deficient in GFAP and vimentin. *Nat. Neurosci.* **6,** 863–868.
221. Akerud, P., Canals, J. M., Snyder, E. Y., and Arenas, E. (2001) Neuroprotection through delivery of glial cell line-derived neurotrophic factor by neural stem cells in a mouse model of Parkinson's disease. *J. Neurosci.* **21,** 8108–8118.
222. Calza, L., Giardino, L., Pozza, M., Bettelli, C., Micera, A., and Aloe, L. (1998) Proliferation and phenotype regulation in the subventricular zone during experimental allergic encephalomyelitis: in vivo evidence of a role for nerve growth factor. *Proc. Natl. Acad. Sci. USA* **95,** 3209–3214.
223. Himes, B. T., Liu, Y., Solowska, J. M., Snyder, E. Y., Fischer, I., and Tessler, A. (2001) Transplants of cells genetically modified to express neurotrophin-3 rescue axotomized Clarke's nucleus neurons after spinal cord hemisection in adult rats. *J. Neurosci. Res.* **65,** 549–564.

Appendix A
Neural Stem Cell Companies

Advanced Cell Technology, Inc.
One Innovation Drive
Biotech Three
Worcester, MA 01605 USA
Phone: +1 508-756-1212
URL: http://www.advancedcell.com/

Advanced Tissue Sciences, Inc.
10933 North Torrey Pines Road
La Jolla, CA 92037 USA
Phone: +1 858-713-7300
URL: http://www.advancedtissue.com/

BioTransplant Incorporated
Building 75, Third Avenue
Charlestown Navy Yard
Charlestown, MA 02129 USA
Phone: +1 617-241-5200
URL: http://www.biotransplant.com/

Clonetics Corporation
PO Box 127
8830 Biggs Ford Road
Walkersville, MD 21793-0127 USA
Phone: +1 800-344-6618
URL: http://www.clonetics.com/

Clonexpress, Inc.
504 E.Diamond Avenue, Suite G
Gaithersburg, MD 20877 USA
Phone: +1 301-869-0840
URL: http://www.clonexpress.com/
Diacrin
Building 96, 13th Street,
Charlestown, MA, 02129 USA
Phone: +1 617-242-9100
URL: http://www.diacrin.com/

From: *Neural Development and Stem Cells, Second Edition*
Edited by: M. S. Rao © Humana Press Inc., Totowa, NJ

Geron
230 Constitution Drive
Menlo Park, CA 94025 USA
Phone: +1 650-473-7700
URL: http://www.geron.com/

Layton BioScience, Inc.
709 East Evelyn Avenue
Sunnyvale, CA 95086 USA
Phone: +1 408-732-5050
URL: http://www.laytonbio.com/

NeuralSTEM Biopharmaceuticals, Ltd.
College Park, MD USA
Phone: +1 301-405-6089
URL: http://www.neuralstem.com/

NeuroSearch A/S
93 Pederstrupvej
DK-2750 Ballerup
Denmark
Phone: +45 44-60-80-00
URL: http://www.neurosearch.com/uk/

NeuroNova AB
Floragatan 5
S-114 31 Stockholm
Sweden
Phone: +46 8-728-00-71
URL: http://www.neuronova.com/

Neuronyx, Inc.
1 Great Valley Parkway, Suite 20
Malvern, PA 19355 USA
Tel: +1 610-240-4150
URL: http://www.neuronyx.com/

Organogenesis Inc.
150 Dan Road
Canton, MA 02021 USA
Phone: +1 781-575-0775
URL: http://www.organogenesis.com/

Osiris Therapeutics, Inc.
2001 Aliceanna Street
Baltimore, MD 21231 USA
Phone: +1 410-522-5005
URL: http://www.osiristx.com/

Proneuron Biotechnology, Ltd.
P.O. Box 277
Ness-Ziona, 74101
Israel
Phone: +972 8-9409550
URL: http://www.proneuron.com/

ReNeuron
Europoint Centre
5-11 Lavington Street
London, SE1 ONZ
United Kingdom
Phone: +44 207-928-1720
URL: http://www.reneuron.com/

Signal Pharmaceuticals, Inc.
5555 Oberlin Drive
San Diego, CA 92121 USA
Phone: +1 858-558-7500
URL: http://www.signalpharm.com/

StemCells, Inc.
525 Del Rey Avenue, Suite C
Sunnyvale, CA 94086 USA
Phone: +1 408-731-8670
URL: http://www.cyto.com/

Titan Pharmaceuticals, Inc.
Post Office Plaza
50 Division Street, Suite 503
Somerville, NJ 08876 USA
URL: http://www.titanpharm.com/

WiCell Research Institute, Inc.
P.O. Box 7365
Madison, WI 53707-7365
Fax: (608) 263-1064
email: info@WiCell.org
https://www.wicell.org/index2.html

Appendix B
Stem Cells and Transplants

Transplants and the Food and Drug Administration

Food and Drug Administration
URL: http://www.fda.gov/
Summary: The Food and Drug Administration (FDA) regulates the use of stem cells for clinical therapy under the provisions of the US Public Health Service Act. Stem Cells fall under the purview of the Center for Biologics Evaluation and Research (CBER), which is the center within the FDA responsible for ensuring the safety and efficacy of blood and blood products, vaccines, allergenics, and biological therapeutics. Newer products, such as biotechnology products, somatic cell therapy and gene therapy, and banked human tissues are also regulated by the same section. However, because most biological products also meet the definition of "drugs" under the Federal Food, Drug, and Cosmetic Act (FD&C Act), they are also subject to regulation under the FD&C Act provisions.

The FDA maintains a comprehensive web-site that can be accessed for detailed information on application procedures, submission requirements and current protocols and policies.

Neural Transplantation Resources

NINDS
URL: http://www.ninds.nih.org/
Summary: The National Institute of Neurological Disorders and Stroke (NINDS), an agency of the US Federal Government and a component of the National Institutes of Health (NIH) and the US Public Health Service, is a lead agency for the Congressionally designated "Decade of the Brain," and the leading supporter of biomedical research on disorders of the brain and nervous system.

Clinical Trials Database
URL: http://clinicaltrials.gov/ct/gui
Summary: The National Library of Medicine at the National Institutes of Health (NIH) has developed a Clinical Trials Database to provide patients, family members, and members of the public with current information about clinical research studies.

Rare Diseases Clinical Research Database
URL: http://rarediseases.info.nih.gov/ord/wwwprot/index.shtml
Summary: This is a searchable database that lists government-funded trials on a variety of CNS and non-CNS disorders.

From: *Neural Development and Stem Cells, Second Edition*
Edited by: M. S. Rao © Humana Press Inc., Totowa, NJ

CenterWatch Clinical Trials Listing Service
URL: http://www.centerwatch.com/
Summary: This is an international listing of clinical research trials containing information about physicians and medical centers performing clinical research and drug therapies newly approved by the FDA.

American Society for Neurotransplantation and Repair
URL: http://www.asntr.org/
Summary: The American Society for Neurotransplantation and Repair (ASNTR) is a society composed of basic and clinical neuroscientists who utilize transplantation and related technologies to better understand the way the nervous system functions and establish new procedures for its repair in response to trauma or neurodegenerative disease.

Cell Transplant Society
URL: http://www.celltx.org/
Summary: The mission of the Cell Transplant Society is to promote research and collaboration in cellular transplantation. The Society publishes a cell transplantation journal that shares information on diverse research topics of interest to transplant researchers.

The Halifax Fetal Transplantation Program
URL: http://www.mcms.dal.ca/dnts/neurotr.html
Summary: As the only program of its kind in Canada, the Halifax Fetal Transplantation Program has been in the forefront of neural transplantation research in this country. Clones of human brain cells are being used in laboratory experiments aimed at repairing, even re-creating, brain areas damaged by injury, disease, and birth defects.

Network of European CNS Transplantation and Restoration
URL: http://www.nectar.org/
Summary: The Network of European CNS Transplantation and Restoration (NECTAR) is aimed at a concerted European effort to develop efficient, reliable, safe and ethically acceptable transplantation therapies for neurodegenerative diseases, in particular Parkinson's and Huntington's diseases.

MRC Cambridge Centre for Brain Repair
URL: http://www.mrc.ac.uk/
Summary: The Brain Repair Centre is an institution of the University of Cambridge. The ultimate aim of work in the Centre is to understand, and eventually, to alleviate and repair damage to the brain and spinal cord, resulting from injury or neurodegenerative disease.

Other Transplant Centers and Sites

Stroke Treatment at the University of Pittsburgh
Summary: The first experimental study of human neuron implantation for patients with paralysis after stroke was conducted here.

Neural Transplantation and Neurotrophin Mechanisms in Experimental Epilepsy
URL: http://www.lu.se/intsek/eaeu/eaeu261.html

The University of Nebraska Medical Center and the Nebraska Health System Transplant Programs
URL: http://www.nebraskatransplant.org/
Summary: The University of Nebraska Medical Center has an active transplant program that includes use of mesenchymal and other stem cells.

Proneuron Biotechnology, Ltd.
URL: http://www.proneuron.com/
Summary: Proneuron has initiated a study that will be conducted in Israel with the approval of the Israel Ministry of Health under a US Food and Drug Administration Investigational New Drug Application. This study is designed to study autologous activated macrophage therapy in approximately eight complete spinal cord injury patients. The investigators will follow their post-treatment course for one year or longer.

Diacrin
URL: http://www.diacrin.com/
Summary: Diacrin has initiated phase I and phase II clinical trials using porcine cells to treat Parkinson's and Huntington's Disease patients.

Layton BioScience, Inc.
URL: http://www.laytonbio.com/
Summary: Layton has recruited twelve stroke patients to undergo human cell transplants (HNT). Transplants will be performed by University of Pittsburgh neurosurgeon Douglas Kondziolka. In 2000 Dr. Kondziolka reported that the patients who received 6 million cells showed much more improvement than those who received 2 million. The first four received 2 million, and the remaining eight received, at random, either 2 million or 6 million cells.

Appendix C
Patents and Stem Cells

The patent situation on stem cells, progenitor cells and differentiated cells for therapy is complex and confusing and more than twenty different patents have issued in the past two years. We have listed some useful searchable sites. The reader is advised to use multiple keywords to obtain a comprehensive listing of patent filings. Given the different requirements for public release in different countries, it is often advisable to search several different databases. Some sites are listed and most other sites can be readily identified using standard search engines.

United States Patent and Trademark Office
URL: http://www.uspto.gov/
Summary: This is the only official web-site of the United States Patent and Trademark Office, a performance-based organization of the government of the United States of America.

US Patents
URL: http://patents.cos.com/
Summary: This is a fully searchable bibliographic database, accessed through the Community of Science, Inc. (COS) web-site, containing all of the approximately 1.7 million U.S. patents issued since 1975.

European Patent Office
URL: http://www.european-patent-office.org/
Summary: This is the official web-site of the European Patent Office, the executive body of the European Patent Organization.

Espacenet
URL: http://www.european-patent-office.org/espacenet/info/access.htm
Summary: Established by the European Patent Office in conjunction with the member states of the European Patent Organization and the European Commission to provide the general public with free patent information.

United Kingdom Patent Office
URL: http://www.patent.gov.uk/
Summary: The role of the UK Patent Office is to help to stimulate innovation and the international competitiveness of industry through intellectual property rights.

From: *Neural Development and Stem Cells, Second Edition*
Edited by: M. S. Rao © Humana Press Inc., Totowa, NJ

Canadian Patent Database
URL: http://patents1.ic.gc.ca/intro-e.html
Summary: The Canadian Patent Database lets you access over 75 years of patent descriptions and images. You can search, retrieve, and study more than 1.4 million patent documents.

Japanese Patent Office
URL: http://www.jpo-miti.go.jp/

Appendix D
Stem Cells and US Federal Guidelines

Currently, US federal law regulates the use of fetal cells and fetal tissue for research or clinical use. Use of neural stem cells, restricted precursors, and more differentiated cells derived from fetal tissue is governed by guidelines established for fetal tissue research. Detailed information on the guidelines that govern fetal tissue research is available from the National Institutes of Health (NIH) web-site.

Adult stem cells and their derivatives are not regulated by the same guidelines that govern fetal research. Individual universities have established Institutional Review Boards (IRBs) that evaluate all applications that involve patient or donor contact. Guidelines for informed consent, donor confidentiality, and donor legal rights have been established. Most universities follow similar guidelines, although minor differences may exist. Researchers can contact their IRB to obtain specific guidelines.

The rules that govern use and isolation of human pluripotent stem cells (hPSCs) or embryonic stem cells (ES cells) have been finalized. Currently, federal law prohibits the Department of Health and Human Services (DHHS) from funding research in which human embryos are created for research purposes or are destroyed, discarded or subjected to greater than minimal risk. In light of this restriction the DHHS Office of the General Counsel sought a legal opinion on whether NIH funds may be used for research utilizing human pluripotent stem cells. DHHS concluded that the Congressional prohibition does not prohibit the funding of research utilizing hPSCs because such cells are not embryos. Thus, NIH funding for research using pluripotent stem cells derived from human embryos is not legislatively prohibited. The legal opinion also clarified that hPSCs derived from fetal tissue would fall within the legal definition of human fetal tissue and are, therefore, subject to federal restrictions on the use of such tissue. NIH funding for research to derive or utilize hPSCs from fetal tissue is permissible, subject to applicable law and regulation.

Final guidelines have been published in the Federal register. A copy of the guidelines obtained from http://www.nih.gov/news/stemcell/stemcellguidelines. htm is appended below. More information on stem cells is available at http://www. nih.gov/news/stemcell/index.htm. Readers are advised to check for updates prior to initiating their experiments. Investigators should also note that different guidelines will apply to deriving new cell lines, use of existing cell lines and use of primordial germ cells.

From: *Neural Development and Stem Cells, Second Edition*
Edited by: M. S. Rao © Humana Press Inc., Totowa, NJ

NATIONAL INSTITUTES OF HEALTH GUIDELINES
FOR RESEARCH USING HUMAN PLURIPOTENT STEM CELLS

Summary

The National Institutes of Health (NIH) is hereby publishing final *National Institutes of Health Guidelines for Research Using Human Pluripotent Stem Cells*. The *Guidelines* establish procedures to help ensure that NIH-funded research in this area is conducted in an ethical and legal manner.

Effective Date

These *Guidelines* are effective on August 25, 2000. The moratorium on research using human pluripotent stem cells derived from human embryos and fetal tissue put in place by the Director, NIH, in January 1999, will be lifted on August 25, 2000.

Summary of Public Comments on Draft Guidelines

On December 2, 1999, the NIH published *Draft Guidelines* for research involving human pluripotent stem cells (hPSCs) in the *Federal Register* for public comment. The comment period ended on February 22, 2000.

The NIH received approximately 50,000 comments from members of Congress, patient advocacy groups, scientific societies, religious organizations, and private citizens. This Notice presents the final *Guidelines* together with NIH's response to the substantive public comments that addressed provisions of the *Guidelines*.

Scope of Guidelines and General Issues

Respondents asked for clarification of terminology used in the "Guidelines" and some commented that the language was not appropriate or was too technical, particularly the informed consent sections. The NIH agrees that these *Guidelines* should be clear and understandable. Changes, including some reorganization of the sections, were made to this end. The *Guidelines* are written primarily for the purpose of informing investigators of the conditions that must be met in order to receive NIH funding for research using hPSCs and, therefore, some technical language is required. The *Guidelines* do not define the precise language that should appear in informed consent documents because these should be developed by the investigator/clinician specifically for a particular study protocol or procedure for which the consent is being sought. Existing regulatory provisions require (45 CFR 46.116) that the language in informed consent documents be understandable to prospective participants in the study.

Respondents suggested that NIH funding for research using hPSCs would be in violation of the DHHS appropriations law and that derivation of hPSCs cannot be distinguished from their use. For this reason, a number of respondents asked that the NIH withdraw the "draft Guidelines." The NIH sought the opinion of the Department of Health and Human Services (DHHS) General Counsel, who determined that "federally funded research that utilizes hPSCs would not be prohibited by the HHS appropriations law prohibiting human embryo research, because such cells are not human embryos." Comments questioning this conclusion did not present information or arguments that justify reconsideration of the conclusion.

Respondents commented that the "Guidelines" are too restrictive or that there is no need for Federal Guidelines for this arena of research. Comments asserted that federally funded research using hPSCs should go forward without formal requirements, in the same manner as in the private sector. In order to help ensure that the NIH-funded research using hPSCs is conducted in an ethical and legal manner, the NIH felt it was advisable to develop and implement guidelines. To this end, the NIH Director convened a Working Group of the Advisory Committee to the Director, NIH (ACD), to advise the ACD on the development of guidelines and an oversight process for research involving hPSCs. The NIH Director charged the Working Group with developing appropriate guidelines to govern research involving the derivation and use of hPSCs from fetal tissue and research involving the use of hPSCs derived from human embryos that are in excess of clinical need.

Respondents commented regarding the sources of stem cells. Some respondents stated that research on hPSCs was unnecessary because stem cells from adults, umbilical cords, and placentas could be used instead. Other respondents asked the NIH to restrict Federal funding for hPSC research to those cells derived from fetal and adult tissue but not embryos. Other respondents asked that the Guidelines encompass research using stem cells from adult tissues. As stated under Section I. Scope of *Guidelines*, the *Guidelines* apply to the use of NIH funds for research using hPSCs derived from human embryos or human fetal tissue. The *Guidelines* do not impose requirements on Federal funding of research involving stem cells from human adults, umbilical cords, or placentas.

Given the enormous potential of stem cells to the development of new therapies for the most devastating diseases, it is important to simultaneously pursue all lines of promising research. It is possible that no single source of stem cells is best or even suitable/usable for all therapies. Different types or sources of stem cells may be optimal for treatment of specific conditions. In order to determine the very best source of many of the specialized cells and tissues of the body for new treatments and even cures, it is vitally important to study the potential of adult stem cells for comparison to that of hPSCs derived from embryos and fetuses. Unless all stem cell types are studied, the differences between adult stem cells and embryo and fetal-derived hPSCs will not be known.

Moreover, there is evidence that adult stem cells may have more limited potential than hPSCs. First, stem cells for all cell and tissue types have not yet been found in the adult human. Significantly, cardiac stem cells or pancreatic islet stem cells have not been identified in adult humans. Second, stem cells in adults are often present in only minute quantities, are difficult to isolate and purify, and their numbers may decrease with age. For example, brain cells from adults that may be neural stem cells have been obtained only by removing a portion of the brain of an adult with epilepsy, a complex and invasive procedure that carries the added risk of further neurological damage. Any attempt to use stem cells from a patient's own body for treatment would require that stem cells would first have to be isolated from the patient and then grown in culture in sufficient numbers to obtain adequate quantities for treatment. This would mean that for some rapidly progressing disorders, there may not be sufficient time to grow enough cells to use for treatment. Third, in disorders that are caused by a genetic defect, the genetic error likely would be present in the patient's stem cells, making cells from such a patient inappropriate for transplantation. In addition, adult stem cells may contain more DNA abnormalities caused by exposure to daily living, including sunlight, toxins, and errors made during DNA replication than will be found in fetal or embryonic hPSCs. Fourth, there is evidence that stem cells from adults may not have the same capacity to multiply as do younger cells. These potential weaknesses may limit the usefulness of adult stem cells.

Respondents were concerned that these are guidelines and not requirements or regulations. Although these are guidelines and not regulations, they prescribe the documentation and assurances that must accompany requests for NIH funding for research utilizing hPSCs. If the funding requests do not contain the prescribed information, funding for hPSC research will not be provided. Compliance with the *Guidelines* will be imposed as a condition of grant award.

Respondents commented that there had not been enough widespread public disclosure/discussion of this research or the "Guidelines". Prior to the development of draft *Guidelines*, there were two Congressional hearings on hPSCs. In a further effort to ensure substantial discussion and comment, the NIH convened a Working Group of the Advisory Committee to the Director, NIH (ACD), to advise the ACD on the development of these *Guidelines*. The Working Group was composed of scientists, patients and patient advocates, ethicists, clinicians, and lawyers. The Working Group met in public session on April 8, 1999, and heard from members of the public, as well as professional associations and Congress. In developing the draft *Guidelines*, the NIH also considered advice from the National Bioethics Advisory Commission (NBAC). *Draft Guidelines* were published for public comment in the *Federal Register* on December 2, 1999, for 60 days, and, in response to public interest, the comment period was extended an additional 28 days. Approximately 50,000 comments were received. NIH issued a national press release announcing the *Federal Register* notice and many of the Nation's newspapers carried articles on this area of research and on the *Guidelines*. Patient groups, scientific societies, and religious organizations convened meetings and discussion groups and disseminated materials about this area of research and about the *Guidelines*.

Comment was received about whether the "Guidelines" apply to hPSC lines developed outside of the United States. The *Guidelines* make no distinction based upon the country in which an hPSC line is developed. All lines to be used in hPSC cell research funded by NIH must meet the same requirements.

Derivation and Use of hPSCs From Fetal Tissue

Respondents made the point that the NIH has specified certain requirements for the use of human fetal tissue to derive hPSCs in addition to those imposed on other areas of human fetal tissue research. These respondents suggested that the section of the "Guidelines" pertaining to fetal tissue sources be omitted. In order to ensure uniformity in NIH's oversight of research using hPSCs, the *Guidelines* were extended to govern hPSCs derived from both human embryos and fetal tissue.

Use of hPSCs Derived From Human Embryos

Respondents suggested that the "Guidelines" refer to "fertility treatment" rather than to "infertility treatment" in order to clarify that they allow the use of human embryos from treatments that employ assisted reproductive technologies to facilitate reproduction in fertile, as well as in infertile, individuals. The *Guidelines* have been changed accordingly.

Respondents suggested dropping the word "early" throughout the document or more clearly defining "early." The word "early" in reference to human embryos has been deleted; the *Guidelines* make it clear that NIH funding of research using hPSCs derived in the private sector from human embryos can involve only embryos that have not reached the stage at which the mesoderm is formed.

Some respondents were concerned that embryos might be created for research purposes. Other respondents stated there should be no distinction between embryos created for research purposes and those created for fertility treatment. Investigators seeking NIH funds for research using hPSCs are required to provide documentation, prior to the award of any NIH funds, that embryos were created for the purposes of fertility treatment. President Clinton, many members of Congress, the NIH Human Embryo Research Panel, and the NBAC have all embraced the distinction between embryos created for research purposes and those created for reproductive purposes.

Respondents were concerned about the creation of a "black market" for human embryos, and expressed concerns that individuals will be coerced into donating embryos. The *Guidelines* state that there can be no incentives for donation and that a decision to donate must be made free of coercion. In addition, the *Guidelines* set forth conditions that will help ensure all donations are voluntary. For example, with regard to hPSCs derived from embryos, research using Federal funds may only be conducted if the cells were derived from frozen embryos that were created for the purpose of fertility treatment and that were in excess of clinical need.

Respondents commented on the requirement that human embryos be frozen in order to qualify for derivation of hPSCs to be used in NIH-funded research. Respondents suggested that the freezing requirement would preclude the use of hPSCs derived from embryos that are genetically and chromosomally abnormal, since such embryos are usually not frozen for reproductive purposes. While the NIH acknowledges that research on hPSCs derived from such embryos could yield important scientific information, limiting research to hPSCs derived from frozen human embryos will help ensure that the decision to donate the embryo for hPSC research is distinct and separate from the fertility treatment.

Financial Issues

Respondents expressed concern regarding the sale of fetal tissue for profit and whether hPSC research would encourage such activity. Respondents also were concerned about whether clinics or doctors would profit from the derivation of hPSCs and/or their sale. Section 498B of the Public Health Service Act prohibits any individual from knowingly acquiring or selling human fetal tissue for "valuable consideration." In addition, the *Guidelines* prohibit any inducement for the donation of human embryos for research purposes. The *Guidelines* also call for an assurance that the hPSCs to be used in NIH-funded research were obtained through a donation or through a payment that does not exceed the reasonable costs associated with the transportation, processing, preservation, quality control and storage of the hPSCs. All grantees must sign an assurance that they are in compliance with all applicable Federal, State, and local laws. Each funded research institution is responsible for monitoring compliance by individual investigators with any such applicable laws.

Respondents questioned the prohibition against embryo donors benefitting financially from their donation. This clause was retained in the final *Guidelines* to help ensure that the donating individuals are offered no inducements to donate and that all donations are voluntary.

Respondents suggested that the "Guidelines" be strengthened to include a waiver of intellectual property rights. This proposed change would be inconsistent with 45 CFR 46.116 of the regulation for the protection of human subjects of research, which provides that no informed consent may include language through which the subject waives or appears to waive any of the subject's legal rights.

Respondents questioned the reference in the requirements for informed consent related to the commercial potential of donated material. The paragraphs providing for disclosure in the informed consent of the possibility that the donated material could have commercial potential were modified. The reference in these paragraphs to "donated material" did not accurately reflect the intent of the provision. The *Guidelines* now make clear that the "results of research on the human pluripotent stem cells may have commercial potential."

Ineligible Research

Respondents objected to the areas of research that the NIH has deemed ineligible, particularly research that is not restricted by statute or regulation, such as research utilizing hPSCs that were derived using somatic cell nuclear transfer, i.e., the transfer of a human somatic cell nucleus into a human egg. The NIH determined that, at this time, research using hPSCs derived from such sources has not received adequate discussion and consideration by the public and is, therefore, ineligible for NIH funding.

Separation of Fertility Treatment and Abortion From Research

Respondents were concerned that hPSC research would encourage abortion. The law and the *Guidelines* guard against encouraging abortion by requiring that the decision to have an abortion be made apart from and prior to the decision to donate tissue.

Respondents objected to the condition in the "Guidelines" that the fertility physician could not be the same person as the researcher deriving stem cells. Some respondents stated that the Institutional Review Board (IRB) or an independent physician would be able to guard against this conflict of interest. The restriction was designed so that the person treating the individuals seeking fertility treatment, who is involved in decisions such as how many embryos to produce, is not the person seeking to derive hPSCs. This separation will help ensure that embryos will not be created in numbers greater than necessary for fertility treatment.

Respondents suggested that the clauses regarding donation of fetal tissue or human embryos for derivation of stem cells for eventual use in transplantation be changed explicitly to prevent directed donation. This change has been made.

Identifiers

Respondents were concerned about removing identifiers. There was concern that the investigator would not be able to document compliance with the "Guidelines" requirements without identifiers, or that the removal of identifiers would make it impossible to conduct certain genetic studies or develop therapeutic materials. The *Guidelines* have been modified to clarify that the term "identifier" refers to any information from which the donor(s) can be identified, directly or through identifiers linked to the donors. However, since information identifying the donor(s) may be necessary if the tissue or cells are to be used in transplantation, the *Guidelines* have also been modified to state that the informed consent should notify donor(s) whether or not identifiers will be retained.

Respondents commented that DNA is an identifier and that all donors of human embryos or fetal tissue should be told that identifiers such as DNA will be retained with the samples. Although DNA can be used to determine the individual from whom a tissue sample was taken, this can be done only when one has a sample from both the tissue in question and the putative donor; it cannot be used to identify an individual out of a population. Moreover, it is difficult to identify a donor using tissue derived from a fetus or embryo, since the tissue is not genetically identical to the donor.

Informed Consent and IRB Review

Respondents asked why investigators were expected to provide documentation of IRB review of derivation from human embryos, but not for derivation from fetal tissue. Respondents suggested that the requirements be changed so that protocols for both sources of hPSCs must be approved by an IRB. The *Guidelines* have been changed to make clear that the IRB review requirements regarding the derivation of cells from fetal tissue and human embryos are the same.

Comment was received expressing concern that the informed consent explicitly state that the donor will have no dispositional authority over derived pluripotent stem cells. The *Guidelines* state that donation of human embryos should have been made without any restriction regarding the individual(s) who may be the recipient of the cells derived from the hPSCs for transplantation. Such a statement is consistent with the statutory provision applicable to the donor informed consent for the use of fetal tissue for transplantation. The *Guidelines* now provide for the inclusion of a statement to this effect in the informed consent.

Respondents urged that the "Guidelines" be revised to remove the prohibition on potential donors receiving information regarding subsequent testing of donated tissue in the situation when physicians deem disclosure to be in the donors' best interest. This change has been made.

Respondents requested clarification regarding the persons from whom consent for donation of embryos for research must be obtained. The *Guidelines* call for informed consent from individual(s) who have sought fertility treatment. Only the individual(s) who were part of the decision to create the embryo for reproductive purposes should have been part of the decision to donate for the derivation of hPSCs.

Respondents urged that fertility clinics should be able to discuss with patients the option of donating embryos for research at the beginning of the IVF process. The *Guidelines* do not delineate the timeframe during which the general option of donating embryos for research can be discussed. However, according to the *Guidelines*, obtaining consent for donation of embryos for the purpose of deriving hPSCs should not occur until after the embryos are determined to be in "excess of clinical need."

Oversight

Respondents stated that the NIH's oversight in this area of research was very important to the legal and ethical conduct of this research, and asked for more information regarding the oversight process. Information about the operations of the Human Pluripotent Stem Cell Review Group (HPSCRG) can be found in the final *Guidelines* and on the NIH Web page.

Respondents were concerned about whether and how NIH would monitor research after a researcher receives NIH funds. Compliance with the *Guidelines* will be largely determined prior to the award of funds. Follow-up to ensure continued compliance with the *Guidelines* will be conducted in the same manner as for all other conditions of all other NIH grant awards. It is the responsibility of the investigator to file progress reports, and it is the responsibility of the funded institution to ensure compliance with the NIH *Guidelines*. NIH staff will also monitor the progress of these investigators as part of their regular duties.

Respondents asked about penalties for not following the "Guidelines." The following actions may be taken by the NIH when there is a failure to comply with the terms and conditions of any award: 1) Under 45 CFR 74.14, the NIH can impose special conditions on an award, including increased oversight/monitoring/reporting requirements for an institution, project or investigator; 2) Under 45 CFR 74.62, if a grantee materially fails to comply with the terms and conditions of the award, the NIH may withhold funds pending correction of the problem or, pending more severe enforcement action, disallow all or part of the costs of the activity that was not in compliance, withhold further awards for the project, or suspend or terminate all or part of the funding for the project. Individuals and institutions may be debarred from eligibility for all Federal financial assistance and contracts under 45 CFR Part 76 and 48 CFR Subpart 9.4, respectively. Because these sanctions pertain to all conditions of grant award, the NIH did not reiterate them in the *Guidelines*.

Respondents suggested that the HPSCRG hold periodic Stem Cell Policy Conferences (similar to the Gene Therapy Policy Conferences conducted by the Recombinant DNA Advisory Committee ("RAC")) in order to solicit and consider public comment from interested parties on the scientific, medical, legal, and ethical issues arising from stem cell research. Members of the HPSCRG will serve as a resource for recommending to the NIH any need for Human Pluripotent Stem Cell Policy Conferences.

Other Changes

Because compliance materials may be made public prior to funding decisions, we have added a sentence requiring the principal investigator's written consent to the disclosure of such material necessary to carry out public review and other oversight procedures.

The draft *Guidelines* required HPSCRG review of proposals from investigators planning to derive hPSCs from fetal tissue. Because the *Guidelines* address proposals for

NIH funding for the use of hPSCs, this requirement has been removed from the *Guidelines*.

The text of the final *Guidelines* follows.

NATIONAL INSTITUTES OF HEALTH GUIDELINES FOR RESEARCH USING HUMAN PLURIPOTENT STEM CELLS

I. Scope of Guidelines

These *Guidelines* apply to the expenditure of National Institutes of Health (NIH) funds for research using human pluripotent stem cells derived from human embryos (technically known as human embryonic stem cells) or human fetal tissue (technically known as human embryonic germ cells). For purposes of these *Guidelines*, "human pluripotent stem cells" are cells that are self-replicating, are derived from human embryos or human fetal tissue, and are known to develop into cells and tissues of the three primary germ layers. Although human pluripotent stem cells may be derived from embryos or fetal tissue, such stem cells are not themselves embryos. NIH research funded under these *Guidelines* will involve human pluripotent stem cells derived 1) from human fetal tissue; or 2) from human embryos that are the result of *in vitro* fertilization, are in excess of clinical need, and have not reached the stage at which the mesoderm is formed.

In accordance with 42 Code of Federal Regulations (CFR) § 52.4, these *Guidelines* prescribe the documentation and assurances that must accompany requests for NIH funding for research using human pluripotent stem cells from: (1) awardees who want to use existing funds; (2) awardees requesting an administrative or competing supplement; and 3) applicants or intramural researchers submitting applications or proposals. NIH funds may be used to derive human pluripotent stem cells from fetal tissue. NIH funds may not be used to derive human pluripotent stem cells from human embryos. These *Guidelines* also designate certain areas of human pluripotent stem cell research as ineligible for NIH funding.

II. Guidelines for Research Using Human Pluripotent Stem Cells that is Eligible for NIH Funding

A. Utilization of Human Pluripotent Stem Cells Derived from Human Embryos

1. Submission to NIH

Intramural or extramural investigators who are intending to use existing funds, are requesting an administrative supplement, or are applying for new NIH funding for research using human pluripotent stem cells derived from human embryos must submit to NIH the following:

a. An assurance signed by the responsible institutional official that the pluripotent stem cells were derived from human embryos in accordance with the conditions set forth in Section II.A.2 of these *Guidelines* and that the institution will maintain documentation in support of the assurance;

b. A sample informed consent document (with patient identifier information removed) and a description of the informed consent process that meet the criteria for informed consent set forth in Section II.A.2.e of these *Guidelines*;

c. An abstract of the scientific protocol used to derive human pluripotent stem cells from an embryo;

d. Documentation of Institutional Review Board (IRB) approval of the derivation protocol;

e. An assurance that the stem cells to be used in the research were or will be obtained through a donation or through a payment that does not exceed the reasonable costs associated with the transportation, processing, preservation, quality control and storage of the stem cells;

f. The title of the research proposal or specific subproject that proposes the use of human pluripotent stem cells;

g. An assurance that the proposed research using human pluripotent stem cells is not a class of research that is ineligible for NIH funding as set forth in Section III of these *Guidelines*; and

h. The Principal Investigator's written consent to the disclosure of all material submitted under Paragraph A.1 of this Section, as necessary to carry out the public review and other oversight procedures set forth in Section IV of these *Guidelines*.

2. Conditions for the Utilization of Human Pluripotent Stem Cells Derived From Human Embryos

Studies utilizing pluripotent stem cells derived from human embryos may be conducted using NIH funds only if the cells were derived (without Federal funds) from human embryos that were created for the purposes of fertility treatment and were in excess of the clinical need of the individuals seeking such treatment.

a. To ensure that the donation of human embryos in excess of the clinical need is voluntary, no inducements, monetary or otherwise, should have been offered for the donation of human embryos for research purposes. Fertility clinics and/or their affiliated laboratories should have implemented specific written policies and practices to ensure that no such inducements are made available.

b. There should have been a clear separation between the decision to create embryos for fertility treatment and the decision to donate human embryos in excess of clinical need for research purposes to derive pluripotent stem cells. Decisions related to the creation of embryos for fertility treatment should have been made free from the influence of researchers or investigators proposing to derive or utilize human pluripotent stem cells in research. To this end, the attending physician responsible for the fertility treatment and the researcher or investigator deriving and/or proposing to utilize human pluripotent stem cells should not have been one and the same person.

c. To ensure that human embryos donated for research were in excess of the clinical need of the individuals seeking fertility treatment and to allow potential donors time between the creation of the embryos for fertility treatment and the decision to donate for research purposes, only frozen human embryos should have been used to derive human pluripotent stem cells. In addition, individuals undergoing fertility treatment should have been approached about consent for donation of human embryos to derive pluripotent stem cells only at the time of deciding the disposition of embryos in excess of the clinical need.

d. Donation of human embryos should have been made without any restriction or direction regarding the individual(s) who may be the recipients of transplantation of the cells derived from the human pluripotent stem cells.

e. Informed Consent

Informed consent should have been obtained from individuals who have sought fertility treatment and who elect to donate human embryos in excess of clinical need for human pluripotent stem cell research purposes. The informed consent process should have included discussion of the following information with potential donors, pertinent to making the decision whether or not to donate their embryos for research purposes.

Informed consent should have included:

(i) A statement that the embryos will be used to derive human pluripotent stem cells for research that may include human transplantation research;

(ii) A statement that the donation is made without any restriction or direction regarding the individual(s) who may be the recipient(s) of transplantation of the cells derived from the embryo;

(iii) A statement as to whether or not information that could identify the donors of the embryos, directly or through identifiers linked to the donors, will be removed prior to the derivation or the use of human pluripotent stem cells;

(iv) A statement that derived cells and/or cell lines may be kept for many years;

(v) Disclosure of the possibility that the results of research on the human pluripotent stem cells may have commercial potential, and a statement that the donor will not receive financial or any other benefits from any such future commercial development;

(vi) A statement that the research is not intended to provide direct medical benefit to the donor; and

(vii) A statement that embryos donated will not be transferred to a woman's uterus and will not survive the human pluripotent stem cell derivation process.

f. Derivation protocols should have been approved by an IRB established in accord with 45 CFR §46.107 and §46.108 or FDA regulations at 21 CFR §56.107 and §56.108.

B. Utilization of Human Pluripotent Stem Cells Derived From Human Fetal Tissue

1. *Submission to NIH*

Intramural or extramural investigators who are intending to use existing funds, are requesting an administrative supplement, or are applying for new NIH funding for research using human pluripotent stem cells derived from fetal tissue must submit to NIH the following:

a. An assurance signed by the responsible institutional official that the pluripotent stem cells were derived from human fetal tissue in accordance with the conditions set forth in Section II.A.2 of these *Guidelines* and that the institution will maintain documentation in support of the assurance;

b. A sample informed consent document (with patient identifier information removed) and a description of the informed consent process that meet the criteria for informed consent set forth in Section II.B.2.b of these *Guidelines*;

c. An abstract of the scientific protocol used to derive human pluripotent stem cells from fetal tissue;

d. Documentation of IRB approval of the derivation protocol;

e. An assurance that the stem cells to be used in the research were or will be obtained through a donation or through a payment that does not exceed the reasonable costs associated with the transportation, processing, preservation, quality control and storage of the stem cells;

f. The title of the research proposal or specific subproject that proposes the use of human pluripotent stem cells;

g. An assurance that the proposed research using human pluripotent stem cells is not a class of research that is ineligible for NIH funding as set forth in Section III of these *Guidelines*; and

h. The Principal Investigator's written consent to the disclosure of all material submitted under Paragraph B.1 of this Section, as necessary to carry out the public review and other oversight procedures set forth in Section IV of these *Guidelines*.

2. Conditions for the Utilization of Human Pluripotent Stem Cells Derived From Fetal Tissue.

a. Unlike pluripotent stem cells derived from human embryos, DHHS funds may be used to support research to derive pluripotent stem cells from fetal tissue, as well as for research utilizing such cells. Such research is governed by Federal statutory restrictions regarding fetal tissue research at 42 U.S.C. 289g-2(a) and the Federal regulations at 45 CFR § 46.210. In addition, because cells derived from fetal tissue at the early stages of investigation may, at a later date, be used in human fetal tissue transplantation research, it is the policy of NIH to require that all NIH-funded research involving the derivation or utilization of pluripotent stem cells from human fetal tissue also comply with the fetal tissue transplantation research statute at 42 U.S.C. 289g-1.

b. Informed Consent

As a policy matter, NIH-funded research deriving or utilizing human pluripotent stem cells from fetal tissue should comply with the informed consent law applicable to fetal tissue transplantation research (42 U.S.C. 289g-1) and the following conditions. The informed consent process should have included discussion of the following information with potential donors, pertinent to making the decision whether to donate fetal tissue for research purposes.

Informed consent should have included:

(i) A statement that fetal tissue will be used to derive human pluripotent stem cells for research that may include human transplantation research;

(ii) A statement that the donation is made without any restriction or direction regarding the individual(s) who may be the recipient(s) of transplantation of the cells derived from the fetal tissue;

(iii) A statement as to whether or not information that could identify the donors of the fetal tissue, directly or through identifiers linked to the donors, will be removed prior to the derivation or the use of human pluripotent stem cells;

(iv) A statement that derived cells and/or cell lines may be kept for many years;

(v) Disclosure of the possibility that the results of research on the human pluripotent stem cells may have commercial potential, and a statement that the donor will not receive financial or any other benefits from any such future commercial development; and

(vi) A statement that the research is not intended to provide direct medical benefit to the donor.

c. Derivation protocols should have been approved by an IRB established in accord with 45 CFR §46.107 and §46.108 or FDA regulations at 21 CFR §56.107 and §56.108.

III. Areas of Research Involving Human Pluripotent Stem Cells that are Ineligible for NIH Funding

Areas of research ineligible for NIH funding include:

A. The derivation of pluripotent stem cells from human embryos;

B. Research in which human pluripotent stem cells are utilized to create or contribute to a human embryo;

C. Research utilizing pluripotent stem cells that were derived from human embryos created for research purposes, rather than for fertility treatment;

D. Research in which human pluripotent stem cells are derived using somatic cell nuclear transfer, i.e., the transfer of a human somatic cell nucleus into a human or animal egg;

E. Research utilizing human pluripotent stem cells that were derived using somatic cell nuclear transfer, i.e., the transfer of a human somatic cell nucleus into a human or animal egg;

F. Research in which human pluripotent stem cells are combined with an animal embryo; and

G. Research in which human pluripotent stem cells are used in combination with somatic cell nuclear transfer for the purposes of reproductive cloning of a human.

IV. Oversight

A. The NIH Human Pluripotent Stem Cell Review Group (HPSCRG) will review documentation of compliance with the *Guidelines* for funding requests that propose the use of human pluripotent stem cells. This working group will hold public meetings when a funding request proposes the use of a line of human pluripotent stem cells that has not been previously reviewed and approved by the HPSCRG.

B. In the case of new or competing continuation (renewal) or competing supplement applications, all applications shall be reviewed by HPSCRG and for scientific merit by a Scientific Review Group. In the case of requests to use existing funds or applications for an administrative supplement or in the case of intramural proposals, Institute or Center staff should forward material to the HPSCRG for review and determination of compliance with the *Guidelines* prior to allowing the research to proceed.

C. The NIH will compile a yearly report that will include the number of applications and proposals reviewed and the titles of all awarded applications, supplements or administrative approvals for the use of existing funds, and intramural projects.

D. Members of the HPSCRG will also serve as a resource for recommendations to the NIH with regard to any revisions to the *NIH Guidelines for Research Using Human Pluripotent Stem Cells* and any need for human pluripotent stem cell policy conferences.

Index

A

A2B5+ cells,
    characterization from E13.5 rat cortex, 160, 161
    differentiation potential, 160–162, 171, 172
    transdifferentiation/dedifferentiation, 253

AD, *see* Alzheimer's disease

Alzheimer's disease (AD), neural stem cell transplantation studies, 383

Apoptosis, *see also* Programmed cell death,
    adult neural stem cells,
        dentate gyrus, 114
        olfactory bulb, 115
    Bcl-2 role, 99, 101
    caspases,
        extrinsic apoptosis pathway, 101, 102
        intrinsic apoptosis pathway, 99–101
        regulation, 99
        types, 98, 99
    extrinsic pathway, 101, 102
    immature neuron death after pathological insult, 111
    intrinsic pathway, 99–101
    morphology, 98
    neural precursor cell death after pathological insult, 108–111

Ara-C, *see* Cytosine arabinoside

Astrocyte,
    central nervous system roles, 144, 171
    coculture for embryonic stem cell neural differentiation induction, 326
    markers, 172

    neurogenic niche in dentate gyrus, 350
    precursor cells, *see* A2B5+ cells; Glial-restricted precursor

Autophagy, programmed cell death, 102

5-Azacytidine, transdifferentiation/dedifferentiation effects, 258

B

Bcl-2,
    apoptosis role, 99, 101
    caspase regulation, 99
    programmed cell death regulation, 106–108
    subfamilies, 99

BDNF, *see* Brain-derived neurotrophic factor

Bmi-1,
    neural stem cell marker, 56
    neural tumor pathogenesis role, 207

BMPs, *see* Bone morphogenetic proteins

Bone morphogenetic proteins (BMPs),
    embryonic neural stem cell lineage regulation, 75, 76
    globose basal cell regulation, 228
    neonatal anterior subventricular zone neurogenic precursor proliferation regulation, 134, 135
    neural crest induction role,
        culture studies, 195, 196
        neural plate border region setup, 193
    neural crest stem cell fate regulation, 200, 202–204
    neuron differentiation role, 5, 15
    oligodendrocyte development in embryonic cortex versus spinal cord, 158–160